1983

Herbert C. Schulberg
Marie Killilea
Editors

The Modern Practice of Community Mental Health

A Volume in Honor of Gerald Caplan

Jossey-Bass Publishers
San Francisco • Washington • London • 1982

THE MODERN PRACTICE OF COMMUNITY MENTAL HEALTH
A Volume in Honor of Gerald Caplan
by Herbert C. Schulberg and Marie Killilea, Editors

433 California Street
San Francisco, California 94104
&
Jossey-Bass Limited
28 Banner Street
London EC1Y 8QE

Library of Congress Cataloging in Publication Data
Main entry under title:

The Modern practice of community mental health.

"A volume in honor of Gerald Caplan"—Copr. p.
Includes bibliographies and indexes.
1. Community mental health services—United States—Addresses, essays, lectures. 2. Mental health policy—United States—Addresses, essays, lectures. 3. Caplan, Gerald—Addresses, essays, lectures. I. Schulberg, Herbert C. II. Killilea, Marie. III. Caplan, Gerald.
[DNLM: 1. Community psychiatry. WM 30.6 M689]
RA790.6.M6 1982 362.2'2'0973 82-48066
ISBN 0-87589-550-6

Manufactured in the United States of America

The paper in this book meets the guidelines for permanence and durability of the Committee on Production Guidelines for Book Longevity of the Council on Library Resources.

JACKET DESIGN BY WILLI BAUM

FIRST EDITION

Code 8238

The Jossey-Bass
Social and Behavioral Science Series

Preface

The bandwagon nature of community mental health, which dominated the field in the late 1960s, has long since passed. Although it is now fashionable in some quarters to emphasize the excesses of the era and the lingering problems left unsolved by a movement that promised so much, major advances were made during that time. Those intimately involved in formulating the theoretical foundations of the community mental health field and in molding its practice can point with pride to profound and wide-ranging innovations whose significance continues into the 1980s. Such well-accepted principles as the organization of population-focused services, whether based on geographic catchment areas or on special populations-at-risk, remain intrinsic to mental health program design. Crisis theory continues to guide both the organization of emergency health and mental health services and interventions in natural disasters. The need to comprehend cultural and subcultural influences on pathology is well recognized, as are the implications of ethnic heritages in seeking and obtaining care for mental disorders. The nature and characteristics of social and community support systems have stimulated a fresh awareness of how people's links to societal networks and social institutions affect their functioning.

Yet, despite these and other indices of meaningful progress, community mental health programs are in a state of crisis. The federal government's leadership and standard-setting role have been radically reduced, resource allocation patterns are being redesigned, and conceptual frameworks more congruent with compacted service systems are being trumpeted. Given these developments, uncertainty and even malaise hover over the field as it seeks to chart a course for the coming decade.

This volume provides a contemporary overview of the community mental health field, fulfilling a need of growing urgency in light of the complex problems and issues facing us in our present environment: The numerous overviews published in the late 1960s and early 1970s have long been outdated. This book provides an integrated statement of the modern practice of community mental health. It should be useful to clinicians and administrators who daily care for the mentally ill in community mental health centers and other caregiving settings and who seek to provide their services in increasingly humane and effective ways. The volume also should be relevant to policy makers at various levels of government who are reevaluating their commitment to social welfare and health services programming.

Our perception of the need for a contemporary appraisal of community mental health was reinforced in October 1978, when Gerald Caplan became professor emeritus of psychiatry at Harvard Medical School and assumed new responsibilities as professor of child psychiatry and head of the Department of Child Psychiatry at Hadassah Medical Organization–Hebrew University in Jerusalem. This milestone in the life of our mentor, colleague, and friend evoked in many of us a renewed appreciation of Caplan's seminal contributions to community psychiatry during the 1952 to 1977 period of his teaching, research, and practice in the United States—a quarter of a century that saw the development of systematic community-based services for the mentally ill and the enactment of major state and federal legislation supporting these services.

This volume was conceived as a fitting acknowledgment of our intellectual and human debts to Gerald Caplan. The authors of the contributed chapters share the common background of having been Caplan's faculty colleagues and students at the Community Mental Health Program, Harvard School of Public Health, and at the Laboratory of Community Psychiatry, Harvard Medical School. Drawing on Caplan's teachings, the authors discuss the theoretical and practical evolutions occurring in their own specialties as well as in the community mental health field. It was not possible, in one volume, to include contributions from all of Caplan's many colleagues and students or to address all issues facing the community mental health movement; nonetheless, we believe this book, in its composite form, succeeds in presenting a wide-ranging analysis of contemporary principles and practices in the field.

Part One begins with a chapter on Gerald Caplan's life work. This biographical chapter offers a brief intellectual history of the times as reflected in Caplan's career development both in the United States and in other countries. Chapter Two integrates ideas from the volume's contributors, focusing on the impact of the community mental health movement on present and future mental health practice. It describes how community mental health has matured to the point where its basic principles and practices are integral to the education and training of all mental health practitioners, and it explores the variety of skills, the domains of professional activity, and the research concerns that are particularly relevant for those choosing to specialize in community mental health practice.

The chapters in Part Two outline advances in such areas as epidemiology, crisis intervention, and support systems. They trace the relationship between early concepts of crisis and contemporary knowledge about how social supports can mediate stress, emphasizing implications for professional practice and the role of mutual help groups. Part Two analyzes the growing interest in and controversy about primary prevention as a framework for reducing the incidence of mental illness. The relative merits of focusing on high-risk populations or on high-risk situations are compared; opportunities for primary prevention in school settings consistent with the former approach and a general disease prevention paradigm consistent with the latter approach are proposed.

The chapters in Part Three emphasize that the environmental context within which community mental health services are delivered is constantly changing. Societal value systems affecting the mentally ill, therefore, are carefully considered in relation to judicial decisions, allocation patterns, and the ideological posture of mental health professionals. Part Three examines implications for the management of community mental health centers and for the ability of executives to exercise needed leadership of the organizational restructuring now occurring in many facilities. Opportunities and strategies for consultation to mental health centers confronting such changes are described.

Community mental health centers are responsible for providing comprehensive services to all catchment area residents, but there is growing concern about how best to meet the needs of populations for whom care has been fiscally, geographically, or psychologically inaccessible. In Part Four, contemporary program models are presented for such groups as the elderly, the chronically mentally ill, the developmentally disabled, disaster victims, and residents of rural areas. Because of the complex diagnostic issues and multiple services required by persons experiencing psychic distress, strategies for linking the health and mental health systems are detailed. And to help meet the need for constant evaluation of the effectiveness of community mental health interventions, Part Four suggests various procedures for designing outcome studies.

The availability of human resources for providing patient care is influenced by training opportunities, regulatory standards, and reimbursement patterns. In Part Five, trends in each of these areas are traced. The substitutability of nonmedical for medical clinicians is examined, as are possibilities for educating nonpsychiatric physicians in the diagnosis and treatment of emotional illness.

The book closes with an epilogue by Gerald Caplan, in

which he reflects on the current state of community mental health and the population orientation at the core of mental health service delivery. Caplan details creative developments in theory and practice and shares his optimism that community mental health programs once again will gain heightened professional and fiscal support.

Preparation of this book was greatly facilitated by the encouragement of many friends and colleagues. We are particularly indebted to Patricia Pricener, Western Psychiatric Institute and Clinic, University of Pittsburgh School of Medicine, for her expert management of the numerous editorial details associated with the book's development.

September 1982

Herbert C. Schulberg
Pittsburgh, Pennsylvania

Marie Killilea
Baltimore, Maryland

Contents

Preface vii

The Authors xvii

Part One: Background

1. Gerald Caplan: The Man and His Work 1
Ruth B. Caplan-Moskovich

2. Community Mental Health in Transition 40
Herbert C. Schulberg and Marie Killilea

Part Two: Principles of Community Mental Health

3. Epidemiology of Mental Disorders 95
Leo Levy

4. Advances and Obstacles in Prevention of Mental Disorders 126
Bernard L. Bloom

5. Relationships of Social Support and Psychological Well Being 148
Robert S. Weiss

6. Interaction of Crisis Theory, Coping Strategies, and Social Support Systems 163
Marie Killilea

7. Role of Support Systems in Loss and Psychosocial Transitions 215
Colin Murray Parkes

Part Three: Changing Contexts of Mental Health Practice

8. Impact of Public Policy on Mental Health Services 230
Dwight Harshbarger and Harold W. Demone, Jr.

9. Effects of Value Systems on Service Delivery 246
Frank Baker

10. Leading and Managing Mental Health Centers 265
Anthony Broskowski

11. Diagnosis and Intervention in Organizational Settings 289
Harry Levinson

12. Consultation to Organizations in Transition 312
Ralph G. Hirschowitz

Part Four: Mental Health Service for Specific Populations

13. Providing Services to the Elderly 334
Robert D. Patterson and Ruby B. Abrahams

14. Serving the Chronically Mentally Ill 358
Norris Hansell

15. Working with the Mentally Retarded and Developmentally Disabled 372
Lewis B. Klebanoff

16. Intervening with Disaster Victims 397
Raquel E. Cohen

17. Brief Family Crisis Therapy 419
Howard J. Parad

18. Primary Prevention of Emotional Disorders in School Settings 445
Helen Z. Reinherz

19. Serving the Underserved Through Rural Mental Health Programs 467
Morton O. Wagenfeld and Lucy D. Ozarin

20. Linking Mental Health and Health Care Systems 486
Anthony Broskowski

21. Evaluating Community Mental Health Programs 514
Herbert C. Schulberg

Part Five: Strengthening Community Mental Health Through Human and Educational Resources

22. Human Resources for Mental Health Services 540
Harold W. Demone, Jr.

23. Social and Behavioral Sciences in Medical School Curriculum 565
James R. Allen

24. Primary Care and Mental Health Training in Community Settings 587
George L. Adams

25. People Helping People: Beyond the Professional Model 611
Phyllis Rolfe Silverman

26. Audiovisuals in Mental Health Education: A Quantum Leap 633
Edward A. Mason

Epilogue: Personal Reflections by Gerald Caplan 650

Chronological Bibliography of Gerald Caplan 667

Name Index 680

Subject Index 693

The Authors

Herbert C. Schulberg is professor of psychiatry and psychology at the University of Pittsburgh School of Medicine and director of the Social and Community Psychiatry Program at Western Psychiatric Institute and Clinic in Pittsburgh. He received his Ph.D. degree in clinical psychology at Columbia University (1960) and his M.S.Hyg. degree at the Harvard School of Public Health (1963). Before joining the University of Pittsburgh in 1976, Schulberg was associate executive director of United Community Planning Corporation in Boston and associate clinical professor of psychology at Harvard Medical School.

Schulberg's interests concern the planning and evaluation of community mental health services. His numerous books and journal publications deal with key issues in both of these realms and have contributed to the advancement of new conceptual strategies for determining program effectiveness. His present research pertains to the treatment of depression in psychiatric and primary medical care programs.

Schulberg is a fellow of the American Psychological Association. He serves on the boards of directors of the American College of Mental Health Administration and of the Association for Mental Health Affiliation with Israel.

Marie Killilea is assistant professor, Department of Mental Hygiene, Johns Hopkins University School of Hygiene and Public Health. Previously, she was for many years assistant director of the Laboratory of Community Psychiatry, Harvard Medical School, a pioneering research and postgraduate training program in community mental health theory and practice.

Killilea is a specialist on social support systems and has extensive experience in teaching community mental health in university graduate and continuing education programs. She served initially as a member and then as staff liaison on the Task Panel on Community Support Systems of the President's Commission on Mental Health. As a citizen volunteer, she has been involved in Mental Health Association work in both Maryland and Massachusetts, and she served for several years on an advisory council for community service and continuing education for the Board of Higher Education in Massachusetts.

Among her publications is a paper, coauthored with Beatrix Hamburg, on social support, stress, illness, and use of health service, as part of the *Surgeon General's Report on Health Promotion and Disease Prevention.* She also coedited with Gerald Caplan *Support Systems And Mutual Help* (1976) and contributed a chapter on mutual help organizations.

Ruby B. Abrahams, M.S., is research associate, University Health Consortium, Brandeis University.

George L. Adams, M.D., is professor of psychiatry and director, Community and Social Psychiatry Programs, Baylor College of Medicine.

James R. Allen, M.D., is professor and chairman, Department of Psychiatry and Behavioral Sciences, University of Oklahoma, Tulsa Medical College, and executive director, Tulsa Psychiatric Center.

Frank Baker, Ph.D., is professor of psychology and of social and preventive medicine, and director, Division of Community Psychiatry, State University of New York at Buffalo.

Bernard L. Bloom, Ph.D., is professor, Department of Psychology, University of Colorado.

Anthony Broskowski, Ph.D., is a practicing psychologist and executive director, Northside Community Mental Health Center, Tampa, Florida.

Gerald Caplan, M.D., is professor of child psychiatry and chairman, Department of Child Psychiatry, Hadassah University Hospital, Ein Karem, Jerusalem.

Ruth B. Caplan-Moskovich, Ph.D., is residing in Jerusalem, Israel.

Raquel E. Cohen, M.D., is associate professor of psychiatry, Harvard Medical School.

Harold W. Demone, Jr., Ph.D., is professor and dean, Graduate School of Social Work, Rutgers–The State University of New Jersey.

Norris Hansell, M.D., is professor of psychiatry, Northwestern University, and head, Department of Psychiatry, Christie Clinic, Champaign, Illinois.

Dwight Harshbarger, Ph.D., is vice-president for human resources, Sealy Incorporated, Chicago.

Ralph G. Hirschowitz, M.D., is assistant clinical professor of psychiatry, Harvard Medical School, and associate, The Levinson Institute, Cambridge, Massachusetts.

Lewis B. Klebanoff, Ph.D., is deputy assistant commissioner (Mental Retardation), Massachusetts Department of Mental Health, Boston.

Harry Levinson, Ph.D., is president, The Levinson Institute, Cambridge, Massachusetts, and lecturer, Department of Psychiatry, Harvard Medical School.

Leo Levy, Ph.D., is professor, Department of Preventive Medicine and Community Health, Abraham Lincoln School of Medicine; and Department of Community Health Sciences, School of Public Health, University of Illinois at the Medical Center.

Edward A. Mason, M.D., is associate clinical professor of psychiatry, Harvard Medical School.

Lucy D. Ozarin, M.D., is assistant director for program development, Division of Mental Health Service Programs, National Institute of Mental Health, Rockville, Maryland.

Howard J. Parad, D.S.W., is professor, School of Social Work, University of Southern California.

Colin Murray Parkes, M.D., Fellow, Royal College of Psychiatry, is senior lecturer in psychiatry, The London Hospital Medical College.

Robert D. Patterson, M.D., is director, Inpatient and Outpatient Mental Health, Waltham Hospital; attending psychiatrist, McLean Hospital; and lecturer, Department of Psychiatry, Harvard Medical School.

Helen Z. Reinherz, M.S.W., Sc.D., is professor of social work and principal investigator, Identifying Preschool Children at Risk, Simmons College School of Social Work.

Phyllis Rolfe Silverman, Ph.D., is associate professor of social work and health, Massachusetts General Hospital Institute of Health Professions, and lecturer, Department of Psychiatry, Harvard Medical School.

Morton O. Wagenfeld, Ph.D., is professor of sociology and of health and human services, Western Michigan University.

Robert S. Weiss, Ph.D., is professor, Department of Sociology, University of Massachusetts, and lecturer, Department of Psychiatry, Harvard Medical School.

The Modern Practice of Community Mental Health

A Volume in Honor of Gerald Caplan

Chapter 1

Gerald Caplan: The Man and His Work

Ruth B. Caplan-Moskovich

The roots of Gerald Caplan's interest in community psychiatry may perhaps be traced to the influence of his father. David Caplan was born to a Chassidic family in Rakishok, a Jewish town in Lithuania. He was an *illuy,* a child prodigy in Talmudic studies. He studied in several non-Chassidic yeshivas (Talmudic seminaries), including Slobodka and Volozhin, which had reputations for breadth of philosophic vision and openness to modern ideas, and he received the first of a number of rabbinical diplomas at the age of seventeen. In 1913, when he was twenty-four, he emigrated to England to embark on a university career. It was characteristic of him that he planned to learn English on the journey. Since he had a photographic memory, he accomplished this by memorizing an English dictionary. When he landed in Britain, however, he was disappointed to find that the natives pronounced their words so strangely that it was impossible to understand them, and he had to start his language studies all over again.

He settled in the midst of closely knit Lithuanian Jewish immigrant communities in Liverpool and later in Manchester, where he taught in yeshivas and worked as a rabbi and cantor. After marrying Sophia Zassman, the daughter of a prominent Liverpool merchant, in 1915, and after the birth of Gerald in

1917, he retired from the rabbinate and went into business as a timber importer in order to earn enough money to establish his family. He continued to officiate for several years on a volunteer basis as a cantor during the annual high holydays, and he operated informally throughout his life as a counselor to people with personal problems, in the pastoral tradition of a Chassidic rabbi. His home was a meeting place for the Zionist intellectuals, Hebrew teachers, and Jewish writers of the area. And he remained deeply involved in religious, educational, and Zionist affairs until he died in 1938 at the age of forty-seven from coronary thrombosis, after suffering for several years from angina pectoris.

The need to make a living for his growing family had forced David to give up his hopes of a university career. Gerald, the only son and the eldest of his four children, was encouraged from an early age to fulfill his father's frustrated ambitions. When he was eleven, he won a much-coveted scholarship to Manchester Grammar School, a famous public school that since its foundation by Henry VIII in 1515 had educated future professionals, academicians, civil servants, colonial administrators, and parliamentary leaders. This school instilled in its students a particular mode of analytic thinking and problem solving, one in which abstraction and generalization always remained close to concrete reality. Theory was not allowed to escape into a rarefied and precious altitude but was kept down to earth and in touch with the affairs of real life, which it was designed to enrich. This intellectual tradition was strikingly similar to that of the yeshivas at which David Caplan had studied, and the development of this style of thinking in the son must have been reinforced simultaneously in school and at home.

In medical school Caplan was usually in the upper quarter of his class, and he obtained a special bachelor of science degree in anatomy and physiology in 1937. His first steps in research were taken at that time when he wrote two theses for this degree, both linked with his father's angina pectoris, concern for which was dominating the family circle: "Investigation of the Nerve Endings in the Pericardium of the Dog" and "Investigation on Muscle Pain in Man." Particularly in working on the latter topic, he began to experience the excitement and joy of research.

Although his academic record at Manchester University was good, Caplan did not spend as much time studying as he had done at Manchester Grammar School. He became active in athletics, got his colors for badminton, and eventually became captain of the university team. He spent most weekends and vacations hiking, cycling, or mountain climbing. He also devoted much time and energy to Zionist work. He organized a University Zionist Society and became chairman of the University Jewish Society. He followed in his father's footsteps in developing an interest in Hebrew language and literature, and while still a teen-ager he became honorary treasurer of a Hebrew-speaking society, most of whose members were two or three times his age.

In his fourth year of medicine Caplan began to move toward choice of a career. He happened to be looking at a book on the psychology shelves of the medical school library when a man standing next to him struck up a conversation. He was E. Howard Kitching, a brilliant young psychiatrist who had just arrived to establish the first psychiatric outpatient clinic at Manchester Royal Infirmary, the main teaching hospital of the medical school. Student and teacher became friends. Kitching was looking for "converts" to his new endeavor. Over the following three years Caplan spent all his spare time in Kitching's clinic, learning about the diagnosis and treatment of neuroses. And, by the end of medical school, Caplan knew that he wanted to be a psychiatrist in the pattern of his mentor.

When Caplan was twenty-one, his father died and the young medical student realized that he must get a job with a good salary as soon as he graduated in order to support his mother and three sisters. He could not afford to do a regular internship and residency because these were too poorly paid. Consequently, after getting his medical degree in June 1940, he did a few months of well-paid temporary jobs in general practice and hospitals, while waiting for an appropriate job in a mental hospital where the pay would be good from the start. Then at the end of 1940 he saw an advertisement in the *British Medical*

Journal asking for applicants for the post of house physician at Winson Green Mental Hospital in Birmingham and offering training in psychiatry but with an annual salary of £200 instead of the usual salary of £350. Caplan decided that this must be a good place since it could apparently afford to offer such poor financial inducement to applicants, and he applied for and got the job. He spent eighteen months at Winson Green before going into military service. Years later J. J. O'Reilly, the Jesuit-educated medical superintendent of Winson Green, confessed that he had baited a trap to recruit a highly motivated and intelligent young man by the careful wording of that advertisement and by offering a substantially lower salary than the going rate.

In Birmingham, Caplan began to learn about major mental illnesses. He quickly realized that even a good hospital like Winson Green was forced (in those years) to be largely custodial because of a lack of effective treatment techniques and because patients were usually admitted late in the course of illness due to the stigma of entering a "lunatic asylum." O'Reilly taught Caplan a good deal about ward and hospital organization and also encouraged him to develop new treatment approaches and new administrative modes. Caplan, with this encouragement and support, reached out to a local general hospital and there established an outpatient clinic along lines Kitching had pioneered at Manchester Royal Infirmary. This clinic quickly attracted a clientele of neurotics and early-stage psychotics who would never have been willing to come directly to the mental hospital.

Caplan also began to experiment with physical therapy—cardiazol injections to precipitate convulsions, insulin therapy, prolonged narcosis, and so on; he also tried faradic shocks with an apparatus he put together, copied from something he read about in an American journal. His first publication was an article about nonconvulsive faradic shock therapy in which he described a case where a defect in his technique had precipitated a convulsion in a depressed patient, with good therapeutic results (Caplan, 1941).

While in Birmingham, Caplan met and married Ann Siebenberg. He volunteered for the Royal Air Force but was discharged after a year for medical reasons. He returned to Winson

Green Hospital as a senior psychiatrist, and over the next year he continued to develop its outpatient clinic in the general hospital.

In 1943, the post of deputy medical superintendent at the Cefn Coed Mental Hospital in Swansea, South Wales became vacant. This had been Kitching's job before he had come to Manchester, and Kitching had often talked of how much he had enjoyed it. Caplan saw this vacancy as an opportunity to follow in the footsteps of his mentor. He applied for the position and was accepted. For two years he worked in Swansea. He learned the rudiments of mental hospital administration; and since part of the hospital was being used as a civilian base hospital for war casualties, he was also able to get experience in general hospital administration. During long periods when the medical superintendent was away, Caplan was in charge—a not inconsiderable challenge to so young a professional.

During his two years in Swansea, Caplan continued his efforts to introduce psychiatric clinics into general hospitals. He took over the clinic at Swansea General Hospital that had been established years earlier by Kitching, and he organized a psychiatric clinic in the general hospital of Merthyr Tydfil, about thirty miles away. By then, electrically induced convulsion therapy had reached Britain, and Caplan had begun to learn the new technique while still in Birmingham. He had become dissatisfied with the cumbersome apparatus that was then available and had begun to consider how to improve it. In Wales, he developed a lightweight electroconvulsive apparatus in collaboration with a local electrical engineer, after which he negotiated with a London electronics firm, the Multitone Company, to market this machine under the name of the Caplan Electroconvulsive Apparatus. For many years, this instrument was widely used in Britain. He also began a series of studies of techniques of electroshock and its complications, which he made the basis of a thesis that he submitted to Manchester University for the degree of M.D., which is an advanced degree in Britain. (The British equivalent of an American M.D. is the M.B.,Ch.B.—a Bachelor's degree.)

Despite the use of electroshock, insulin, prolonged narcosis, and milieu therapy in mental hospitals and psychotherapy in general hospital outpatient clinics, Caplan was still not happy with the results that could be obtained in established clinical cases, and he set out to find methods of early treatment and prevention of mental disorder. He began to consider intervention earlier in the life cycle and thus to experiment with the treatment of psychiatric disturbances in children. He quickly discovered, however, that his knowledge and skills, developed with adults, were not adequate for treating children. He therefore decided to go to London for training in child psychiatry and at the same time to undertake training in psychoanalysis, which his reading had by then persuaded him was the most valid basis for developing both therapeutic and preventive psychosocial understanding and techniques. Since the war was coming to an end, he could easily leave his administrative responsibilities at the Cefn Coed mental hospital and the military hospital, and so he moved with his wife and daughter to London in 1945.

In London, Caplan trained in child psychiatry with John Bowlby at the Tavistock Clinic. Anna Freud and her group at the Psychoanalytic Institute offered him training in psychoanalysis. The adult department of the Tavistock Clinic gave him an honorary staff position to work with Walter Bion and John Rickman in developing methods of group psychotherapy. Because no salary was available, Caplan went into private consulting practice in Harley Street. Within a few months he succeeded in establishing a reputation as a specialist in ambulatory electroshock treatment of patients suffering from depression, and over the next three years his income from this source was sufficient to allow him and his family to live in comfort, while he was pursuing his studies in psychoanalysis, child psychiatry, and group psychotherapy.

Until the move to London, Caplan had been largely self-taught, although he owed much to the stimulation and support of Kitching and O'Reilly. In London he had a number of excellent teachers: Bowlby, J. R. Rees, Bion, Rickman, and Eric Trist at the Tavistock Clinic; and Anna Freud, Kate Friedlander, Michael Balint, and Willie Hoffer at the Psychoanalytic Institute. In those years, the Tavistock Clinic was a most exciting place. Its senior staff had just returned from the army, where they had worked out innovative psychosocial and social system ideas and techniques with a population orientation. They were now trying to adapt these methods to civilian conditions in such fields as education and industry, as well as to patients in more traditional clinic settings. Bowlby had recently written his World Health Organization monograph, *Maternal Care and Mental Health* (Bowlby, 1951), showing the etiological importance of mother-child separation in hospitalized and institutionalized children and recommending relevant methods of primary prevention. Friedlander was Caplan's analyst. She was developing psychoanalytically oriented child guidance methods, as well as ways of preventing and treating child delinquency. Bion and Rickman were developing psychoanalytic group therapy. Anna Freud was the control analyst of Caplan's first psychoanalytic treatment case, and Balint controlled his second case. Balint was developing his method of group discussion with general practitioners to help them become more sophisticated in handling mental health aspects of patients in general practice.

The year 1946 was to mark a turning point in Caplan's career. J. R. Rees had been in charge of army psychiatry during the war, and on demobilization had led his senior staff back to the Tavistock Clinic, of which he had been the prewar director. Asked to organize the first postwar International Congresses of Mental Health and Child Psychiatry in London in 1948, Rees invited Bowlby to organize the Child Psychiatry Congress, and Bowlby suggested that this job be entrusted to Caplan, despite the latter's youth. Rees agreed. Caplan became secretary general of the child psychiatry organizing committee and then secretary general of the newly established International Association of Child Psychiatry. He remained a member of its executive committee until he was made its honorary president in 1970, in which office he continues to this day. Over many years, he also served as honorary treasurer. He helped build up the organization and obtain funds from foundations and governments to finance its four yearly international congresses. He became expert in the administrative and political aspects of building and running a large international organization. He also got to know personally the leading child psychiatrists of the world, as well as learning the techniques of dealing with audiences of thousands at international congresses.

During the years 1945-1948, Caplan also played a prominent role in English Zionism. He was a member of the executive committee of the English Zionist Federation; was elected to the Board of Deputies, the representative body of British Jewry; and continued in the London area what he had started in Swansea and Birmingham—traveling round to Rotary Clubs and churches to give Zionist information lectures to non-Jews. He also helped to organize Professional and Technical Workers For Alyah (PATWA), an organization to promote immigration to Israel of professional and technical workers, and in 1947 he became its chairman. So it was natural that when the State of Israel was established in 1948 and the War of Independence started, he should be invited to come to Israel to help in the war effort. And it was natural that he should immediately sell his home and practice and get on the first available plane to answer the call.

From 1948 until 1952 Caplan lived in Israel. During his first year he worked as a civilian in the Israeli army and was put in charge of army psychiatry in the northern region of the country. During this period he also undertook the job of senior adviser in mental health to the Ministry of Health and organized the first Department of Mental Health in the State of Israel. The British, on their departure, had left the country with only 200 state mental hospital beds; thus, one urgent task was to discover and acquire buildings to house the thousands of mentally ill who were wandering the streets. While this search was going on, Caplan opened two psychiatric inpatient units in general hospitals in Haifa, which he directed. He started a school for psychiatric nurses, began to train psychiatrists in active treatment methods inside the general hospital psychiatric units, and pioneered methods of outreach consultation to new immigrant camps. He negotiated with the authorities of the Greek Orthodox church to acquire a disused monastery in Jerusalem with the idea of turning this into a government mental hospital that would be linked with the Hadassah Hebrew University Medical School. He was to be the first director of this teaching hospital.

At this point there was a political reorganization in the Israeli government. A new minister of health was appointed. He in turn appointed a new director general. The latter arbitrarily closed Caplan's general hospital unit in Haifa and replaced Caplan as acting head of the projected mental hospital in Jerusalem with his own candidate. Caplan resigned from the ministry. He was then approached by Hadassah Hebrew University Medical School and invited to organize a child guidance clinic within its framework in Jerusalem. He accepted and went on to develop the Lasker Mental Hygiene and Child Guidance Center during the years 1949-1952.

At the Lasker Center, Caplan began to build a program of preventive child psychiatry, focusing mainly on the first years of life. He soon discovered that by the time emotionally disturbed small children were referred to a clinic, even one established in a public health framework where there was minimal stigma, they were already long-term treatment problems. So he began to search for even earlier points of intervention. He began to work with pregnant women within the framework of maternal and childcare centers in Jerusalem, which were at that time administered by Hadassah. He investigated factors in pregnancy that were predictive of possible later disorders in mother-infant relationships. He developed methods of preventive intervention through discussion groups with expectant mothers and trained public health nurses to run these group meetings so that it would be possible to affect the lives of a large number of people. He realized that this would be essential if effective methods of prevention were to be achieved.

He was able to recruit a team of social workers and psychologists with English and American training. With these, he began to study ways of identifying disturbed mother-child relationships in the populations of well-baby clinics in collaboration with public health nurses and pediatricians. He wanted to find ways of persuading mothers with disturbances that seemed pathogenic to enter short, focused treatments, so that these disturbances could be remedied before they led to disorders in the young children. He also trained pediatricians and nurses to become more sophisticated in dealing with the mental health aspects of their daily work. They might then be able to prevent psychopathology in their child patients by influencing the psychological aspects of mothers and their childrearing practices.

By 1952, however, Caplan was beginning to question the value of intervention early in the life cycle. As he moved from intervention in adults to intervention in older children to intervention in younger children to intervention in mother-infant relationships to intervention in pregnancy, he discovered that many women were being influenced as mothers by personality traits they had developed in their formative years of childhood in their relationships with their own parents. There was an obvious limit to tracing etiology back to previous generations and of using a model of prevention that required earlier and earlier intervention in the natural history of a disorder in an individual. Focus on an individual patient could reveal by retrospective anamnesis the crucial turning points in the early history of the child, the mother, the grandmother, and so on. But how could such understanding be used in a feasible prospective program, particularly with the large numbers of cases involved?

Caplan began to grope toward a possible answer to this question, and a possible new model of prevention, in work carried out from 1950 in a program of the Lasker Center in Youth Aliya, an immigrant children's organization. At that time, Youth Aliya was dealing with about 18,000 new immigrant children, aged ten to sixteen, who were being educated in residential centers throughout Israel, many of them in kibbutzim (collective settlements). The Lasker Center signed a contract with Youth Aliya to handle the mental health aspects of this program. At first, the Lasker Center staff traveled round the residential centers and investigated individual disturbed children. Staff members made diagnostic formulations and recommended administrative disposition and treatment plans. But there were never less than 1,000 disturbed children being referred in a year, and although a small number could be treated at the Lasker Center or in branches that were set up in Haifa and Tel Aviv, no treatment facilities adequate to make a dent in this large number were available. Nor could three therapeutically oriented treatment institutions run by Youth Aliya cope with more than a fraction of those children who were too disturbed for continued care in an ordinary Youth Aliya educational setting.

In this program, Caplan and his colleagues were forced to face the implications of responsibility for a total population by an organization with limited resources—a responsibility that could be evaded when working in community agencies such as child guidance clinics and well-baby clinics that recruited cases from the general community. What began to emerge was a new practice modality and a new conceptual model. Caplan and his colleagues began to develop a method they first called *counseling the counselors*—namely, educating and supporting the staff members of the ordinary residential institutions of Youth Aliya to understand the special needs of disturbed children and to try to satisfy these without removing the children from their natural setting or sending them for specialized therapy. This technique, which when it was first described in 1954 in the *American Journal of Orthopsychiatry* (Rosenfeld and Caplan, 1954) had come to be known as *staff consultation,* was based on the finding that the difficulties of a problem child were often influenced by idiosyncratic problems in the adults caring for him and in the social system of the residential institution. Children with objectively similar problems were referred for consultation in some institutions and by certain childcare staff but apparently were adequately handled by other staff members or other institutions. Caplan began to realize that not infrequently the crux of the difficulty was the *disturbing* child rather than the inherently *disturbed* child. This led to focusing the consultation on the relative shortcomings of the childcare worker and his institution in that particular case rather than investigating and diagnosing the disturbance of the child and then making a treatment recommendation that in practice usually could not be implemented.

The new focus led to developing techniques for understanding and modifying the problems of the counselor or teacher and the institution in coping with emotional problems or behavior deviations in certain classes of children. It was then discovered that requests for consultation often came when there was an acute upset in the equilibrium between child and institution.

This upset could be triggered by some recent change in the child or by some disequilibrium in the mental economy of the child-care worker or in the social system of the institution.

At this stage Caplan began to feel the need for new knowledge and skills that would enable him to get a better grasp on the problems of dealing with the interpenetration of psychosocial and sociocultural factors of the individual in his social setting and of understanding the meaning of disequilibrium or crisis in both. He wanted to know how these ideas might be used to develop a new conceptual model of prevention that would not be pinned to an early intervention approach in an individual.

In 1951, the World Federation of Mental Health, which was one of the organizations that had been established at the 1948 London congress, held an international congress in Mexico City, to which Caplan was invited and at which he gave a paper about his preventive work with new immigrants in Israel. In connection with this congress, Caplan, along with several other speakers, was invited to be part of a "flying seminar" that would conduct a lecture tour in several psychiatric centers in the United States. Caplan gave lectures in New York, Chicago, Topeka, San Francisco, Los Angeles, and Boston, and there met many of the leaders of American psychiatry. In particular, he found that Franz Alexander and John French at the Chicago Psychoanalytic Institute and Erich Lindemann at Harvard were thinking along lines similar to his. The former were experimenting on modifications in psychoanalytic psychotherapy to develop short methods of treatment of the kind that might be used in preventive intervention. And in Boston, Erich Lindemann, at the Harvard School of Public Health, had recently organized the Wellesley Human Relations Service, where he was accepting responsibility for the mental health of a total community. Lindemann was developing methods of prevention based on offering consultation to clergymen, teachers, family doctors, and other "caretakers" to enable them to help their clients master current life crises. This approach had emerged from Lindemann's study (1944) of the crisis of bereavement in victims of the Coconut Grove fire, a tragic fire in a Boston night club in which dozens of people died.

Caplan and Lindemann, who had not known of each other's work before, discovered that over the previous few years they had been converging on similar concepts and techniques and had even begun to develop an almost identical terminology. Caplan was impressed to discover how much Lindemann's ideas had been enriched by what he was learning from his public health colleagues at the Harvard School of Public Health, as well as from the social scientists at Harvard's Department of Social Relations. He decided that he would take a year off from his work in Jerusalem and accept Lindemann's invitation to spend a sabbatical with him at Harvard.

On his return to Jerusalem, Caplan's request for leave was refused by his Hadassah superiors. They would not give him either sabbatical leave or leave without pay, since he had worked in Hadassah for only three years. The director of Hadassah issued an ultimatum: If Caplan persisted in his plans to go to Harvard, his job at Hadassah would be terminated. At the end of a year, if his post had not been filled, an application by Caplan for reinstatement would be considered. Nevertheless, Caplan took his family to Boston for a year. At the end of that period, Lindemann and the Harvard School of Public Health authorities asked him to stay on for a second year. Since he had no job in Jerusalem, he agreed. The following year Lindemann moved to Harvard Medical School as head of the Department of Psychiatry at the Massachusetts General Hospital, and Caplan was asked to replace him as head of the Community Mental Health Program at the Harvard School of Public Health, with the academic title of associate professor of mental health. He accepted. By then he had begun to come to terms with his mixed feelings about leaving Israel, since he continued to identify with Zionist ideology and missed being personally involved in the development of the new state. In later years he came to the retrospective conclusion that had he not lost his Hadassah position in 1952, he would almost certainly have returned to Jerusalem at the end of the first year in Boston, and his subsequent career at Harvard would have been aborted.

During his first three years in Boston, Caplan continued his work along the lines he had been developing between 1949 and 1952 in Israel. He worked with Grete Bibring at the Beth

Israel Hospital on developing a psychiatric consultation service in the Department of Obstetrics. He continued his work with pregnant women at the Boston Lying-in Hospital, where he became a member of a multidisciplinary team of the Harvard School of Public Health and the Boston Children's Medical Center, called the Harvard Family Health Clinic. This team included obstetricians, pediatricians, nurses, social workers, and nutritionists. It cared for pregnant women and their husbands, conducted prenatal clinics, and followed the woman during the birth and lying-in period. Later, the same workers cared for the child in a well-baby clinic and offered guidance to the parents on childcare during the first years of the child's life.

Caplan also worked with George Gardner at the Judge Baker Clinic in supervising psychotherapy carried out by child psychiatry and child psychology residents. He collaborated with Dane Prugh in the psychiatric department of the Children's Medical Center, mainly in offering consultation to pediatricians working in the child health division. He spent much of his time with Lindemann at the Wellesley Human Relations Service, where for the first time he had the experience of working collaboratively with anthropologists and sociologists in investigating the structure and culture of a community—in this case a middle-class suburban population—and in trying to build a preventively oriented mental health program. The latter was, in certain respects, a model for the community mental health center programs that were to be developed some ten years later.

During this period Caplan also continued his own training in line with the plan formed when he first came to Boston. He wished to acquire the conceptual models of public health and some of its techniques of research and practice and to modify them for use in the mental health field. At the Harvard School of Public Health, the community mental health program was part of the Department of Public Health Practice, directed by Hugh R. Leavell, a world leader in public health. Caplan learned a great deal from him, both formally by attending his lectures to postgraduate public health students and informally by discussing with him matters of joint responsibility. He also learned much from Franz Goldman, another senior colleague in the department, who at that time was laying the foundations of specifically formulated programs of medical care. John Gordon, professor of epidemiology, and Benjamin Paul, professor of medical anthropology, were also valuable sources of information.

Influenced by these authorities, as well as by Lindemann, Caplan began to evolve a new model of prevention. He began to conceptualize prevention of mental disorder along public health lines by dividing it into primary, secondary, and tertiary prevention and by moving the focus of preventive efforts from individuals to populations. He now saw the goal of preventive programs as that of changing community rates of disease rather than as interrupting a pathogenic process in a particular individual. He was thus able to discard the approach of early intervention in the natural history of the unfolding of disease in an individual in favor of crisis intervention at any stage of the history of disease in populations. This advance in theory was beginning to develop in Caplan's mind during those early formative years at the Harvard School of Public Health. It eventually crystalized in his book, *Principles of Preventive Psychiatry* (1964a), which represented the first major statement of his new conceptual model.

During his first years in Boston, while studying public health, Caplan also continued, and eventually completed, his training in psychoanalysis. When he had unexpectedly left London in 1948, he had not yet finished his training at the British Psychoanalytic Institute. In a desultory fashion, he had tried to continue this in Israel. But when he came to Boston, and when it became clear that he would stay in that city for several years, he entered the Boston Psychoanalytic Institute. He underwent a second personal analysis with Joseph J. Michaels, and he treated two adult patients under the supervision of Grete Bibring and Helen Tartakoff. He also attended theory and practice seminars at the institute. In 1955, he completed this training and was admitted to the British Psychoanalytic Society as an associate member, eventually being accepted as a full member in 1977. Thus, while he was developing his population-oriented theories and techniques, Caplan was continuing to practice individual psychoanalysis and psychoanalytically oriented psychotherapy. Until 1970, when his traveling made this impossible, he usually had three or four patients in five-times-a-week psychoanalysis and another four to six patients whom he saw two or three times a week, in addition to several cases in more superficial psychotherapy. This explains the fundamental psychoanalytic underpinnings of his population-oriented theories and techniques, along with the fact that their ultimate referent is the promotion of the well-being of individuals, based on an understanding of, and sensitivity to, their personal needs and psychology.

In 1953, Caplan established a Harvard School of Public Health field training laboratory at the Whittier Street Health Center of Boston's Health Department. In this setting, he organized a research and community practice unit, modeled in part on the Lasker Center of Hadassah in Jerusalem. The focus was on building day-to-day collaborative relationships with the public health nurses and pediatricians who staffed well-baby clinics and offered preventive health care in the neighborhood. The innovation in Boston was that the unit provided a setting for the training in mental health of postgraduate public health students and that its research projects were designed to produce material that could be used in lectures and seminars for this student body in the Harvard School of Public Health.

The Whittier Street mental health team comprised psychiatrists, psychologists, social workers, and social scientists, some of whom were attending the Harvard School of Public Health to obtain degrees in public health with community mental health as their area of specialization. The team sponsored a series of studies of crises in individuals and families, such as crises precipitated by the birth of a premature baby or by the diagnosis of pulmonary tuberculosis in a family member. Out of these investigations emerged the model of crisis as a central fulcrum for primary prevention. The emphasis was on the crisis period as one in which individuals are more open to outside influence and hence to short-term interventions by nonspecialist counselors using a "human helping hand" approach. Moreover, these studies revealed the regularly occurring patterns of crisis behavior among normal people. They mainly utilized a natural history or descriptive approach—interviewing a random sample of ordinary people drawn from the regular clientele of the health center and categorizing the details of their responses to the particular crisis situations.

The studies identified the generic responses that could be expected in most crises, the specific sequence of problems to which people probably would have to adapt in particular crises, and the range of their expectable reactions. The last were studied from the point of view of the basic human response, irrespective of its coloring by idiosyncratic personality traits or the effects of individual experience. Findings could thus be used to develop methods of anticipatory guidance and preventive intervention with general application. This approach was also geared to developing methods of prevention that might be used on a widespread scale by such nonspecialist professional caregivers as public health nurses, pediatricians, and public health physicians, as well as by nonprofessional helpers and supporters, including family members, friends, neighbors, and informal community caregivers. Even as early as 1954, the concept began to emerge of the "supporters" who might exert a helpful influence on individuals in crisis and who might in turn be a target group to be identified, recruited, and educated by community mental health specialists as line workers in a widespread program of primary prevention. It was not until twenty years later that these ideas were refined to become the basis for support systems theory and practice, but the conceptual seeds can clearly be found in Caplan's analysis of the results of his empirical studies of crisis that were started in Whittier Street in the early 1950s (Caplan, 1974).

The second main area of exploration in Whittier Street was the development, description, definition, and evaluation of techniques of mental health consultation. Public health nurses were the main consultees in the early years: those working within the framework of the City of Boston Health Department, and also those who did bedside nursing in the home, as staff members of the Boston Visiting Nurse Association, with which organization Caplan and his unit signed a consultation agreement in 1955. The consultation method became the cornerstone of community mental health practice. It was the main skill that was taught in a supervised practicum and in practice-oriented seminars to the community mental health students in Caplan's program at the Harvard School of Public Health.

The latter program began to take shape in 1954, after Lindemann left to take up his duties as professor of psychiatry of Harvard Medical School at the Massachusetts General Hospital and Caplan replaced him as head of the community mental health program at the Harvard School of Public Health. In the ten years that Lindemann worked at this school, and during Caplan's first years there, the focus of their efforts was on the introduction of lectures, seminars, and field training opportunities in mental health for public health students, so that everyone who graduated would have received minimal education in mental health as part of his public health studies. But when Caplan took over the program, he added the element of specialized training for psychiatrists, psychologists, social workers, nurses, and social scientists, who came to the school for one or two years to obtain a degree in public health with mental health as a speciality. The first group of three mental health specialist students graduated in 1955. By the time Caplan left the Harvard School of Public Health in 1964, sixty-two specialist students had completed courses of training there. Some of them had received the degree of master of public health, others the master of science in hygiene, and three the doctor of science in hygiene degree. Among those graduates were many specialists who later became leaders in community mental health, key administrators in federal and state programs, and professors in medical schools, university departments of psychology, and schools of social work and nursing. Their students, and in certain cases the students of their students, have developed and spread Caplan's original ideas throughout America and Europe.

Active involvement in the multidisciplinary teams at Wellesley Human Relations Service, the Harvard Family Health Clinic, and the Whittier Street Field Training Program aroused Caplan's interest not only in solving the problems of interdisciplinary cooperation but also in trying to understand the particular contributions of the different professions. Those were linked with the workers' own definition of their role, a definition that in turn is based on their community-prescribed domain and the culture and traditions of their guild, as well as on their image in the eyes of their clients, which provides them with special opportunities and constraints. The results of this interest have been recorded in a series of lectures, articles, and books by Caplan that have appeared over the years. The first of these, a lecture Caplan delivered at the annual convention of the National League of Nurses in 1953, was entitled "The Mental Hygiene Role of the Nurse in Maternal and Child Care" (Caplan, 1954). This was the first public statement of Caplan's ideas on primary prevention through anticipatory guidance and crisis intervention by community caregiving professionals who are not mental health specialists.

The second publication was more ambitious. It was a book-length transcript (Caplan, 1959a) of a series of lectures that Caplan delivered to an institute for social workers over a three-day period at the School of Social Welfare of the University of California at Berkeley in June 1955. Topics included "Ingredients of Personality and Personality Development," "Epidemiological Ideas Regarding Mental Health and Mental Ill-Health," "Emotional Implications of Pregnancy," "Origins and Development of Mother-Child Relationships," "Mother-Child Relationships During the First Year of Life," and "Consultation." An important chapter in this book was the text of a lecture Caplan had delivered a few days earlier at a meeting in San Francisco of the American Association of Medical Social Workers entitled "The Role of the Social Worker in Preventive Psychiatry for Mothers and Children." This was the analogue of the lecture delivered two years earlier to the National League of Nurses. Caplan challenged the social workers to return to their traditional role of specializing in the psychosocial and sociocultural aspects of ameliorating the environmental forces that influence the mental health of individuals rather than placing their top professional priority on modifying intrapsychic forces by psychoanalytically oriented psychotherapy or casework.

The San Francisco and Berkeley lectures led to an interesting development: Caplan was invited to return to the School of Social Welfare in Berkeley annually for eight years to lead two- or three-day institutes with a group of leading social workers from the western states and Hawaii. These institutes were sponsored by the U. S. Children's Bureau and by the California State Health Department. The membership of the institutes remained remarkably stable from year to year, and it was discovered that there was considerable continuity in the discussions. Participants developed into a reference group with a shared philosophy and vocabulary; they molded their practice throughout the year along similar lines, and they reported to the institute at its annual meetings how their experiences had validated or required changes in Caplan's conceptual and methodological ideas. All concerned discovered that the organizational format of this advanced postgraduate educational project fostered the orderly development of systematic learning with a minimal expenditure of time and effort. The interval of a whole year between the meetings did not interrupt personal relationships among students or between them and their teacher, nor did it prevent the development of sustained in-depth discussion of significant issues. On the contrary, the year-long interruptions maximized learning by providing opportunities for field exploration and the working through in practice of theoretical and methodological ideas that could then be shared with other students and with the teacher at the meetings of the institute.

A third lecture in this series was delivered by Caplan in 1957 in Hawaii. Entitled "Practical Steps for the Family Physician in the Prevention of Emotional Disorder," it was subsequently published in the *Journal of the American Medical Association* (Caplan, 1959b). A fourth lecture was delivered in 1962 on "Opportunities for School Psychologists in the Primary Prevention of Mental Disorders in Children" (Caplan, 1963b), and a fifth contribution in 1964 took the form of a chapter on "The Role of Pediatricians in Community Mental Health (with Particular Reference to the Primary Prevention of Mental Disorders in Children)" (1964b).

In each paper in this series, Caplan first presented his evolving ideas about primary prevention. He then analyzed the implications of these ideas for preventive action by community caregivers in general and for the special contribution by the profession to which that paper was being addressed. The series as a whole attempted to increase each profession's understanding of the potential contributions of members of other professions and to catalyze communication among them. Caplan believed that their domains would inevitably overlap and that they would thus very often deal with similar clients and similar problems, often by similar methods. Nevertheless, each profession would develop a specialized orientation and particular focal interests, so that their combined work might optimally enrich one another and the well-being of their clients.

During the period 1955-1960, Caplan began to go further afield in his consulting and teaching activities to communicate his developing ideas and to submit them to critical scrutiny by colleagues working in other settings. The style of his teaching activities was much influenced by his experience in California. His lectures usually concentrated on the crisis model as a basis for primary prevention; the family as a system, with particular reference to the reactions of "healthy" and "unhealthy" families to crisis; methods of mental health consultation, anticipatory guidance, and preventive intervention; methods of gaining entry into a community and of collecting relevant data about factors influencing the mental health of its members and the pattern of its mental health services; and methods of community organization and development to improve such services, based on Caplan's experience in Wellesley and Whittier Street, as well as on what he had learned from his public health practice and health education colleagues at the Harvard School of Public Health. Institutes were organized for key public health and mental health workers in Norway, Holland, and Denmark; and in the two former countries they were repeated at intervals and exerted a significant effect on the development of national health policy and on the patterns of local community mental health practice.

Caplan continued this educational work in a modified form at the Tavistock Clinic in London, where in 1964 he began a series of seminars for leaders in public health and eventually also for psychiatrists, social workers, psychologists, and other caregivers such as probation officers, health visitors, and nurses. These seminars, each lasting for two or three days, were repeated annually for six years and eventually were attended by almost a thousand participants.

His developing interest in patterns of organization of community mental health services and also in administrative consultation led Caplan during the same period to become involved in a series of consultations in the United States and overseas to state or regional agencies that sought his help in reorganizing their mental health programs. These included the Health Department of Hawaii, the Indian Health Service in Arizona, the Native Health Service of Alaska, and the health authorities in the Republic of Ireland, Norway, Holland, the Virgin Islands, and Puerto Rico. Caplan was guided in this program-centered administrative consultation by a philosophy that departed from the traditional approach of organizing a number of service facilities that would cater to a range of patients with special needs and for whom responsibility would be assumed only during the course of their contact with the clinic or hospital. Instead, Caplan advocated accepting responsibility for a circumscribed population, both sick and well, and developing preventive, treatment, and rehabilitation facilities designed to satisfy its needs.

This approach involved keeping abreast of the felt needs of the population, flexibility in developing innovative programs and methods to satisfy needs, and in-service training of staff to equip them to operate with maximum effectiveness in dealing with large numbers of people. This philosophy implied that mental health workers must collect information about what was happening to the persons for whom they accepted responsibility before and after contact with them in a service facility and that staff members must spend a significant part of their working day outside the walls of mental health institutions—in schools, public health facilities, churches, work places, and the like. Here, the focus of specialist mental health endeavor would be to "sanitize" the human environment in order to promote mental health and counteract pathogenic factors, as well as to offer education and consultation to community caregivers and to help them better handle people with established psychopathology, both in their community setting and by referral to specialized mental health facilities.

Caplan was to have two opportunities to turn this population-oriented philosophy into a practical reality and also to learn how to influence mental health specialists to change their traditional patterns and to train them on a widespread scale in the relevant new concepts and skills. The first of these opportunities occurred when he became involved in shaping state mental health policy in Massachusetts, the second when he was appointed senior psychiatric consultant in the Peace Corps, shortly after its inception in 1961. Over the following nine years, but most intensively during the first five of these, Caplan worked with Joseph English, Leonard Duhl, Robert Leopold, and many other leading young psychiatrists to develop an imaginative program of anticipatory guidance and support in the field for the tens of thousands of Peace Corps volunteers who spent a two-year period of service in the developing countries of the world. There, these young people were exposed to unfamiliar cultures and to considerable physical and occupational stress. Caplan and his colleagues succeeded in helping mental health specialists influence the policies and the patterns of operation of administrative, educational, and medical staff of the organization to improve support for volunteers in the field. This was accomplished by promoting peer contacts among volunteers, particularly at recurrent times of expectable crisis, and by preventive and supportive intervention by local administrative staff. These measures were buttressed by regular and on-demand field visits by headquarters staff, including psychiatrists and psychologists.

Caplan gave a series of seminars to all new Peace Corps psychiatrists, who were mainly recruited from the middle echelons of academic departments of psychiatry throughout the country and who were then deployed in local or regional selection and training programs for Peace Corps volunteers. These seminars had a double goal: First and most obvious, their aim was to communicate Caplan's preventive and population orientation and to provide participants with a framework for acquiring new skills in consultation and community organization. Second, by focusing on a group of key psychiatrists from training programs, the seminars attempted to spread this approach widely throughout residency programs in the country in order to influence the next generation of psychiatrists.

Two documents epitomize Caplan's contribution to the Peace Corps. The first was "Adjusting Overseas: A Message to Each Peace Corps Trainee," written by Caplan and a journalist colleague, Vivian Cadden, with an introduction by Sargent Shriver, the first director of the Peace Corps (Caplan and Cadden, 1964). This describes expectable stresses overseas and states that signs of psychological strain should be expected even in psychologically healthy volunteers. It notes that the Peace Corps is committed to an active program of helping volunteers to adapt, in the expectation that with such support most people will overcome their difficulties and, despite temporary periods of unavoidable discomfort and confusion, will be able to function effectively. The second document, a *Manual for Psychiatrists Participating in the Peace Corps Program* (1963a), was Caplan's first systematic monograph-length presentation of the theoretical basis of his approach and of the techniques to be employed by psychiatrists in grappling with expectable problems in the selection, training, and support of volunteers overseas.

The years 1961-1964 were a period of major change in American psychiatry. The Joint Commission on Mental Illness and Mental Health, established by the Mental Health Study Act of 1955, presented its findings and its recommendations in 1961. The findings demonstrated that current services for the mentally ill were grossly inadequate. The recommendations, molded mainly by the vested interest groups of traditional psychiatry and allied professions, demanded increased governmental resources to improve existing clinical institutions but did not ask for significant changes in the organization of services.

A group of population-oriented psychiatrists led by Robert H. Felix, director of the National Institute of Mental Health, and supported by program analysts of the Bureau of the Budget, opposed these recommendations and urged a revolutionary shift in federal policy toward a community preventive approach. This group prevailed. On February 5, 1963, President Kennedy delivered a message to Congress that called for a focus on the total population of the mentally disordered and on the development of locality-based interlocking services that would identify and satisfy the whole range of a population's needs. This would reverse the past policy of providing distant institutions to which certain individuals would be admitted in order to remedy particular aspects of their problems. Congress responded the following year by passing the Community Mental Health Centers Act, P.L. 88-164, which provided for federal funding to finance the development of a country-wide network of community mental health centers, each of which would be responsible for satisfying the preventive, treatment, and rehabilitation needs of its surrounding catchment-area population of from 75,000 to 200,000.

The shaping of the Community Mental Health Centers legislation and regulations owed much to the influence of Caplan, who over the previous few years had played important roles as theoretician and methodologist through his widely read publications, through his lectures and consultations, and through the graduates of his training program, several of whom occupied key positions in Washington. In October-November 1963, the National Institute of Mental Health organized a series of regional institutes on training in community psychiatry in Chicago, Dallas, Berkeley, and New York that were designed to develop support for the emerging program among the country's leading psychiatrists. Their further goal was to begin a process of training in such population-oriented skills as consultation, preventive intervention, and community organization, which would be needed by psychiatrists operating outside the walls of their traditional hospitals and clinics.

Caplan was asked to give the keynote lecture for each of these institutes. His presentations were not, however, unanimously acclaimed. In fact, they sparked active, and sometimes acrimonious, debate, because they were correctly interpreted by traditionalists as advocating a radical new approach that would upset the established hierarchy by demanding the acquisition of new conceptual models and the learning of new techniques. Caplan took a leading part in these debates and succeeded in influencing many participants, particularly the younger psychiatrists, several of whom he had already helped to win over to a population orientation in the Peace Corps. Other psychiatrists who rallied round the banner of community mental health during these debates and who were active in molding national policy in Washington were the members of the Committee on Preventive Psychiatry of the Group for Advancement of Psychiatry, to which Caplan had been introduced by Lindemann in 1954. Caplan was chairman of that important committee during the crucial years 1957-1961, at the end of which it published a learned report on the problems of estimating changes in the frequency of mental disorders in the population (Committee on Preventive Psychiatry, 1961). The underlying thesis was that methods were available from epidemiology and public health practice that could be used by psychiatrists to measure changes in rates of mental disorder in populations as a result of planned community intervention by mental health workers and other professional caregivers.

In 1964, there appeared Caplan's *Principles of Preventive Psychiatry* (Caplan, 1964a), which was described by Felix in the foreword as "a primer for the community mental health worker [that] should be read by every psychiatric resident and mental health worker in training, as well as by those who are engaged in community mental health programs " (p. vii). To this day, the book continues to be used as a basic text in the field. This was the third of Caplan's books that had been published by Basic Books under the direction of Arthur Rosenthal. The first two, *Emotional Problems of Early Childhood* (Caplan, 1955) and *Prevention of Mental Disorders in Childhood* (Caplan, 1961), had been edited versions of lectures given at congresses of the International Association for Child Psychiatry and Allied Professions.

In 1964, at the height of the campaign to promote community mental health, Caplan moved his work base from the Harvard School of Public Health to the Harvard Medical School, under circumstances that were interestingly parallel to what had happened when he left Hadassah twelve years earlier. In 1961, the old order at the School of Public Health was replaced. Dean Symonds, who had fostered and encouraged an appropriate balance between the laboratory scientists and the public health practice faculty at the school, retired and was replaced by a microbiologist who had little sympathy for the "practitioners." Leavell retired. Goldman and Paul took positions elsewhere. The school became an arena for disputes between the two feuding groups of its faculty and was no longer a setting where Caplan's philosophy was highly valued. Then a new head of the Department of Public Health Practice was appointed, a young man who wanted to impose strict managerial controls on the several semiautonomous units that made up his department, including the community mental health program. Caplan was at that time asked by the Peace Corps to travel to Nigeria to help support the volunteers and their administrators there, since they were having problems with the host country's authorities. The new department head did not feel that this journey fitted his priorities, and he opposed it. Caplan failed to persuade him but decided to fulfill his urgent obligations to the Peace Corps anyway. The department head reported this to the dean as an act of insubordination; on his return Caplan tendered his resignation.

Jack R. Ewalt, professor of psychiatry of Harvard Medical School at the Massachusetts Mental Health Center, then offered Caplan a job to establish and direct a new institute, to be called the Laboratory of Community Psychiatry, that would act as a center for research and training in community mental health. Its mission would be to provide the theoretical and methodological ideas needed by the new national community mental health center program, based on P.L. 88-164, and to train its leaders. Caplan accepted and was given an academic appointment as clinical professor of psychiatry at Harvard Medical School. When the necessary funds were made available in 1970, Caplan received a tenure appointment as professor of psychiatry, which he held until he retired from Harvard in 1978 to become professor of psychiatry emeritus.

Caplan never regretted his move to the medical school.

Ewalt provided him with the freedom to build his new center according to his own ideas. As a department head Ewalt never interfered; he was always ready to provide support; and when, for instance, in 1969, Caplan began to spend half of every year in Jerusalem, studying how to reduce tension between Arabs and Jews, Ewalt not only did not question the prolonged absences from Boston but added his own voice strongly to that of the dean of the Medical School in approving this project as one of crucial importance to Harvard University. Both administrators felt that it represented not only an opportunity for important scientific exploration, the results of which might be as applicable in Boston as in Jerusalem, but also a contribution of Harvard University to the solution of an international problem.

Caplan did not go alone to Harvard Medical School. He took his entire staff with him, along with four specialist students in community mental health, not to mention his furniture and equipment. This wholesale transfer was made possible because Caplan persuaded the financial sponsors of his program to agree to move their grants from the School of Public Health to Harvard Medical School. These grants totaled some $600 thousand and included a sizable grant for multidisciplinary community mental health specialist training and a "center" grant for a broadly defined research program into preventive psychiatry. By that time Caplan was skilled in "grantsmanship" and had become highly successful in raising training and research funds from the National Institute of Mental Health and from several private foundations, particularly the Commonwealth Fund, the Grant Foundation, and later the Falk Fund and the Stone Foundation. Since these grants covered all salaries, including his own, and training stipends, as well as outlays for furniture, equipment, and administrative costs, Harvard Medical School did not lose financially by the transfer. Ewalt made available an old three-storied wooden house at 58 Fenwood Road next to the Massachusetts Mental Health Center, and this became the headquarters of the new Laboratory of Community Psychiatry. Fenwood Road was lined with similar old houses, which had been vacated over the years by their original Irish-American owners. This situation allowed for expansion as the laboratory grew, because apartments or entire houses could easily be rented. At the School of Public Health the size of the unit had been limited in recent years not only by the restrictions placed upon it by an ambivalent administration but also by the very real limitations of space in the school buildings. At the medical school, with the radical change in both these factors, the unit quickly grew. Within five years its annual budget approached $2.5 million, and its student body increased to an average of fifteen to twenty students each year. A comprehensive one-year curriculum of public health and community mental health was soon developed for these students.

At the laboratory, the first priority was to establish it as a freestanding semiautonomous unit of Harvard Medical School. In this work, which went smoothly because of the helpfulness of Ewalt, Caplan was greatly assisted by an enthusiastic staff, especially by his administrative assistants, Marie Killilea, who coordinated the training program and the rapidly increasing number of research units, and Joyce Brinton, who managed the finances and integrated the laboratory within the Harvard University system.

Even while he was setting up the Laboratory of Community Psychiatry, Caplan was developing a plan to provide an educational program for the faculties of the country's psychiatric training programs, so that they might reorient themselves to impart the ideas and skills needed to work in the new community mental health centers. To this end he organized the Harvard Visiting Faculty Seminar, which was modeled on his Berkeley institutes for social workers, but with important modifications. After convening a representative group of sixteen full professors or associate professors of psychiatry from different parts of the country, each of whom was responsible for a major psychiatric residency program, he invited them to participate in a residential seminar at Harvard, which would meet eight times for two-week sessions over three years. Caplan organized this seminar as a group of peers who would together plan their curriculum and conduct their studies of topics that they felt to be central to the field of community mental health and preventive psychiatry. Caplan by design did not accept the status of teacher to his colleagues, some of whom were already very experienced in community work and would rightly have resisted being cast into a student role. Still, his special expertise and his leadership were accepted by all his colleagues, or they would not have agreed to participate. Caplan structured the seminars as meetings to which carefully chosen outside experts were invited. These experts were not asked to give formal lectures but to be interviewed by the chairman and by the rest of the group as a basis for informal discussions, usually lasting an entire day, during which the focal topic might be systematically explored. Caplan had perfected this technique while teaching at the Harvard School of Public Health and used it whenever he invited visiting speakers to provide specialized input for his courses. At the seminars, it usually led to a stimulating discussion and ensured that the remarks of the visiting expert would fit in with the current preoccupations of his audience.

The atmosphere of these seminars can be appreciated in an excerpt from Caplan's report to the dean of the Harvard Medical School following the first two-week session:

> The whole of the second week was devoted to increasing our understanding of community life by looking at the ongoing life of Boston "through the window" of examining the operations of its urban renewal program. We interviewed Mayor Collins; the redevelopment administrator, Mr. Logue; the directors and staffs of Action for Boston Community Development and the United Community Services; and a number of "grass-roots" workers involved in dealing with social and health problems of relocation. These interviews afforded us an opportunity of getting an inside view of the political, social, and psychological forces involved in the dynamics of decision making and social change in Boston, and also of getting to know a number of dedicated and vibrant people, each of whom was making his contribution according to his own individual style. Part of the enthusiasm which gripped our group during the second week was undoubtedly related to the

> dramatic impact of this human documentary which we were privileged to observe. For all of us it demonstrated the value of such privileged observation of exciting current events and personalities in action as a basis for productive learning.

Over the sixteen weeks of the seminar, sessions focused on the entire range of research, theory, and practice issues of relevance to community mental health. Despite the fact that each of the participants was a busy person in his home setting, nobody was absent for more than one day from the eight sessions. Enthusiasm remained at a uniformly high level, and everyone felt that he had learned a great deal that could immediately be utilized in his current psychiatric residency program, as well as in developing new elements in the community service program of his department.

At the end of the three-year period, the participants, who by then had become welded together into a cohesive reference group, decided to organize a second training program on a wider scale. Under Caplan's leadership, and with the assistance of Marie Killilea as executive director, they organized the Inter-University Forum for Educators in Community Psychiatry. Six regional centers were established, at each of which fifteen to twenty senior psychiatric educators were enrolled to attend residential seminars for seven to ten days twice a year for four years. This endeavor was also successful; by 1972, senior teachers from most of the leading psychiatric residency training programs of the country had been given the opportunity to learn the essentials of research, theory, and practice in community psychiatry.

Caplan's commitment to "spreading the word" about community mental health theory and practice also led him to increase his peripatetic consultations and three-day institutes, particularly in semirural and small-town settings where the need for instruction was most urgently felt. In addition, he organized, with the help of Killilea, a series of three-day institutes at Harvard. These were attended over the following years by almost a thousand key workers and teachers in the fields of psychiatry, psychology, social work, education, social science, general medical practice, corrections, and public welfare. These one-time institutes catered to about fifty participants each. Caplan gave many of the lectures, and the rest were given by other laboratory faculty. Lectures were invariably interspersed with small-group discussions, mainly led by the specialist students of the laboratory, who were thus enabled to study at firsthand the problems and techniques of interprofessional continuing education, as well as to obtain vivid current information about the doings and preoccupations of community workers in a variety of settings.

After Lindemann left the School of Public Health, and until he retired from Harvard in 1970, Caplan maintained close links with him. From 1954 to 1964 they used to meet once a week over lunch, and each used to consult the other about current problems in his own department. Particularly in regard to the development of crisis theory and the consultation model, Caplan owed much to these talks with Lindemann. After the establishment of the laboratory in Ewalt's Harvard department, these contacts became less regular, but Caplan continued his friendly relationship with Lindemann until the latter's death in 1974 and wrote his obituary notice in the *American Journal of Psychiatry*.

Within the Laboratory of Community Psychiatry itself, Caplan and his colleagues continued the research they had started at the School of Public Health on the reactions of individuals and families to crises. The crisis of conjugal bereavement, for example, became a major focus of study, and a series of publications reported on the expectable reactions of widows and widowers during the years following the death of a spouse. As had become traditional with Caplan, such studies usually led to the development of methods and services for preventive intervention and rehabilitation.

In his first years at the medical school, Caplan also devoted much effort to refining techniques of mental health consultation, and this work was eventually published as *The Theory and Practice of Mental Health Consultation* (Caplan, 1970). This book dealt almost entirely with consultation to individuals, but even before its publication Caplan began to explore modification of the method for use with groups. As usual, his methodological concepts were derived from his immersion in a particular practice setting. In this case, his opportunities for field exploration were derived from a program of mental health consultation that he developed in the Episcopal church. This has been described by Ruth Caplan in *Helping the Helpers to Help* (1972). The program had two main elements. First, faculty and specialist students of the laboratory provided consultation on a regular weekly basis in Boston to groups of parish clergy of the diocese of Massachusetts; this consultation dealt with their handling of the human problems of their parishioners. This group consultation was supplemented by Caplan's individual consultation to the bishop of Massachusetts in which he focused on the bishop's problems in providing for the human needs of his parish clergy, as well as on other psychosocial aspects of his role as bishop. The second element of the program was consultation provided by Caplan to the national House of Bishops of the Episcopal church to develop ways of supporting bishops in their diocesan work. This led to the establishment of a consultation training program by Caplan for senior bishops to teach them techniques of offering collegial consultation to new bishops during the first years of their episcopate to help them deal with the human relations problems of their diocesan role.

Both elements of this program were successful. The consultations with clergymen in Boston added much to the knowledge and skills of the psychiatrists in group consultation. And Caplan's work in the House of Bishops, which led over a six-year period to his training more than half its members in techniques of individual consultation, showed that the skills of this method can be learned by sophisticated people who are not mental health specialists and that these skills can be modified for providing significant peer support inside an organization. These findings, along with an analysis of the way that the House of Bishops eventually incorporated his ideas and used them creatively to help new bishops deal with the human relations aspects of their role, added important insights to Caplan in his development of his theory of support systems, as it began to emerge in the mid 1970s.

Paradoxically, Caplan's work in the medical school gradually focused more on social planning and community service patterns and on interinstitutional factors than it had while he was at the School of Public Health. In the latter setting he had relied on his colleagues in the relevant specialist departments of epidemiology, biostatistics, and especially public health practice to provide his community mental health specialist students with essential teaching in these fields. In the medical school, he was forced to deal with these issues himself or to recruit appropriate specialists to do so; thus, he added to his teaching faculty and to his research staff lawyers, political scientists, a historian, environmental analysts, architects and town planners, in addition to the psychiatrists, psychologists, nurses, sociologists, and anthropologists who had been members of his core staff in the School of Public Health. This led the laboratory to focus on helping populations at mental health risk in metropolitan areas and on developing intervention strategies for schools, hospitals, religious organizations, and community action programs. The laboratory also focused on the legal system and on program and social policy development, especially on working out mechanisms for modifying the life conditions of slum dwellers and other populations at risk because of deprivation, prejudice, or community conflict.

Among the two dozen studies of the interface between mental health and societal factors that Caplan helped to organize at the Laboratory of Community Psychiatry over the period 1964-1977, he concentrated his personal efforts on four areas of exploration:

First, he collaborated with his daughter Ruth, an intellectual historian, on her study of the history of preventive community psychiatry in the twentieth century (Caplan and Caplan, 1967). He also wrote an epilogue to her *Psychiatry and the Community in Nineteenth-Century America* (Caplan, 1969) in which he analyzed the parallels between the historical forces operating during the nineteenth and twentieth centuries. This led Caplan to make specific predictions about the future of the community mental health center movement that have turned out to be remarkably accurate and to propose social policies to deal with some of the difficulties that he predicted would occur.

Second, Caplan organized a multidisciplinary staff seminar on Human Relations and the Law at Harvard Law School. This seminar met once a month over three years, and on the basis of legal case discussions and descriptions of community conflict situations, the social scientists, mental health specialists, and lawyers analyzed the role of the lawyer and the possible contribution of the legal system in resolving or managing individual and community conflicts.

Third, Caplan explored the contribution of community mental health specialists to the management of community conflicts in situations where it was inadvisable or impractical to energize formal legal mechanisms. *Theory and Practice of Mental Health Consultation* (Caplan, 1970, chap. 14) describes Caplan's attempts to prevent an incipient race riot between black parents and white administrators of the Boston School Department, and also his offer of support to state government officials in confrontation with rebelling welfare recipients in a sit-down strike in the Massachusetts State House.

Finally, Caplan continued this line of development in a seven-year study in Israel of the intercommunity conflicts of Arabs and Jews in Jerusalem. There he explored the possibility that someone skilled in community psychiatry could help the conflicting parties to communicate with each other and to reduce to a minimum the psychosocial dissonances that would interfere with their daily lives. In *Arab and Jew in Jerusalem*, Caplan describes the possibilities and limitations of a community mental health worker acting both as a mediator in community conflicts and as a change agent and community organizer in trying to develop institutions to satisfy ongoing needs of populations for human services in situations of dissonance between the would-be providers of service and the potential recipients (Caplan and Caplan, 1980).

During his final years at the Laboratory of Community Psychiatry, Caplan devoted his main thinking to the development of support systems theory and practice. His ideas grew naturally from his work with the crisis model and from his experiences in helping people master stress. While he continued to value the crisis intervention approach to prevention, he gradually came to appreciate the limitations of that model. From the beginning he had emphasized the importance of "informal caregivers" in helping people in crisis deal adaptively with their predicaments, and for several years he had tried to educate such informal caregivers, who in the nature of things were not easily identifiable, by writing articles in such journals as *Redbook* and *McCall's,* which he had reason to believe included many such key persons in their regular readership. In the laboratory's "widow-to-widow" project, Caplan made an attempt to organize such nonprofessional caregivers to act as a mechanism for prevention, and this led him to the "discovery" of the mutual help groups that exist on a widespread scale in most communities (Caplan and Killilea, 1976). He then became interested in some unexpected developments in his program in the Episcopal church. He had originally based this program on the consultation model. He had trained senior bishops to offer formal consultation to inexperienced colleagues. Before long, however, bishops who had been trained as consultants began on their own to meet informally in pairs or in small groups and to help each other with their diocesan problems. They then began to transform part of the regular meetings of the House of Bishops into organized peer support groups. As Caplan studied these spontaneous developments that had been set in motion by his consultation seminars, he began to appreciate the attractiveness and the power of support systems and to build an explicit model that had clear implications for preventive action.

In *Support Systems and Community Mental Health* (1974), Caplan traced the development of his concept of support systems by reanalyzing a number of his previous lectures. And two years later in *Support Systems and Mutual Help* (Caplan and Killilea, 1976), Caplan and his Harvard colleagues published a comprehensive statement of the new theory and of the practice prescriptions that emerge from it. In some of his later papers Caplan reviewed empirical researches that demonstrate persuasively that exposure to high stress in the absence of social support is associated with increased vulnerability to mental and bodily disease, whereas adequate social support seems to prevent increased vulnerability in people exposed to similar levels of stress. These articles provide guidelines for organizing support systems in the community to prevent physical and mental disorder in individuals exposed to acute, as well as to long-term, stress (Caplan, 1980, 1981).

In 1977, when he was sixty, Caplan took early retirement from Harvard and settled in Jerusalem. He decided to devote the remainder of his working life to using his population-oriented ideas and experience in developing child psychiatry services there. He organized a new Department of Child Psychiatry within the Hadassah-Hebrew University Hospital in Jerusalem and has written a number of papers that extend the boundaries of the crisis model to the support systems model and of the method of consultation to the methods of collaboration. He has also been taking every opportunity to enjoy the company of his three young grandsons.

At the time this chapter was written, Caplan had just returned from an American lecture tour, during which he gave lectures and one-day institutes in Boston, Baltimore, Raleigh, Dayton, Chicago, Toronto, New York, and New Haven. His new ideas on mastery of stress, support systems, and methods of collaboration were enthusiastically received by large audiences in each place—a reception that indicates that his creativity and his energy to generate and disseminate pioneering concepts and methods have, if anything, increased following his "retirement."

References

Bowlby, J. *Maternal Care and Mental Health.* New York: Columbia University Press, 1951.

Caplan, G. "A Convulsion During Nonconvulsive Faradic Shock Therapy." *British Medical Journal,* 1941, *1,* 479.

Caplan, G. "The Mental Hygiene Role of the Nurse in Maternal and Child Care." *Nursing Outlook,* 1954, *2,* 14-19.

Caplan, G. (Ed.). *Emotional Problems of Early Childhood.* New York: Basic Books, 1955.

Caplan, G. *Concepts of Mental Health and Consultation: Their Application in Public Health Social Work.* Children's Bureau Publication No. 393. Washington, D.C.: Department of Health, Education, and Welfare, 1959a.

Caplan, G. "Practical Steps for the Family Physician in the Prevention of Emotional Disorder." *Journal of the American Medical Association,* 1959b, *170,* 1497-1506.

Caplan, G. (Ed.). *Prevention of Mental Disorders in Childhood: Initial Explorations.* New York: Basic Books, 1961.

Caplan, G. *Manual for Psychiatrists Participating in the Peace Corps Program.* Washington, D.C.: Medical Program Division, Peace Corps, 1963a.

Caplan, G. "Opportunities for School Psychologists in the Primary Prevention of Mental Disorders in Children." *Mental Hygiene,* 1963b, *47,* 525-539.

Caplan, G. *Principles of Preventive Psychiatry.* New York: Basic Books, 1964a.

Caplan, G. "The Role of Pediatricians in Community Mental Health (with Particular Reference to the Primary Prevention of Mental Disorders in Children)." In L. Bellak (Ed.), *Handbook of Community Psychiatry and Community Mental Health.* New York: Grune & Stratton, 1964b.

Caplan, G. *The Theory and Practice of Mental Health Consultation.* New York: Basic Books, 1970.

Caplan, G. *Support Systems and Community Mental Health.* New York: Behavioral Publications, 1974.

Caplan, G. "An Approach to Preventive Intervention in Child Psychiatry." *Canadian Journal of Psychiatry,* 1980, *25,* 671-682.

Caplan, G. "Mastery of Stress: Psychosocial Aspects." *American Journal of Psychiatry,* 1981, *138,* 413-419.

Caplan, G., and Cadden, V. "Adjusting Overseas: A Message to Each Peace Corps Trainee." In G. Caplan, *Principles of Preventive Psychiatry.* New York: Basic Books, 1964.

Caplan, G., and Caplan, R. B. "Development of Community Psychiatry Concepts." In A. M. Freedman and H. I. Kaplan (Eds.), *Comprehensive Textbook of Psychiatry.* Baltimore, Md.: Williams and Wilkins, 1967.

Caplan, G., and Caplan, R. B. *Arab and Jew in Jerusalem: Explorations in Community Mental Health.* Cambridge, Mass.: Harvard University Press, 1980.

Caplan, G., and Killilea, M. (Eds.). *Support Systems and Mutual Help: Multidisciplinary Explorations.* New York: Grune & Stratton, 1976.

Caplan, R. B. *Psychiatry and Community in Nineteenth-Century America.* New York: Basic Books, 1969.

Caplan, R. B. *Helping the Helpers to Help: Mental Health Consultation to Aid Clergymen in Pastoral Work.* New York: Seabury Press, 1972.

Committee on Preventive Psychiatry, Group for the Advancement of Psychiatry. *Problems of Estimating Changes in Frequency of Mental Disorders,* Report No. 5a. New York: Group for the Advancement of Psychiatry, 1961.

Lindemann, E. "Symptomatology and Management of Acute Grief." *American Journal of Psychiatry,* 1944, *101,* 141.

Rosenfeld, J. M., and Caplan, G. "Techniques of Staff Consultation in an Immigrant Children's Organization in Israel." *American Journal of Orthopsychiatry,* 1954, *24,* 45-62.

Chapter 2

Community Mental Health in Transition

Herbert C. Schulberg
Marie Killilea

Almost two decades have passed since President Kennedy's historic 1963 message to Congress about the need to redirect and intensify this nation's commitment to the mentally ill. In the subsequent years, we have witnessed the growth of numerous strategies aimed at prevention and treatment of mental illness. Psychiatric conditions long considered to be chronically dysfunctional have yielded to pharmacological, social, and/or psychological interventions. The American mental health system has been profoundly altered as the locus of care has shifted from large distant state hospitals to smaller mental health centers located in the midst of dense populations. Public acceptance of the mentally ill, although far from ideal, has significantly improved. And yet, despite these and other indexes of meaningful progress, community mental health programs are in a state of crisis. A persistent malaise and uncertainty hover over the field as it seeks to chart a course for the coming decade. On the one hand, early and ardent supporters confess in apologetic terms about the excesses of the 1960s and 1970s; they embarrassedly seek to explain the misplaced zealotry invested in efforts to reform "pathological" societies. Some advocate the rejuvenation of institutional care for persons who had been discharged to community residences. On the other hand, even those who consider community mental health programs successful acknowledge that periodic alterations in course are intrinsic to the delivery of human services and that priorities and practices need significant refocusing if they are to be relevant in the 1980s. Although no apologies are offered by the latter group for strategies that have proven less than optimal, they, too, urge renewed vigor so that community mental health can maintain earlier gains.

Regardless of which perspective one assumes about the recent history of community mental health, it is clear that the field now is facing a major, if not fundamental, transition. The federal government's leadership and standard-setting role have been radically reduced, resource allocation patterns are being redesigned, and conceptual frameworks more congruent with compacted service systems are being trumpeted. These and similar developments require careful analysis and deliberation if the planning process is to be progressive rather than regressive. This chapter reviews key issues affecting the design and operation of community mental health programs. The contributions of the present volume's succeeding chapters to the resolution of critical conceptual, organizational, and personnel issues will be particularly highlighted.

Community Mental Health Legislation

For the past twenty years, the scope and parameters of psychiatric care have been determined as much by governmental legislation as by scientific advances. The historic Community Mental Health Centers Act of 1963 (P.L. 88-164) and its amendments were instrumental in determining that public as well as private recipients of federal funds must provide at least five essential services to all residents of their catchment areas. This precept fundamentally altered service delivery patterns during the ensuing years. While the precise nature of the act's implementation has created awkward dilemmas and provoked unnecessary power struggles between providers and governmental administrators, continuity of care improved and service fragmentation was diminished. Systems of comprehensive care were designed under the pressure of federal and state legislation, and mental health centers assumed vital roles in their community's human services network. In general, the legislative thrust during the period from 1963 to 1975 was toward expanded services (twelve rather than five essential ones) and toward inclusive rather than exclusive requirements in serving patients (embracing children, the elderly, and special-need populations). Details of P.L. 88-164, its subsequent extensions, and its amendments are analyzed by Bloom (1977).

Widespread national support existed in the mid 1970s for community mental health legislation; for example, Congress overwhelmingly overrode President Nixon's 1975 veto of the extension of P.L. 94-63 (a later version of P.L. 88-164). Nevertheless, a ground swell of concern was simultaneously emerging in public and professional arenas with regard to how mental disorders could best be prevented and treated. Public officials were disquieted about the mounting unit costs of health services, including psychiatric care, at a time when the country's fiscal resources were no longer expanding. By 1978, 731 community mental health centers assisted by federal funds were providing services to 47 percent of the U.S. population (Sharfstein, 1979), but Congress and mental health planners had begun to question whether the community mental health center model was in fact applicable throughout the country. Center directors and clinicians were dismayed by the stringent regulations imposed by federal bureaucrats, the unmet needs of patients being discharged from institutional settings to local communities, and the massive efforts required of "graduate" centers to replace federal staffing funds with other income sources (Weiner and others, 1979). Sharfstein (1978) concluded that the rigid service and accountability requirements of P.L. 94-63 made it a complex and inflexible piece of legislation that had produced a dinosaur incapable of coping with environmental stresses.

A troublesome issue for community mental health practitioners is what Borus (1978) has described as the boundary problem. Not only were mental health centers explicitly mandated to serve all catchment area residents with defined mental illnesses, but the centers were also implicitly assigned responsibility to prevent mental illness in high-risk groups and to improve the mental health of all other citizens living in the area. While these latter mandates generated creative collaboration and consultation ventures with diverse community groups, Borus notes that they also deceived mental health professionals into believing that they could solve social ills. Public disillusionment was inevitable when community mental health centers failed to perform the impossible. During much of the late 1970s, therefore, the nature of contracted but realistic program boundaries became the subject of intense controversy and extensive debate at the local and national levels.

Several themes recurred in the course of these lengthy deliberations; two warrant specific mention because of their impact upon legislative actions. The first is the responsibility of community mental health practitioners to care for the seriously ill, a mission that Zusman and Lamb (1977) consider the field's prime reason for existing. They assert that failure to implement community treatment of the long-term, severely ill has not resulted from a lack of knowledge about how to care for such persons. Instead, community mental health practitioners have preferred to treat the "healthy but unhappy" patient experiencing existential dilemmas and problems in living. This misplaced priority is directly related to the dilemmas of deinstitutionalization, a problem whose dimensions will be analyzed in greater detail later in this chapter.

The second recurrent theme pertains to the campaign for "remedicalization" of mental health services. While sharing the previously described concern about misplaced priorities and the neglect of persons with serious psychiatric illnesses, Langsley (1980) and others have stressed that psychiatrists must function as more than prescription signers. They deride the drift of mental health centers toward a social services model and the frittering of scarce resources upon unproven preventive interventions; they urge that medical practice be elevated in the diagnosis and treatment of patients. It is important to recognize that efforts by the profession of psychiatry to forge closer ties with other realms of medicine have been spurred by research findings from biological psychiatry, the neurosciences, and psychopharmacology, as well as by the continuing debates about criteria for inclusion of mental health care under governmental and commercial health insurance plans. While the scientific impetus for remedicalization is intended to improve the quality of treatment, remedicalization stimulated by fiscal concerns would have the opposite effect of reducing the growing array of treatment choices available to those seeking care.

Additional implications of the medical model are analyzed by Bursten (1979) and Adler (1981). Noting that mental health centers engage in medical as well as rehabilitative, societal-legal, and educative-developmental tasks, Adler distinguished the psychiatrist's differing role in each. He concluded that the clinical medical model is appropriate to all four task areas even though the primacy of authority in some areas will be nonmedical, for example, in the disposition of forensic psychiatry cases.

Converging professional concerns about the future of community mental health programs and President Carter's commitment to improved treatment of mental disorders led in February 1977 to establishment of the President's Commission on Mental Health. By executive order, the commission was authorized to review the nation's mental health needs and to recommend to the president how they might best be met. Public hearings were held throughout the country, and task panels composed of hundreds of knowledgeable professionals and volunteers produced reports for the commission's consideration. In contrast to the 1961 report of the Joint Commission on Mental Illness and Health that called for a basic reorganization of America's mental health system, the report of the President's Commission on Mental Health (1978) concluded that, despite shortcomings and inequities in this system, the foundation existed for providing high-quality services at reasonable cost to all who need them. Nevertheless, the commission urged that a new national priority be established to meet the needs of chronically mentally ill persons; that services be specifically targeted to special-need populations such as children, adolescents, and the elderly; that mental health services be better coordinated with general health and other human services; and that states be assigned primary responsibility for developing federally supported services. Of particular interest was the commission's emphasis on the mental health value of personal and community support systems that strengthen individuals, neighborhoods, and communities.

Translating these recommendations and others into enabling legislation was a time-consuming, complex, and periodically even stormy process. Nevertheless, in October 1980—the final days of the Carter administration—Congress passed the Mental Health Systems Act (P.L. 96-398). Among its provisions were funds for special-need populations and the delegation of increased authority to state agencies in administering grant programs. While the National Institute of Mental Health (NIMH) was still drafting the regulations needed to implement the Mental Health Systems Act, Congress repealed the legislation in 1981 at President Reagan's behest. Community mental health center funds were substantially reduced and included in a block grant to states for mental health, alcohol abuse, and drug abuse programs. The twelve essential services included in P.L. 96-398 were reduced to five, and no funds are to be used for inpatient care—a major departure from the initial 1963 Community Mental Health Centers Act.

The effect of block grant allocations and of other forms of the New Federalism that alter mechanisms for allocating funds to community mental health programs remains to be seen. It already is evident, however, that these legislative actions will increase competition between rival constituencies, produce greater program diversity, alter service priorities, and complicate the enforcement of standards for quality care. There is also concern as to whether changes that minimize the number of core services required of community mental health centers will adversely affect continuity of care and threaten the systems of comprehensive care developed so painstakingly over many years. Not surprisingly, then, many observers share Goldman's (1981) lament that trends under the Reagan administration are "extremely demoralizing." Fearing that even well-intentioned states will not assume responsibility for neglected minorities and the chronically mentally ill, Goldman predicts that many of the steps pursued earlier to create a quality mental health system will have to be retraced during the coming years.

Concepts of Community Mental Health

The viability and growth of any human service program depend upon its capacity for continuously producing fresh intellectual capital. When such enrichment is lacking, practices become outdated, services become irrelevant, and fossilization impends. Given this vital need, how adequately have community mental health programs generated the concepts crucial to their contemporary functions? How ably can practitioners in the field, relying on the present state of knowledge, cope with diminished resources and the increased demands of previously neglected special-need populations and of persons with serious mental illnesses?

Since value judgments strongly affect such determinations, these questions are not readily answered. Nevertheless, we conclude that in recent years the community mental health field has not properly met this need for fresh intellectual capital. Caplan's (1964) seminal work on *Principles of Preventive Psychiatry* certainly stimulated diverse activity, its tenets permeate countless variations in community mental health practice, and, as Caplan notes in the Epilogue to the present volume, no static dogma has come to dominate the field. Caplan's successors, however, have channeled their theoretic and investigative efforts in fairly specialized directions, and wide gaps still exist in the field's scientific foundation. Leighton, commenting in an interview about failures of the community mental health movement, observed that despite the large number of beliefs, convictions, opinions, and theories about the nature of mental illness, there still is an insufficient factual underpinning for public policy purposes (Curtis and Yessian, 1981). Ironically enough, a survey by Lounsbury and others (1979) of the community mental health literature between 1965 and 1977 revealed a decrease in "think pieces," while articles on administrative issues and personal concerns more than doubled in this time period. Despite these continuing limitations in the conceptual framework of community mental health practice, progress nevertheless can be identified in several domains, and it will be considered in the sections that follow.

Epidemiological Strategies. Given the wide-ranging, even contradictory, demands placed upon community mental health centers, it is vital that administrators utilize cogent priority-setting procedures in the allocation of scarce resources. Such strategies may range from the grossly impressionistic to the highly objective. When the latter are based upon epidemiological indexes of incidence, prevalence, and severity, a quantitative approach is possible. In his interview, Leighton suggested that researchers and clinicians investigate a population's prevalence rates for different mental illnesses and then determine the percentage of persons who are disabled and which categories of disorder are most treatable (Curtis and Yessian, 1981).

While it is unlikely that epidemiological measures alone will determine planning decisions, given increased consumer choice and other factors that have a strong political component, it is realistic to expect them to have a profounder influence than has been true thus far. There are many reasons for earlier failures to utilize epidemiological data, but certainly a key factor has been psychiatry's difficulty in defining a case of mental disorder. As Levy notes in Chapter Three, the absence of biological markers for most psychiatric illnesses has left diagnostic decisions essentially to the judgment of observers. Earlier studies found reliability to vary considerably and to be significantly influenced by the sociodemographic characteristics of those being diagnosed. Not surprisingly, then, prevalence rates have been the subject of much conjecture and confusion. In its report to the President's Commission on Mental Health, the Task Panel on the Nature and Scope of the Problems (1978) concluded that although 10 percent of the population is commonly estimated as needing some form of mental health care, fresh evidence indicates that this proportion may be closer to 15 percent. Ambiguities in case definition have also obscured the issue of where mentally ill persons obtain treatment and have thus impeded priority-setting procedures. Again, based on less than reliable diagnostic categories, Regier, Goldberg, and Taube (1978) have estimated that 54 percent of the identified mentally ill are treated in the primary medical care sector while only 15 percent receive treatment in the specialty mental health sector.

Recognizing the limitations imposed by poor case definition, epidemiologists and clinicians have struggled to refine objective criteria for psychiatric diagnoses. Their efforts culminated in the development of the third edition of *Diagnostic and Statistical Manual of Mental Disorder* (DSM-III), a multiaxial evaluation system that formulates diagnoses with significantly improved reliability (Spitzer, Williams, and Skodol, 1980; American Psychiatric Association, 1980). While the construct and predictive validity of this latest nomenclature still remain to be demonstrated, DSM-III already serves as the conceptual framework within which virtually all epidemiological research is now being conducted. DSM-III has also led to the construction of the Diagnostic Interview Schedule (DIS), a highly structured questionnaire capable of minimizing the error variance due to differing interview styles (Robins and others, 1981). The DIS can be administered by persons without clinical experience, and it presently is being utilized in the NIMH-supported Epidemiologic Catchment Area Program, a multisite research endeavor that seeks to determine incidence and prevalence rates of specific mental disorders (Eaton and others, 1981). The great potential of such highly structured epidemiological investigations for clarifying a community's mental illness patterns can be seen in Myers and Weissman's (1980) earlier study in which the Schedule for Affective Disorders and Schizophrenia (Endicott and Spitzer, 1978)—a semistructured predecessor of the Diagnostic Interview Schedule—was administered to New Haven residents.

While the development and testing of a highly operationalized diagnostic system represent considerable progress, much work still is required before epidemiological data can serve as the bedrock foundation for community mental health planning and priority setting. As Levy notes in Chapter Three, the relationship between clinical diagnosis and need for treatment remains unclear; not all persons obtaining a psychiatric diagnosis necessarily require therapeutic intervention. Srole and Fischer (1980) similarly question whether the Diagnostic Interview Schedule, which was largely developed with identified psychiatric patients, can be validly utilized in epidemiological surveys of nonpatient populations residing in the community. Furthermore, even valid incidence and prevalence rates serve only to identify populations at risk without thereby dictating the treatment of choice. The latter is affected by differing clinical orientations, as well as by fiscal, political, and social factors. Nevertheless, it is fair to conclude that these recent epidemiological developments significantly advance the state of the art. An operationalized diagnostic system can provide a primary data base that, although still far from perfect, is more conceptually valid for planning purposes than secondary information bases such as social area analysis (Piasecki and Kamis-Gould, 1981), which is ambiguous in meaning and potentially subject to the confounding of correlation and causation.

Primary Prevention. There probably is no community mental health activity that has stimulated so much optimism but also provoked so much controversy as primary prevention. Utilizing the well-established public health paradigm of altering factors in the host, agent, or environment that contribute to the development of a disorder, community mental health specialists have attempted to apply this model with the goals of reducing the incidence of specific mental illnesses and/or improving mental health. This quest is not a new one; it had been attempted during the 1920s and 1930s through such undertakings as mental health education. However, primary prevention was raised to a new prominence in the 1970s—partially as the result of larger societal efforts to eliminate the pathological influences in the environment but also because of refinements in the concepts of crisis theory, psychosocial transitions, and social support systems. The heightened level of recent interest in primary prevention activities has led to the holding of the annual Vermont Conference on the Primary Prevention of Psychopathology and numerous other meetings, initiation of the *Journal of Prevention* in 1981, and establishment of the National Association of Prevention Professionals by those identifying themselves as working in this field. The field's dynamic quality is also evident in descriptions by Klein and Goldston (1977), Vayda and Perlmutter (1977), Matus and Nuehring (1979), Glasscote (1980), and Reinherz (Chapter Eighteen) of numerous direct and indirect efforts to improve emotional well-being, build social competence, create stimulating environments, and so on. Vayda and Perlmutter's survey of forty-three community mental health centers found that half of the centers' consultation and education services were devoted to primary prevention interventions at both the individual and institutional levels. Detailed analyses of the primary prevention programs sponsored by six selected community mental health centers are provided by Glasscote. After reviewing activities of the previous decade and estimating the field's future potential, the President's Commission on Mental Health (1978) recommended helping children as the nation's first priority in primary prevention. The commission's recommendation that a Center for Prevention be established at NIMH was enacted as an amendment to section 235 of the Public Health Service Act. Although other initiatives were abrogated by repeal of the Mental Health Systems Act, NIMH remains formally responsible for primary prevention activities.

Given this range of contemporary practice that has buoyed the spirit of those committed by theory and ideology to strategies of primary prevention, it is important to consider the conceptual trends guiding such activities. The first is what Caplan in the Epilogue characterizes as a movement away from vague global frameworks to more precise guidelines for interventive actions. His own work is now based on a conceptual model that incorporates biopsychosocial risk factors, the individual's complex of experiential and constitutional traits, his or her repertoire of learned skills for solving interpersonal and physical problems, and the social supports available at times of stress. The model's relevance to reducing childhood psychopathology is described by Caplan (1980); its validity can possibly be assessed within the research paradigm utilized by Mednick, Schulsinger, and Venables (1979) in their primary prevention studies with children at high risk for schizophrenia.

The second conceptual trend is evident in Bloom's thesis

in Chapter Four that precise definitions and delimited disease entities of known etiology are exceptional rather than the rule in the mental health field. Those conditions that can be prevented through specific biological or genetic interventions make up but a fraction of mental disorders. In contrast to Caplan's espousal of more precise guidelines for interventive actions, Bloom's thesis leads him to propose a "general disease prevention paradigm" based upon established associations between stress and increased risk of illness. This paradigm postulates that psychosocial stressors are unlikely to be etiologically specific to a particular disease; attention, therefore, should be shifted from predisposing to precipitating factors. Researchers and practitioners should focus upon high-risk situations rather than high-risk populations, and far greater emphasis should be devoted to ameliorating adverse environmental conditions, enhancing life-style practices, and improving the organization of health care. Earlier applications of this ecological perspective to community mental health are described by Holahan and others (1979). Given these successful precedents of comprehensive rather than narrow interventive approaches, Bloom (1981) notes that the Reagan administration ironically "has decided to biologize the mental health field while primary care physicians are accelerating their attempts to psychologize medicine. The hope that the key to controlling the major, currently unpreventable, disorders lies exclusively in our biology seems not only illusory but defies an overwhelming amount of evidence" (p. 841).

While the Reagan administration is thought to have rejected nonbiological prevention strategies for essentially political reasons, it must be recognized that many mental health professionals have adopted an identical position for clinical reasons. For example, Lamb and Zusman (1979, 1981) question the wisdom of those who minimize genetic factors in the etiology of mental disorders while emphasizing social ones. In the absence of strong evidence favoring social factors, Lamb and Zusman view a major investment in the social arena as hazardous at best. At worst, Lamb and Zusman fear that environmentally oriented activities will become a glamorous rationalization for avoiding the direct treatment of difficult mental illnesses. Some of community mental health's overzealous ventures into social engineering in the late 1960s and early 1970s serve as a rueful reminder of how ineffective political, sociological, and educational activities can divert limited resources from meeting the needs of chronically mentally ill persons and other troubled populations.

Debate will continue for some time about the clinical and epidemiological significance of primary prevention's recent momentum, the validity of its various conceptual paradigms, the proportion of scarce personnel and funds to be expended for these activities, and so on. Nevertheless, consensus has existed for some time about the need to improve research into primary prevention models and practices. Heller, Price, and Sher (1980) analyze the conceptual and methodological obstacles to these investigations and conclude with "guarded optimism" that high-quality research is possible despite the ambiguities that have retarded the generation of crisply defined independent and dependent variables and of valid cause-effect relationships. Along these lines, Gruenberg (1980) suggests the strategy of preventive trials analogous to clinical trials. In such research, the preventive intervention would be harmless, socially acceptable and not frightening to subjects, and conceptually plausible in its mode of preventing disorder.

Social Support Systems. The critical functions of social support for sustaining mental health have been recognized for many years. In the past decade, however, we have witnessed a veritable explosion of interest in the structures, functions, and processes of social networks and mutual help systems (Caplan and Killilea, 1976; Gartner and Riessman, 1977; Katz and Bender, 1976; Lieberman, Borman, and Associates, 1979; Gottlieb, 1981). This recent attention in both professional and lay circles is exemplified by the recommendation of the President's Commission on Mental Health (1978) that "a major effort be developed in the area of personal and community supports which will recognize and strengthen the natural networks to which people belong and on which they depend [and] improve the linkages between community support networks and formal mental health services" (p. 15).

Cynics have asserted that the present prominence of social support systems is intended to obscure the fact that government is reducing the funds for trained mental health clinicians. Nevertheless, even professionals acknowledge that social support systems make a unique, positive contribution to their patients' psychological well-being. Mueller's (1980) analysis of the social environment's relationship to psychiatric disorder, Henderson and others' (1980) epidemiological study of social networks and neurosis, Dean, Lin, and Ensel's (1981) research on social support systems and depression, Hammer, Makiesky-Barrow, and Gutwirth's (1978) review of social networks and schizophrenia, and so on consistently suggest that a person's pattern of social relationships plays a crucial role in the etiology, process, and/or resolution of mental disorders. Given this postulate, how sophisticated is our present conception of social support systems and what further refinements are needed for this construct to become a valid cornerstone of community mental health practice?

The underlying rationale for how and why social support systems manifest their influence resides in such diverse theoretical bases as epidemiology, biology, psychoanalysis, anthropology, and sociology. However, the principles of crisis theory have perhaps most directly sensitized community mental health practitioners to the purposes and applications of social supports. The early work in crisis theory and in crisis intervention contained many of the elements that a decade later became central to social support systems theory—for example, the individual's signaling of distress in order to mobilize help from significant others; the individual's expectation that help will be forthcoming; and the individual's accessibility to help from formal and informal caregivers. Killilea states in Chapter Six that while crisis theory focuses upon the individual, short-term events, and current influences, the support systems model enlarges the framework to include social aggregates, continuing socioenvironmental influences, and communication patterns. Both models, however, focus on coping and mastery.

Through what processes do social ties enhance psychological well-being? Weiss (Chapter Five) suggests that social ties provide functional, informational, and emotional support that can be obtained in varying degrees from close and intimate relationships as well as from friends and family. Pioneering studies on the social ties of separated and divorced persons led Weiss to distinguish the specific contributions to well-being made by (1) relationships of attachment that foster feelings of security and comfort, (2) affiliative relationships based on shared interests or similarity of circumstances, (3) kin-type alliances organized around bonds of loyalty, (4) collaborative relationships that are work related, (5) nurturant relationships in which the investment is in another's well-being, and (6) help-receiving relationships within which one comfortably accepts support and guidance. Caplan's (1981) review of recent research on the mastery of stress led him to conclude that a high level of social support significantly reduces vulnerability to physical and mental illness by lowering emotional tension and supplementing eroded cognitive and problem-solving capacities. In the Epilogue, Caplan also emphasizes that while this conception of social support and stress mastery does not negate the importance of crisis intervention, it significantly widens the preventive field by concerning itself with long-term as well as acute stress.

The relevance of support system concepts to the reduction of prolonged stress has been recognized for some time with regard to bereavement and psychosocial transitions. Noting that some losses cannot be resolved despite anticipatory guidance and grief, Parkes in Chapter Seven describes the characteristics of posttransition guidance that are crucial for persons seeking new roles and relationships. He emphasizes that grief cannot be suppressed with drugs and that effective counseling methods are needed to help replace disintegrated social support systems. While random assignment studies have investigated the efficacy of professional interventions, Parkes is concerned that the efficacy of the burgeoning mutual help groups has not yet been subjected to similar scientific evaluation.

Definitive assessments may still be lacking, but evaluative studies nevertheless are becoming more commonplace. Thus, psychiatric and social science researchers have begun to investigate whether social supports play an independent or mediating role in reducing the effects of stress on health and well-being (Hirsch, 1979). This distinction has crucial implications for etiological models of emotional and physical illness, as well as for the design of pertinent intervention models. As research on social support has progressed, investigators have sought to operationalize the quantitative and qualitative characteristics of social networks. Thus far, they have fared better in refining the structural indexes of a network's size, membership, density, duration, and so on, although the reliability of such data remains unduly low (Killworth and Bernard, 1976). Less progress has been made in measuring psychological processes and contributions to social functioning. Furthermore, a myriad of scales appear in the literature, since each investigator has devised unique data-gathering instruments to reflect his or her conception of a social network's composition and its instrumental and expressive purposes. Such disorganization typifies most new fields of intellectual inquiry. However, if generalizations are to emerge from this growing body of research, consensus must soon be reached about social network concepts and measures. When this occurs, a high-priority study would be the causal relationship between social support and stress, including longitudinal comparisons of groups varying in their use of such support during stressful periods. Killilea (Chapter Six) also suggests that preventive trials and demonstration intervention projects be designed that would assess whether social and community supports have a beneficial effect at times of high stress and in chronic deficit situations.

The Environment and Community Mental Health Centers

Mental health services are delivered through a variety of health and social welfare agencies. While only past and present recipients of federal operational funds have been bureaucratically designated as community mental health centers (CMHCs), in practical terms this classification is equally applicable to the numerous other human service organizations providing multiple types of interventions for mental disorders. Regardless of which classificatory scheme is used, CMHCs now are undergoing major changes in their mode of operation. They are assigning new priorities for the allocation of limited resources and redesigning clinical structures in the face of shifting judicial standards of proper treatment, alterations in both the source and level of public funding, ambiguous third-party payment patterns, and so on. The following section reviews the contemporary program models that are emerging to meet the needs of specific patient populations. It first is necessary, however, to consider the generic environmental forces that Harshbarger and Demone describe in Chapter Eight as affecting the structure and administration of all CMHCs, whether they are federally funded or not.

Ideology and Social Values. The several revolutions that have occurred in psychiatric care during the past 150 years have been heavily influenced by the ideologies of mental health practitioners and public policy makers. Their orientations to the control of social deviance have been as significant as scientific theory and findings in molding the nature of care for persons defined as mentally ill. Schulberg and Baker (1969) have emphasized that in the absence of scientific knowledge, belief systems provide a common rationale to guide the behavior of a group's members. Not surprisingly, ideology is as influential in natural support systems as in professional service delivery systems. The common beliefs of members of peer therapy groups serve as cognitive antidotes to discrepant experiences and maintain the members' unity of purpose. This does not mean that the relationship between attitudes and behavior is simple and direct. Rather, it is a complex one whose vicissitudes must be studied in relation to other social situational variables capable of affecting behavior.

The mental health system has constantly been marked by what Baker (Chapter Nine) describes as a "strain toward revision," that is, a conviction that fresh ideas and practices surpass preceding ones even though evidence for this is lacking. In climates of innovation, novelty in itself provides the requisite validity. However, even well-accepted novel approaches will soon falter unless their effectiveness can be demonstrated, and they inevitably will be succeeded by fresh innovative practices more congruent with contemporary social values. Tracing the ebb and flow of ideologies that have affected psychiatric practice over the past three decades, Baker indicates that during the 1960s the Great Society's cultural norm of social engineering provided a supportive ethos within which community mental health innovations could be pursued. The community mental health ideology prevailing in the 1960s was succeeded by the human services ideology of the 1970s, which in turn has been succeeded by disparate belief systems seeking to impose their mark upon the 1980s.

We had noted previously that members of the psychiatric establishment are seeking to "remedicalize" mental health services and to return the administration and delivery of clinical care to the confines of the medical model. This orientation focuses upon serious mental disorders rather than problems in living and views professionals as having little, if any, role in alleviating adverse social conditions. A markedly contrasting orientation is evident in Nevid and Morrison's (1980) "Libertarian Mental Health Ideology," which considers mental illness an antiquated metaphor. This ideology regards deviant conduct in terms of psychological, cognitive, or existential antecedents and rejects the medical treatment model.

Still another ideological orientation that is hoping to influence service delivery in the 1980s is described by Hollander (1980) as the consumer alternative to professional domination. This ideology espouses an egalitarian relationship between consumer and professional, contending that expert knowledge should contribute to the helping process but not dominate it—a perspective reinforced by legal decisions over the past decade. This ideology is rooted in various intellectual sources, but a key one within the community mental health field is the concept of maximizing citizen and consumer participation. Windle and Cibulka (1981) trace efforts over the past two decades to implement this principle, and they identify progress and failure in terms of who should participate, the functions citizens and consumers should fulfill, and the powers they should be assigned. Windle and Cibulka conclude that conflicting social trends in the early 1980s leave the future of citizen and consumer participation in community mental health programs uncertain. Although faltering citizen and community involvement may portend renewed professional domination, the judicial developments to be considered next are likely to have a mediating effect for at least the next several years.

Judicial Decisions. One of the most profound ways in which a society's values are manifested is through the actions of its judicial system. Ennis (1978) indicates that as recently as the late 1960s, a few pages would have sufficed to discuss court involvement in the public practice of psychiatry; today the subject could not be adequately reviewed even in several volumes. The dramatic increase of judicial activity is meaningful in its own right, but even more crucial is the libertarian tenor of decisions handed down in the last fifteen years. In fact, Ennis feels the pressures experienced by psychiatrists recently from the judiciary are insignificant compared to those to be confronted in the years to come. What societal values are inherent, then, in these court decisions, and how are they affecting community mental health practice?

The judiciary's policies and principles were analyzed by Stone (1975), who concluded that each landmark decision in the 1960s and early 1970s spoke to the same underlying principle of freedom. The courts have consistently held that loss of freedom in civil commitment is at least as grievous as criminal confinement; indeed, when misused, civil commitment may be even more injurious. This ideology has produced stringent standards for determining dangerousness to self or others if a person is to be committed. The tensions that have resulted between psychiatrists and judges by the application of these standards have been heightened by what Ennis (1978) considers to be the judiciary's growing recognition that psychiatry is an art, not a science. Within this perspective, judges may consider the clinical decisions of not always neutral mental health professionals to be unduly influenced by subjective judgments. In the short run at least, Ennis considers judicial insistence on dangerousness, as evidenced by an overt act, a sensible method for limiting psychiatric abuse of the commitment power.

Not surprisingly, intense controversy has been provoked by the discrepant views of psychiatrists who perceive themselves as exercising the noble societal function of *parens patriae* when hospitalizing unstable individuals and the views of civil libertarians who consider psychiatrists to be exercising excessive police powers by restricting the freedom of individuals through hospitalization. The depth of these differences has spawned a wide variety of legal advocacy programs whose major purpose is the protection and enhancement of human rights. The direction of the continuing bitter debate between psychiatrists and libertarians as they are reflected in commitment practices is reviewed by Roth (1980). He believes that there will be no compromise between the sharply differing value systems of psychiatry and the law until more scientifically valid data exist about the precise impact of mental disorder upon human behavior, and until society expends the resources necessary to ensure a better standard of care for committed persons. Such scientific data and societal concern are unlikely to emerge for some time to come. In the interim, community mental health centers will continue to grapple with the clinical consequences of judicial decisions, among the most provocative and far reaching of which are "the right to the least restrictive environment" and "the right to refuse treatment."

The community mental health movement has long implicitly, if not explicitly, espoused the humanitarian concept of least restrictive environment that the President's Commission on Mental Health (1978) defined as "maintaining the greatest degree of freedom, self-determination, autonomy, dignity, and integrity of body, mind, and spirit for the individual while he or she participates in treatment or receives services." A decade has passed since this concept was legally established in the 1972 *Wyatt* v. *Stickney* decision, and yet, as Bachrach (1980a) emphasizes, empirical criteria for its implementation still are lacking. The resulting problems are perhaps most evident with regard to the movement of chronically ill persons from institutional to community settings. Bachrach suggests that for some individuals, the institution may well be the least restrictive environment if available community settings fail to enhance well-being. Perversions of this principle have even led to the death of former inpatients who were placed in group homes and nursing facilities that lacked adequate fire protection. Deinstitutionalization efforts have been plagued by other unwarranted assumptions and confusions about how to provide the least restrictive environment. Bachrach suggests, therefore, that we instead focus on its polar opposite, that is, the "most therapeutic environment"—a concept that emphasizes the patient's ever-changing level of functioning rather than the locus of care.

The pioneering court decisions of *Rouse* v. *Cameron* (1966), *Wyatt* v. *Stickney* (1972), and *O'Connor* v. *Donaldson* (1975), which established the various circumstances under which patients have a right to treatment, interfered very little with clinical practice. It is unlikely that more or differing treatment is provided to hospitalized patients as a result of these rulings. But the 1979 decisions of *Rennie* v. *Klein* and *Rogers* v. *Okin,* which established a patient's right to *refuse* treatment under specified conditions, have triggered a fire storm of protest among psychiatrists who consider themselves placed in a double bind. Delaying such treatment as medication until legal procedures are implemented causes discomfort for the patient and staff; conversely, forcing treatment on the patient undermines his or her sense of autonomy and may interfere with constitutional rights (Ford, 1980; Appelbaum and Gutheil, 1980). This dilemma has led to a profound legal and ethical debate about the nature of informed consent and true freedom. The need for an accommodation between abstract constitutional concepts and the practical realities of mental illness is evident. In 1982, however, the U.S. Supreme Court declined to issue a definitive ruling and remanded earlier appeals to lower courts for reconsideration. In its action, the Supreme Court implied that professional judgment warrants more attention than it had been given in previous federal court decisions.

Diminishing Resources and Administrative Solutions. The recession pervading America's economy in the early 1980s is taking its toll on the human services. Community mental health centers have suffered from federal funding cutbacks in terms of both substantial reductions of appropriations and the shift to block grant mechanisms. Many state appropriations are being reduced as well. Moreover, the savings potentially to be generated from reduced federal regulations conceivably could be matched by the costs of newly imposed state-level regulations. As a consequence of these troubling developments, mental health administrators have become acutely sensitive to the negative economic environment within which their centers are functioning.

While always susceptible to adverse fiscal developments, program priorities and organizational strategies more than ever must be formulated in relation to basic economic principles. McGuire and Weisbrod (National Institute of Mental Health, 1981) suggest that efforts by community mental health centers to resolve budgetary problems and to control expenditures are likely to founder unless they critically examine the following: (1) local and national influences upon the demand for care by patients and their agents, (2) forces affecting the supply of mental health resources, (3) the consequences of regulating labor and capital in the mental health industry, (4) problems in adequately caring for the chronically mentally ill, and (5) the cost-benefit ratios of alternative treatment approaches. Frank (1981) notes that while cost-benefit analysis has been used since the late 1950s, for conceptual and practical reasons it has yet to be broadly applied in the mental health field. Nevertheless, its utility is likely to become increasingly apparent to public policy analysts who need to make decisions about the allocation of social resources when the private market fails.

The present economic environment of diminishing resources has focused attention on the containment of costs and on strategies for "managing with less" (Ashbaugh, 1981; Curtis, 1981). In Chapter Ten, Broskowski urges that CMHCs use this adverse milieu to clarify, perhaps even redefine, long-range goals. Discouraging fiscal and political trends leave a CMHC with the options of planning a series of cutbacks, some of which may improve efficiency; replacing lost "markets" with new ones so as to maintain present program levels; and engaging in selective cutbacks and expansion of clinical service in well-targeted areas. The management of service cutbacks clearly differs from the management of growth since CMHCs cannot be dismantled in the same sequential manner in which they were created. Instead, administrators are faced with the dilemma of whether to utilize equity or efficiency criteria in their budgetary decisions.

Broskowski indicates that staff participation in these deliberations can lead to meaningless reductions because of self-serving staff needs.

CMHCs attempting to expand into new domains of service delivery while contracting existing ones are increasingly resorting to corporate configuring, a strategy long utilized in the profit-making sector. By establishing related nonprofit corporations, CMHCs can take advantage of highly specific funding opportunities, avoid regulatory disincentives, and shelter the parent corporation from undue fiscal risk. The legal and administrative intricacies facing CMHCs interested in corporate configuring are outlined by Broskowski. Another organizational strategy increasingly utilized by CMHCs seeking to respond flexibly to shifting environmental demands is the matrix design (White, 1978). An alternative to classical bureaucratic or pyramidal administrative structures, the matrix organization superimposes task-oriented project teams upon existing departmental lines.

If the economic environment within which CMHCs operate continues to require that they simultaneously impose cutbacks and explore growth opportunities, the cognitive and emotional resources of administrators will be severely taxed. Leadership in these circumstances requires exceptional skills; the training of administrators has therefore become a topic of major concern to educators, bureaucrats, and clinicians. Emphasizing that mental health administration is still in its formative stages, the Report of the National Task Force on Mental Health/Mental Retardation Administration (1979) recommends a model training curriculum covering these major areas: (1) the functions and skills of generic administration, (2) the substance of clinical care, (3) the symbiotic relationship between program and administration, and (4) the values and characteristics of the CMHC's environment.

With the growth of the CMHC movement, executive positions have been assumed in many local and state programs by professional managers who lack clinical training. Feldman (1981) fears that this will lead to the triumph of administrative process over patient needs, but he also recognizes that clinicians promoted to middle- and upper-management positions often experience difficulty coping with role-inherent power. They must learn to reconcile the need for peer approval with the responsibility of critically reviewing colleagues' behavior (Feldman, 1980). In the process of resolving the dilemmas associated with managerial functioning, clinician-executives must be as careful as lay administrators not to be overwhelmed by their organization's anxiety-provoking fiscal needs and thus to become insensitive to the needs of patients.

The critical role of leaders in managing the transition of CMHCs to meet the complex needs of the 1980s will afford unique opportunities for consultation to changing organizations. Concerned that administrators often seek help only when system dysfunction is advanced and even then with ambivalence, Levinson (Chapter Eleven) and Hirschowitz (Chapter Twelve) offer their conceptions of how consultants can promote healthy organizational adaptation. Levinson builds upon Caplan's (1970) framework of consultee-centered consultation and offers a comprehensive approach to organizational diagnosis. Factual data are assembled through a highly detailed case-study outline and analyzed within an ego psychology model to determine how effectively the CMHC is adapting to market conditions, personnel needs, and so on. Since the CMHC and the consultant are actively engaged with each other, the process necessarily is both diagnostic and interventive.

Hirschowitz suggests that consultation to changing organizations be based on four concepts. First, all change involves loss and transitional tasks must be accomplished; second, defensive behavior is normal during the early stages of change but it must not become frozen as resistance; third, transitional tasks are promoted when staff receive supportive, mastery, and modeling supplies; and fourth, leadership processes alternate between the arousal of staff distress and the provision of alleviating support. Once change has occurred, the consultant can help the leader explore buried psychological meanings, legitimate grief, and restore program continuity. Additional conceptions of the consultation process during periods of organizational transition are offered by Goodstein (1978), Berlin (1979), and Hausman and Prosen (1981).

Program Models

A major principle of community mental health ideology is the provision of comprehensive services to those requiring multifaceted care. Before the era of community mental health services, organizational capability rather than patient needs often dictated the nature of treatment since agencies specialized in a particular service, for example, inpatient or outpatient service. Continuity of care was difficult to maintain when the patient's clinical needs changed. Community mental health centers have been required to provide a minimum of five essential services so as to be more responsive to patient needs and to facilitate patient movement through the differing services required during an episode of illness. Caplan in the Epilogue credits the framers of community mental health legislation with the wisdom of permitting flexible, alternative patterns of service delivery. Thus, the obligatory functions of a comprehensive program may be provided through a single CMHC or spread among several community agencies linked by formal affiliative agreements.

While obstacles to appropriate treatment and continuity of care persist for such patient groups as the chronically mentally ill, the manner in which most psychiatric patients are treated has changed markedly over the past quarter of a century. Taube, Regier, and Rosenfeld (1978) report that outpatient services in organized care settings increased almost 1,000 percent per 100,000 population between 1955 and 1975, while inpatient episodes increased only 10 percent per 100,000 population during this period. Treatment that once was predominantly long term and inpatient is now, therefore, primarily acute and ambulatory. Furthermore, the locus of care has shifted markedly since 1950 from state hospitals to various community-based facilities (Kramer, 1977). The number of persons in homes for the aged and dependent has increased dramatically while the resident population of state hospitals is significantly lower. Much of this change has resulted from the growth of private and governmental insurance plans that now provide reimbursement for inpatient and outpatient services at local facilities. In particular, Medicare and Medicaid have shifted residential care of the elderly from state hospitals to nursing homes.

Pardes and Pincus (1980) reviewed the developments of the 1970s and concluded that while this decade seemed to contain no revolutionary shifts in treatment, closer analysis reveals several developments that may have sown the seeds for profound change during the 1980s. The following trends are deemed particularly significant by Pardes and Pincus: continued expansion of the therapeutic armamentarium, refinements in existing therapies, greater focus on negative effects of therapies, and strengthening of the scientific knowledge base for therapeutic interventions. With regard to the refinement of existing treatments, much attention is being directed to whether unique interventions can be specified for given diagnoses or conditions. In 1980, the American Psychiatric Association established a commission to produce a comprehensive manual with specific treatment guidelines for every DSM-III category of disorder. This comprehensive undertaking is considered premature by Frances and Clarkin (1981), given the present state of knowledge about many psychiatric illnesses, but they nevertheless offer a framework of seven covarying dimensions for determining which particular psychotherapeutic modality is most suited to a given clinical situation.

The ultimate specification of which treatment is most validly prescribed for which illness undoubtedly will constitute major progress, but services must still be organized and delivered on the basis of existing knowledge while this quest continues. In the Epilogue, Caplan suggests that from the community mental health perspective, it remains as necessary as ever to maintain a population focus and not just a concern for patients who seek care and are accepted for treatment. This public health orientation differs significantly from the individual-patient orientation and manifests itself in the type of programs designed for high-risk groups.

A key debate in the early 1980s has been whether the population focus should continue its concentration on specified geographic catchment areas or shift in its orientation to delimited, high-risk groups, for example, children, the elderly, minority groups, and the chronically mentally ill. In the following section, we will briefly analyze several program models that exemplify efforts to meet the needs of specific populations. Procedures for linking the health and mental health care systems and organizing the diverse range of human services required by the chronically mentally ill are at the center of this recent thrust and they will be highlighted.

General Health and Mental Health Linkages. Efforts to reemphasize the medical component of community mental health practice have provoked controversy between psychiatrists and other mental health professionals. Nevertheless, all disciplines acknowledge that the relationship between general health and mental health must be reexamined because of advances in biological psychiatry, the neurosciences, and behavioral medicine; epidemiological findings about the prevalence of emotional disorders in medical patients and medical illnesses in psychiatric patients; federal initiatives in the organization and financing of health care; cost-offset studies demonstrating the savings to be gained by substituting psychiatric care for more expensive medical interventions; and so forth. The report of the President's Commission on Mental Health (1978) emphasized the interdependence between physical and psychological disorders and called for cooperative arrangements between general health care settings and CMHCs. What issues are to be resolved in negotiating such linkages, and what directions are being pursued by the planners and administrators of such ventures?

Concern about how to move the general health and mental health systems more closely together is but the most recent focus of those studying the interorganizational behavior of human service agencies caring for the mentally ill. O'Brien (1980) reviews these dynamics within the framework of open systems concepts and presents a generic typology of interorganizational linkages. The growth of neighborhood health centers, health maintenance organizations, and other forms of primary medical care during the 1970s offered a unique opportunity to experiment with general health and mental health linkages, and a sizable literature reports on these experiences (for example, Borus, 1976; National Institute of Mental Health, 1980; Broskowski,

Marks, and Budman, 1981). Indicating that linkages of the general health and mental health systems benefit patients through improved case finding and diagnosis, comprehensiveness of services, and continuity of care, Broskowski offers several models in Chapter Twenty for coordinating these diverse clinical entities. He urges that linkage development proceed slowly and focus on well-defined goals, since a multiplicity of forces can promote or inhibit this complex process. A related scheme for analyzing the ties between mental health and primary medical care practice is presented by Pincus (1980). He suggests that a given model be chosen in terms of the people to be served and their needs, the nature of the community, the administrative structure to be implemented, financing mechanisms, philosophy of care, and the types and levels of settings to be linked.

A more specialized direction for promoting the growth of mental health linkages is in the general hospital setting (Pardes, 1981). Psychiatric units were still exceptional in the late 1950s, but growing recognition of their clinical efficacy and fiscal viability was accelerated by the 1963 Community Mental Health Centers Act. It established inpatient care as an essential service that in many communities could be provided most efficiently within general hospitals. Such psychiatric units are now commonplace. Keill (1981) suggests that a general hospital's easy accessibility and comprehensive medical and psychosocial services make it, in fact, the proper core for a mental health services system. While this role may be feasible in many instances, Bachrach (1981b) cautions that the general hospital's capacity to deliver psychiatric services is still undergoing change. Issues requiring resolution include the boundaries of the hospital's responsibility relative to those of other human service agencies, the target populations that can be most effectively treated, and the service that can be most appropriately provided. Of pressing concern is the extent of the general hospital's responsibility for chronically mentally ill persons residing in the community as the result of deinstitutionalization.

Community Care of the Chronically Mentally Ill. The failure of health and human service agencies to provide the care needed by chronically mentally ill persons to live in the community has been noted earlier in this chapter. Community mental health centers, in particular, have been charged with shirking their responsibility to this group despite some evidence to the contrary (Goldman and others, 1980). A full review of the problems associated with community care of the chronically mentally ill and recent remedial actions would require a book of its own. The following analysis, therefore, is limited to a brief consideration of key developments in the past decade.

Several etiological models now exist to explain schizophrenic illnesses, but no model would contend that these illnesses can ever be fully eradicated as a public health problem. Hansell in Chapter Fourteen, for example, views them as genetically transmitted, basic cellular system impairments that will recur even in the face of successful primary prevention programs. It is vital, therefore, to improve strategies of secondary and tertiary prevention; indeed, for the past three decades remarkable gains have been achieved in both these realms. With regard to reducing schizophrenia's long-term debilitating consequences, planners and clinicians have come to realize that many are iatrogenic in nature. To a significant degree, the chronic social breakdown syndrome can be prevented through improved linkages between hospital and community services; it need not be a standard outcome of the disease process (Gruenberg, 1967). Hansell views schizophrenia as radically interfering with the individual's capacity for bonding with others, but he also considers properly structured social support systems an effective means for reducing the isolation and interpersonal fragility so often experienced by persons with this illness. From this perspective, it is critical that such hospitalizations as are unavoidable be for brief periods in a local facility so that the person's tenuous social affiliations may be preserved and continuity of care maintained.

Research demonstrating that the chronically mentally ill could function in the community under proper supportive conditions led policy makers and administrators to pursue alternatives to large-scale, state hospital care. Deinstitutionalization was carried out on a massive scale during the 1970s, producing both an altered service delivery system and a sociopolitical movement (Bachrach, 1976). By the mid 1970s, however, evidence had begun to mount that deinstitutionalization had generated deleterious as well as salutary effects, and the needs of the chronically mentally ill were rescrutinized by governmental and professional bodies. In the succeeding years, a stream of reports was published by the General Accounting Office (1977), the Group for the Advancement of Psychiatry (1978), the American Psychiatric Association (Talbott, 1978), and the U.S. Surgeon General's Office (DHHS, 1980). After analyzing the programmatic components of the surgeon general's report, Talbott (1981) concluded that the most recent "national plan" for the chronically mentally ill is based on three assumptions. First, deinstitutionalization has replaced the imperfect system of state hospital care with a "nonsystem" of community care. Second, most of the chronically mentally ill need not be hospitalized if comprehensive human services are available in the community. Third, financing mechanisms must be redesigned so as to reduce the number of persons being placed in nursing homes rather than in more therapeutic and more cost-effective alternative community settings. How valid are these assumptions and what steps are being taken to act upon them?

A sizable body of evidence clearly indicates that society's commitment to providing the chronically mentally ill with properly organized, community-based human services is ambivalent at best. The legal and moral responsibility traditionally assumed by the states for this population has eroded, in some instances almost to the vanishing point, without other public, voluntary, or private entities stepping into the breach. The difficulties in planning for the human service needs of the chronically mentally ill under this condition are severe. It is true that high-quality, comprehensive programs have been designed in the wake of deinstitutionalization, but such undertakings have been the exception rather than the rule. Because of her concern that exemplary programs of the type reviewed by Stein and Test (1978) could not be readily reproduced or generalized, Bachrach (1980b) called for strategies that would translate model-derived knowledge into systems-related action.

The most focused, if meagerly funded, attempt to stimulate comprehensive, standardized services for the chronically mentally ill is the NIMH Community Support Program (CSP). It involves broad-scale, multilevel interventions aimed at the chronically mentally ill, their families, agency personnel, and the communities within which the chronically mentally ill reside (Turner and Ten Hoor, 1978). Intrinsic to a CSP are carefully organized networks of human services that include elements of the medical, rehabilitation, and social support models. CSPs are especially concerned with the unique continuity of care required by chronic patients (Bachrach, 1981a), and they have highlighted the case manager's function in meeting this need. Whether the CSP model is effective and efficient remains to be determined. Even if the findings are positive, however, there is no indication as yet that the Reagan administration will maintain a federal role in stimulating such endeavors. If this priority is dropped at the national level, it is doubtful whether states, under the block grant mechanism, will meaningfully address the needs of the chronically mentally ill. Such a development would be most unfortunate at a time when data from better designed research are suggesting that community alternatives to hospital-based care are clinically effective (Braun and others, 1981) and generate comparable cost-benefit ratios (Weisbrod, Test, and Stein, 1980).

With regard to the financing of services required by the chronically mentally ill, the U.S. Surgeon General's proposed "national plan" describes five major federal programs presently offering fiscal assistance to this population (Rubin, 1981). Medicaid is recommended as the primary program through which short-term changes could be achieved; numerous incremental reforms are also recommended both to fill gaps in the present service delivery system and to expand coverage to more individuals. Long-term financing options include a structured services program operated by the public sector, a benefit-voucher program to increase the individual's capacity to purchase private sector services, and a cash transfer program with few restrictions for people meeting certain categorical tests. The Reagan administration will likely choose immediate and distant fiscal solutions within the philosophy of decentralizing responsibility to the states. However, the New Federalism policy set forth by President Reagan in early 1982 would return the Medicaid program to the national level while transferring public welfare programs to the states. Since the chronically mentally ill are dependent upon care administered through both these domains, contradictory program pursuits are conceivable should the New Federalism legislation be enacted at some future time.

Community Care of the Mentally Retarded. The mentally retarded experience many of the same functional disabilities as the chronically mentally ill. Not surprisingly, they share related problems in obtaining human services and have struggled with similar legal, fiscal, and attitudinal obstacles to shifting the service delivery system from institutional to community settings. Klebanoff (Chapter Fifteen) reviews the history of psychiatric involvement in providing therapeutic, educational, and habilitative services to the mentally retarded. He concludes that educational components linked to CMHCs grew quite rapidly in the 1960s but that clinical services lagged far behind. By the early 1970s, legislation coalescing mental retardation with other developmental disabilities became a rallying point for strong parent advocacy groups, an effort that Klebanoff notes was spurred by the willingness of professionals to assign whatever diagnostic label would entitle a child to needed services. As retarded persons became newly eligible for care in various medical and social welfare agencies, the tenuous commitment of CMHCs to this population became even weaker.

At this point in time, the psychiatric needs of the mentally retarded are met by CMHCs in only a marginal way, despite the intent of federal and state planners that this group be treated in them. A 1979 survey of CMHCs in the state of Washington, for example, revealed that they were treating only 1,500 of 22,500 retarded individuals with a potential for mental disorder (West and Richardson, 1981). The reluctance of CMHCs and other human service agencies to serve the retarded has led parent groups to organize and operate their own programs. Klebanoff emphasizes that where this occurs, ironically, the advocacy function becomes subservient to the need for government financing, and the risk of co-optation is high.

The struggle to establish community services for the mentally retarded is very much linked to the deinstitutionalization movement described earlier in this chapter. However, the discharge of state school residents to the community started later and has proceeded more gradually than was the case with the chronically mentally ill. Boggs (1981) outlines a variety of factors such as public perception, case management techniques, and the use of specialized private residential settings that she considers associated with the more successful manner in which this transition has occurred for the retarded. Additionally, many of the major class action suits noted earlier in this chapter, for example, *Wyatt* v. *Stickney,* have also enabled retarded persons residing in state schools to receive community care. More recently, the Pennhurst suit brought against the commonwealth of Pennsylvania specifically espoused the right of the retarded to treatment in the least restrictive environment. The U.S. Supreme Court rejected this view in a 1981 decision, but it affirmed the state's obligation to provide habilitation. The progressive court decisions of recent years may now have ground to a halt. If so, litigation will need to be replaced by legislative and administrative strategies for advancing the rights of the retarded to proper care. The fiscal implications of several such options are analyzed by Braddock (1981).

The Elderly. In contrast to prevailing stereotypes, the elderly are a heterogenous group whose human service needs cover a broad spectrum, ranging from life enrichment opportunities for those who are well to medical, psychiatric, and social services for the frail. While most elderly are well, increased longevity is producing an increased incidence of chronic health and mental health problems (Gruenberg, 1977; Kramer, 1980). In Chapter Thirteen, Patterson and Abrahams emphasize that professional intervention is required primarily by persons over age seventy-five with general health and mental health problems. Given the sensitivity of elderly persons to environmental changes, an ecological perspective is useful for determining the degree to which symptoms represent the interaction between waning personal abilities and adverse environmental stimuli. Patterson and Abrahams urge that CMHCs utilize a population focus and seek to reduce destabilizing forces in the environment. Unfortunately, the record of CMHC involvement in policy-oriented concerns, as well as in direct clinical interventions with regard to the elderly, is a poor one.

While the role of the CMHC and other components of formal caregiving systems remains to be developed, the ability of informal support systems to provide social support and practical assistance is increasingly recognized. Mutual support groups are particularly valuable in helping families endure the prolonged tensions associated with the care of a severely impaired relative. Patterson and Abrahams note that there is also a growing self-advocacy, self-help, and self-care movement among the elderly that is based on the premise that self-actualization occurs during old age as well as during other periods of life. This movement has considerable potential for stimulating beneficial preventive ventures.

Primary Prevention in Schools. Caplan's (1964) seminal work on the potentialities of primary prevention has found fertile ground in school systems since they afford a unique institutional structure for impacting upon all children, including those potentially at risk for developing emotional disorders. In most communities, the school's traditional role as the major gatekeeper to mental health care has been furthered by the Education for All Handicapped Act (P.L. 94-142), which provides for the special needs of all handicapped children. By using Caplan's concept of mental health/illness as ranging from positive well-being to emotional disorder, school-based programs may enhance the youngster's competency and/or alter environmental stresses. In Chapter Eighteen, Reinherz presents a framework in which children are part of a larger ecological system; the primary prevention target is selected from among students, school personnel, parents, and the school environment.

Much of the work focused on students emerges from Ojemann's (1961) demonstration that youngsters can be taught causal thinking and alternative solutions to interpersonal conflicts. This finding has generated numerous programs that aim to improve student behavior and peer acceptance as well as to enhance self-awareness and the scope of personal abilities. Caplan's (1964) work on crisis theory has also stimulated primary prevention programs with student groups who are vulnerable to expectable psychosocial or biological transitions—for example, entering the first grade or adolescence. Among such programs are those that see children as capable of helping themselves and their peers (Gartner, Kohler, and Reissman, 1971; Hamburg and Varenhorst, 1972).

School personnel can be the target of primary prevention efforts since they have considerable contact with youngsters and the potential for influencing them in positive directions. Reinherz states that Caplan's (1970) model for consultation between mental health professionals and teachers continues to be commonly utilized. Its objectives are to heighten the teacher's self-awareness and to improve his or her ability to manage classroom behavior. While the role of school administrators in sanctioning primary prevention programs is critical, consultation models with this personnel group are less well refined. Parents are another possible target for primary prevention, on the assumption that appropriate efforts to alter the family environment will improve the child's social interaction and self-understanding. The school environment is a still further potential target, but Reinherz considers changes at this level difficult to achieve; social and physical engineering requires an activist stance and political sophistication. Environmental change is also impeded by the difficulty of specifying precisely which social or physical variables contribute to or detract from the fit between student and school. Among the few efforts to intervene at both the individual and socioenvironmental levels was the Woodlawn Project in Chicago, which operated from a community mental health center with significant neighborhood support (Kellam and others, 1975).

Disaster Intervention. A significant body of research depicting the profound psychological consequences of a community disaster has led to greater public awareness of its mental health consequences. State and local governments have designed increasingly sophisticated intervention strategies, and the federal Disaster Relief Act of 1974 authorized fiscal support for crisis counseling programs to prevent the development of chronic problems. Precise cause-effect relationships in the etiology of postdisaster psychiatric symptoms are yet to be demonstrated, but it is widely thought that interventions should be focused upon high-risk populations. Since time-consuming need assessments are unfeasible in the aftermath of a disaster, planners and clinicians should have previously identified a community's vulnerable subgroups so that limited resources can be expended effectively and efficiently.

With regard to the mental health professional's specific role in disaster intervention, Cohen in Chapter Sixteen stresses that he or she must be capable of functioning within the context of other human services whose scope and pace often are established by governmental priorities. Community mental health theory relevant to this role includes knowledge about loss and mourning and the progression of crisis reactions. Techniques of crisis resolution suggested by Caplan (1964) are highly pertinent, including short-term treatment, counseling with couples and families, and the use of social support systems. Despite the effectiveness of crisis intervention strategies, for some persons the consequences of a disaster can linger long after the catastrophe. In these cases, adaptation is a slower, if not impossible, process. The symptoms displayed may be at a clinical level sufficient to warrant the DSM-III diagnosis of posttraumatic stress disorder, chronic or delayed type, and techniques for coping with long-term stress will be needed.

Rural Mental Health Services. Despite the predominantly urban character of the United States, almost one quarter of its population continues to reside in rural or semirural areas that differ on such dimensions as geography, economic resources, and ethnic and religious characteristics. Furthermore, the traditional impression that rural mental illness rates are lower than urban ones is being increasingly questioned; Wagenfeld (1982) contends that they are higher in the rural areas. Regardless of which prevalence rates are higher, psychiatric care in rural regions is generally considered inadequate in terms of both quality and quantity. In Chapter Nineteen, Wagenfeld and Ozarin identify the following five factors as critical to "culturally syntonic" rural service delivery, that is, care that is consonant with the needs, perceptions, and values of those being treated:

1. Transportation. Given the sizable area covered by a rural CMHC, fixed or movable satellites are often needed. Transportation systems shared with other human service agencies may also be required.
2. Personnel Recruitment and Retention. Professionals prefer to practice in urban settings, although persons raised in rural regions tend to gravitate back to their earlier residences. Staffing patterns must take into account the limited number of professionals and the fact that they will require continuing education and opportunities for peer interaction if burnout is to be avoided.
3. Interagency Collaboration. Informal rather than formal exchanges are the norm in rural areas. Particularly noteworthy are linkages that have developed between general health and mental health agencies in sparsely settled areas.
4. Governmental Regulations. While all human service agencies are constrained by bureaucratic rules, rural CMHCs perceive themselves as the object of discriminatory standards. Whether the governmental regulations established to administer block grants will alter this situation remains to be seen.
5. Community Advocacy. Citizen support is central to any CMHC's viability. However, such support is more difficult to sustain in a rural area where fewer residents have mental illness as a strongly felt concern. If CMHC boards are to advocate successfully for needed resources, professionals must supply them with adequate information and technical support.

Community Mental Health Technologies. Earlier sections of this overview have considered legislative, administrative, and programmatic developments affecting community mental health practice. Another dimension pertinent to this analysis involves the technologies utilized by staff to achieve CMHC goals. During the past two decades, numerous biological, psychological, behavioral, and social interventions have been introduced and refined for general psychiatric practice (Arieti and Brodie, 1981). We will restrict ourselves here to the consideration of "brief family crisis therapy" and mental health consultation because of their specific relevance to a CMHC.

In Chapter Seventeen, Parad describes how Caplan's (1964) formulation of crisis theory and intervention opened new vistas for those concerned with the treatment of populations rather than individuals. It permitted staff to shift their efforts from long-term therapies while still strengthening a patient's adaptive and integrative capacities. The burgeoning of short-term treatment strategies (Budman, 1981) has renewed interest in crisis intervention, and Parad details a framework for linking these related orientations in the treatment of families. Initially applied in studies of how families cope with the stress related to the birth of a premature infant, "brief family crisis therapy" has been increasingly utilized in community care of the mentally ill as well. If this treatment is to grow, Parad urges that staff be provided with needed training and that administrative changes be initiated so as to accommodate the therapy's unique requirements within organizational practice.

Most mental health technologies involve direct contact between the professional and the patient. Consultation, however, is an indirect service widely championed by those espousing community mental health ideology. The 1963 Community Mental Health Centers Act designated consultation as one of five essential services, thus establishing it as a mandated component of CMHC practice. The applications of this technology range across all levels of prevention and include clinical, programmatic, and policy concerns (Caplan, 1970). For numerous proper and improper reasons, consultation has also been perceived as synonymous with primary prevention.

Now in the 1980s, prospects for consultation's future growth appear unclear. Paradoxically, as the process of consultation is becoming increasingly sophisticated, funding for its practice is becoming less stable. With regard to refinements in the consultation process, on the one hand, a voluminous literature continues to clarify the varied models and approaches used by consultants, to portray the settings within which they are practiced, and to analyze the subtleties of the process (Rogawski, 1979; Grady, Gibson, and Trickett, 1981). On the other hand, it must be recognized that over the past years only about 6 percent of CMHC staff hours have been expended on this service. Furthermore, consultation services were among the first to be reduced as federal staffing monies diminished since, unlike direct services, they do not generate income. Finally, vague federal guidelines have made it difficult to establish consultation units with a clearly understood mission; staff have been inadequately trained; and there has been a lack of evaluation research demonstrating consultation's efficacy. While these issues certainly are troublesome, many practitioners want to maintain consultation as a viable CMHC activity. Ketterer (1981) and Bergner (1981) analyze the organizational, administrative, and fiscal requirements for consultation's survival and suggest strategies to achieve this goal.

Program Evaluation. Our review of the future design and delivery of mental health services must consider the accountability mechanisms for assessing the effectiveness and efficiency of these systems. In Chapter Twenty-One, Schulberg analyzes the strategies being pursued at various levels of program activity. He emphasizes that the major evaluative focus remains at the level of effort assessment although effectiveness studies are being undertaken more frequently. A theoretical model of how programs impact upon patients is particularly crucial for the latter investigations since it affects the choice of research design, target and comparison populations, and outcome indexes. Repeal of the Mental Health Systems Act in 1981 halted the development of performance measures and other evaluation requirements that had been included in this federal CMHC legislation. Despite this setback, the need for accountability remains unchallenged, and there are growing indications that evaluation will assume increased centrality at the state level, where allocations from block grants to service programs are now being made. If such a trend grows, responsibility for establishing program standards and monitoring their achievement will be decentralized from the federal to the state level. While this eventuality has many potential virtues, it also raises profound concerns about how a national biometric and epidemiological data system can be maintained in the future if each state utilizes idiosyncratic indexes of program effort and effectiveness.

Resource Development

During the 1950s and 1960s, community mental health programs were faced with the problem of how to recruit an adequate number of competent professional staff. Expanding the supply of such personnel, therefore, became a central goal of federal and state manpower development efforts. These strategies were highly successful; by the 1970s, personnel shortages were regarded as selective rather than absolute. Federal planners turned their attention to strategies for reducing the training funds that had become so vital to academic institutions, redistributing personnel from surplus to shortage areas, and enlarging the pool of minorities and women in the mental health professions.

Supply and production trends of recent years are analyzed by Demone (Chapter Twenty-Two), and he points to the ambiguities underlying the several projection models upon which present federal training policies are based. Supply and demand estimates, manpower to population ratios, health needs assessments, and service targeting are fraught with complexities that Demone thinks seriously impair their usefulness in estimating personnel needs. For example, the number of psychiatrists required in the future, according to Pardes (1979) and Liptzin (1979), will depend not only on the preceding factors but also on such additional ones as the functions of other medical and nonmedical disciplines, the restructuring of service delivery systems, technological advances, and the third-party reimbursement structure for psychiatric services. At this time, classical economic principles in which patient demand for services would determine the supply of a given discipline have not been properly tested in the mental health marketplace. It, therefore, is of great interest that freedom of choice laws enacted by thirty-one states in the 1970s and early 1980s are demonstrating that competition affects pricing structure and consequently the supply of psychiatrists needed relative to psychologists (Frank, 1982). Against the background of these overall trends in resource development, we now will consider manpower patterns in CMHCs, the role of nonpsychiatric physicians in the medical sector in providing care to mentally disordered persons, and the contributions of mutual help groups.

CMHC Staffing Patterns. The number and types of personnel employed by a human services facility are usually determined by licensing and certification requirements, program priorities, the clientele to be served, funding sources, staff recruitment and retention patterns, and so on. Given the evolving scope of CMHC responsibilities and the changing environments within which they function, how well have staffing patterns mirrored these shifts and how ready are present personnel to function within the priorities of the 1980s?

Over the past decade, the most marked trend in CMHC staffing patterns is the diminishing amount of psychiatric time and the growing amount of psychologist and social worker time utilized in the operation of these facilities. A recent NIMH manpower study by Bass (1981) reveals that between 1974 and 1978 full-time equivalent (FTE) professionals in all core disciplines increased by 11 percent. However, the number of FTE psychiatrists dropped 13 percent, while psychologists increased 15 percent and social workers increased 23 percent. The degree to which these altered staffing patterns reflect cost-containment strategies, that is, substitution of higher-paid personnel by lower-paid ones, was studied by McGuire (1980), who concluded that cost containment indeed was operative. It is interesting to note that the 1974-1978 decline in the number of psychiatrists per CMHC was part of a larger trend affecting all organized mental health settings; Veterans Administration and private psychiatric hospitals were the only facilities not affected by it.

What are the implications of reduced psychiatric participation in CMHC patient care activities? Winslow (1979), Fink and Weinstein (1979), and Berlin and others (1981) decry the resulting drop in the quality of clinical care and the deprofessionalization that they perceive as accompanying diminished psychiatric availability. They emphasize the unique contributions to assessment and treatment that can only be made by staff with medical training—a theme intrinsic to the remedicalization movement discussed earlier in this chapter. There is no question that skilled psychiatrists are vital to the operation of a CMHC, but unfortunately the renewed emphasis upon the medical model of practice also often betokens a desire to shift CMHCs away from the public health model that guided their early development. The continuing need to integrate medical skills and public health principles to ensure high-quality patient care is particularly evident with regard to the chronically mentally ill—a high-risk population with which many psychiatrists and other professionals have been loathe to become involved. Procedures for training psychiatric residents during their formative years in the knowledge and attitudes required to work with this patient group are described by Cutter, Bloom, and Shore (1981) and Nielsen and others (1981).

Medical Sector. The manpower shortages described earlier have led to the increased production of mental health specialists, as well as to the training of nonpsychiatric physicians in psychiatric principles and techniques. This latter development is part of the present national health policy that assigns primary care settings and practitioners a high priority in the organization and delivery of health services. It also recognizes that a person's life-style can be significantly related to physical illness and to adherence to medical regimens. The key role of nonpsychiatric physicians in assessing and treating emotional problems has also led to heightened interest by general hospital psychiatrists in consultation-liaison services. Refinements in consultation practice and applications of systems theory are thus producing medical care that is increasingly holistic rather than fragmented. In the light of these trends in policy and practice, Allen outlines in Chapter Twenty-Three the behavioral and social concepts that he thinks should be taught in a medical school curriculum. He considers it ironic that at a time when behavioral and social concepts finally are infiltrating the general field of health care, psychiatry is eschewing a broader psychosocial approach to mental disorders and emphasizing narrower biomedical strategies instead.

Concern about how to provide continuous, coordinated, and holistic treatment that would link primary care practitioners with mental health specialists led to the establishment in 1976 of the Houston Primary Care Mental Health Training Consortium. In Chapter Twenty-Four, Adams describes the consortium's efforts at providing interdisciplinary training to residents in psychiatry, pediatrics, and internal medicine, as well as to graduate students in psychology, social work, and nursing. A key issue for such a program is the determination of which curricular elements can be taught generically and which are best taught in a discipline-specific manner. Adams concludes that each discipline's unique needs cannot be met through a generic mental health curriculum. He, therefore, recommends that the interdisciplinary training of health and mental professionals emphasize patient care issues rather than abstract concepts, and that learning occur in field training sites rather than in classrooms.

Regardless of where this or other training occurs, modern audiovisual technology has produced major changes in pedagogical techniques. Mason (Chapter Twenty-Six) observes that with present electronic equipment, virtually every professor can be a filmmaker and every institution a producer. He views the key issues confronting users of audiovisual techniques as those of how to evaluate the flood of new materials, select needed hardware, and protect the confidentiality of persons filmed or videotaped. Most frequently used for clinical supervisory purposes, audiovisual materials are now being designed for such other educational purposes as patient and public education.

Mutual Help Groups. Simultaneous with the development of new strategies for linking professional caregivers, there has been an exponential growth of self-help groups whose ideology often conforms to the egalitarian precepts described by Hollander (1980) and whose practices cover the range portrayed by Killilea (Chapter Six). In Chapter Twenty-Five, Silverman distinguishes mutual help and mental health service systems on the dimensions of how services are organized, the consumer's relationship to the system, and criteria for selecting helpers. Silverman emphasizes that the two systems are not competing modalities; each is uniquely appropriate for different purposes. Nevertheless, a growing number of consumers are seeking "humanized" support and assistance from mutual help groups. For example, families of chronically mentally ill persons dissatisfied with professional services in 1979 founded the National Alliance of Families of the Mentally Ill, a relatives' counterpart to the Mental Patients Liberation Front established by the mentally ill themselves more than a decade earlier.

Despite lingering reservations among more cautious professionals about the value of mutual help, there is growing appreciation of the significant ways in which groups of this type help meet an individual's and community's human service needs. This latter awareness led the President's Commission on Mental Health (1978) to recommend that CMHCs develop meaningful linkages to mutual help groups and other community support programs.

This overview has attempted to portray the transition facing CMHCs in the early 1980s and to analyze the internal and external forces likely to mold their future shape. Program models developed in the two decades since the initial 1963 federal legislation are being altered to conform with technological advances and fiscal stringencies, and patient populations usually afforded a low service priority are being targeted for special interventions. Administrative structures and personnel patterns that became solidified with the passage of time are being unraveled while fiscal criteria are receiving increased emphasis in the making of key organizational decisions. Like all developmental transitions, the one now being experienced by CMHCs is generating inevitable anxiety and even concern for their survival.

Despite the present tensions, we agree with Caplan in the Epilogue that CMHCs have become sufficiently entrenched in the mental health service delivery system to remain viable for many years to come. In the immediate future, modified program priorities and altered organizational structures are likely, as pressures to meet patient needs and generate revenue are accommodated. Closer ties will be forged with the medical sector, and links to other human service agencies will be maintained. Nevertheless, the challenges of establishing primary prevention from a CMHC base will attract mainly those committed to the public health model.

We conclude with the classic principle of crisis theory, that is, the present crisis contains both dangers and opportunities. With the courage to withstand ideological and fiscal onslaughts, wisdom to recognize the inevitability of periodic transitions, and foresight to lay new foundations for the future, the community mental health field can readily surmount the dangers and capitalize on opportunities for improved patient care and future growth.

References

Adler, D. "The Medical Model and Psychiatry's Tasks." *Hospital and Community Psychiatry,* 1981, *32,* 387-392.

American Psychiatric Association. *Diagnostic and Statistical Manual of Mental Disorders.* (3rd ed.) Washington, D.C.: American Psychiatric Association, 1980.

Appelbaum, P., and Gutheil, T. "Drug Refusal: A Study of Psychiatric Inpatients." *American Journal of Psychiatry,* 1980, *137,* 340-346.

Arieti, S., and Brodie, H. (Eds.). *American Handbook of Psychiatry.* (2nd ed.) Vol. 7. New York: Basic Books, 1981.

Ashbaugh, J. "The Containment of Mental Health Center Costs." *Administration in Mental Health,* 1981, *9,* 46-56.

Bachrach, L. *Deinstitutionalization: An Analytical Review and Sociological Perspective.* Department of Health, Education, and Welfare Publication No. (ADM) 76-351. Washington, D.C.: U.S. Government Printing Office, 1976.

Bachrach, L. "Is the Least Restrictive Environment Always the Best? Sociological and Semantic Implications." *Hospital and Community Psychiatry,* 1980a, *31,* 97-102.

Bachrach, L. "Overview: Model Programs for Chronic Mental Patients." *American Journal of Psychiatry,* 1980b, *137,* 1023-1031.

Bachrach, L. "Continuity of Care for Chronic Mental Patients: A Conceptual Analysis." *American Journal of Psychiatry,* 1981a, *138,* 1449-1456.

Bachrach, L. "General Hospital Psychiatry: Overview from a Sociological Perspective." *American Journal of Psychiatry,* 1981b, *138,* 879-887.

Bass, R. "Trends Among Core Professionals in Organized Mental Health Settings: Where Have All the Psychiatrists Gone?" National Institute of Mental Health, Division of Biometry and Epidemiology Statistical Note No. 160. December 1981.

Bergner, L. "The Making of a Consultation Program: Administrative Issues and Strategies." *Administration in Mental Health,* 1981, *8,* 237-247.

Berlin, I. "Resistance to Mental Health Consultation Directed at Change In Public Institutions." *Community Mental Health Journal,* 1979, *15,* 119-128.

Berlin, R., and others. "The Patient Care Crisis in Community Mental Health Centers: A Need for More Psychiatric Involvement." *American Journal of Psychiatry,* 1981, *138,* 450-454.

Bloom, B. *Community Mental Health: A General Introduction.* Monterey, Calif.: Brooks/Cole, 1977.

Bloom, B. "The Logic and Urgency of Primary Prevention." *Hospital and Community Psychiatry,* 1981, *32,* 839-843.

Boggs, E. "Contrasts in Deinstitutionalization." *Hospital and Community Psychiatry,* 1981, *32,* 591.

Borus, J. "Neighborhood Health Centers as Providers of Primary Care." *New England Journal of Medicine,* 1976, *295,* 140-145.

Borus, J. "Issues Critical to the Survival of Community Mental Health." *American Journal of Psychiatry,* 1978, *135,* 1029-1035.

Braddock, D. "Deinstitutionalization of the Retarded: Trends in Public Policy." *Hospital and Community Psychiatry,* 1981, *32,* 607-615.

Braun, P., and others. "Overview: Deinstitutionalization of Psychiatric Patients, A Critical Review of Outcome Studies." *American Journal of Psychiatry,* 1981, *138,* 736-749.

Broskowski, A., Marks, E., and Budman, S. (Eds.). *Linking Health and Mental Health.* Beverly Hills, Calif.: Sage, 1981.

Budman, S. (Ed.). *Forms of Brief Therapy.* New York: Guilford Press, 1981.

Bursten, B. "Psychiatry and the Rhetoric of Models." *American Journal of Psychiatry,* 1979, *136,* 661-666.

Caplan, G. *Principles of Preventive Psychiatry.* New York: Basic Books, 1964.

Caplan, G. *The Theory and Practice of Mental Health Consultation.* New York: Basic Books, 1970.

Caplan, G. *Support Systems and Community Mental Health: Lectures on Concept Development.* New York: Behavioral Publications, 1974.

Caplan, G. "An Approach to Preventive Intervention in Children." *Canadian Journal of Psychiatry,* 1980, *25,* 671-682.

Caplan, G. "Mastery of Stress: Psychosocial Aspects." *American Journal of Psychiatry,* 1981, *138,* 413-420.

Caplan, G., and Killilea, M. (Eds.). *Support Systems and Mutual Help: Multidisciplinary Explorations.* New York: Grune & Stratton, 1976.

Curtis, W. *Managing Human Services with Less: New Strategies for Local Leaders.* Rockville, Md.: Project Share, Human Services Monograph Series, No. 26. 1981.

Curtis, W., and Yessian, M. "The Editors Interview Alexander H. Leighton." *New England Journal of Human Services,* 1981, *1,* 6-14.

Cutter, D., Bloom, J., and Shore, J. "Training Psychiatrists to Work with Community Support Systems for Chronically Mentally Ill Persons." *American Journal of Psychiatry,* 1981, *138,* 98-101.

Dean, A., Lin, N., and Ensel, W. "The Epidemiological Significance of Social Support Systems in Depression." In R. Simmons (Ed.), *Research in Community and Mental Health.* Vol. 2. Greenwich, Conn.: JAI Press, 1981.

Department of Health and Human Services Steering Committee on the Chronically Mentally Ill. *Toward a National Plan for the Chronically Mentally Ill.* Washington, D.C.: U.S. Government Printing Office, 1980.

Eaton, W., and others. "The Epidemiologic Catchment Area Program of the National Institute of Mental Health." *Public Health Reports,* 1981, *96,* 319-325.

Endicott, J., and Spitzer, R. "A Diagnostic Interview: The Schedule for Affective Disorders and Schizophrenia." *Archives of General Psychiatry,* 1978, *35,* 837-844.

Ennis, B. "Judicial Involvement in the Public Practice of Psychiatry." In W. Barton and C. Sanborn (Eds.), *Law and the Mental Health Professions.* New York: International Universities Press, 1978.

Feldman, S. "The Middle-Management Muddle." *Administration in Mental Health,* 1980, *8,* 3-11.

Feldman, S. "Leadership in Mental Health: Changing the Guard for the 1980s." *American Journal of Psychiatry,* 1981, *138,* 1147-1153.

Fink, P., and Weinstein, S. "Whatever Happened to Psychiatry? The Deprofessionalization of Community Mental Health Centers." *American Journal of Psychiatry,* 1979, *136,* 406-409.

Ford, M. "The Psychiatrists' Double Bind: The Right to Refuse Medication." *American Journal of Psychiatry,* 1980, *137,* 332-339.

Frances, A., and Clarkin, J. "Differential Therapeutics: A Guide to Treatment Selection." *Hospital and Community Psychiatry,* 1981, *32,* 537-546.

Frank, R. "Cost-Benefit Analysis in Mental Health Services: A Review of the Literature." *Administration in Mental Health,* 1981, *8,* 161-176.

Frank, R. "Freedom of Choice Laws: Empirical Evidence of Their Contribution to Competition in Mental Health Care Delivery." *Health Policy Quarterly,* June 1982.

Gartner, A., Kohler, M., and Riessman, F. *Children Teach Children.* New York: Harper & Row, 1971.

Gartner, A., and Riessman, F. *Self-Help in the Human Services.* San Francisco: Jossey-Bass, 1977.

General Accounting Office. *Returning the Mentally Disabled to the Community: Government Needs to Do More.* Washington, D.C.: U.S. Government Printing Office, 1977.

Glasscote, R. *Preventing Mental Illness: Efforts and Attitudes.* Washington, D.C.: Joint Information Service, 1980.

Goldman, H., and others. "Community Mental Health Centers and the Treatment of Severe Mental Disorder." *American Journal of Psychiatry,* 1980, *137,* 83-86.

Goldman, W. "Mental Health Services in '82: A Dismal Scenario." *Roche Report: Frontiers of Psychiatry,* November 15, 1981, p. 14.

Goodstein, L. *Consulting with Human Service Systems.* Reading, Mass.: Addison-Wesley, 1978.

Gottlieb, B. (Ed.). *Social Networks and Social Support.* Beverly Hills, Calif.: Sage, 1981.

Grady, M., Gibson, M., and Trickett, E. *Mental Health Consultation Theory, Practice, and Research 1973-1978. An Annotated Reference Guide.* Department of Health and Human Services Publication No. (ADM) 81-948. Washington, D.C.: U.S. Government Printing Office, 1981.

Group for the Advancement of Psychiatry. *The Chronic Mental Patient in the Community.* New York: Group for the Advancement of Psychiatry, 1978.

Gruenberg, E. "Social Breakdown Syndrome–Some Origins." *American Journal of Psychiatry,* 1967, *123,* 1481-1489.

Gruenberg, E. "The Failures of Success." *Health and Society,* 1977, *55,* 3-24.

Gruenberg, E. "Epidemiology." In H. Kaplan, A. Freedman, and B. Sadock (Eds.), *Comprehensive Textbook of Psychiatry.* (3rd ed.) Baltimore, Md.: Williams and Wilkins, 1980.

Hamburg, B., and Varenhorst, B. "Peer Counseling in the Secondary Schools." *American Journal of Orthopsychiatry,* 1972, *42,* 566-581.

Hammer, M., Makiesky-Barrow, S., and Gutwirth, L. "Social Networks and Schizophrenia." *Schizophrenia Bulletin,* 1978, *4,* 522-545.

Hausman, W., and Prosen, H. "The Mental Health Administrator as Organizational Consultant." *Administration in Mental Health,* 1981, *8,* 177-184.

Heller, K., Price, R., and Sher, K. "Research and Evaluation in Primary Prevention: Issues and Guidelines." In R. Price and others (Eds.), *Prevention in Mental Health: Research, Policy, and Practice.* Beverly Hills, Calif.: Sage, 1980.

Henderson, S., and others. "Social Relationships, Adversity, and Neurosis: A Study of Associations in a General Population Sample." *British Journal of Psychiatry,* 1980, *136,* 574-583.

Hirsch, B. "Psychological Dimensions of Social Networks: A Multimethod Analysis." *American Journal of Community Psychology,* 1979, *7,* 263-277.

Holahan, C., and others. "The Ecological Perspective in Community Mental Health." *Community Mental Health Review,* 1979, *4,* 1-9.

Hollander, R. "A New Service Ideology: The Third Mental Health Revolution." *Professional Psychology,* 1980, *11,* 561-566.

Katz, A., and Bender, E. (Eds.). *The Strength in Us: Self-Help Groups in the Modern World.* New York: Franklin Watts, 1976.

Keill, S. "The General Hospital as the Core of the Mental Health Services System." *Hospital and Community Psychiatry,* 1981, *32,* 776-778.

Kellam, S., and others. *Mental Health and Going to School.* Chicago: University of Chicago Press, 1975.

Ketterer, R. *Consultation and Education in Mental Health.* Beverly Hills, Calif.: Sage, 1981.

Killworth, P., and Bernard, H. "Informant Accuracy in Social Network Data." *Human Organization,* 1976, *35,* 269-286.

Klein, D., and Goldston, S. *Primary Prevention: An Idea Whose Time Has Come.* Department of Health, Education, and Welfare Publication No. (ADM) 77-447. Washington, D.C.: U.S. Government Printing Office, 1977.

Kornberg, M., and Caplan, G. "Risk Factors and Preventive Intervention in Child Psychopathology: A Review." *Journal of Prevention,* 1980, *1,* 71-133.

Kramer, M. *Psychiatric Services and the Changing Institutional Scene, 1950-1985.* Department of Health, Education, and Welfare Publication No. (ADM) 77-433. Washington, D.C.: U.S. Government Printing Office, 1977.

Kramer, M. "The Rising Pandemic of Mental Disorders and Associated Chronic Diseases and Disabilities." *Acta Psychiatrica Scandinavica Supplement 285,* 1980, *62,* 382-397.

Lamb, H., and Zusman, J. "Primary Prevention in Perspective." *American Journal of Psychiatry,* 1979, *136,* 12-17.

Lamb, H., and Zusman, J. "A New Look at Primary Prevention." *Hospital and Community Psychiatry,* 1981, *32,* 843-848.

Langsley, D. "The Community Mental Health Center: Does It Treat Patients?" *Hospital and Community Psychiatry,* 1980, *31,* 815-819.

Lieberman, M., Borman, L., and Associates. *Self-Help Groups For Coping With Crisis: Origins, Members, Processes, and Impact.* San Francisco: Jossey-Bass, 1979.

Liptzin, B. "The Psychiatrist Shortage. What's the Right Number." *Archives of General Psychiatry,* 1979, *36,* 1416-1419.

Lounsbury, J., and others. "An Analysis of Topic Areas and Topic Trends in the *Community Mental Health Journal* from 1965 Through 1977." *Community Mental Health Journal,* 1979, *15,* 33-40.

McGuire, T. "Markets for Psychotherapy." In G. VandenBos (Ed.), *Psychotherapy: Practice, Research, Policy.* Beverly Hills: Sage, 1980.

Matus, R., and Neuhring, E. "Social Workers in Primary Prevention: Action and Ideology in Mental Health." *Community Mental Health Journal,* 1979, *15,* 33-40.

Mednick, S., Schulsinger, F., Venables, P. "Risk Research and Primary Prevention of Mental Illness." *International Journal of Mental Health,* 1979, *7,* 150-164.

Mueller, D. "Social Networks: A Promising Direction for Research on the Relationship of the Social Environment to Psychiatric Disorder." *Social Science and Medicine,* 1980, *14,* 147-161.

Myers, J., and Weissman, M. "Use of a Self-Report Symptom Scale to Detect Depression in a Community Sample." *American Journal of Psychiatry,* 1980, *137,* 1081-1084.

National Institute of Mental Health. *Use of Health and Mental Health Outpatient Services in Four Organized Health Care Settings.* Series DN No. 1. Department of Health and Human

Services Publication No. (ADM) 80-859. Washington, D.C.: U.S. Government Printing Office, 1980.

National Institute of Mental Health. *Economics and Mental Health.* Series EN No. 1. Department of Health and Human Services Publication No. (ADM) 81-114. Washington, D.C.: U.S. Government Printing Office, 1981.

Nevid, J., and Morrison, J. "Attitudes Toward Mental Illness: The Construction of the Libertarian Mental Health Ideology Scale." *Journal of Humanistic Psychology,* 1980, *20,* 71-85.

Nielsen, A., and others. "Encouraging Psychiatrists to Work with Chronic Patients: Opportunities and Limitations of Residency Education." *Hospital and Community Psychiatry,* 1981, *32,* 767-775.

O'Brien, G. "Interorganizational Behavior." In S. Feldman (Ed.), *The Administration of Mental Health Services.* (2nd ed.) Springfield, Ill.: Thomas, 1980.

Ojemann, R. "Investigations on the Effects of Teaching an Understanding and Appreciation of Behavior Dynamics." In G. Caplan (Ed.), *Prevention of Mental Disorders in Children.* New York: Basic Books, 1961.

Pardes, H. "Future Needs for Psychiatrists and Other Mental Health Personnel." *Archives of General Psychiatry,* 1979, *36,* 1401-1408.

Pardes, H. "Mental Health-General Health Interaction: Opportunities and Responsibilities." *Hospital and Community Psychiatry,* 1981, *32,* 779-782.

Pardes, H., and Pincus, H. "Treatment in the Seventies: A Decade of Refinement." *Hospital and Community Psychiatry,* 1980, *31,* 535-542.

Piasecki, J., and Kamis-Gould, E. "Social and Area Analysis in Program Evaluation and Planning." *Evaluation and Program Planning,* 1981, *4,* 3-14.

Pincus, A. "Linking General Health and Mental Health Systems of Care: Conceptual Models of Implementation." *American Journal of Psychiatry,* 1980, *137,* 315-320.

President's Commission on Mental Health. *Report to the President.* Vol. 1. Washington, D.C.: U.S. Government Printing Office, 1978.

Regier, D., Goldberg, I., and Taube, C. "The De Facto U.S. Mental Health Services System: A Public Health Perspective." *Archives of General Psychiatry,* 1978, *35,* 685-693.

Report of the National Task Force on Mental Health/Mental Retardation Administration. *Administration in Mental Health,* 1979, *6,* 267-323.

Robins, L., and others. "National Institute of Mental Health Diagnostic Interview Schedule." *Archives of General Psychiatry,* 1981, *38,* 381-389.

Rogawski, A. S. (Ed.). *New Directions for Mental Health Services: Mental Health Consultations in Community Settings,* no. 3. San Francisco: Jossey-Bass, 1979.

Roth, L. "Mental Health Commitment: The State of the Debate, 1980." *Hospital and Community Psychiatry,* 1980, *31,* 385-396.

Rubin, J. "The National Plan for the Chronically Mentally Ill: A Review of Financing Proposals." *Hospital and Community Psychiatry,* 1981, *32,* 704-713.

Schulberg, H., and Baker, F. "Community Mental Health: Belief System of the 1960s." *Psychiatric Opinion,* 1969, *6,* 14-26.

Sharfstein, S. "Will Community Mental Health Survive in the 1980s?" *American Journal of Psychiatry,* 1978, *135,* 1363-1365.

Sharfstein, S. "Community Mental Health Centers: Returning to Basics." *American Journal of Psychiatry,* 1979, *136,* 1077-1079.

Spitzer, R., Williams, J., and Skodol, A. "DSM-III: The Major Achievements and an Overview." *American Journal of Psychiatry,* 1980, *137,* 151-164.

Srole, L., and Fischer, A. "Debate on Psychiatric Epidemiology." *Archives of General Psychiatry,* 1980, *37,* 1421-1423.

Stein, L., and Test, M. (Eds.). *Alternatives to Mental Hospital Treatment.* New York: Plenum, 1978.

Stone, A. *Mental Health and the Law: A System in Transition.* DHEW Publication No. (ADM) 75-176. Washington, D.C.: U.S. Government Printing Office, 1975.

Talbott, J. (Ed.). *The Chronic Mental Patient: Problems, Solu-*

tions, and Recommendations for Public Policy. Washington, D.C.: American Psychiatric Association, 1978.

Talbott, J. "The National Plan for the Chronically Mentally Ill: A Programmatic Analysis." *Hospital and Community Psychiatry,* 1981, *32,* 699-704.

Task Panel on the Nature and Scope of the Problems. *Report Submitted to the President's Commission on Mental Health.* Vol. 2. Appendix. Washington, D.C.: U.S. Government Printing Office, 1978.

Taube, C., Regier, D., and Rosenfeld, A. "Mental Disorders." In *Health, United States, 1978.* Washington, D.C.: U.S. Public Health Service, 1978.

Turner, J., and Ten Hoor, W. "The NIMH Community Support Program: Pilot Approach to a Needed Social Reform." *Schizophrenia Bulletin,* 1978, *4,* 319-348.

Vayda, M., and Perlmutter, F. "Primary Prevention in Community Mental Health Centers: A Survey of Current Activity." *Community Mental Health Journal,* 1977, *13,* 343-351.

Wagenfeld, M. "Psychopathology in Rural Areas: Issues and Evidence." In P. Keller and J. Murray (Eds.), *Handbook of Rural Community Mental Health.* New York: Human Sciences Press, 1982.

Weiner, R., and others. "Community Mental Health Centers and the 'Seed Money' Concept: Effects of Terminating Federal Funds." *Community Mental Health Journal,* 1979, *15,* 129-138.

Weisbrod, B., Test, M., and Stein, L. "Alternative to Mental Hospital Treatment, II. Economic Benefit-Cost Analysis." *Archives of General Psychiatry,* 1980, *37,* 400-405.

West, M., and Richardson, M. "A Statewide Survey of CMHC Programs for Mentally Retarded Individuals." *Hospital and Community Psychiatry,* 1981, *32,* 413-416.

White, S. "The Community Mental Health Center as a Matrix Organization." *Administration in Mental Health,* 1978, *6,* 99-106.

Windle, C., and Cibulka, J. "A Framework for Understanding Participation in Community Mental Health Services." *Community Mental Health Journal,* 1981, *17,* 4-18.

Winslow, W. "The Changing Role of Psychiatrists in Community Mental Health Centers." *American Journal of Psychiatry,* 1979, *136,* 24-27.

Zusman, J., and Lamb, H. "In Defense of Community Mental Health." *American Journal of Psychiatry,* 1977, *134,* 887-890.

Chapter 3

Epidemiology of Mental Disorders

Leo Levy

Epidemiology is the fundamental research method that undergirds the field of public health and as such relates to a broad array of issues, starting with traditional conceptions of bona fide disease and extending in the end to any set of human behaviors that are capable of accurate definition. Epidemiology is thus seen as a subcategory of human ecology that relates to states of health and social adaptation and may be formally defined as the study of the rate of occurrence, the distribution in time and space, and the social, personal, and environmental correlates of specified human afflictions. Historically, epidemiology gave priority to acute infectious diseases, as in Snow's classic work on cholera (1855), and to nutrition-related diseases, as in Goldberger's definitive studies of pellagra (1914). As our comprehension of the etiology, prevention, and treatment of infectious disease grew, it was inevitable that investigators would increasingly turn their attention to chronic diseases and to mental illness as a subset of chronic illnesses.

The basic methods of epidemiology have wide applica-

Note: The author wishes to express his gratitude to Allen N. Herzog for his critical reading of and many helpful comments on this manuscript.

tion; indeed, they constitute a well-systematized method for the study of a wide variety of human conditions, which extend easily into the realm of psychosocial phenomena quite apart from disease entities in themselves. Appropriate application of epidemiological methods may be made to such diverse phenomena as suicide, divorce, and delinquency and extended into such realms as the planning of community mental health and other human services and their evaluation (Monroe, Klee, and Brody, 1967; Mikawa, 1975; Schwab and others, 1979). This is not to suggest that classical epidemiological methods are the sole means of providing useful insights or explanations into the extensive complex of relevant factors that impinge upon the planning, assessment, evaluation, delivery, and use of community mental health programs. The more traditional techniques of randomized experimental clinical trials (Gilbert, Light, and Mosteller, 1975) and nonexperimental case control methods (Anderson and others, 1980) also have their contributions to make. Similarly, the increasingly popular, if perhaps less well understood and more esoteric methods of goal attainment scaling (Kiresuk and Lund, 1978), cost-benefit analysis (Weisbrod and Helming, 1980; Goldberg and Jones, 1980), controlled family genetic-environmental inheritance studies using path analysis (Reich and others, 1980), aggregated time-series models (Brenner, 1973; Dooley and Catalano, 1980), and the like also have their uses.

Nevertheless, it seems likely, from the practical perspective of the program director of the community mental health center that to the extent that community mental health continues to deal with populations at risk in clearly defined geographical catchment areas and with the patterned interactions between social structure (class, status, income, power) and individual mental disability, the simpler traditional epidemiological methods will prove most useful. This is so because the chief purpose of social epidemiological studies is to attain a fuller understanding of the "true" distribution of mental illness and of the social-structural factors associated with this distribution, toward the practical end of eventually preventing or reducing the incidence of mental disability, providing effective treatment, forecasting future community needs, and planning to meet such needs within expected resource constraints. Having said this, one must caution that this research method, particularly as applied to psychiatric disorders, encounters several serious problems.

Case Definition

First and foremost of these is the problem of case definition. It is generally true of medical diagnosis that there is, to one degree or another, a reliability problem. Psychiatry, however, is unique in clinical medicine in that diagnosis relies almost exclusively on judgments made by an observer about human behavior. From this fact alone, one would expect substantial chaos to result and, indeed, one often finds it. Dohrenwend and Dohrenwend (1974) analyzed seventy reports of surveys of treated and untreated prevalence of mental illness and reported rates of mental illness in examined populations that ranged from a low of .84 percent to a high of 69 percent. Studies of reliability of diagnosis, by authors favorably inclined toward existing diagnostic paradigms (Spitzer and Fleiss, 1974), and in which diagnoses were made under good training and control conditions for fairly common and broad diagnoses, show wide variability estimates. Average Kappa coefficients for six or fewer studies are .77 for organic brain syndrome, .57 for schizophrenia, .41 for affective disorder, .40 for neurosis, and .53 for sociopathy. (Kappa, which is closely related to the more familiar intraclass correlation, is a measure of the distance or disagreement between two raters adjusted for chance agreement, and it may be extended to multiple raters and to estimate partial associations; see Fleiss, 1973.) In community mental health center settings and state mental hospitals, measures of diagnostic agreement are likely to be even lower.

We have, as yet, no generally accepted definition of mental health or illness, and the criteria for establishing any specific diagnosis such as schizophrenia are vague to begin with and often socially judgmental, conditions that further weaken their reliable application. Hollingshead and Redlich (1958), in their study of the distribution of New Haven psychiatric patients by social class, discovered that both diagnosis and treatment varied systematically as a function of social class membership. The use of custodial and physical treatment, along with diagnoses of psychotic conditions, predominated for lower-class patients, whereas those from higher classes more often received individual therapy and were more often diagnosed as neurotic.

Scheff (1966) and Schur (1980) have carried this observation further by exploring the concept of "labeling" as a societal means for defining and stigmatizing mental illness as deviance and for using such arbitrary diagnoses as a means of political control. Labeling people as mentally ill not only classifies them but also changes their behavior. Although there is much controversy about this sociological interpretation of mental illness diagnosis (Gove, 1980), it is of importance in the setting of a community mental health center to be aware of how both the patient's and the therapist's social class may significantly influence treatment and diagnosis. It is difficult to see how this field can proceed with its business until some breakthrough occurs in this area. The core problem is that we have, at present, no other choice but to rely on behavioral criteria for diagnosis. In the absence of objective, value-neutral signs, preferably laboratory tests, for specified mental disorders, the reliability of psychiatric diagnosis will remain a major roadblock to definitive studies.

However, objective indexes of schizophrenia and manic-depressive psychoses are likely to emerge. Some significant progress has recently been made, or at least is asserted to have been made (Regier, 1980), under the impetus of the Division of Biometry of the National Institute of Mental Health (NIMH), on the problem of standardizing interviewing and classification of mental disorders using the Feigner criteria (Feigner and others, 1972) and the Research Diagnostic Criteria (RDC) (Spitzer, Endicott, and Robins, 1978). Myers and Weissman (1980), for example, in their 1975-1976 longitudinal resurvey of 515 New Haven residents used the Spitzer, Endicott, and Robins Categorical Schedule for Affective Disorders and Schizophrenia (SADS-RDC) (1975). The SADS, on which the American Psychiatric Association *Diagnostic and Statistical Manual* (DSM-III) is partly based, is a structured interview guide that records data on the interviewee's symptomatology and functioning and provides a means for classifying persons for most major psychotic, neurotic, and personality disorders. The method claims to reduce the systematic and error variance due to variable interviewing styles and coverage and provides current, five-year, and lifetime diagnostic assessments. When it was employed in conjunction with RDC, which provides operationally defined criteria for differential diagnosis, Myers and Weissman note that two nonpsychiatric interviewers became excellent diagnosticians with only three months of training. The implication of improved diagnostic interviewing by staff members of community mental health centers who are nonpsychiatrists, as well as the provision of such methods to other caretakers (general physicians, social workers, and so on) in case finding and service provision should be obvious.

Nevertheless, given the expense of large-scale community surveys to ascertain "true" mental disability prevalence, efforts are being made to simplify the interviewing procedures so that lay interviewers with less training can provide sufficient information to use the DSM-III categories with the design of the Diagnostic Interview Schedule (DIS). Regier (1980) writes that "the ability to use lay interviewers to determine the presence of specific mental disorders on a large scale is necessary in order to realize the potential of epidemiological method as postulated by Morris twenty years ago. [He noted that it can be used for] 'community diagnosis, the historical study of a community's health, monitoring the workings of the health system, estimating risks, completing the clinical picture, identifying the syndromes, and ultimately searching for the causes of disorders' " (Morris, 1957, p. 7).

Connected with the development of DIS, the NIMH in 1978 instituted an Epidemiological Catchment Area (ECA) research program. This program is designed to use DIS for case identification of mental disorders in a population of at least 200,000 by surveys of both institutionalized and noninstitutionalized persons. Once the population is identified, a cohort of 3,000 will be followed for at least one year to determine incidence of new disabilities, diagnostic changes, social functioning, and the use of specialty mental health, medical, and other human services. An analysis of risk factors, barriers to care, and the consequences of mental illness to the ill person, his family, and the community will also be made. However, one must be cautious of government-sponsored research. Given the wide variety of disagreement, both philosophical (Szasz, 1974; Schur, 1980) and conceptual, as to the appropriate model for mental illness, it is perhaps too early to embrace without misgivings the psychiatrist's rosy expectations of a rigorous methodological future; reliable labels that reflect systematic bias may well fail to achieve construct validity.

In this connection it is important to be aware, as Spitzer and others (1980) have emphasized, that psychiatric epidemiological assessment instruments do not need to be highly reliable when used for the purpose of case identification. In their reply to the criticism by Dohrenwend and others (1978) of the adequacy of the Psychiatric Status Schedule (PSS), they note that instruments with low reliability such as PSS can nonetheless be useful for the identification of extreme cases and thus have psychometric construct validity useful for epidemiologic surveys, even while having moderate to low internal reliability. In the same manner, instruments of high reliability may have little value because of the low construct validity resulting from systematic bias (Zeller and Carmines, 1980). With regard to the diagnosis of psychoneurosis and personality disorders, it appears that we will not proceed beyond behavioral symptomatic criteria and that epidemiological studies will likely remain primitive. This means that studies of these disorders are not likely to progress beyond the point where studies of the major psychoses are today, which is by no means a hopeless state of affairs. Behavioral symptoms are definable with standardized interview techniques, symptom checklists, and application of computer logic. Through these means adequate, though far from perfect, reliability may be attained—reliability that will permit useful scientific investigation.

Resolution of the diagnostic problem in the absence of

firm biological indicators will await certain other developments. We must come to grips with the problem of disentangling true states of disease from everyday problems in living. On the one hand, it is too facile and most probably incorrect to label the whole of psychiatric illness as myth and to refer to the entire spectrum of behavior disorders as "problems in living," as Szasz does (1974). On the other hand, one must pay careful attention to the issue, for example, of differentiating unhappiness with one's lot in life with resultant dysphoric mood from clinical depression. Community surveys of mental illness such as the Midtown Manhattan study (Srole and others, 1962) and the Nova Scotia study (Leighton and others, 1963) are generally conceded to have produced overestimates of the extent of psychiatric disorder in the community.

One major contribution to this inflation of discovered psychopathology is the inability of survey instruments to differentiate between persons undergoing transient reactions to stressful situations (problems in living) and stable psychopathology. Further, these instruments, while finely tuned to potentially pathological symptoms, are far less attentive to coexisting strengths in personality and to the constellation of supportive networks in which individuals are embedded. A given level of symptomatology in one person by these measures makes him equivalent to another person exhibiting the same level and quality of symptomatology. This is an error because one individual may have a better constellation of coping mechanisms and/or a better, more developed system of social support than another. Indeed, one may speculate that this latter difference may account for the difference in help-seeking behavior between two persons with identical symptom levels and presumed discomfort. One may seek treatment and indeed may be more disabled by his symptoms than the other, who may not seek help and may in fact function well in the presence of a high level of symptomatology. Fuller discussion of the controversial nature of selecting appropriate diagnostic criteria in psychiatric epidemiology may be found in a recent series of Letters to the Editor in the *Archives of General Psychiatry* (1980), as well as in the papers by various authors (Cancro, Shapiro, and Kesselman,

1979) on the multiaxial diagnostic system for the schizophrenias and the affective disorders. A favorable review of the considerable potentialities of DSM-III for longitudinal cohort and repeated representative sampling studies in community-based psychiatric epidemiology may be found in Murphy (1980).

Another noteworthy problem in psychiatric diagnosis involves the value judgments inherent in behavioral assessment. Erroneous assignment of the diagnosis of schizophrenia in unclear or borderline cases to members of cultural groups foreign to the diagnostician is very likely a partial explanation for the overrepresentation of this diagnosis in poor people and in blacks (see Levy and Rowitz, 1973; Cooper and others, 1972). An even greater abuse of this diagnosis on similar grounds is represented in the flagrant misuse of schizophrenia as a label for political dissidents in the Soviet Union (Bloch and Reddaway, 1977). As long as behavioral norms are tied to middle-class, white conventions of conduct, observer bias will function in the assessment of such items as propensity for "acting out," attitudes toward work and family life, appropriate mood, rational behavior, presence of delusions, adequate cognitive functioning, and a host of other common criteria for establishing psychiatric diagnosis. A psychiatrist observing what he perceives to be aggressive behavior is some distance from a physician who observes a broken limb or an infected wound. The latter observation is relatively value free; the former is inevitably culture- and value-related.

Defining the Point of Onset

Critical to the definition of incidence is the issue of the point of onset of disorder. Let us say that a case of schizophrenia has been identified by careful assessment of symptoms. When did it begin? Mental illness in general, and schizophrenia in particular, are characterized as having an insidious onset. Where does one turn to establish the beginning point? The patient, his parents, spouse, employer, family doctor, and friends will often furnish widely discrepant answers. The epidemiologist has only one realistic option, that is, to accept the criterion of first admission to treatment as his operational definition of point of onset. This is hardly an ideal solution. A person may have been suffering with a condition for months, years, or all his life before finally appealing for psychiatric assistance. Furthermore, what of the minor or more subtle forms of mental illness such as neurosis or personality disorder where admission to a hospital seldom occurs and where even admission to outpatient treatment occurs in only a minority of cases? Thus it is not surprising that community surveys frequently deal only with the issue of prevalence and ignore the problem of incidence.

In the future, however, the previously described ECA research program may be helpful in providing some evidence on incidence. One should also mention some recent longitudinal resurveys that also address this issue. In 1973, Schwab and others (1979) conducted a three-year follow-up study of about one third of their 1970 Florida Health Study in Alachua County, utilizing the Health Opinion Survey (HOS), which was the standardized scale originally used in the Sterling County studies of Leighton and others (1963). They found that the three-year incidence for risk for mental disorder as measured by HOS caseness scores was 14.1 percent; the three-year remission rate was 29 percent. Those who changed from low to high risk tended to be those over forty-five, the black, the poor, the widowed or separated. Remission tended to occur most often among whites, respondents aged twenty-three to twenty-nine, and those in the middle or highest socioeconomic status (SES). Incidence was mainly associated with physical illness and low SES.

Similarly, Srole's (1975) twenty-year follow-up of the Midtown Manhattan study started in 1954 found, as Schwab and others (1979, p. 185) note, that the prevalence of serious impairment rose only 2.2 percent between 1954 and 1974 and that the twenty-year incidence of "less favorable mental health" was 22 percent. Since both these studies utilize scales of mental impairment, which are subject to all the difficulties so often ascribed to them, they are at best suggestive. They do not provide an adequate basis for determining incidence.

Population at Risk

Except in special instances such as postpartum psychosis, the answer to the question "Who is the population at risk?" also presents difficulties. In schizophrenia the answer is frequently given as persons of either sex between the ages of fifteen and forty-five. The lower end of this age spectrum derives more from theory than satisfactory empirical evidence, that is, dementia praecox is defined as a disorder of adolescence and early adulthood, thus establishing a diagnostic bias against finding schizophrenia in prepubescent children or in persons in middle or old age. One nevertheless finds descriptions of childhood schizophrenia, and it is not unknown to observe a first-time episode of schizophrenia in an older person. In involutional melancholia the at-risk population presumably includes members of either sex between the ages of forty and sixty. But is this not again a superimposition of theory? Any person having a first-time reported depression in this age span is simply assumed to be depressed due to involution. The population at risk for this disorder was once assumed to be women exclusively based on the menopausal change of life. One wonders how many persons are diagnosed as having senile dementia simply because they show some behavioral symptoms after the age of sixty-five. The point is that both the numerator and the denominator, in equations defining the incidence and prevalence rates of mental illness, are very difficult to establish with precision.

Correlation and Causation

If the ancient methodological caution that "correlation does not imply causation" is true, we may wonder why it is so often ignored in practice. If we were to follow this principle, analytical epidemiological methods, which are observational and normally nonexperimental, would be without any scientific force. The fact is, of course, that the saying is misleading in several ways.

First, correlational inference (Kenny, 1979) is indeed possible through the application of the usual multivariate statistical methods, provided we first formulate a well-defined structural model that relates all the relevant variables required for explaining our dependent variables. Correlation means no more than specifying a statistical relationship between a set of variables, none of which need be experimentally manipulated. Statistical inference means confirmation or disconfirmation of the hypotheses implied by the statistical model, which is assumed to have generated the observations. To claim, for example, that A causes B, we only make the claim that A must precede B or (with cross sectional data) that A and B are in equilibrium, that there is a functional relationship between A and B, and that any other variables that influence A and B are included in the equation either directly or indirectly. Experiments, through randomization or using the Bayesian concept of "exchangeability," can often be used to eliminate the necessity for measuring and controlling the multitude of extraneous variables (C, D, and so on) in estimating the effect of the variable of interest.

When models are improperly specified, moreover, we often get disparate conclusions. For example, the broad consensus of research findings on the inverse relationship of social class to the prevalence of mental illness suggests that we may proceed from this statistical datum to the more interesting inference that poverty causes mental illness. Unfortunately, there are also empirical studies on first admissions for schizophrenia that tend to refute the notion that poverty causes schizophrenia (see Levy and Rowitz, 1973; Dunham, 1965). The problem is that the simple association found between poverty and schizophrenia reflects specification error; not all the relevant variables that would adjust for the possibility of selection, drift, and other potential confounding factors have been included in the model.

A similar and, for many, a more perplexing problem is the ongoing controversy over what has been termed the *ecological fallacy*. The issue here is that correlations or regression parameter estimates derived from aggregated data (ecological correlations) will not always accord with correlations and regressions derived from similar measures made on the individuals whose aggregate measures are used in the analysis. For example, Robinson (1950), using data grouped by state, found that the aggregate relationship between illiteracy and race was strong but that the individual-level correlation was weak. Hanushek, Jackson, and Kain (1974) showed that by improving the specification of the micromodel, one could reduce the aggregation bias of the unstandardized regression coefficients computed from aggregate data. Using data grouped by state, they found that the bivariate unstandardized regression coefficient of illiteracy on race was .22. Due to the concentration of nonwhites in states with low literacy rates among both whites and blacks, the estimate is biased, since relevant variables have been excluded in the misspecified model. Controlling for the percent of school-age population, they produced a less biased estimate, which agreed closely (.17 versus .14) with the micromodel, because the effects of race on illiteracy were no longer confounded with the effects of schooling on illiteracy.

Langbein and Lichtman (1978) discuss this and other problems associated with aggregation and model misspecification errors, as well as possible solutions to them. Their moral seems to be that we should construct consistent testable theories, formulate fully specified statistical models appropriate to the data, and attempt to disconfirm these models, using proper multivariate statistical methods with a wide range of carefully collected data. The use of aggregate data is obviously appropriate for purposes of mental health planning and evaluation if such data are used to explore the behavior of groups themselves rather than the individuals making up the groups. For example, it is perfectly legitimate to explore the impact of different welfare policies in states or counties on state or county admission rates to mental health facilities. However, when aggregate data are used as a surrogate or substitute for a model of individual-level behavior, a good deal of caution is necessary. Where, for example, spatial patterning is a variable influencing the aggregate model, it will be necessary to include some proxy to account for this effect if the variable is irrelevant to the micromodel. Thus, for example, one must take explicit account of how people sort themselves into groups. Suppose we want to determine how crowding influences rates of mental illness in community areas (groups of census tracts). Since community area undoubtedly has a direct relation with both mental illness and crowding, we must include other characteristics of areas, such as median income and percent of population over sixty-five, which are correlated with our variables of interest. This will reduce aggregation bias, which would produce misleading estimates if not included (Levy and Herzog, 1974).

Dooley and Catalano (1980) have recently reviewed a large number of studies of individual and aggregate cross sectional and longitudinal models on the relationship of economic change to behavioral disorder. A detailed examination of the studies brought to light many of the model misspecification problems associated with attempting to consistently integrate diverse models of data analysis. Dooley and Catalano found that individual-level longitudinal research is generally consistent with the results from aggregate time-series findings. In general they found that most studies show undesirable economic change (for example, unemployment) to have a positive association with undesirable behavioral change.

Rate of Mental Disorder in the General Population

Much effort has been expended in attempts to offer a satisfactory answer to this elementary epidemiologic question. One crucial step forward in this endeavor has been the development of highly reliable standardized interview techniques and computer strategies for making diagnostic judgments (Spitzer and others, 1964; Spitzer and Endicott, 1968; Wing, Cooper, and Sartorius, 1974, 1977; Wing and Sturt, 1978). The studies of cross-national diagnostic differences between the United States and England have done much to explain and reduce the observed discrepancy in the rates of diagnosis of schizophrenia in those two countries (Cooper and others, 1972). Detailed community survey instruments have been developed by Srole and others (1962) in their Midtown Manhattan study and by Leighton and others (1963) in their Nova Scotia study. Psychiatric case registers have been established and are now functioning in many parts of the world (Bahn and others, 1966; Baldwin and others, 1965; Gardner and others, 1963; Krupinski and Stroller,

1962; Wing and others, 1967, 1968). While these deal with treated incidence and prevalence, they still furnish much help in establishing estimates of the true rates of disorder and are really our only source of reliable information on incidence through first-admission statistics. Many community surveys have been reported, and useful summaries of their findings have been assembled (Lin and Standley, 1962; Plunkett and Gordon, 1960; Shepherd and others, 1966; Dohrenwend and Dohrenwend, 1974). What, then, can one conclude about the rates of incidence and prevalence of mental disorder divided into the categories of affective disorders, schizophrenia, and nonpsychotic disorders (psychoneurosis and personality disorders)? (I will make no attempt here to cover the senile psychoses, drug addiction, mental retardation, or the spectrum of childhood mental disorders.)

Affective Disorders. The bulk of the disorders in this category involve depressed mood. Bipolar manic-depressive psychosis is comparatively rare and unipolar mania exceedingly rare. Incidence studies based on case registry data from Aarhus, Denmark and from London yield annual incidence figures of mania of 2.6 per 100,000 general population, with men predominating over women by a ratio of three to two. When this figure is corrected using an appropriate age group (eighteen to sixty) as the denominator, the figure increases for Aarhus to 4.4 and for London to 4.7 (Leff, Fischer, and Bertelsen, 1976). These figures, being based on inpatient admissions, are probably low estimates of true incidence. Some hypomanics undoubtedly are treated on an outpatient basis and still others go untreated. Still, one may assume that mania is an infrequently occurring disease. Depressive disorders, by contrast, are quite common. Brown and Harris (1978), in their survey of women in the Camberwell area of London, showed 15 percent suffering from a definite affective disorder in the three months preceding the interview. About half of these were onset cases who had developed the disorder in the year preceding the interview, and practically all were depressed. Weissman and Myers (1978), based on their U.S. community survey, set the point prevalence of definite major and minor depression in the mid 1970s at 5.7

percent. Figures for treated depression from Scandinavia suggest an annual incidence figure of .36 percent (Juel-Nielsen and others, 1961). Thus, one may conclude that depression is exceedingly common, particularly in women, and to a large extent is untreated, at least by psychiatrists.

While there does not appear to be any remarkable relationship of depression with age, interesting relationships emerge by sex, social class, and marital status. Depression is twice as common in women as in men. Brown and Harris (1978) list as risk factors for depression: being a working-class woman with young children (three or more children under fourteen), loss of mother (but not father) before age eleven, and lacking a confiding tie with husband or boyfriend. The presence of severe life events involving long-term threats will act to increasingly provoke depression as these risk factors are present. According to Paykel (1978), stressful life events increase substantially the risk of depression (sixfold for the more stressful classes of events).

Schizophrenia. Estimates of the "true" annual incidence of schizophrenia are given by Lemkau and Crocetti (1958) as falling between .05 percent and .15 percent. Mischler and Scotch (1963) estimate the incidence figure at .15 percent. Figures on treated incidence predictably run much lower as, for example, from the Camberwell (London) registry, where the recorded first-admission rate for schizophrenia annually is .012 percent to .015 percent (Wing and Fryers, 1976). It would appear axiomatic that cases of psychiatric disorder of all varieties are to be found among community members who avoid the psychiatric treatment network. Estimates of lifetime prevalence of schizophrenia now run around 1 percent. The vast difference between incidence and prevalence figures for this disorder reflects the chronicity of the disease.

As indicated earlier, the generally held conception of schizophrenia is that onset is usually in late adolescence or early adulthood, but it is difficult to estimate whether a true age relationship exists. The illness appears to have no relationship to gender. Most of the admissions to mental hospitals with a diagnosis of schizophrenia are single persons, but it is unclear to what extent this is conditioned by relatively early onset and/or by the general social withdrawal associated with the schizophrenic illness. In at least two large U.S. urban centers (Chicago and New York), blacks are assigned this diagnosis with greater frequency than whites (Levy and Rowitz, 1973; Cooper and others, 1972). This racial difference is seen to arise from cultural differences between the usually white, upper-middle-class credentials of the diagnostician and the black, usually lower-class social credentials of the patient. There is no basis for positing a racial link with schizophrenia (as there is with sickle-cell disease). As we have indicated in our Chicago study (Levy and Rowitz, 1973), the incidence of schizophrenia as reflected in hospital first-admission statistics does not vary by social class. The prevalence, however, does vary by social class, and the consensus of the research on this relationship indicates an inverse one (Dohrenwend and Dohrenwend, 1969). Although the argument is not finally settled, the reasons for this accumulation of schizophrenics in the lower social strata appear to be downward social drift or failure to rise because of the effects of the disorder and less adequate care of first episodes of schizophrenia in poor people.

Eaton (1980) has recently developed a simple stochastic transitional probability model in which he shows that selection and drift (mobility) together form a sufficient explanation for the class differential in rate of schizophrenia. He further notes that if some kinds of stress affect the development of schizophrenia, such stress is not necessarily related to social class, but would be constant between social classes and might even involve stressful events related to the economy as a whole. Also, as indicated before, schizophrenia lends itself to ideological and socially judgmental interpretations, and thus poor persons, persons culturally distant from the diagnostician, and, at least in the Soviet Union, political dissidents may be misdiagnosed as schizophrenics.

Rabkin's critical review (1980) of the results and methodological shortcomings of numerous studies on the relationship between stressful life events and schizophrenia concluded that schizophrenics do not report more stressful events than other diagnostic groups. Also, the differences between schizophrenics and normals in these studies are inconsistent. However, schizophrenics who had relapsed after recovery from a first episode reported more stressful events than those who had not. This indicates a weaker relationship between life events and onset of schizophrenia than the clinical literature suggests. Since in the DSM-III occurrence and severity of recent stressful life events together constitute one of the five multiaxial dimensions on which patients are described and since they are favorable prognostic indicators, the evidence reviewed must cast some doubt on the usefulness of such indicators in diagnosis. The further difficulty of determining the cause-effect directionality of life-stress rating scales is a related and more difficult problem to resolve (Dohrenwend and Dohrenwend, 1980).

Nonpsychotic Disorders. As we proceed from the more dramatic and, at least in the past, frequently hospitalized disorders of manic-depressive illness and schizophrenia to the less extreme and perhaps less clearly defined behavior problems, we are on even softer ground in estimating rates of prevalence and incidence. There is a clear general consensus that these constitute the bulk of psychiatric disorder in the community at large and that, in the main, they go undetected and untreated.

General estimates of total mental disorder in the population have been growing. Dohrenwend and Dohrenwend (1969) indicate that studies published prior to 1950 show a median prevalence rate of mental illness of 2.1 percent as opposed to a rate of 15.6 percent in studies published after 1950. Srole and others (1962), based on the Midtown Manhattan survey, rated 23.4 percent of the survey sample as "definitely psychiatrically impaired," and Leighton and others (1963) in their Nova Scotia study counted 31 percent of the study sample as "definitely psychiatrically impaired." For a variety of reasons, both of these estimates are probably misleadingly high. Such counts are based on rating instruments that are heavily weighted with physical symptoms presumed to reflect psychosomatic illnesses such as asthma, migraine, colitis, and ulcers–illnesses that may or may not reflect psychiatric impairment. Further, such counts include many persons undergoing transient stress reactions who would look considerably different if surveyed a few weeks later.

Also, as Dohrenwend (1970) has pointed out in a New York City study, there appears to be a vast difference between those diagnosed as mentally ill who are in treatment and those similarly diagnosed who are not. In the Midtown Manhattan study, three fourths of the "cases" uncovered have never been treated by a mental health professional. Again, we are here back to the root problem of the definition of mental disorder, a problem to which there is presently no satisfactory solution. Suffice it to say that, from the viewpoint of psychiatry, minor mental illness abounds and is generally estimated at 15 percent of the total population. Much of it is potentially treatable, but very little is actually treated in professional mental health settings.

In Western societies psychoneurotic disorder is more often associated with women and personality disorders more often with men. This would appear to reflect in part culturally defined stereotypes of passivity and aggression as sex-linked characteristics. Age does not appear to be a highly relevant variable with either disorder. Social class is inversely related with both the incidence and prevalence of personality disorders, but here again a cultural bias is probably at work. There is no demonstrated relationship between the rate of neurosis and social class.

Dohrenwend and others (1980), under the egis of the President's Commission on Mental Health, have again and more fully summarized the published data on the prevalence of mental disabilities in the United States. In the concluding chapter a succinct summary of their most recent assessment is provided; it disagrees little with the preceding review. Using the Dohrenwend and others (1980) table 3A.2 of rates of psychopathology, one can be better than 95 percent confident that the median for all types of psychopathology lies between 13.8 and 28.2 percent, for neuroses between 6.5 and 13.3 percent, for psychoses between .26 and 1.47 percent, for affective disorders between .4 and 7.7 percent, and for personality disorders between 1.8 and 9.3 percent (Dixon and Massey, 1969). Furthermore, they hypothesize that about 13 percent of the U.S. population shows severe psychological and somatic distress that is not accompanied by clinical psychiatric disorder. Following Frank's (1973) characterization, they call this the rate of "demoralization." Finally, they estimate that only about one fourth of those with clinically significant functional disorders have ever received treatment from mental health professionals.

Planning and Evaluation of Mental Health Services

It would appear reasonable to assume that prevalence figures, and treated prevalence figures for mental illness in particular, would be useful in planning mental health services. The problem is that there is still controversy over which disorders are to be treated in outpatient rather than inpatient facilities, and in certain instances over what mode of treatment is to be employed and for how long a period of time. To complicate matters still further, treatment decisions are not purely professional decisions but are tied up with political and general social considerations. Should schizophrenia, for example, be treated in or out of hospital? Convincing scientific evidence has been present for some time (Pasamanick, Scarpitti, and Dinitz, 1967) that outpatient treatment for schizophrenia is not only possible but indeed preferable to other modes of treatment. Yet, at least for the acute phase, hospitalization is still the route preferred by most psychiatrists. Families of schizophrenic patients will often press for hospitalization simply because they feel that they cannot cope with odd and difficult behavior. Since government funds are most frequently involved in the treatment of mental disorder, expensive hospital treatment is not an attractive option to state and local authorities. The message of the community mental health movement in the United States has been seized upon widely by state governments to create pressure to empty the hospitals and restrict the building of new hospital beds. Thus, leaving aside the preferences of the individual patient, one sees that the decision to hospitalize the schizophrenic is conditioned in part by available scientific evidence, prevailing professional practice, family preference, and the willingness of government to build and maintain beds.

Similarly, the treatment of neurosis, if left to the psychiatrist, would most often involve long-term intensive psychotherapy. Because of the expense involved in this approach, short-term crisis-oriented treatment or, alternatively, long-term non-intensive, supportive treatment is often combined with the use of medication. Both of these approaches require less professional time and are obviously attractive alternatives in terms of cost. Another option is to deemphasize treatment of less troublesome disorders such as neuroses and concentrate available resources on the more disabling disorders such as psychoses. Political and monetary considerations assume all the more importance in the light of the substantial controversy that still abounds about all aspects of the diagnosis and treatment of mentally ill persons—a controversy that results from the fact that a solid scientific knowledge base in the area of mental health is only being slowly built up.

Even a relatively straightforward problem such as the optimal ratio of mental hospital beds to population is not simply solved. The application of treatment according to the philosophy of community care, vigorously pursued, would reduce hospital beds drastically and close mental hospitals. At a time when many countries were still planning mental hospital beds on a formula of 3 to 4 beds per 1,000 general population, the Saskatchewan plan was calling for a ratio of .8 beds per 1,000 and bravely asserting on principle that no custodial chronic care was necessary. That is, all the care for inpatients would be accomplished in district hospitals (LeFave, Stewart, and Grunberg, 1968). Similarly, by emphasizing a community-based system of services in a two-county catchment area of 235,000 persons in Illinois, Hansell (1967) found that he could service all mental health casualties from the area with 30 beds, whereas over 420 beds had been required when a traditional state hospital system was in use. Current standards in Great Britain reflect this emphasis on care in the community but add some caution regarding chronic and geriatric patients (Department of Health and Social Security, 1975):

- .5 acute beds in district hospitals per 1,000 population
- .17 new long-term hospital beds per 1,000 population

- .65 places in day hospitals per 1,000 population
- 2.3-3.0 dementia beds per 1,000 population aged sixty-five and over
- 2.0-3.0 places in daycare centers per 1,000 population aged sixty-five and over

The number of beds planned will obviously reflect the availability of other modes of treatment such as day hospital care, outpatient care, halfway houses, and so on. The final solution will be arrived at under the influence of prevailing economic and sociopolitical considerations, as well as scientific and professional ones.

In performing program evaluation, epidemiology offers an obviously useful research strategy for evaluation studies. Stated simply, effective preventive programs should reduce incidence, and effective treatment programs should reduce prevalence. The same experimental and quasi-experimental strategies that apply to drug trials in general apply to the evaluation of psychotropic drugs. The various research strategies used to good advantage in general epidemiology apply conceptually to psychiatric epidemiology. Many excellent evaluative studies have been done, and no attempt will be made to systematically survey this literature. The few studies mentioned here are presented as examples of work in this area that I feel have important implications for the field of mental health.

As indicated above, Pasamanick, Scarpitti, and Dinitz (1967) have demonstrated that schizophrenia can be successfully treated at home and, in fact, that medication plus outpatient supportive care provide a better method of treatment than inpatient care. Gruenberg, Snow, and Bennett (1969), after defining the "social breakdown syndrome," showed that its prevalence could be halved by the development of a community service. Similar encouraging findings concerning institutionalism in hospitalized schizophrenic patients are reported by Wing and Brown (1970). They demonstrate that changes in hospital environment in three U.K. hospitals were related to increases and decreases in the rate of symptoms of chronic schizophrenia. Hansell (1967) found that severely disturbed psychiatric patients were best treated with very short hospital stays, if hospitalization was required at all. In a study by Fenton, Tessier, and Struening (1979), 155 patients destined for inpatient psychiatric care were randomly assigned to home care (76) and hospital care (79). Symptoms, role functioning, and psychosocial burden on the family were similar in the two groups at admission and at one, three, six, and twelve months. The patient sample was composed of 41.9 percent schizophrenics, 30.3 percent other functional psychoses, and 27.8 percent neuroses. Here, as in the other studies, community care was demonstrated to be an effective alternative to hospital care.

From this small group of studies, one may conclude that the treatment of schizophrenia is possible outside a hospital and that what has been variously referred to as the social breakdown syndrome, institutionalism, and chronic schizophrenia is to some extent a hazard of psychiatric hospitalization. Moreover, community-based services are at least as effective as traditional mental hospital services in achieving prompt and stable remission of symptoms and lessen considerably the dangers of untoward iatrogenic effects of hospitals. Finally, factors that encourage the untoward iatrogenic effects of hospitals may be identified and altered to good effect, thus lessening the danger of institutionalism if hospitalization is deemed important to treatment of a given patient. Herz (1979), for example, on the basis of several carefully controlled studies writes: "For the great majority of schizophrenic patients, comprehensive and continuous community treatment is essential. We must reorient our thinking away from the belief that the hospital is the primary modality of treatment. Instead, we should utilize a variety of other treatment modalities, including daycare, various outpatient therapies, pharmacotherapy, social and vocational rehabilitation, and sheltered living, in the comprehensive treatment of what is, for most patients, a chronic illness" (p. 96).

The successful execution of evaluation research depends upon:

1. A clear definition of the condition to be treated or prevented.

2. A clear statement of the outcome desired, together with objective measures of the outcome variables.
3. A clear operational definition of the strategies employed to effect the desired outcome.
4. A reasonable time span in which to allow the desired outcome to become manifest.

The assessment of needs in the community is believed by planners to be one of the primary steps in the planning and evaluation process of the community mental health center, for it is the foundation on which services are developed and delivered. Techniques for such assessment have varied. The easiest method is to extrapolate or prorate someone else's prevalence study to one's own catchment area. The trouble here is that prevalence studies often employ different methods and produce widely varying estimates. This leads often to another slightly more expensive but equally indirect approach, namely, census tract analysis (Rosen and others, 1975). In census tract analysis, census data are used to locate geographical areas that are high risk with respect to mental health problems. High risk is defined in terms of conditions in which true prevalence or aggregate data analysis models have been found to be associated with mental health problems in various research studies. Of particular interest are indexes of community instability based on migration, mobility, divorce, and crime rates.

Unfortunately, however, such indicators are at best only very rough indicators of need. They tell nothing about the link between need and true prevalence and provide no specific way to link resource investment to need. This is one reason that the ECA program to provide standardized tools for true prevalence and incidence assessment of mental illness is now being promoted by the National Institute of Mental Health. Only a proper epidemiological community data base can effectively be employed for sensitive evaluation of programs and for planning for future programs. Aggregate geographical profiles of community needs inform the planner of relative need but fail to provide the hard data with which to plan service delivery or assess program impact. Only given such basic data can evaluative research proceed effectively and produce unambiguous results. Whether these results will affect prevailing policy and feed back into the planning cycle is conditioned upon a whole other set of political, social, and monetary considerations.

Summary

As a consequence of vigorous research in psychiatric epidemiology during the last fifty years, a good deal has been discovered about the rate, nature, and distribution of psychiatric disorders and other psychosocial phenomena. To accomplish this, techniques of measurement have had to be markedly improved. Given the problems inherent in behavioral assessment, the techniques developed appear to be quite good. Tightening of the criteria for diagnosis is crucial to successful research efforts, epidemiological and other, and it has had a generally salutary effect on the field of clinical psychiatry. The necessity of making highly accurate diagnoses in clinical practice has become increasingly critical because specific treatments are being developed for specific disorders. Thus, lithium is specific for bipolar manic-depressive psychosis and for unipolar mania, while phenylthiazine is specific for schizophrenia. Obviously it is crucial to be able to tell the disorders apart.

Having said this about diagnosis, one must add that the progress noted is relative to the rather bad state of affairs that existed in the past. For research to become fully effective in establishing the etiology, prevention, and treatment of mental disorders, further progress will have to be made in rendering diagnosis a completely valid and reliable objective process. This would mean the relegation of behavioral criteria to a secondary role in the formulation of psychiatric diagnosis. Only then can definitive work on genetic, biochemical, and cross-cultural factors, natural life history, and treatment effectiveness proceed. In this, analytical epidemiology will play an important role as it has for all other diseases.

Finally, what about applications of epidemiological findings to the process of planning and evaluating mental health services? Even if one solves the scientific problems inherent in such research, one is still faced with formidable social, political, and economic forces that will ultimately decide the fate of even the clearest and most unequivocal research findings. This is not a unique problem for scientists, but one that must be noted and rationally assessed in each context.

References

Anderson, S., and others. *Statistical Methods for Comparative Studies: Techniques for Bias Reduction.* New York: Wiley, 1980.

Bahn, A. K., and others. "Admissions and Prevalence Rates for Psychiatric Facilities in Four Register Areas." *American Journal of Public Health,* 1966, *56,* 2033-2051.

Baldwin, J. A., and others. "A Psychiatric Case Register in North-East Scotland." *British Journal of Preventive and Social Medicine,* 1965, *19,* 38-42.

Bloch, S., and Reddaway, P. *Psychiatric Terror: How Soviet Society is Used to Suppress Dissent.* New York: Basic Books, 1977.

Brenner, M. H. *Mental Illness and the Economy.* Cambridge, Mass.: Harvard University Press, 1973.

Brown, G. W., and Harris, T. *Social Origins of Depression: A Study of Psychiatric Disorder in Women.* London: Tavistock, 1978.

Cancro, R., Shapiro, L. E., and Kesselman, M. (Eds.). *Progress in the Functional Psychoses.* New York: Spectrum, 1979.

Cooper, J. E., and others. *Psychiatric Diagnosis in New York and London.* Oxford, England: Oxford University Press, 1972.

Department of Health and Social Security. *Better Services for the Mentally Ill.* London: H. M. Stationery Office, 1975.

Diagnostic and Statistical Manual of Mental Disorders (3rd ed.) Washington, D.C.: American Psychiatric Association, 1980.

Dixon, W. J., and Massey, F. J., Jr. *Introduction to Statistical Analysis.* (3rd ed.) New York: McGraw-Hill, 1969.

Dohrenwend, B. P. "Psychiatric Disorder in General Populations: Problem of the Untreated 'Case.' " *American Journal of Public Health,* 1970, *60,* 1052-1064.

Dohrenwend, B. P., and Dohrenwend, B. S. *Social Status and*

Psychological Disorder: A Causal Inquiry. New York: Wiley Interscience, 1969.

Dohrenwend, B. P., and Dohrenwend, B. S. "Social and Cultural Influences on Psychopathology." In M. R. Rosenzweig and L. W. Porter (Eds.), *Annual Review of Psychology,* 1974, *25,* 417-452.

Dohrenwend, B. P., and Dohrenwend, B. S. "Psychiatric Disorders and Susceptibility to Stress." In L. N. Robins, P. J. Clayton, and J. K. Wing (Eds.), *The Social Consequences of Mental Illness.* New York: Brunner/Mazel, 1980.

Dohrenwend, B. P., and others. "The Psychiatric Status Schedule as a Measure of Dimensions of Psychopathology in the General Population." *Archives of General Psychiatry,* 1978, *35,* 731-737.

Dohrenwend, B. P., and others. *Mental Illness in the U.S.: Epidemiological Estimates.* New York: Praeger, 1980.

Dooley, D., and Catalano, R. "Economic Change as a Cause of Behavioral Disorders." *Psychological Bulletin,* 1980, *87,* 450-468.

Dunham, H. W. *Community and Schizophrenia.* Detroit: Wayne State University Press, 1965.

Eaton, W. W. "A Formal Theory of Selection for Schizophrenia." *American Journal of Sociology,* 1980, *86,* 149-156.

Feigner, J. P., and others. "Diagnostic Criteria for Use in Psychiatric Research." *Archives of General Psychiatry,* 1972, *26,* 57-63.

Fenton, F. R., Tessier, L., and Struening, E. L. "A Comparative Trial of Home and Hospital Psychiatric Care." *Archives of General Psychiatry,* 1979, *36,* 1073-1079.

Fleiss, J. L. *Statistical Methods for Rates and Proportions.* New York: Wiley, 1973.

Frank, J. D. *Persuasion and Healing.* (Rev. ed.) Baltimore, Md.: Johns Hopkins University Press, 1973.

Gardner, E. A., and others. "All Psychiatric Experience in a Community—a Cumulative Survey: Report of the First Year's Experience." *Archives of General Psychiatry,* 1963, *9,* 369-378.

Gilbert, J. P., Light, R. J., and Mosteller, F. "Assessing Social

Innovations: An Empirical Base for Policy." In C. A. Bennet and A. Lumsdaine (Eds.), *Evaluation and Experiment: Some Critical Issues in Assessing Social Programs.* New York: Academic Press, 1975.

Goldberg, D., and Jones, R. "The Cost and Benefits of Psychiatric Care." In L. N. Robins, P. J. Clayton, and J. K. Wing (Eds.), *The Social Consequences of Psychiatric Illness.* New York: Brunner/Mazel, 1980.

Goldberger, J. "The Cause and Prevention of Pellagra." *Public Health Reports,* 1914, *29,* 2354.

Gove, W. R. (Ed.). *The Labeling of Deviance.* (2nd ed.) Beverly Hills, Calif.: Sage, 1980.

Gruenberg, E. M., Snow, H. B., and Bennett, C. L. "Preventing the Social Breakdown Syndrome." In F. C. Redlich (Ed.), *Social Psychiatry.* Baltimore, Md.: Williams and Wilkins, 1969.

Hansell, N. "Patient Predicament and Clinical Service: A System." *Archives of General Psychiatry,* 1967, *17,* 204-210.

Hanushek, E. A., Jackson, J. E., and Kain, J. F. "Model Specification, Use of Aggregate Data, and the Ecological Correlation Fallacy." *Political Methodology,* 1974, *1,* 87-106.

Herz, M. I. "Brief Hospitalization of Schizophrenic Patients." In R. Cancro, L. E. Shapiro, and M. Kesselman (Eds.), *Progress in the Functional Psychoses.* New York: Spectrum, 1979.

Hollingshead, A. B., and Redlich, F. C. *Social Class and Mental Illness.* New York: Wiley, 1958.

Juel-Nielsen, N., and others. "Frequency of Depressive States Within Geographically Delimited Population Groups: 3. Incidence." (The Aarhus County Investigation) *Acta Psychiatrica Scandinavica Supplement,* 1961, *162,* 69-80.

Kenny, D. A. *Correlation and Causality.* New York: Wiley, 1979.

Kiresuk, T. J., and Lund, S. H. "Goal Attainment Scaling." In C. C. Attkisson, W. A. Hargreaves, and M. J. Horowitz (Eds.), *Evaluation of Human Service Programs.* New York: Academic Press, 1978.

Krupinski, J., and Stroller, A. "A Statistical System Introduced for the Evaluation of the Epidemiology of Psychiatric Disorders in Victoria." *Australia Health Bulletin,* 1962, *27,* 3.

Langbein, L. I., and Lichtman, A. J. *Ecological Inference.* Beverly Hills, Calif.: Sage, 1978.

LeFave, H. G., Stewart, A., and Grunberg, F. "Community Care of the Mentally Ill: Implementation of the Saskatchewan Plan." *Community Mental Health Journal,* 1968, *4,* 37-45.

Leff, J. P., Fischer, M., and Bertelsen, A. "A Cross-National Epidemiological Study of Mania." *British Journal of Psychiatry,* 1976, *129,* 428-437.

Leighton, D. C., and others. *The Character of Danger.* New York: Basic Books, 1963.

Lemkau, P. V., and Crocetti, G. M. "Vital Statistics of Schizophrenia." In L. Bellak (Ed.), *Schizophrenia: A Review of the Syndrome.* New York: Logos Press, 1958.

Letters to the Editor. *Archives of General Psychiatry,* 1980, *37,* 1421-1427.

Levy, L., and Herzog, A. "The Effects of Population Density and Crowding on Health and Social Adaptation in the Netherlands." *Journal of Health and Social Behavior,* 1974, *15,* 228-240.

Levy, L., and Rowitz, L. *The Ecology of Mental Disorder.* New York: Behavioral Publications, 1973.

Lin, T., and Standley, C. C. "The Scope of Epidemiology in Psychiatry." *Public Health Papers,* No. 16. Geneva: World Health Organization, 1962.

Mikawa, J. K. "Evaluation in Community Health." In P. McReynolds (Ed.), *Advances in Psychological Assessment III.* San Francisco: Jossey-Bass, 1975.

Mischler, E. G., and Scotch, N. A. "Sociocultural Factors in the Epidemiology of Schizophrenia." *Psychiatry,* 1963, *26,* 315-351.

Monroe, R. R., Klee, G. D., and Brody, E. B. *Psychiatric Epidemiology and Mental Health Planning.* Psychiatric Research Reports, No. 22, Washington, D.C.: American Psychiatric Association, 1967.

Morris, J. N. *The Uses of Epidemiology.* Edinburgh: E. S. Livingstone, 1957.

Murphy, J. M. "Continuities in Community-Based Psychiatric Epidemiology." *Archives of General Psychiatry,* 1980, *37,* 1215-1223.

Myers, J. K., and Weissman, M. N. "Psychiatric Disorders and Treatment: A Community Survey." In L. N. Robins, P. J. Clayton, and J. K. Wing (Eds.), *The Social Consequences of Psychiatric Illness.* New York: Brunner/Mazel, 1980.

Pasamanick, B., Scarpitti, F. P., and Dinitz, S. *Schizophrenia in the Community: An Experimental Study in the Prevention of Hospitalization.* New York: Appleton-Century-Crofts, 1967.

Paykel, E. S. "Contribution of Life Events to Causation of Psychiatric Illness." *Psychological Medicine,* 1978, *8,* 245-253.

Plunkett, R. J., and Gordon, J. E. *Epidemiology and Mental Illness.* New York: Basic Books, 1960.

Rabkin, J. G. "Stressful Life Events and Schizophrenia: A Review of the Research Literature." *Psychological Bulletin,* 1980, *87,* 408-425.

Regier, D. A. "Research on the Social Effects of Mental Disorders." In L. N. Robins, P. J. Clayton, and J. K. Wing (Eds.), *The Social Consequences of Psychiatric Illness.* New York: Brunner/Mazel, 1980.

Reich, T., and others. "The Contributions of Affected Parents to the Pool of Affected Individuals: Path Analysis of the Segregation Distribution for Alcoholism." In L. N. Robins, P. J. Clayton, and J. K. Wing (Eds.), *The Social Consequences of Psychiatric Illness.* New York: Brunner/Mazel, 1980.

Robinson, W. S. "Ecological Correlations and the Behavior of Individuals." *American Sociological Review,* 1950, *15,* 351-357.

Rosen, B. M., and others. *Mental Health Profile System Description: Purpose, Contents, and Sampler of Uses.* Department of Health, Education, and Welfare Publication No. (ADM) 76-263. Washington, D.C.: U.S. Government Printing Office, 1975.

Scheff, T. J. *Being Mentally Ill.* Hawthorne, N.Y.: Aldine, 1966.

Schur, E. M. *The Politics of Deviance: Stigma Contest and the Uses of Power.* Englewood Cliffs, N.J.: Prentice-Hall, 1980.

Schwab, J. J., and others. *Social Order and Mental Health: The Florida Health Study.* New York: Brunner/Mazel, 1979.

Shepherd, M., and others. *Psychiatric Illness in General Practice.* Oxford, England: Oxford University Press, 1966.

Snow, J. *On the Mode of Communication of Cholera.* (2nd ed.) London: J. Churchill, 1855.

Sorensen, A., and Stromgren, E. "Frequency of Depressive States Within Geographically Delimited Population Groups. 2. Prevalence." (The Samso Investigation) *Acta Psychiatrica Scandinavica Supplement,* 1961, *162,* 62-68.

Spitzer, R. L., and Endicott, J. "Diagno: A Computer Program for Psychiatric Diagnosis Utilizing the Differential Diagnostic Procedure." *Archives of General Psychiatry,* 1968, *18,* 746-756.

Spitzer, R. L., Endicott, J., and Robins, E. "Research Diagnostic Criteria." *Archives of General Psychiatry,* 1978, *35,* 773-782.

Spitzer, R. L., and Fleiss, J. L. "A Reanalysis of the Reliability of Psychiatric Diagnosis." *British Journal of Psychiatry,* 1974, *125,* 341-347.

Spitzer, R. L., and others. "The Mental Status Schedule: Rationale, Reliability, and Validity." *Comprehensive Psychiatry,* 1964, *5,* 384-395.

Spitzer, R. L., and others. "The Psychiatric Status Schedule for Epidemiological Research." *Archives of General Psychiatry,* 1980, *37,* 1193-1197.

Srole, L. "Measurement and Classification in Sociopsychiatric Epidemiology: Midtown Manhattan Study (1954) and Midtown Manhattan Restudy (1974)." *Journal of Health & Social Behavior,* 1975, *16,* 347-364.

Srole, L., and others. *Mental Health in the Metropolis: The Midtown Manhattan Study.* New York: McGraw-Hill, 1962.

Szasz, T. S. *The Myth of Mental Illness.* (Rev. ed.) New York: Harper & Row, 1974.

Weisbrod, B. A., and Helming, M. "What Benefit-Cost Analysis Can and Cannot Do. The Case of Treating the Mentally Ill." In E. W. Stromsdorfer and G. Farkas (Eds.), *Evaluation Studies Review Annual.* Vol. 5. Beverly Hills, Calif.: Sage, 1980.

Weissman, M. M., and Myers, J. K. "Affective Disorders in a United States Urban Community. The Use of Research Diagnostic Criteria in an Epidemiological Survey." *Archives of General Psychiatry,* 1978, *35,* 1304-1311.

Wing, J. K., and Brown, G. W. *Institutionalism and Schizophrenia: A Comparative Study of Three Mental Hospitals, 1960-1968.* Cambridge, England: Cambridge University Press, 1970.

Wing, J. K., Cooper, J. E., and Sartorius, N. *The Description and Classification of Psychiatric Symptoms: An Instruction Manual for the PSE and CATEGO System.* Cambridge, England: Cambridge University Press, 1974.

Wing, J. K., and Fryers, T. *Psychiatric Services in Camberwell and Salford.* London: Medical Research Council Social Psychiatry Unit, Institute of Psychiatry, 1976.

Wing, J. K., and Sturt, E. *The PSE-ID-CATEGO System: A Supplementary Manual.* London: Institute of Psychiatry, 1978.

Wing, J. K., and others. "Further Developments in the PSE and CATEGO System." *Archiv für Psychiatrie und Nervenkronkheiten,* 1977, *224,* 151-160.

Wing, L., and others. "The Use of Psychiatric Services in Three Urban Areas: An International Case Register Study." *Social Psychiatry,* 1967, *2,* 158-167.

Wing, L., and others. "Camberwell Cumulative Psychiatric Case Register. Part B: Aims and Methods." *Social Psychiatry,* 1968, *3,* 116-122.

Zeller, R. A., and Carmines, E. G. *Measurement in the Social Sciences: The Link Between Theory and Data.* New York: Cambridge University Press, 1980.

Chapter 4

Advances and Obstacles in Prevention of Mental Disorders

Bernard L. Bloom

Until very recently, it was generally believed that at any given moment 10 percent of the population was at least partially disabled by an emotional or psychiatric disorder. Indeed, the phrase "one out of ten" has been the long-time rallying cry of those citizens who have organized themselves as advocates for expanded services for the mentally ill. Yet tragically, in spite of the continually expanding capacity of the American mental health service delivery system to provide mental health care, it is now estimated that 15 percent of the American population suffers from some form of emotional disorder and that of these thirty-two million persons, nearly seven million receive no care of any kind (Regier, Goldberg, and Taube, 1978).

These facts are illustrative of the public health axiom that major disorders can be controlled only by prevention, not by providing treatment services. In the United States, at least, there

Note: This paper is a revision and updating of Bloom (1979). I wish to thank the publishers for their permission to draw on that paper in the preparation of this manuscript.

seems to be no alternative other than to conclude that emotional disorders are out of control and are likely to remain so until more resources are put into effective preventive intervention programs. Albee (1980) has suggested that the growing interest in primary prevention has many of the characteristics of a revolution, one that will challenge both the authority of the mental health establishment and the current disproportionately large allocation of mental health resources to the provision of treatment services for persons who are already emotionally disordered. While the rationale for expanded preventive programs seems unobjectionable, the issues that are raised as one discusses prevention can quickly become very complex and controversial. Part of this complexity results from inadequate understanding of some basic concepts relevant to the field of prevention (see Caplan, 1961, 1964; DeWild, 1981).

Basic Concepts and Definitions

With regard to the control of any disorder—emotional or physical—two types of interventions exist. The first seeks to reduce the number of persons suffering from the disorder, that is, to decrease the *prevalence* of that disorder. The second seeks to reduce the severity, discomfort, or disability associated with the disorder. This latter kind of intervention is formally known as *tertiary prevention* but is better known as *rehabilitation.* With lifelong disorders, rehabilitation programs generally have little effect on prevalence. Indeed, a well-run rehabilitation program may actually increase the prevalence of these disorders because it may increase life expectancy. Unfortunately, within the context of our current knowledge, many emotional disorders appear to be lifelong or nearly lifelong illnesses.

Because the prevalence of any disorder is a function of its duration and the rate at which new cases are produced, two approaches to reducing the actual prevalence of a disorder are commonly employed. The first seeks to reduce prevalence by reducing the duration of the disorder, usually through the development of some form of early case finding combined with the prompt application of effective treatment. Techniques for the control of any disorder that focus on early case finding and on prompt, effective treatment, that is, techniques that seek to reduce the prevalence of a disorder by reducing its duration, are formally called *secondary prevention.* Secondary prevention efforts are preventive only in the sense that systematic early case finding brings with it the possibility that the duration of the disorder may be reduced.

Should a technique for the early identification of some disorder be developed and employed without the concomitant development of more effective treatment procedures, a paradoxical increase in the prevalence of that disorder would occur. Gruenberg has commented that "without an effective treatment, early diagnosis only provides more work for clinicians without changing the prevalence of the disorder" (1980, p. 1323). For example, an increase in the duration and prevalence of diabetes has occurred because of improved techniques for its early identification. A similar increase in the duration and prevalence of Down's syndrome has occurred as a consequence of the medical advances that have taken place in the development of antibiotics. In this case, however, the death rate from secondary causes among persons with that syndrome has been significantly reduced (Gruenberg, 1977).

The alternative approach to prevalence reduction is to reduce the rate at which new cases of a disorder develop. This approach, which seeks to reduce prevalence by reducing *incidence,* is formally designated as *primary prevention.* This is the concept that most closely matches lay use of the term *prevention.* Effective primary prevention programs actually prevent disorders from occurring or reduce the likelihood that a disorder will occur in a particular population (Perlmutter, Vayda, and Woodburn, 1976).

The concept of primary prevention requires that the intervention take place in a population free of the disorder in question. It might be appropriate to consider the development of a primary prevention program for schizophrenia aimed at a sample of neurotics. As long as it is thought that acute and chronic schizophrenia are part of a single continuum, however, it would be incorrect to suggest that effective treatment services provided for acute schizophrenics constitute a primary prevention program for chronic schizophrenia. Such programs, while critically important, are in fact secondary prevention; that is, they seek to reduce the duration of a disorder already present. In contrast, physical rehabilitation and consciousness-raising programs provided for postmastectomy patients can quite legitimately be examined in terms of the extent to which they serve a primary prevention function for emotional disorders (Goldston, 1977).

One additional important distinction should be made, that is, the distinction between disease prevention and health promotion (McPheeters, 1976). Some disorders can be prevented by highly specific procedures—procedures that do not appear to be effective in preventing anything other than that specified disease. Malaria can be prevented by destroying the breeding grounds of a particular type of mosquito. There is no evidence that any other disease is thereby prevented. Drinking of fluoridated water results in a dramatic reduction in the incidence of dental caries, but no other disorder is reduced by fluoridated water. These are examples of specific forms of disease prevention. Although the mechanisms that give rise to specific diseases or disorders may not be completely understood, many such illnesses may be prevented by the application of specific procedures. And, as will be seen, this disease-specific prevention strategy has been very effectively employed in the case of several psychiatric disorders.

In contrast, a variety of nonspecific practices—for example, the provision of crisis intervention services or social support during times of stress—may have a positive effect on health in general and may, in fact, prevent a variety of forms of disordered behavior. Those practices that have a generally salutary but unspecifiable effect on health are referred to as health promotion strategies. Eisenberg similarly defines health promotion strategies as those activities that "contribute to resistance to disease, even when the disease agents are not known or beyond control" (1981, p. 5). One of the most influential recent reports on ways of improving the general level of health of a population by both disease prevention and health promotion strategies was prepared by the Canadian minister of National Health and Welfare (Lalonde, 1974). In this report, Lalonde introduced the concept of the health field and its four components: human biology, environment, life-style, and health care organization.

Human biology refers to aspects of health that are developed within the human body and are related to the organic nature of the individual, including the individual's genetics. The environment refers to those matters outside the body over which the individual has little if any control but that can have an effect upon health. Included in this category would be food and water purity, air pollution, safe disposal of sewage, noise control, and road and vehicular safety. Life-style refers to decisions people make about those aspects of their behavior over which they have considerable control and that can have an effect upon their health, for example, overeating, smoking, the abuse of alcohol and drugs, insufficient exercise, or careless driving. Finally, the health care organization refers to the quality, quantity, and distribution of health-related services in any community.

Using the health field concept, it is possible to examine morbidity or mortality rates in an effort to determine to what extent these rates could be reduced. In the case of traffic deaths, for example, it has been estimated that 75 percent of them can be accounted for by pathological life-styles, 20 percent by the environment, and 5 percent by defects in the health care organization. Similarly, it has been estimated that self-destructive life-styles account for about half of all deaths that occur before age seventy and that 20 percent of those premature deaths may be attributed to just two life-style habits—cigarette smoking and excessive use of alcohol.

Since the publication of this Canadian report, there has been a growing interest in examining life-styles and their role in illness and premature death. As part of this interest in health promotion, mental health professionals are beginning to examine various aspects of life-styles in terms of their roles in predisposing people to emotional disorders or to precipitating such disorders in populations that are vulnerable but not disordered. The explicit objective in this examination is to develop programmatic strategies for the prevention of emotional disorders before they start.

Preventable Psychiatric Disorders

There is by now a well-established knowledge base regarding the role of specific interventions in preventing specific psychiatric disorders. The American Public Health Association (1962) has identified five categories of mental disorders that are preventable, in part because they are all disorders of known etiology. While these disorders do not constitute a large proportion of all mental disorders, nearly all result in chronic brain syndromes, many are lifelong in their effects, and they represent, in total, an enormous cost to society as well as to the victims and their families (also see Gruenberg, 1980; Kornberg and Caplan, 1980).

The first group of preventable disorders includes those related to poisoning. These disorders are typically subdivided into acute poisoning (disorders that are the result of intentional or accidental ingestion of drugs, inhalants, or solvents) and chronic poisoning (disorders that are most commonly caused by prolonged exposure to industrial toxins or by prolonged use of medications or addicting drugs). There are over 250,000 chemicals and drugs that can be poisonous, including, for example, acetone, arsenic, barbiturates, carbon monoxide, cyanides, DDT, kerosene, morphine, and turpentine. Poisonings account for about 3,000 deaths every year and another 3,000 survivors who are left with chronic brain syndromes. Prevention requires changes in the environment, in life-styles, and in the health care system; specifically, it requires more prudent prescribing, dispensing, and storage of drugs, more careful control over drug prescriptions and their renewal, reduced exposure to industrial poisons, better safety standards in industrial and agricultural settings, better labeling of industrial and household products, and prompt, accurate diagnosis and treatment. Health education can play an important role in achieving these objectives, as can changes in laws and regulations and the development of a network of readily accessible poison control centers.

The second category of preventable disorders includes those that result from infectious agents that can invade the central nervous system and leave permanent brain damage. Infections during the fetal period, such as those caused by rubella, syphilis, and toxoplasmosis, can produce severe mental retardation, epilepsy, perceptual and cognitive defects, and difficulty in impulse control. Rubella can be prevented by the administration of gamma globulin to women who have not previously had the disease. Successful treatment of syphilis in the mother prevents the development of fetal syphilis. Prompt treatment of toxoplasmosis can prevent the transmission of this disease during pregnancy. Infectious diseases during childhood, such as pertussis, influenza, measles, meningitis, mumps, and tuberculosis, can also produce permanent brain damage and thus lead to defects in sensory, motor, and intellectual development. Many of these infectious processes can be prevented by immunizations, yet substantial proportions of young children are not completely immunized against these diseases (Eisenberg, 1981, pp. 9-10).

The third category of preventable disorders includes those that are brought about by a genetic process. Among these conditions are Tay-Sachs disease, phenylketonuria, galactosemia, tuberous sclerosis, and Huntington's chorea. Phenylketonuria and galactosemia, both of which can produce severe mental retardation, can be prevented by special dietary intake. In the case of most genetic disorders, carriers can be identified or risks estimated on the basis of family studies. Under these circumstances, genetic counseling can help reduce the number of vulnerable children.

In the fourth category of preventable mental disorders are those produced by nutritional deficiencies, including beriberi, Wernicke's encephalopathy, kwashiorkor, pellagra, and anoxemia. These prolonged nutritional deficiencies during childhood appear to have a considerable general impact on mental development and to increase the risk of mental retardation, epilepsy, and a variety of perceptual and cognitive disorders. In addition, there is considerable evidence that general nutritional deficiencies increase vulnerability to infections. Nutritional dietary supplementation combined with nutritional education can prevent these disorders.

The fifth category of preventable mental disorders includes those that are the result of injuries to the central nervous system, including falls, gunshot wounds, and vehicular accidents. The incidence of such injuries can be dramatically reduced by making the sources, such as guns, less readily available, by encouraging the use of protective equipment, such as motorcycle helmets and seat belts, and by improving the safety of motor vehicles and roads. The fifth category of preventable mental disorders also includes general systemic disorders that can produce chronic brain syndromes, such as erythroblastosis fetalis, hyperthyroidism, cretinism, intracranial masses, toxemia of pregnancy, or prematurity. With respect to the knowledge base used in the treatment of these five categories of mental disorders, additional investigation is required only when it appears that an effective procedure is not being applied. For example, why in view of their clear effectiveness in reducing automobile accident injuries, do drivers and passengers persist in failing to wear seat belts; or why is a substantial proportion of the population not immunized against diseases that can sometimes, as in the case of measles, have profoundly harmful effects upon central nervous system functioning?

Current studies of the effectiveness of motorcycle helmets in reducing both injury and mortality rates are unusually interesting because the laws governing their use are in a very fluid state. In addition, these studies are worth examining because they are illustrative of the controversy that is often generated in the discussion of prevention when health-related values appear to be in conflict with economic considerations.

More than 4,000 persons were killed and 350,000 persons injured in motorcycle accidents in 1977, representing a rate seven times higher than in the case of automobile accidents. Head injuries were the major cause of those deaths and were far less frequent among persons wearing protective helmets than among those who did not. As a consequence of these findings, when federal funds became available in 1967 for state highway safety programs, states were required to enact motorcycle helmet use laws in order to qualify for the funds. By 1975, virtually all states had enacted laws requiring motorcycle riders to wear helmets, and studies of the effectiveness of these laws showed that both mortality rates and the degree of severity of nonfatal injuries subsequently decreased—in the case of fatalities by about 30 percent (Watson, Zador, and Wilks, 1980). There was thus an annual reduction of more than 1,000 in motorcycle fatalities and of many times that number in the case of nonfatal injuries.

In 1976, Congress removed the financial penalty for noncompliance with the helmet law provisions, influenced in part by the lobbying efforts of organizations such as the American Motorcyclist Association that are opposed to this requirement. Between 1976 and 1978, a total of twenty-six states repealed their motorcycle helmet use laws. Studies in those states showed substantial increases in motorcycle fatalities and injuries following the repeal of these laws. In 1979, nearly 5,000 motorcyclists died in crashes (Watson, Zador, and Wilks, 1981).

Watson, Zador, and Wilks (1980) found a 38 percent increase in motorcycle fatalities in those states in which helmet laws had been repealed when contrasted with geographically and demographically similar states in which the laws had not been repealed. Of the twenty-six states in which the helmet law was repealed, fatality rates increased in all but three. Noting that the mortality rate was twice as high among unhelmeted riders as among helmeted riders, Watson, Zador, and Wilks concluded that "the repeals of motorcycle helmet laws have been one of the most tragic decisions made recently in the U.S.A. from the standpoint of public health" (1980, p. 583). In a related study, Muller (1980) ascertained that more than $60 million could be saved annually if all motorcyclists were to wear helmets. In spite of these studies, current efforts to reenact motorcycle helmet laws at the state level are generally unsuccessful.

Paradigm Shift in Primary Prevention

Even if every preventable psychiatric disorder were prevented, however, we would still be left with a very large number of psychiatric casualties in our communities. The following paradigm for specific disease prevention, which has worked so well for the past 200 years in the prevention of infectious and nutritional diseases, has also been applied to psychiatric disorders:

1. Identify a disease of sufficient importance to justify the development of a preventive intervention program. Develop reliable methods for its diagnosis so that people can be divided with confidence into groups according to whether they do or do not have the disease.
2. By a series of epidemiological and laboratory studies, identify the most likely theories of that disease's path of development.
3. Mount and evaluate an experimental preventive intervention program based on the results of those research studies.

This, in somewhat oversimplified form, is the paradigm we assume whenever we think about the prevention of a specific disorder. The paradigm has been remarkably effective for a broad array of communicable diseases—smallpox, typhus, cholera, typhoid fever, the plague, malaria, diphtheria, tuberculosis, tetanus, and, more recently, sexually transmitted diseases, rubella, polio, and an equally impressive list of what are now known to be nutritional diseases—scurvy, beri-beri, pellagra, rickets, kwashiorkor, endemic goiter, and dental caries.

All these diseases have one attribute in common. For each, there is an identified necessary, although not always sufficient, biological precondition for its appearance—lack of niacin or vitamin B, protein deficiency, invasion of a particular bacillus, lack of fluoride, and so on. Because of this necessary precondition, we can talk about the "cause" of a particular disease. In keeping with this tradition, active research has been underway for some time in an effort to identify the biological bases of specific psychiatric disorders.

In an effort to understand the development and prevention of currently unpreventable disorders, however, researchers have developed a new paradigm within the past decade or so. It is a paradigm that does not begin with the assumption that every specific disorder has a single or even a multiple necessary precondition. Rather, this paradigm, which is based upon the clearly established association of stress with increased risk of illness, assumes that we are all variously vulnerable to stressful life experiences and that "almost any disease or disability may be associated with these events" (Dohrenwend and Dohrenwend, 1974, p. 314). Four vulnerable persons can face a stressful life experience, perhaps the collapse of their marriages or the loss of their jobs. One person may become severely depressed; the second may be subsequently involved in an automobile accident; the third may become clinically alcoholic; and the fourth may develop a psychotic thought disorder or coronary artery disease. In the most recent report of the surgeon general (U.S. Department of Health and Human Services, 1980), one important goal that has been articulated for promoting health and preventing disease is the more effective control of stress.

On the basis of this paradigm, preventive intervention programs can be organized for the purpose of reducing the incidence of particular stressful life events, whenever possible, or of facilitating their mastery once they occur. In either case, one need not be overly concerned with prior specification of the forms of disability that might thereby be prevented; that is, this new paradigm begins by abandoning at the outset the search for a unique cause or set of causes for each disorder. In contrast to the classic paradigm that we have already described, the new paradigm has the following sequence of steps:

1. Identify a stressful life event that appears to have undesirable consequences. Develop procedures for reliably identifying persons who have undergone or who are undergoing that stressful experience.
2. By traditional epidemiological and laboratory methods, study the consequences of that event and develop hypotheses related to how one might go about reducing or eliminating the negative consequences of the event.
3. Mount and evaluate experimental preventive intervention programs based on these hypotheses.

This *general* disease prevention paradigm, which has turned our attention from long-standing predisposing factors in psychopathology to much more recent precipitating factors, is part of an even broader phenomenon. It has long been known that biological, psychological, and sociological factors differentially predispose persons to emotional disorders. With few exceptions, however, efforts to develop effective preventive services based on attempts to modify these distal predisposing factors have been unsuccessful. Eisenberg has recently commented that "measurement of distant outcome places a terrible burden of proof on childhood interventions; they must be powerful indeed to be able to show a clear effect despite the vicissitudes of subsequent life experience" (1981, p. 4). Furthermore, psychotherapeutic strategies that focus on developing greater understanding and acceptance of these predisposing factors in the case of casualties have not been conspicuously successful, and even when successful have demanded unrealistically large proportions of our resources.

There is every reason to believe that preventive programs linked to stressful life events can be effective, particularly when we set about to build on what is already known about crisis theory and crisis intervention (Bloom, 1975, pp. 134-172; Caplan, 1964, pp. 34-54; Mann, 1978; Parad, 1965; Parad, Resnik, and Parad, 1976). Our own applied research program at the University of Colorado concerns itself with separation and divorce as stressful life events. But other critical precipitating factors that are receiving increasing attention include school entrance, parenting, retirement, and widowhood. It should be noted that these events are all common, many are becoming more common, and few sustained and comprehensive services exist within our society to assist people in mastering any of them.

Once mental health professionals and social scientists became interested in stress, their initial approach was to examine the possibility that each type of stressful experience was associated with a particular stress disease. Cassel makes a persuasive case that "there is serious doubt as to the utility or appropriateness of both of these notions. It is most unlikely that any given psychosocial process or stressor will be etiologically specific for any disease, at least as currently classified" (1976, p. 109; also see Cassel, 1973, 1974). Cassel's own research, as well as his review of the studies of others, led him to conclude that although psychosocial processes enhance susceptibility to disease, the clinical manifestations of this enhanced susceptibility would not be functions of the particular psychosocial stressor. If we then keep in mind these two developments—the growing interest in precipitating crisis events rather than in predisposing developmental variables and the growing acceptance of general as well as disorder-specific preventive interventions—we can better appreciate much of the recent research literature.

Two particularly compelling concepts that have been introduced to link individual disorders with the stressful properties of the social system are the concepts of social competence and competence building, on the one hand, and of social support, on the other. Much human misery appears to be the result of a lack of competence—that is, a lack of control over one's life and a lack of effective coping strategies—and the lowered self-esteem that accompanies these deficiencies (Ryan, 1971; Shure, 1979). A substantial body of research from a variety of domains appears to converge on social competence building as one of the most persuasive preventive strategies for dealing with individual and social issues.

The second line of recent research links the absence of social support systems to vulnerability to disease. Caplan has provided a valuable analysis of the nature of support systems, those "continuing social aggregates that provide individuals with opportunities for feedback about themselves and for validations of their expectations about others, which may offset deficiencies in these communications within the larger community context" (1974, pp. 4-5). Cassel's (1973) review of the research suggested that people are likely to have increased susceptibility to disease when they find themselves in an unfamiliar environment or when there is considerable social disorganization. Cassel also noted that susceptibility to disease is greater in those persons who are subordinate rather than dominant in a society and in persons who are deprived of meaningful social contacts and social supports. He concluded that a high level of disease in general might be anticipated under conditions of social change and social disorganization and that "preventive action in the future should focus more directly on attempts at modifying these psychosocial factors, on improving and strengthening social supports, and reducing the circumstances which produce ambiguities between actions and their consequences" (1973, p. 547; also see Berkman and Syme, 1979; Gottlieb and Todd, 1979; and Kagey, Vivace, and Lutz, 1981).

The links between these areas of research and conceptualization are striking and make a persuasive case for competence assessment and competence building at the individual and aggregate community level (Iscoe, 1974) as a high-priority objective of community mental health programs. In summary, these studies suggest that we may be able to make significant progress in the prevention of emotional disorders by (1) rephrasing the primary prevention question to ask about the prevention of mental disorders in general, (2) identifying stress-producing and crisis-precipitating events in our environments, and (3) developing systematic and multidimensional interventions to help in the mastery of these stresses. Included among these strategies might well be the development of strengthened sources of social support and of improved social competencies.

While these two orientations to health promotion appear to be unusually promising, they do not exhaust the list of potential approaches. The American Public Health Association has suggested a number of other strategies, including prevention of maternal deprivation, improvement of childrearing practices, better prenatal care, reduction of radiological exposure, and genetic counseling (1962, pp. 57-61). More recently, Gruenberg (1980) has suggested additions to this list—improved nutrition, improved dental health, and improved medical care.

Immediate Future of Primary Prevention

Evaluation of the status of primary prevention programs in a typical community will generally show that preventable disorders continue to occur, that only a small proportion of the population is functioning at maximal potential, and that insufficient resources are allocated to extending the frontiers of knowledge that might serve to diminish the incidence of emotional disorders. Because those disorders are rarely fatal and express their impact primarily in terms of high morbidity rather than mortality, communities face unmet needs in their efforts to treat the already ill and are often reluctant to divert scarce resources away from that important humanitarian task (see, for example, Lamb and Zusman, 1979). Yet the public is not unwilling to seek preventive services. It has recently been estimated (Cypress, 1981) that 17 percent of the visits to physicians' offices during 1977-1978 took place primarily in the interest of preventive care.

Clearly, however, a number of barriers exist that make it difficult to enlarge upon primary prevention activities in the field of emotional disorders. First, no national policy exists with regard to the enhancement of mental health, although the President's Commission on Mental Health (1978) proposed steps toward such a policy. This lack of national policy is reflected in a wide variety of phenomena. No one seems to be in charge of health maintenance or promotion. Responsibilities are fragmented even when assigned, and coordination among agencies is often impossible to achieve.

A second barrier relates to the difficulty in extending our knowledge regarding effective approaches to primary prevention. Excellent research is now being undertaken and reported, however (see, for example, Albee and Joffe, 1977; Bond and Rosen, 1980; Forgays, 1978; Kent and Rolf, 1979; and Price and others, 1980). But continuing to extend our knowledge base will require both increased numbers of skilled and dedicated scientists and expanded research support. Eisenberg has noted that "when one considers that the entire investment in the basic and applied research and the field trials that made the poliomyelitis vaccine possible was less than the cost of the illness burden from a single epidemic year of the disease, pursuit of the same strategy for other disorders is immensely appealing" (1981, p. 4). It may require a decade or longer to determine the extent to which preventive services have been effective. These longitudinal studies need not be prohibitively expensive in any one year, but there needs to be a stable and predictable support base over a relatively long period of time.

Gruenberg has recently commented about the need for better research in the field of primary prevention:

> A special group of prevention advocates share three critical assumptions about the interventions they advocate. They assume that the interventions are harmless; socially acceptable and not frightening to the subjects; and able to prevent some disorders on some reasonable basis. Whether or not they actually prevent a disorder is best found out by starting with a planned preventive trial. It is extraordinary that many of the fashionable mental health prevention programs have these characteristics, yet none of them have produced a preventive trial. Such programs as widow-to-widow counseling to prevent extended depression; correction of low self-esteem in pregnant women to prevent neurotic symptom formation in their daughters; and enhancing the coping skills of mentally retarded parents and of their children to prevent mental retardation in the children are excellent examples of hypotheses that are best tested in the first instance by a carefully prepared preventive trial. If such educational and counseling methods actually have large effects, they deserve to become more widespread. If they do not, other preventable causes must be found to lower the incidence of these disorders [1980, pp. 1323-1324].

A third barrier lies in our failure to act on our growing realization that monoetiological theories do not really explain the development of most forms of psychiatric disorder (Weissman and Klerman, 1978) and that the concept of health is itself multidimensional. Effective preventive efforts will require the active collaboration of many professions, many agencies, and many social systems. These efforts will demand the active involvement of teachers, parents, clergy, nutritionists, economists, architects, and so on. Although this sentiment is often subscribed to in theory, it is rarely adopted in practice.

Most activities in the field of primary prevention appear

to equate health with the absence of disease and thus see their goal as the enhancement of health by means of the reduction of disease. For more than 2,000 years, however, an alternative view of health has had its adherents—a view that equates health with those "natural laws which will ensure . . . a healthy mind in a healthy body" (Dubos, 1959, p. 111). From this point of view, health is not a state; it is a process, a way of life. It is from this point of view that Williamson and Pearse described health as "intrinsically and distinctively a positive process not definable in terms of 'absence' of disease and/or disorder; hence not attainable through a 'preventive' approach necessarily directed to securing the absence of disease and disorder" (1966, pp. 293-294). This broad continuum in the concept of health brings with it an equally broad array of appropriate objectives, ranging from primary prevention activities that are designed to maintain a disease-free status quo to those activities that are designed to promote growth and wholeness and to help persons make maximum use of their potential, independently of whether a disease process might be present.

Some preventive interventions can be effective if made available to individuals singly or in groups. Other interventions must be directed at social systems in order to have a significant effect on individuals. In part, this issue relates to the theory to which one subscribes regarding a particular type of stress and appropriate strategies for intervention. Just as theories and strategies may vary, so may levels of intervention. Some years ago, Mills (1959) proposed a distinction between troubles, when an individual's values are seen as being threatened, and issues, when a society's values are seen as being threatened. Reiff (1977) makes use of this distinction when contrasting the instability of an individual marriage—a personal trouble—with the larger social world in which 50 percent of marriages end in divorce. In this latter case, Reiff suggests, "there is something beyond the intrapsychic and interpersonal, something beyond the situation, and something in the social structure that accounts for these personal troubles" (1977, p. 49). The clear implication of this line of reasoning is that any intervention that stops short of a thoroughgoing examination of the societal conditions that are producing this much disruption may very well fail.

A final barrier that should be noted lies within the mental health establishment itself; this barrier is reflected in the characteristics of contemporary practice and its underlying societal values. First, as Albee (1979) has noted, our society is oriented toward quick solutions to current problems, and mental health professionals are rarely enthusiastic about long-term planning aimed at long-term goals. Second, most members of the mental health establishment have been socialized into believing that treatment is a far more valued activity than prevention. Third, the mental health establishment is unprepared, either by training or ideology, to push for needed social change in an effort to prevent mental disorders. Finally, members of the mental health establishment are part of a larger third-party reimbursement procedure that legitimizes little more than the provision of treatment for diagnosed diseases. In such a fiscal environment, there is little motivation to develop preventive programs that are neither fundable nor reimbursable.

It may be necessary to develop an agency solely concerned with primary prevention—an agency that would serve the healthy for the purpose of maintaining and enhancing their robustness. At one time, the public health agency played that role. Perhaps local health departments need to be encouraged to resume that responsibility in a late twentieth-century version of a once-esteemed community service. Such an agency must deal with the entire spectrum of preventive services. It must recognize that health is a social as well as a biological phenomenon and that there are healthy ways of being sick just as there are unhealthy ways of being well. It must legitimize and encourage holistic as well as specialized views of the process of health and of a healthy life, and it must attend to the entire range of contemporary stress, from the biological and the psychological to the sociological and the cultural. It must take a broad view of health as not only the absence of disease but also as the presence of joy in living and hope in the ultimate resolution of life's conflicts.

References

Albee, G. W. "Primary Prevention." *Canada's Mental Health,* 1979, *27,* 5-9.

Albee, G. W. "The Fourth Mental Health Revolution." *Journal of Prevention,* 1980, *1,* 67-70.

Albee, G. W., and Joffe, J. M. (Eds.). *The Issues: An Overview of Primary Prevention.* Hanover, N.H.: University Press of New England, 1977.

American Public Health Association. *Mental Disorders: A Guide to Control Methods.* New York: American Public Health Association, 1962.

Berkman, L. F., and Syme, S. L. "Social Networks, Host Resistance, and Mortality: A Nine-Year Follow-up Study of Alameda County Residents." *American Journal of Epidemiology,* 1979, *109,* 186-204.

Bloom, B. L. *Community Mental Health: A General Introduction.* Monterey, Calif.: Brooks/Cole, 1975.

Bloom, B. L. "Prevention of Mental Disorders: Recent Advances in Theory and Practice." *Community Mental Health Journal,* 1979, *15,* 179-191.

Bond, L., and Rosen, J. (Eds.). *Competence and Coping During Adulthood.* Hanover, N.H.: University Press of New England, 1980.

Caplan, G. (Ed.). *Prevention of Mental Disorders in Children: Initial Explorations.* New York: Basic Books, 1961.

Caplan, G. *Principles of Preventive Psychiatry.* New York: Basic Books, 1964.

Caplan, G. *Support Systems and Community Mental Health: Lectures on Concept Development.* New York: Behavioral Publications, 1974.

Cassel, J. "The Relation of the Urban Environment to Health: Implications for Prevention." *Mount Sinai Journal of Medicine,* 1973, *40,* 539-550.

Cassel, J. "Psychosocial Processes and 'Stress': Theoretical Formulation." *International Journal of Health Services,* 1974, *4,* 471-482.

Cassel, J. "The Contribution of the Social Environment to Host Resistance." *American Journal of Epidemiology,* 1976, *104,* 107-123.

Cypress, B. K. "Office Visits for Preventive Care, National Ambulatory Medical Care Survey: United States, 1977-78." *Na-*

tional Center for Health Statistics Advanced Data, No. 69. Department of Health and Human Services Publication No. (PHS) 81-1250. Washington, D.C.: U.S. Government Printing Office, 1981.

DeWild, D. W. "Toward a Clarification of Primary Prevention." *Community Mental Health Journal,* 1981, *16,* 306-316.

Dohrenwend, B. S., and Dohrenwend, B. P. (Eds.). *Stressful Life Events: Their Nature and Effects.* New York: Wiley, 1974.

Dobus, R. *Mirage of Health.* New York: Harper & Row, 1959.

Eisenberg, L. "A Research Framework for Evaluating the Promotion of Mental Health and Prevention of Mental Illness." *Public Health Reports,* 1981, *96,* 3-19.

Forgays, D. (Ed.). *Primary Prevention of Psychopathology: Environmental Influences.* Hanover, N.H.: University Press of New England, 1978.

Goldston, S. E. "An Overview of Primary Prevention Programming." In D. C. Klein and S. E. Goldston (Eds.), *Primary Prevention: An Idea Whose Time Has Come.* Washington, D.C.: U.S. Government Printing Office, 1977.

Gottlieb, B. H., and Todd, D. M. "Characterizing and Promoting Social Support in Natural Settings." In R. F. Muñoz, L. R. Snowden, J. G. Kelly, and Associates, *Social and Psychological Research in Community Settings: Designing and Conducting Programs for Social and Personal Well-Being.* San Francisco: Jossey-Bass, 1979.

Gruenberg, E. M. "The Failures of Success." *Milbank Memorial Fund Quarterly/Health and Society,* 1977, *55,* 3-24.

Gruenberg, E. M. "Mental Disorders." In J. M. Last (Ed.), *Maxcy-Rosenau Public Health and Preventive Medicine.* (11th ed.) New York: Appleton-Century-Crofts, 1980.

Iscoe, I. "Community Psychology and the Competent Community." *American Psychologist,* 1974, *29,* 607-613.

Kagey, J. R., Vivace, J., and Lutz, W. "Mental Health Primary Prevention: The Role of Parent Mutual Support Groups." *American Journal of Public Health,* 1981, *71,* 166-167.

Kent, M. W., and Rolf, J. E. (Eds.). *Promoting Social Competence in Children.* Hanover, N.H.: University Press of New England, 1979.

Kornberg, M. S., and Caplan, G. "Risk Factors and Preventive Intervention in Child Psychopathology." *Journal of Prevention,* 1980, *1,* 71-133.

Lalonde, M. *A New Perspective on the Health of Canadians.* Ottawa: Canadian Government Printing Office, 1974.

Lamb, H. R., and Zusman, J. "Primary Prevention in Perspective." *American Journal of Psychiatry,* 1979, *136,* 12-17.

McPheeters, H. L. "Primary Prevention and Health Promotion in Mental Health." *Preventive Medicine,* 1976, *5,* 187-198.

Mann, P. A. *Community Psychology: Concepts and Applications.* New York: Free Press, 1978.

Mills, C. W. *The Sociological Imagination.* Oxford, England: Oxford University Press, 1959.

Muller, A. "Evaluation of the Costs and Benefits of Motorcycle Helmet Laws." *American Journal of Public Health,* 1980, *70,* 586-592.

Parad, H. J. (Ed.). *Crisis Intervention: Selected Readings.* New York: Family Service Association of America, 1965.

Parad, H. J., Resnik, H. L. P., and Parad, L. G. (Eds.). *Emergency and Disaster Management.* Bowie, Md.: Charles Press, 1976.

Perlmutter, F. D., Vayda, A. M., and Woodburn, P. K. "An Instrument for Differentiating Programs in Prevention–Primary, Secondary, and Tertiary." *American Journal of Orthopsychiatry,* 1976, *46,* 533-541.

President's Commission on Mental Health. *Report to the President.* Vol. 1. Washington, D.C.: U.S. Government Printing Office, 1978.

Price, R. H., and others. *Prevention in Mental Health: Research, Policy, and Practice.* Beverly Hills, Calif.: Sage, 1980.

Regier, D. A., Goldberg, I. D., and Taube, C. A. "The De Facto U.S. Mental Health Services System." *Archives of General Psychiatry,* 1978, *35,* 685-693.

Reiff, R. "Ya Gotta Believe." In I. Iscoe, B. L. Bloom, and C. D. Spielberger (Eds.), *Community Psychology in Transition.* Washington, D.C.: Hemisphere, 1977.

Ryan, W. *Blaming the Victim.* New York: Random House, 1971.

Shure, M. B. "Training Children to Solve Interpersonal Problems: A Preventive Mental Health Program." In R. F. Muñoz, L. R. Snowden, J. G. Kelly, and Associates, *Social and Psychological Research in Community Settings: Designing and Conducting Programs for Social and Personal Well-Being.* San Francisco: Jossey-Bass, 1979.

U.S. Department of Health and Human Services. *Promoting Health/Preventing Disease: Objectives for the Nation.* Washington, D.C.: U.S. Government Printing Office, 1980.

Watson, G. S., Zador, P. L., and Wilks, A. "The Repeal of Helmet Use Laws and Increased Motorcyclist Mortality in the United States, 1975-1978." *American Journal of Public Health,* 1980, *70,* 579-585.

Watson, G. S., Zador, P. L., and Wilks, A. "Helmet Use, Helmet Use Laws, and Motorcyclist Fatalities." *American Journal of Public Health,* 1981, *71,* 297-300.

Weissman, M. M., and Klerman, G. L. "Epidemiology of Mental Disorders: Emerging Trends in the United States." *Archives of General Psychiatry,* 1978, *35,* 705-712.

Williamson, G. S., and Pearse, I. H. *Science, Synthesis, and Sanity.* Chicago: Contemporary Books, 1966.

Chapter 5

Relationship of Social Support and Psychological Well Being

Robert S. Weiss

Two perplexing questions, perhaps the central questions of social psychology, are those of the determinants and consequences of social bonding. Why do we maintain links with others? And, given that we do maintain such links, with what benefit or harm?

American social science has since its inception emphasized the benefits of social ties and has suggested, generally implicitly, that individuals establish social ties in order to gain these benefits. Cooley, in his *Social Organization* (1909), proposed that close face-to-face relationships enhanced individual functioning by providing socially sanctioned understandings with which to make sense of the complexities of reality. Furthermore, he wrote, close face-to-face relationships helped sustain individuals'

Note: Work on this paper and the pilot study referred to in it was facilitated by a fellowship from the John Simon Guggenheim Memorial Foundation.

morale. Others who were near contemporaries of Cooley's and who had very similar views of social relationships included Mead (1934) and Dewey (1922). This school of thought argued that the German armed forces maintained their effectiveness as long as their constituent groups remained intact (Shils and Janowitz, 1948), and that industry would do well to acknowledge the governing role in workers' behavior of the close face-to-face associations they formed with fellow workers (Homans, 1950). It is a continuation of this tradition that views social ties as likely to sustain the functioning of stressed individuals (House, 1981; Cobb, 1976; Caplan, 1974).

In contrast, European examination of the functioning of social ties has given more attention to their negative potentials. European writers have more often than American seen the individual as needing to defend himself against burdensome relations with others. They do not see individuals as seeking others because of the positive value of association so much as they see individuals caught up in a web of exchanges from which sentiments arise willy-nilly (Simmel, 1950) or almost passively carried along by the social world in which they are immersed (LeBon, 1896). It was within this tradition that Freud (1930) wrote: "Suffering comes from three quarters: from our body, which is destined to decay and dissolution . . . ; from the outer world which can rage against us with the most powerful and pitiless forces of destruction; and finally from our relations with other men" (p. 28). Surprisingly, Freud does not in this passage speak of that source of suffering to the elucidation of which he gave his career: our inner conflicts. But it is clear that in his view "relations with other men" are potential sources of distress, whatever their potential for gratification.

Empirical research tends to find, as might be expected, that the quality of relationships is critically related both to well-being and to distress. Campbell, Converse, and Rogers (1976) correlated general life satisfaction, as reported in a national sample survey, with satisfaction with particular areas of life. They found that life satisfaction most strongly correlated with satisfaction with family life and marriage. While life satisfaction was next most strongly correlated with satisfaction with the situational characteristics of finances and housing, it also correlated with the largely relational "satisfaction with job" and the entirely relational "satisfaction with friendships." Similar results were reported by Bradburn and Caplovitz (1965). In a survey of residents of four Illinois communities, they found that marital tensions, along with job dissatisfactions, reliably produced negative feelings strong enough to make for a generally unhappy mood.

Research on social support (as distinguished from research on happiness or well-being) has generally given attention only to the positive potential of social ties. That relationships may also induce discomfort and distress has tended to escape notice. Nor has there been acknowledgment that relationships may make demands on time and other resources, may draw on limited energies, and inevitably involve opportunity costs in that other activities must be forgone so that relationships can be maintained. Instead, attention has been restricted to the ways in which social ties may contribute to well-being.

There appear to be three quite distinct ways in which social ties can be supportive of well-being; to use terms suggested by House (1981), these are functional, informational, and emotional contributions. *Functional support* refers to the provision of tangible help: services, material resources, money. *Informational support* refers to the provision of knowledge, experience, and advice. The nature of *emotional support,* however, seems difficult to specify.

One kind of emotional support, provided by counselors and other professional helpers, has been described by Burnand (1969) as the assurance of an emotional alliance with a figure of unquestionable effectiveness. The counselor, by communicating a willingness to commit his or her skills and energies to the pursuit of the client's goals, provides the client with a basis for optimism and encourages the client to act with assurance. But a relationship of this sort hardly seems to represent all the relationships that provide emotional support, nor does its particular provision seem to sum up the various forms emotional support may take.

Indeed, virtually every social relationship would seem to

have some potential for providing emotional support. Friendships offer the augmentation of a peer, while work relationships may foster a sense of competence. It would seem that to understand the nature of emotional support is a task not very different from that of understanding the nature of the provisions of relationships, simply because so large a proportion of relational provisions have some element of emotional support. Insofar as the provisions made by a relationship are emotionally valuable, they would constitute emotional support. Thus, we might rephrase the question about the forms of emotional support in this way: Neglecting, for the time being, the negative potentials of relationships, what are the different emotionally important provisions of social relationships? What are the different ways in which relationships contribute to emotional well-being?

Provisions of Social Relationships

Cooley (1909) proposed that relationships could be divided into two classes. One class would include "primary relationships," face-to-face relationships developed between individuals who are irreplaceable to one another, sustaining of emotion and "we-feeling." The other class would include "secondary relationships," relationships entered into for instrumental purposes, to get something accomplished, but otherwise without emotional importance. Primary relationships, Cooley proposed, help establish the shared understandings necessary for functioning in a social world and also help maintain individuals' morale. These are the relationships, it might seem, that provide emotional support.

Observation of actual relationships suggests that Cooley's scheme is flawed in two ways. First, the category of secondary relationships turns out to be virtually empty, in that no interchange, however bureaucratized or fleeting, is without exchange of perceptions and impact on feelings. True, some relationships are much more nearly "secondary" than others, but this is a different way of viewing the matter. The second flaw in Cooley's scheme is that it groups together, in the category of primary relationships, relationships that are quite different from each other. In one demonstration of this, individuals who had in their lives a close, security-fostering, intimate relationship—marriage or a relationship near to it in emotional quality—but who were removed from any community of friends or colleagues as a result of change of residence, complained, when interviewed, that they suffered from social isolation. The marriage or marriagelike relationship they maintained, good as it may have been, did not substitute for the absence of a community in which they had a place. Conversely, individuals who were without a close, security-fostering, intimate relationship such as marriage complained of emotional isolation, even though they belonged to communities of friends or colleagues (Weiss, 1974a, 1974b). In the one instance the presence of a close relationship did not compensate for the absence of community; in the other the availability of community did not compensate for the absence of a close relationship. Here are two primary relationships that each provided something different.

If we reject the idea that relationships are basically of two forms, in only one of which emotional support takes place, how can we develop a more realistic appraisal of the types of social relationships and the provisions they make? Is there a way of *developing* theory from empirical study?

One approach is to use survey methods. Here we might, in the same interview, learn about the presence or absence of particular social ties in respondents' lives and also about the quality of respondents' functioning or well-being. Correlations between the absence of particular ties and diminished well-being would suggest a causal relationship. Still more effective would be a longitudinal survey study in which we would ask what were the effects on well-being in a subsequent interview of presence or absence of particular ties in an earlier interview. Henderson (in press) has done just this by correlating presence or absence of relationships at Time 1 with reported well-being at Time 2. He found that both very close relationships, as well as relationships that might provide a sense of community, serve to protect well-being despite adversity. This study goes far toward establishing the independent importance of these relationships as sources of emotional support.

A different approach to identifying the provisions of social relationships would invite individuals to describe the relationships they maintain and also the ways in which these relationships express themselves. Whereas the survey approach relies on a statistical demonstration of a connection between respondents' descriptions of relationships and the quality of respondents' functioning, this second approach utilizes respondents' descriptions of the processes by which relationships provide emotional support. The argument that a particular relationship provides emotional support would then be based on a detailed description of how it does so. The survey approach can demonstrate statistically that there is a connection between a relationship and its provisions; detailed interviewing can make evident the nature of that connection.

In pilot work I conducted for a detailed interview study of the functioning of social ties in response to stress, it was found that men who could call on their wives for support when their work became stressful emphasized in interviews that their wives were in touch with them. One respondent said he felt there was resonance between himself and his wife. Several said that they felt "in tune" with their wives. One respondent who felt that his wife failed to provide emotional support, despite her attempts to be helpful, believed that the problem was an absence of just this sense of her being in touch with him, his feelings, and his needs. The support provided by close relationships, as established by the correlational approach, is shown by detailed interviewing to involve a feeling that there is someone who is not only sympathetic but also truly in touch.

In this example an association identified in survey work was extended through process-focused interviewing. Conversely, theory based on process-focused interviewing may be disciplined by the findings of survey work. In an interview study of the character and functioning of social ties among single parents, it appeared that six types of social ties might be identified (Weiss, 1973, 1974a). In this study, a "type" was distinguished if it provided elements to well-being not available from other "types" of relationships. Henderson's work, however, makes it appear more reasonable to propose that there are just four distinct types of social ties (Henderson, in press).

The empirical question of how many "types" of relationship may be usefully distinguished leads quickly to the theoretical question of what would be the essential characteristic of relationships of the same type. And here we quickly encounter terminological difficulties. The terms we use in characterizing relationships in ordinary speech may not exactly match the essential properties of the relationships. This is most evident, perhaps, with the term *friend.* A friend may be an intimate companion, an occasional companion toward whom there are feelings of loyalty and affection, or a kind of ally in the battles of everyday life who is now and again called on for help. The term *friend* means that a tie exists not based on kinship or collaboration, but only on positive feelings—and these feelings may be of different sorts.

Ordinary speech uses social-structure terms to refer to relationships. The social basis for our relationship is what is indicated by the terms *brother, colleague,* and *friend.* What actually holds us together, however, is only imperfectly specified by these terms. My brother and I may work together, or we may not; we may serve as companions to one another, or we may not; we may or may not be intimates. We need another set of terms to refer to the bonds that unite each participant in the relationship.

Relationships and Bonds

Observation supports the very reasonable surmise that the bonds that maintain relationships are roughly associated with the social-structural characterization of relationships. The bond in friendships is likely to be the expectation of gratifying companionship, developed from the belief that a community of interests exists. The bond in work relationships is likely to be linked to responsibilities based on commitment to some joint project. But there is no necessary association between relationships, understood in social-structure terms, and bonds. In most marriages, one of the bonds is emotional attachment, an emotional organization such that the other's accessibility fosters feelings of security. But even apart from marriages of convenience, there are marriages—not many, to be sure—in which husbands and wives, while fond of each other, live entirely independent lives; and there are new marriages in which one or both of the spouses have emotionally not yet left home.

Bonds would seem to have four important characteristics. The first is the basis for engagement in the relationship that is associated with them. Bonds would appear to vary in the degree to which this basis is motivational. Work-related collaboration tends, for example, to be largely prescribed, whereas friendships are usually maintained because the participants want to maintain them. Insofar as the basis is motivational, it might be expected to vary with the character of the bond. The motivation for maintaining friendships would be different from the motivation for maintaining work relationships.

Second, bonds have associated with them assumptions regarding the nature of the relationship. These assumptions include beliefs about the feelings and behaviors appropriate to the relationship, beliefs about the requests each participant can appropriately make of the other, and beliefs about the provisions each participant can reasonably expect to receive.

Third, different bonds give rise to different relational events, the specific happenings between the participants. The content of one relationship will be different from that of another. The steady, unconstrained companionship of a friendship is a development different from the occasional companionable episodes that occur in a work relationship. Relationships organized around different bonds are likely to have different histories and to follow different courses from beginning to end.

Finally, we might expect that different bonds will make available different provisions. In some measure the motivations for engaging in relationships are grounded in expectations of gains from the relationships, and so there is a linkage between provisions and the reasons for engagement. But there are provisions made by particular bonds not closely related to the reasons for engagement. For example, work relationships, engaged in for instrumental reasons, also provide support for a sense of competence and worth and confer the benefits of companionship.

Clearly there are many discrete bonds, many bases for engaging in social relationships. But not all these bonds fit together well. The bonds linking parent to child, including as they may parental identification with the child, sense of the child as an extension of self, as well as some measure of companionship, do not intermesh well with the bonds linking friend to friend, which include focus on common interests, sense of shared membership in a larger community, feelings of mutual loyalty, and many other elements. There are elements in common, to be sure—but the cluster is quite different.

We might now ask what different clusters of bonds can be identified or, in other words, what "types" of relationships? (It is, of course, part of this question to ask whether types can be usefully identified, that is, whether bonds do cluster in particular ways rather than associating themselves randomly.) A first attempt at answering this question was the study of individuals who had close relationships but were without community ties and individuals who had community membership but were without close relationships. This study found that individuals whose marriages had ended and who were in consequence without a close and intimate relationship to another adult were lonely, even though they had active, effective friendship ties. It was also found that nonworking wives whose marriages were intact but who, because of change of residence, were without access to an accepting community of friends or family tended to feel isolated and lonely, although their loneliness was different from that of the separated or divorced (Weiss, 1974b). A conclusion drawn from these observations was that the provisions of close and intimate relationships are distinct from those of the community of friends or family (or the community found at work) and that each makes an independent contribution to well-being. To put this another way, the bonds to be seen at work in close, intimate relationships (such as marriage) are different from those that sustain ties to the community, whether it is the community of friends or family or the community found at work. Our respondents found the provisions of each sort of bond essential to their well-being.

With this demonstration that in the instance of these two relationships (one close, intimate; the other a relationship with someone who is a fellow member of a community) there seemed not to be overlap in provisions and, therefore, in some essential bonds, it seemed reasonable to try to identify other relationships in which distinct bonds might be found. I proposed a set of six relationships that were distinct, each from the others, in the bonds they contained. These were:

1. *Relationships of attachment:* Relationships that were organized around a bond that was itself a development of early attachment to parents, now marked by its being established with someone understood as a peer and characterized by the presence of the other, its fostering of feelings of comfort and security.
2. *Affiliative relationships:* Relationships organized around a bond of alliance based on recognition of shared interests or similarity of circumstance. Associated with this bond might often be bonds of mutual acceptance and mutual loyalty.
3. *Kin-type alliances:* Relationships organized around bonds of loyalty in which shared interests play secondary roles or none at all.
4. *Collaborative relationships:* Relationships organized around work-related bonds—bonds whose premise is shared commitment to the achievement of some goal.
5. *Nurturant relationships:* Relationships organized around investment in another's well-being.
6. *Help-receiving relationships:* Relationships organized around acceptance of the other figure as a source of support and guidance.

Henderson's recent survey study (in press) made it possible for him to examine the independent contribution of the first four of these relationships to well-being. A factor analysis of his data conducted by his colleague Duncan-Jones suggested strongly that affiliative relationships, kin-type alliances, and collaborative relationships could be considered a single category without significantly affecting the study's findings. This suggests, in turn, that affiliative relationships and kin-type alliances may simply be different ways of establishing linkages to a community: Affiliative relationships base such linkages on common interest or concern and carry with them limited commitments to continuity, while kin-type alliances for the most part base such linkages on family membership and carry with them virtually unlimited commitment to continuity.

But what of work relationships? Here, pilot work already alluded to has been useful. It would appear that work, insofar as it takes place within a large organization, provides a social world parallel to that of the nonwork community, a social world in which the same bonds may enter into new relationships. Almost all work relationships, however, include among their bonds the sense of membership in the community of the organization. Working in a large organization brings with it linkages to a community—based, now, not on common interest or on family membership, but simply on shared membership in the organization.

In the world of work—insofar as work takes place within large organizations—bonds appear in contexts and combinations different from those with which they are associated in the nonwork world. In consequence, the relationships they establish are quite different. Of special significance in the world of work is the relationship with the boss. Here the underlying bond in the relationship is, initially, a hierarchical imposition: Having a boss comes with the job. But rather quickly, it would seem, this fosters in many individuals the kind of transference feeling that is the primary bond in help-receiving relationships, that is, relationships with counselors or other professional helpers. The different context, however, produces a quite different relationship.

Transference feelings, in help-receiving relationships, are feelings based on early experiences with awesomely powerful parents. In adults' relationships with figures they understand to be more capable than they—possessed of greater knowledge and power—feelings appropriate to early relationships with parents are elicited. In the presence of priests, counselors—or bosses—adults may display deference, feel uncertain, and become somewhat awed. In relationships with counselors, where there is the understanding that the counselor is committed to the realization of the clients' goals, transference feelings may foster feelings of security: Someone of special competence is on the clients' side. But in relationships with bosses, where there may be no such understanding, subordinates' transference feelings may foster insecurity as well as security. Here, everything depends on whether the boss is believed to be an ally or a real or potential enemy. Indeed, if a boss seen as strong and effective is also considered hostile, the work situation may become nearly intolerable.

In most work situations bosses are seen as conditional allies: on an individual's side only as long as the individual does a good job. In consequence, some individuals, to win the boss's approval, are driven to prodigies of effort. They come early and leave late, skip lunch hours, and take work home. They are not working merely for a raise or promotion; rather, they are working for the emotional security that is obtainable by having the boss as ally. For this, any amount of effort is justifiable. (There are, of course, other reasons for working hard, for example, interest in the work.)

Where there is no boss, or where the boss is seen as without power, but there is available a coherent and potentially sustaining community of similarly placed others, affiliative relationships may become the primary source of security. In this circumstance the work group can assume great power. Maintaining membership in the community of fellow workers would then be of critical importance for security at work. Work relationships might be continued off the job, might extend into after-work coffees or beers, and might even turn into friendship commitments of individuals' nonwork lives. Work relationships might well become the basis for social life.

Conclusions About Emotional Support

First, we might surmise that there are four—not six—types of relationships, each different from the others in the bonds that constitute its core. There are (1) relationships organized around attachments; (2) relationships organized around linkages to a community, whether it be a community of friends, of family, or of fellow workers; (3) relationships organized around investments in the well-being of another, ordinarily one's own children; and (4) relationships organized around a transference-associated acceptance of someone as a valid source of support and guidance. Second, in this list of conclusions, we might surmise that the work within organizations provides an inventory of potential relationships within any of which particular bonds may be established, but that it is likely that while relationships with most co-workers will be organized around bonds of shared interest, rather in the manner of friendships, relationships with bosses are likely to be organized around the transference-associated bond established with security-controlling figures.

Emotional support is a term that can refer to many different elements that are likely to be found in many different relationships. Not only do different relationships sustain different bonds, but any particular relationship is likely to carry within it more than a single bond and so to provide more than a single form of emotional support. Friends provide a sense of augmentation, insofar as their efforts are supportive of one's own, but they also provide reassurance of worth, by their acceptance, and provide affirmation by their listening and responding; relationships with one's children provide a rationale for one's continued striving, a sense of continuity through time, an opportunity for reliving and mastering unsatisfactory early experiences of one's own, and so on. Furthermore, different social milieu—the contrast of the world of work and the world of home and family is a contrast of milieu—make for different kinds of relationships in which particular bonds may be combined differently. In the world of work, for example, the transference-associated bond is not necessarily associated with a sense of fundamental alliance, as tends to be the case in the nonwork world.

From this perspective, to explain how social ties provide emotional support is tantamount to explaining what social ties are and how they function. There is, however, another and somewhat more restricted way of thinking about emotional support. This is to ask what relationships are appealed to when individuals find themselves under extraordinary stress. Here a relationship would provide "emotional support" only insofar as the relationship could be relied on to maintain or to reestablish the equilibrium of individuals under stress.

Yet even here, relationships of many sorts may be seen as providing emotional support. Relationships organized around attachment,especially marriage, are, of course, appealed to. The spouse ordinarily knows both the individual and the context of the stress, is felt to be allied with the individual, can provide reassurance and, by displaying empathy, a sense of being augmented. It should be noted, however, that not all spouses prove effective as providers of emotional support: Some are not sufficiently "in tune" with their partners to foster a sense of augmentation. In addition to the spouse, individuals under stress may call on affiliative figures, especially, it would seem, old friends with whom they feel themselves to be going through life, as well as figures with whom transference feelings are associated, such as counselors.

Even in this more limited view of the meaning of emotional support, it turns out to be a demanding task to describe the ways in which emotional support may be provided by social ties. It is wrong to suppose, as has sometimes been done, that social ties of any sort provide some unitary benefit that can be called *emotional support.* In addition, to focus simply on emotional support is to neglect that very important and as yet largely unexplored aspect of relationships: their costs. This, too, must at some point be studied.

References

Bradburn, N., and Caplovitz, D. *Reports on Happiness.* Hawthorne, N.Y.: Aldine, 1965.

Burnand, G. "The Natue of Emotional Support." *British Journal of Psychiatry,* 1969, *115,* 139-148.

Campbell, A., Converse, P., and Rogers, W. *The Quality of American Life.* New York: Russell Sage Foundation, 1976.

Caplan, G. *Support Systems and Community Mental Health.* New York: Behavioral Publications, 1974.

Cobb, S. "Social Support as a Moderator of Life Stress." *Psychosomatic Medicine,* 1976, *38* (5), 300-314.

Cooley, C. H. *Social Organization.* New York: Scribner's, 1909.

Dewey, J. *Human Nature.* New York: Holt, Rinehart and Winston, 1922.

Freud, S. *Civilization and Its Discontents.* (J. Riviere, Trans.) New York: Cape and Smith, 1930.

Henderson, A. S. "Social Relationships, Adversity, and Neurosis: Evidence for a Protective Effect in a Prospective Study." *British Journal of Psychiatry,* in press.

Homans, G. *The Human Group.* New York: Harcourt Brace Jovanovich, 1950.

House, J. S. *Work Stress and Social Support.* Reading, Mass.: Addison-Wesley, 1981.

LeBon, G. *The Crowd.* New York: Macmillan, 1896.

Mead, G. H. *Mind, Self, and Society.* Chicago: University of Chicago Press, 1934.

Shils, E. A., and Janowitz, M. "Cohesion and Disintegration of The Wehrmacht in World War II." *Public Opinion Quarterly,* 1948, *12,* 280-315.

Simmel, G. *The Sociology of Georg Simmel.* (K. H. Wolff, Ed. and Trans.) New York: Free Press, 1950.

Weiss, R. S. "The Contributions of an Organization of Single Parents to the Well-Being of its Members." *The Family Coordinator,* July 1973, pp. 321-326.

Weiss, R. S. *Loneliness: The Experience of Emotional and Social Isolation.* Cambridge, Mass.: M.I.T. Press, 1974a.

Weiss, R. S. "The Provisions of Social Relationships." In Z. Rubin (Ed.), *Doing Unto Others.* Englewood Cliffs, N.J.: Prentice-Hall, 1974b.

Chapter 6

Interaction of Crisis Theory, Coping Strategies, and Social Support Systems

Marie Killilea

Contemporary social support system theory has emerged from several streams of research and clinical practice, including psychoanalysis, studies on the psychology and strategies of coping, general system theory, and studies on stress, its effects on health and the development of the general disease prevention paradigm. Crisis theory and crisis intervention contributed knowledge now considered integral to social support system theory and practice. This convergence of crisis theory and social support system theory has extended the conceptual boundaries and significant parameters of crisis theory and practice in dealing with situations of acute stress and periods of psychosocial transition to include the management of chronic deficit situations.

In the 1980s there has been a veritable explosion of programs utilizing social support system concepts in health promotion and health education activities and in the clinical management of illness. This chapter will provide a historical perspective, along with a selective analysis, synthesis, and reconceptualization, of the evolution and interaction of these complex bodies of knowledge. It will also discuss their implications for program strategies to be initiated by professionals. Descriptions of recent innovative uses of social support systems in community mental health practice will be given, and future directions for research on the structure, processes, and functions of social support will be outlined. Of most importance, an action-research, evaluative intervention paradigm for testing various hypotheses about social support theory and community support systems programming in the management of chronic illness will be presented. In deficit situations such as chronic illness, this paradigm hypothesizes that cognitive resources, both individual and community, in conjunction with instrumental support will be relatively more effective than affective support in bettering the quality of life. The findings of such research efforts will provide enormously valuable information for refining our conceptual understandings of the mechanisms of social support and guiding the deployment of scarce professional and public resources in health and mental health services.

Crisis Theory

The idea of crisis as a period of upset is probably as old as time itself; the first recorded use of the term was in 1543. According to the *Oxford English Dictionary* (1971), a crisis is "the point in the progress of the disease when a change takes place which is decisive of recovery or death, also any marked or sudden change of symptoms" (p. 605). Caplan gives the most encompassing definition of crisis (1963) and the one most commonly used by mental health professionals, which can be summarized as: Crisis is a period of disequilibrium accompanied by psychological and physical distress of a relatively limited duration which temporarily taxes a person's ability to cope competently or to achieve mastery. Crises can be predictable or unpredictable. Some predictable crises are marriage, the birth of a child, and retirement. Some unpredictable crises are loss of a spouse, an accident, and change to a new job.

Crisis has situational elements that often predominate over the personality characteristics of the individual. The context of the event and its social components are as important as the biological and psychological components. The principle of homeostasis (Cannon, 1935) has been fundamental to an understanding of reactions to crises. Return to equilibrium sometimes comes spontaneously through the individual's own efforts, sometimes through intervention by family and friends, sometimes through intervention by a professional. Crises involve a time element that varies with each individual and situation but is usually of limited duration. The preexisting coping strategies of the individual are brought into play in a crisis. At the same time, people become open to influence; there is opportunity for leverage, for good or ill. However, professionals skilled at crisis intervention prefer to work through others rather than to assume immediate responsibility for the care of the affected individual. The desirable way of managing crisis is to maintain the individual in his or her ordinary social environment, building on the individual's psychological and social assets. The outcome of crisis can be positive and growth promoting or may have negative consequences for the individual.

Development of Theory and Practice. Of the many contributions of psychoanalytic theory to crisis theory, the most important have been the work of Bowlby (1952, 1969, 1973, 1977a, 1977b) on attachments and separation, Erikson (1950) on the "eight stages of man," and Erikson (1959) on the developmental and accidental crises throughout the life cycle.

Thomas (1909), an early pioneer in sociology, was interested in the relation between social organization and social personality. He identified the concept of crisis as an organizing idea for understanding individuals and their behavior in society. He cited control as the object of all purposeful activity and attention as "the mental attitude which takes note of the outside world and manipulates it; it is the organ of accommodation. It is associated with *habit* on the one hand and *crisis* on the other. . . . When habits are running smoothly, attention is relaxed; . . .

when something happens to disturb the run of habit, the *attention* is called into play and devises a new mode of behavior which will meet the crisis. That is, the attention establishes new and adequate habits, or it is its function to do so" (pp. 3-18). Thomas categorized several classes of crises as developmental and accidental, and as internal and external to the individual:

1. Exhaustion of game, intrusion of outsiders, defeat in battle, floods, drought.
2. Incidents of birth, death, adolescence, marriage.
3. Shadows, dreams, epilepsy, intoxication, swooning, sickness.
4. Conflict between individuals, and individual and group.

Thomas stated that crisis produces specialized occupations that represent classes of persons who have or profess special skill in dealing with crises: the medicine man, the priest, the lawgiver, the judge, the ruler, the physician, the teacher, the artist.

Much of the early work in developing crisis theory and intervention at the individual and community levels emerged from clinical work that dealt with situations of loss—for example, individual life crises such as bereavement and large-scale community crises such as polio epidemics, fires, and natural disasters. The earliest systematic research on loss of a spouse as a critical life crisis seems to have been done by Becker (1927) and Eliot (1930, 1932) at the University of Chicago. Eliot's work is of particular importance. Based on empirical studies of bereaved people, it established the loss of a spouse and the consequent bereavement and mourning reactions as a legitimate area of research. This pioneering work outlined both normal and pathological patterns of grief. Lindemann's classic analysis (1944) of the symptomatology and management of acute grief came out of his work with survivors, and the families of casualties, of the Coconut Grove fire in Boston. He identified the situational aspects of the disaster rather than the idiosyncratic characteristics of the affected persons as most important to the expression of their distress. Like Eliot, and in very similar terms and scope, Lindemann categorized and described normal and morbid patterns of grief reactions. The essential task for the psychiatrist in the management of grief, according to Lindemann, is to provide for the sharing of grief work by the individual, utilizing "auxiliary workers" such as social workers and clergy when necessary.

In addition to Thomas's ideas on crisis and the importance of the situation or context, other concepts pertinent to crisis theory include Park's views (1928) on the person in migration who is trying to live in two diverse cultural groups; Mannheim's (1943) concept of "crisis in valuation"; Ames' (1951) and Cantril's concepts (1950) of "the assumptive form world" —an individual's presently existing assumptions that serve as guides to action—of "hitches," and of "action" that leads to revisions of current value systems (also see Ittleson and Cantril, 1954); and Wallace's (1956) empirical studies on ambiguous and disorienting situations that can lead to rapid personality changes. These earlier contributions formed the conceptual models for Tyhurst's (1957) description of the dynamics of transition states. Tyhurst studied situations of intense, often sudden change—migration, retirement, civilian disaster, and so forth—in the lives of individuals. From his studies of individual responses to community disaster, he identified three phases, each with its own manifestations of distress and attempts at control: (1) a period of impact, (2) a period of recoil, and (3) a posttraumatic period of recovery. Appropriate intervention is phase specific. Among the principles outlined by Tyhurst for management of individuals in transitional states were to avoid removing the individual from his or her life situation whenever possible (a practice used in military psychiatry); and to intervene within a social system, that is, within a network of relationships.

Rediscovering lessons learned by Salmon and others (1929) in World War I and refined during World War II and the Korean War, military psychiatry elaborated many of the principles of community psychiatry that were later to be incorporated into civilian community mental health services. These principles were based implicitly on what has come to be known as crisis theory and crisis intervention and, as we now recognize, on social support systems theory and practice. They can be summarized (Talbott, 1969; Glass, 1971) as:

1. *Proximity:* "Treat 'em where they lie."
2. *Immediacy:* "Treat 'em right away."
3. *Expectancy:* "Expect rapid recovery and prompt return to duty." Diagnostic labels can exert significant influence on outcome; hence the origin of the terms *combat fatigue* and *exhaustion.* Situations of extreme stress will produce high casualties in normal persons as well as in those whose personalities may predispose them to break down.
4. *Community:* "A problem is often a group problem and not an individual problem." Recognizing that command is responsible for social and situational factors in military settings, psychiatrists as advisers to commanders attempted to alter the conditions under which soldiers trained, lived, worked, and fought.

Analogous lessons from experience with health and mental health casualties in a very different organization emerged from research done in the early years of the Peace Corps. A consistent pattern of adjustment by Peace Corps volunteers was identified:

1. *The crisis of arrival* in the host country, during the first month; *successful resolution:* reduction of anxiety through beginning work at place of local assignment.
2. *The crisis of engagement,* usually from the third to sixth month of volunteer service; *successful resolution:* a new sense of mastery after grappling with depression and with recognition of the naiveté of expectations.
3. *The crisis of acceptance,* about the eleventh to the thirteenth month; *successful resolution:* a new sense of self, providing a sense of fulfillment, after dealing with anger and boredom and after coming to understand and respect persons volunteer was dealing with.
4. *The crisis of re-entry,* usually beginning about three months before the end of service; *successful resolution:* volunteers began to look forward to discovering in their own society back home equally meaningful challenges after dealing with separation anxiety and depression about work undone.

The Peace Corps also found a consistent pattern of casualties occurring during the same time periods as the crisis phases. As an organizational entity, from its beginning, the Peace Corps recognized a responsibility to study the predictable psychological problems that a volunteer would experience overseas and to design support systems that would help volunteers to cope successfully, without early return to this country because of adjustment problems or psychiatric disorders (Menninger and English, 1965; English and Colmen, 1966).

Tyhurst (1957) mentions two other concepts that are of significance to both crisis theory and support system theory: the importance of ritual and of transitional communities. Van Gennep ([1908], 1961) analyzed ceremonies that accompany life crises; he was interested in their underlying pattern and order and in their function in people's lives. He identified three major types of ceremonies: those for transition (for example, betrothal), those for incorporation (marriage), and those for separation (funerals). There are ceremonials that announce and enact changes in the person's position in the life cycle and those that strengthen the identity of the group, reinforce beliefs, and reaffirm the social and political order. Curle (1947; Curle and Trist, 1947) describes transitional communities as mechanisms to help people deal with change and promote social reconnection. His examples are taken from the rehabilitation of prisoners of war.

Writing on the transition from engagement to marriage, Rapoport (1964) says, more generally, that major social role transitions are points at which the evolution of personality systems is linked to social processes and that such transitions provide new social environmental contexts within which the individual can relate to others. She conceptualizes a series of tasks specific to each role transition; accomplishment of these tasks affects the outcome of the transition. Parkes (1971) considers psychosocial transitions as natural experiments, with grief as the mediating factor. Thus, in psychosocial transitions as distinct from maturation, aging, and accidents, the need arises for the individual to restructure his ways of looking at the world and his plans for living in it, with the crucial factor being the way that the individual copes with the process of change. In his research on the processes of transition resulting from amputation, Parkes was puzzled by the great interest shown by some amputees in those who were worse off. He concluded that this interest was not sadistic but rather a source of encouragement that it is possible to cope well and cheerfully; the less well-off others were role models.

Weiss (1975, 1979) examined the social and psychological effects of ending a marriage and trying to manage alone in its aftermath. Persons in this situation often lack an intimate connection to another adult and often are burdened with the special demands and constraints of unshared responsibility for children. Many people learn to cope by relying on alternative support systems: family, friends, counselors, and organizations of peers in the same situation.

Thus, over time there has been an elaboration of crisis theory to include distinctions among:

1. *Acute crisis periods* of sudden onset, limited duration, and usually of considerable severity and distress that have an expectation upon resolution of a return to a stable identity and to the same precrisis environment.
2. *Transition periods* that disrupt previously maintained relationships, involving movement from one status to another, resulting in a changed identity and a changed assumptive world.
3. *Chronic deficit situations* in which a relational provision important to well-being is unattainable, with periodic acute upsets (Weiss, 1976).

Crisis Intervention Programs. From the beginning, theoreticians and practitioners in the crisis field have been interested in looking at individuals in crisis as part of family systems. There have been explorations of families under stress (Koos, 1946; Hill, 1949); a conceptual framework presented to study families in crisis (Parad and Caplan, 1960); patterns of parental adjustment to premature birth (Caplan, 1960; Kaplan and Mason, 1960; Caplan, Mason, and Kaplan, 1965); preventive intervention in individual and family crisis situations (Klein and Lindemann, 1961; Rapoport, 1963); normal crises, family structure, and mental health (Rapoport, 1963); and the treatment of families with mentally ill members (Langsley and Kaplan, 1968). Of particular interest is Caplan's (Rosenfeld and Caplan, 1954) work with Israeli children undergoing the stress of immigration and adaptation to a new country. In this work, Caplan and his colleagues began to develop techniques of mental health consultation, that is, a process of interaction between two professionals, a mental health specialist (the consultant) and a non-mental health specialist (consultee)—teacher, public health nurse, or social worker. The consultations centered on a current work problem, with the aim of improving the consultee's ability to handle the mental health dimensions of that and similar problems (Caplan, 1970). Coleman (1947, 1953, 1956) in the United States was developing a similar model.

Distinct from the development of specific crisis intervention techniques was the establishment of crisis intervention facilities organized independently or as designated components of other facilities, staffed by mental health professionals, and offering early access and brief treatment to all types of nonhospitalized persons (Jacobson, 1974). The Wellesley Human Relations Service was a laboratory organized in 1948 by Erich Lindemann to test in a community the concepts of crisis theory and techniques of crisis intervention, as well as the mental health consultation model of Caplan, Lindemann, and their colleagues. The Wellesley program was an early prototype of the community mental health center proposed under the 1963 federal community mental health center legislation, with its requirements, among others, of emergency services and consultation for and education of community caregivers and agencies. The theoretical model of crisis theory and the techniques of crisis intervention and mental health consultation, within a stated frame of reference of primary, secondary, and tertiary prevention (Caplan, 1964, 1970), were the underpinnings of the new national thrust of community-based services.

Coping

Coping is a process of dealing with and attempting to overcome threat, stressful situations, and problems in such a way as to be protective of comfort and health. People develop from their own experience a repertoire of coping skills. These coping skills may draw on an individual's inner psychological resources or may serve to mobilize external social resources.

Over the years a number of investigators have made substantial contributions to our understanding of the tasks and challenges that are posed by life transitions and crises. There is now a framework for conceptualizing the field, and there are also systematic coping inventories. These inventories include descriptions of (1) the tasks embedded in life transitions and crises; (2) feasible strategies for coping; (3) ways to implement these strategies that have some degree of specificity; (4) the role of the social environment, especially of naturally occurring social supports as critical variables in determining the effectiveness of coping efforts.

The broad tasks for coping with a range of stressful circumstances have been outlined (Hamburg, 1981) as the ability to contain distress within limits that are personally tolerable, to maintain self-esteem, to preserve interpersonal relationships and a sense of belonging to a valued group, to meet the conditions and demands of the new situation, and to prepare for the future. For each of these major tasks, multiple strategies must be employed. The particular array of strategies chosen will reflect not only the developmental and family history of the person but also the specific circumstances surrounding each crisis or major psychosocial transition. Cultural and subcultural influences also play a role (White, 1974; Hamburg and Killilea, 1979).

Development of Theory and Practice

Freud ([1915], 1957) described "the work of mourning" after loss. Janis (1951, 1958), in his development of the techniques of emotional inoculation in situations of threat and danger, proposed an analogous concept, "the work of worry." The adequacy of "worry work" is affected by both environmental conditions, for example, exposure to information about the impending danger, and personality predisposition elements, for example, the individual's motivation to pay attention to warnings. When worry work is successful, it leads to action and mastery. Janis used these ideas in his work on the in-hospital management of acute stress in patients about to undergo surgery. Hahn's educational methods of character building (James, 1957) extended the capacity of individuals to withstand stress and master future crises. These methods proved effective in increasing the survival at sea of British mariners whose ships were sunk during World War II and were also the founding principles of Outward Bound (an organization formed to teach youth survival skills in the wilderness, which could then be applied to their everyday lives). Caplan and Cadden (1964) developed a pamphlet for Peace Corps volunteers that emphasized principles of anticipatory guidance in managing problems of adjustment overseas. Egbert and others (1964) demonstrated the differential utility of affective support and cognitive guidance in patients' recovery from surgery. Lazarus (1966) and Lazarus, Averill, and Opton (1974) delineated the psychology of coping and the importance of cognitive coping mechanisms in adaptation to stress, including the costs and benefits of denial—"working fictions" (Lazarus, 1981).

Studies of hospital wards with burn patients (Hamburg, Hamburg, and de Goza, 1953) and polio patients (Visotsky and others, 1961) identified consistent patterns for coping with severe illnesses and their resulting deficits. Coping was accomplished through a variety of means, with each stage of illness and disability having a number of strategies specific to it. Most persons had good psychological recovery over several years, with an interplay between physical progress and the use of psychological, family, and community resources. In problems of severe disability, group membership—for example, in a family, a ward group of other patients and staff, or a home community, especially a community of close friends—was an important factor in their resolution. The patterns of involvement varied for any one individual over time and from individual to individual.

This work with illness and disability led to research that developed typologies of coping strategies for specific normal life situations, for instance, entering early adolescence, entering high school, or moving away from home to go to college or to take a first job (Hamburg and Adams, 1967; Hamburg, 1974; Hamburg, Adams, and Brodie, 1976).

In studies of coping, crisis theory, and crisis intervention, cognitive processes have been identified as critical to successful adaptation to stress. The principal mechanisms can be summarized as:

1. Appraisal and reappraisal, especially in situations of threat and danger.
2. Seeking of new information specific to the task and situation, development of new perspectives and new alternatives for dealing with the situation, learning through the pooling of information from others.
3. Seeking appropriate role models whose behavior can be adopted or adapted.
4. Referring to analogous past experiences that have been mastered in order to gain reassurance that they are similar to the new experience that can also be mastered.
5. Seeking to link the stressful new event and present self-image with past functioning and social competencies.
6. Obtaining reliable feedback about behaviors, plans, and goals.
7. Modifying level of aspiration, acquisition of growth-promoting skills (Hamburg and Killilea, 1979).

An individual's cognitive resources thus include internalized value systems, the capacity to send and receive signals for help, inner psychological resources such as memories and imagination, the capacity to accomplish worry work, information regarding the problem or predicament, information regarding alternative coping mechanisms and the location of technical assistance, perceptions of the availability of positive emotional and instrumental support, perceptions of the adequacy of psychological and social resources to present need, and knowledge about and social competence in the mobilization and use of social resources. An additional cognitive resource would be the capacity to use the self in service to others, thereby reinforcing one's own identity and gaining support for behavior change and maintenance of effort.

In situations of everyday stress and strain Pearlin and Schooler (1978, 1979) identify the following types of coping responses (perceptions, behaviors) in marriage, parenting, and work: (1) responses that modify the situation by direct action, including self-reliance and seeking the advice of others; (2) responses that control the meaning of the problem or situation, including the use of positive comparisons with others, selective ignoring of certain elements in the problem, and substitution of rewards; and (3) responses that seek to manage the stress and minimize the resulting discomfort, including a reliance on cultural beliefs that convert endurance of unavoidable hardship into a moral virtue, passive forbearance, and optimistic faith. Pearlin and Schooler found that coping mechanisms in which persons interact with others to solve problems were most effective in the intimate roles of spouse and parent. Coping mechanisms of psychological distancing from the problem were less efficacious, although commonly used, in dealing with more impersonal problems over which people perceived themselves as having little control, that is, problems growing out of their roles in the larger environment (for example, the workplace).

Folkman and Lazarus (1980), in an analysis of coping in a community sample of middle-aged persons, found consistent patterns of both emotion-focused and problem-focused coping strategies for dealing with stressful events of daily living. The context of the event and how the event is appraised were the most important influences on the individual's choice of coping mechanisms. Caplan (1981), reviewing a large body of data on the mastery of stress and its implications for the prevention of physical and mental illnesses, identified the main benefits of external social support resources as the lowering of emotional tension and the supplementation of a stressed individual's eroded cognitive and problem-solving capacities.

Social Support Theory

Some people can readily tolerate what for others is overwhelming stress (Engel, 1968). Factors that influence the impact of stress include: (1) a person's biological and psychological characteristics; (2) an individual's coping strategies; and (3) the social and environmental context of the life event (Hamburg and Killilea, 1979).

Current approaches to the study of stress and illness are founded on the classic contributions of Cannon (1929) on bodily changes in pain, hunger, fear, and rage; of Selye (1946) on the general adaptation syndrome and the diseases of adaptation; and of Wolff (1950) on life stress and bodily disease. Building on this work, Cassel (1974a, 1974b), a social epidemiologist and major theoretician in the development of concepts of social support, postulated that while psychosocial processes could be stressors, they could also be buffers against the effects of stress and, therefore, could be protective and beneficial. In his Wade Hampton Frost lecture on the contribution of the social environment to host resistance to disease, Cassel (1976) presented an enlarged concept of the environment: Moving from a concern with the physical and microbiological alone, he set forth a view of the environment that also includes the social, particularly the presence or absence of members of the same species. In this view of the environment, subgroups become important as communicators of information that can act to buffer the individual from the ill effects of stress generated in strange, complex, and often hostile situations. Cassel pointed out the nonspecificity of cause and effect in stress-related illnesses and the importance for the individual of the interaction between high stress and social support. He urged that basic research be conducted on this interaction rather than on the unilateral effects of stress and that research be initiated on intervention strategies to increase social support for individuals in high-stress situations.

Reviews by Cobb (1976), Kaplan, Cassel, and Gore (1977), Dean and Lin (1977), the President's Commission on Mental Health (1978), and Hamburg and Killilea (1979) of research findings conclude that social support may play a major role in modifying the deleterious effects of stress on health, in influencing the use of health services, and in affecting other aspects of health behavior such as adherence to medical regimens. The mechanisms by which social support exerts its effects are as yet unclear. Among several hypotheses are those that postulate that social support has (1) a direct effect on health; (2) a buffering or mediating effect on the impact of stress; (3) enhances the development of coping strategies that promote social competence in dealing with stressful situations.

Development of Theory and Practice. There are currently two main operational definitions of social support: one given by Gerald Caplan and another by Sidney Cobb. In a book on the utility of support systems in community mental health practice, Caplan (1974) states that social support systems are attachments between individuals and between individuals and groups that promote mastery; offer guidance about the field of relevant forces, expectable problems, and methods of dealing with them; and provide feedback about behavior that validates identity and fosters improved competence. Cobb (1976), in a paper on social support as a moderator of the ill effects of life stress on the health of individuals, states that social support is information that tells a person that he or she is loved, valued, and part of a network of communication and mutual obligation. The operative words in Caplan's definition are *attachments, guidance,* and *mastery*; the emphases are structural and functional. The operative words in Cobb's definition are *network, communication,* and *mutual obligation*; the emphases are on the processes of social support.

Attachment theory, a major conceptual foundation of social support theory, states that positive interaction with trusted others is essential for well-being (Bowlby, 1969, 1973, 1977a, 1977b). Hansell (1976) states that a person's seven essential attachments are to:

1. Food, oxygen, and information of requisite variety.
2. A clear concept of self-identity held with conviction.
3. Persons, at least one, in persisting interdependent contact, which occasionally approximates intimacy.

4. Groups, at least one, comprised of individuals who regard this person as a member.
5. Roles, at least one, that offer a context for achieving dignity and self-esteem through performance.
6. Money or purchasing power to participate in an exchange of goods and services in a society specializing in such exchanges.
7. A comprehensive system of meaning, satisfying sets of notions that clarify experience and define ambiguous events.

Weiss similarly postulates (1969, 1974) that each person typically requires a set of relationships, of varying degrees of intensity during different phases of life, that provides not only meaningful attachment to significant others but also social integration in a network of common-interest relationships, an opportunity to nurture, reassurance of individual worth gained through the performance of a valued social role, a sense of reliable alliance with kin, and access to the obtaining of guidance from a trustworthy and authoritative person in times of stress. Weiss's formulation of the provisions of social ties as contributory to well-being, along with Bowlby's theory of mother-child attachment extended to adult relationships, was the theoretical grounding for an Australian epidemiological study of social support and neurosis (Henderson, 1977; Henderson and others, 1978; Henderson and others, 1981).

A major contributing stream of theory and research on social support has been the largely European anthropological and sociological studies, particularly from the University of Manchester, on the structure, processes, and functions of personal social networks. These include Barnes' study (1954) of class and committees in a Norwegian island parish, Bott's analysis (1957) of the division of labor in marriage as a function of embeddedness in different types of social networks, and Mitchell's research (1969) on the utility of social networks as adaptation mechanisms for tribal Africans migrating to urban centers.

The structural characteristics of social networks vary along several dimensions, such as size, strength of ties, number of independent contacts among persons in the network, clustering, symmetry (reciprocity), congruence of values, and reachability of members (their nearness, distance, availability for mobilization). These dimensions have been increasingly studied as factors contributing to well-being or ill health for individuals in specific situations and life predicaments. The number of studies is formidable; a representative sample of recent studies would include Gottlieb (1975) on natural support systems of subgroups of adolescent males; Tolsdorf (1976) on social networks in an adult male schizophrenic population; Hammer, Makiesky-Barrow, and Gutwirth (1978) on social networks and schizophrenia; Colletta (1979) on support systems after divorce; Berkman and Syme (1979) on social networks, host resistance, and mortality; Lin and others (1979) on social networks in a Chinese-American population; Mueller (1980) on social network characteristics and psychiatric disorders, particularly depression; Cochran and Brassard (1979) on child development and personal social networks of parents; Colletta and Gregg (1981) on adolescent mothers' social networks and their vulnerability to stress; Gerstel and Riessman (1981) on social networks of the separated and divorced; Goldberg (1981) on social networks of older married women; McQueen and Celentano (1981) on social support and problem drinking among women; Belle (1982) on the context of the lives of women in stress and on its relationship to depression.

Hammer (1979) distinguishes social support (function) from social network (structure). She advocates the study of structural variables in personal social networks—the complex patterns of connection among individuals in the network—rather than simply the context or the quality of the relationships. Pattison (1977, 1979), on the basis of empirical social science research and clinical intervention studies, identified three types of networks: essentially normal, neurotic-type, and psychotic-type. They could be distinguished on the parameters of number of persons, types of actors involved (family members, friends, neighbors, colleagues), and links among them; positive or negative feelings generated by interactions; instrumentality of interactions; and degrees of reciprocity.

Kahn (1979) describes the social network as a "social

convoy," changing over the life cycle and with the needs of the situation. Social networks can be both a source of direct help and a source of linkage to other resources. Tolsdorf (1976) conceptualized the idea of "network orientation," that is, the individual's set of beliefs, attitudes, and expectations concerning the usefulness of network members in helping him or her cope with a life problem. In crises, a small, dense network with strong ties may be most valuable. At times of psychosocial transition, a low-density network with relatively weak ties–identified by Granovetter (1973) as "the strength of weak ties"–may be most useful (Walker, MacBride, and Vachon, 1977). Social ties can also support undesirable behavior or be burdensome and preventive of change. It remains unclear whether it is better to have many diverse relationships or whether a single, intimate, confiding relationship is sufficient to be protective of well-being (Brown, Bhrolchain, and Harris, 1975; Henderson and others, 1978; Porritt, 1979). Weiss (1976), in his ongoing attempt to understand the role of social ties in people's lives and to suggest appropriate kinds of help in the absence of one or more kinds of social relationships, states that "crisis occurs on first awareness of imminence of loss; if loss cannot be avoided, then transition ensues; transition may in part give rise to a life organization which is in some respect deficient" (p. 215). In crisis situations, according to Weiss, general support from a person not in crisis who allies himself with the distressed individual is probably most helpful; in transition states, in addition to general support, orientation, guidance, and access to an accepting community are probably best; in deficit situations, people seem to need a continuing, problem-focused, social support system to help them deal with specific problems resulting from inadequacies in their life organization.

From these and other studies, the processes of social networks have been classified as emotional, cognitive, and instrumental, based on reciprocity and exchange. The functions of social networks have been identified as maintaining social identity, providing emotional support, providing material aid and tangible services, providing access to information, and providing access to new social contacts and new social roles (Walker,

MacBride, and Vachon, 1977). In addition to personal social networks, other structures that provide social support functions in our lives are families (Caplan, 1976a); neighborhood helping networks—including natural helpers; mutual help groups; "alternative" services, often provided by those who are veterans of the problem or predicament; and community institutions with other primary societal functions such as schools, churches, workplaces, and hospitals (President's Commission on Mental Health, 1978; Hamburg and Killilea, 1979).

The development of social support systems theory and practice has also been stimulated by the following diverse bodies of knowledge:

- Sociometric study of small groups (Moreno, 1941), theory and research on social structure (Merton, 1949), and structural anthropology (Lévi-Strauss, 1963, 1969).
- Field theory (Lewin, 1935, 1951) and the concept of ecology that focuses on transactions between, and the reciprocal influences of, the individual and his environment (Murray, 1938; Barker, 1968; Bronfenbrenner, 1977).
- Research in the workplace on the person-environment fit, that is, the goodness of fit between the needs of the person and the supplies of the person's environment, and between the abilities of the person and the demands of the environment (French and Kahn, 1962; Kahn and others, 1964; Kahn and Quinn, 1970; French, 1973; French, Rodgers, and Cobb, 1974; LaRocco, House, and French, 1980).
- Research on the impact of stressful life events on health and well-being (Meyer, 1951; Holmes and Rahe, 1967; Maddison and Walker, 1967; Paykel and others, 1969, 1980; Dohrenwend and Dohrenwend, 1974, 1981; Rabkin and Struening, 1976; Brown and Harris, 1978); the effects of social support (Nuckolls, Cassel, and Kaplan, 1972; Meyers, Lindenthal, and Pepper, 1975; Eaton, 1978; Andrews and others, 1978; Lin, Dean, and Ensel, 1979; Frydman, 1981; Eckenrode and Gore, 1981); and the development of instruments to provide contextual measures of life events (Brown and Harris, 1978; Brown, 1981), of social interaction (Henderson, Byrne, and

Duncan-Jones, 1981), and of social behavior and social performance and their effects on the household (Gruenberg and Sluss, 1980; Platt and others, 1980).

- Studies of social space: therapeutic communities (Jones, 1953); human adaptation, human milieus, and social climate (Moos, 1974); networks and places (Fischer and others, 1977); and the neighborhood context of helping networks (Wellman and Leighton, 1979; Warren, 1981).
- Studies that have examined health status in relation to a community's level of social and economic stability/instability and of social integration/disorganization (Stout and others, 1964; Bruhn and others, 1966; Nesser, Tyroler, and Cassel, 1972; James and Kleinbaum, 1976).
- Epidemiological research on the availability of social support and mortality (Berkman and Syme, 1979) and on social support and neurosis, the major finding in the latter being the importance of the perceived adequacy of support (Henderson, Byrne, and Duncan-Jones, 1981).
- Research on the pathways to care and factors affecting utilization of health services, particularly the influence of the lay referral and lay treatment network (Freidson, 1960, 1961; Liberman, 1965; McKinlay, 1973; Gottlieb, 1976) and the self-care movement (Levin, Katz, and Holst, 1976).
- Identification of the helper therapy principle (Riessman, 1965) and of the non-role related "natural helper" in communities (Collins, 1973).
- Research and programming on informal helpers and the kinds of help they offer (Katz, 1965, 1970; Silverman, 1966, 1967, 1970; Shapiro, 1969, 1971; Collins and Pancoast, 1976; Salber, Beery, and Jackson, 1976; Leutz, 1977; Vallé and Mendoza, 1978; Vallé and Vega, 1980; Froland and others, 1981).
- Research on the prevention of chronic disability in mental disorders through the reorganization of services, linking the hospital and the community—preventing the chronic social breakdown syndrome. The concept of the social breakdown syndrome looks for causes in a person's social relationships. This syndrome differs from deterioration due to chronicity

and from institutional neuroses (MacMillan, 1957; Milbank Memorial Fund, 1958; Gruenberg, 1967; Gruenberg and Archer, 1979).

- The use of personal and social networks in psychiatric practice, including family therapy, and in the design of mental health services (Fine, 1973; Speck and Attneave, 1973; Erickson, 1975; Hansell, 1976, 1977; Tolsdorf, 1976; Garrison, Kulp, and Rosen, 1977; Garrison, 1978; Pattison, 1977; Pattison and others, 1979; Bordow and Porritt, 1979).
- Research on social networks as coping resources in emergency situations, for everyday support, and for the management of chronic illness (Litwak and Szelenyi, 1969; Nuckolls, Cassel, and Kaplan, 1972; Crogg, Lipson, and Levine, 1972; de Araujo and others, 1973; Finlayson, 1976; Capildeo, Court, and Rose, 1976; Bordow and Porritt, 1979).
- Family and community management of schizophrenia in collaboration with professionals and institutions (Fairweather, Sanders, and Maynard, 1969; Sanders, 1972; Test and Stein, 1976a, 1976b; Budson, 1978; Turner and Ten Hoor, 1978; Hatfield, 1979).

Social and Community Support System Programming. The early pioneers in crisis theory and crisis intervention were probably not aware that their work ultimately would contribute to development of a social support systems model. For example, buried in Lindemann's paper (1944) on grief was a key concept that later became a critical component of the continuing Harvard work on bereavement: "He [the bereaved person] will have to find persons around him whom he can use as 'primers' for the acquisition of new patterns of conduct" (p. 147). This key social support systems concept was the cornerstone of the Boston widow-to-widow program (Silverman, 1967). In offering mental health consultation to some bishops of the Episcopal Church, Caplan developed the Bishop-to-Bishop program in which an experienced bishop became a consultant to a new bishop, the consultee. In reviewing the implementation of the program with these bishops, Caplan discovered the spontaneous occurrence among some of them of a complementary role reversal, each taking turns at the consultant and consultee roles. Taking advantage of this serendipitous happening, Caplan developed, within the House of Bishops, a systematic intraorganizational support system (Caplan, 1972).

Silverman's development (1970, 1976) of the person-to-person (veteran widow reaching out to new widow in the community) approach to helping people deal with the problems of bereavement and the transition to a new life organization was also influenced by the experience of such self-help and mutual help groups as Alcoholics Anonymous, which was founded as long ago as 1935. Mutual help groups as coping resources have proliferated in recent decades in the health field—for example, Recovery, Inc., for "nervous" people and mental patients; Mended Hearts, for persons who have had open heart surgery; TOPS (Take Off Pounds Sensibly), for overweight persons; and Make Today Count, for the terminally ill and their families (Killilea, 1976; Levy, 1976; Gussow and Tracy, 1976). According to Silverman (1978), these and other mutual help groups have been a response to:

1. The lack of socially sanctioned coping strategies—a lack that has resulted from dislocations in a time of rapid social change; for example, La Lêche League (breastfeeding), Widow-to-Widow, and C.O.P.E. (Coping with the Overall Pregnancy Experience).
2. Professional or institutional failure to meet the needs of particular client or patient groups, for example, Alcoholics Anonymous and National Alliance for the Mentally Ill (families of adult chronic schizophrenics).
3. The consequences of technological advances that prolong life in persons with chronic deficits without parallel attention to the quality of life, for example, Ostomy groups, Stroke Clubs, and Alzheimer's Senile Dementia Family Groups.

Mutual help groups make possible person-to-person exchanges that provide identification and reciprocity, access to a body of specialized information, an opportunity to share coping techniques based on realistic expectations for optimal functioning, an increased sense of worth by focusing on how *like* the members are to others in the same situation, reinforcement for change and maintenance of effort (feedback on performance), and an arena for advocacy and social change empowerment (subgroup activity is powerful in confronting stigma and choosing activity over passivity in the face of adverse conditions). These groups also provide an opportunity for educating others with similar problems, along with professionals and the public, and an opportunity to help others by giving concrete aid and serving as role models.

Some of the reasons for the increase in the number of mutual help groups concerned with chronic illnesses include the unknown etiology of many diseases, the rising prevalence of chronic diseases, the unpredictable course of some illnesses; ineffective or unreliable specific treatments, residual dysfunctions that limit an individual's activities, increased familial burdens, and gaps in or barriers to and/or inappropriate professional services.

Given the proliferation of mutual help groups, a look at the first mutual help effort in the medical care field might be instructive. In 1905, Joseph Pratt organized "classes" for tuberculosis patients in Boston. These were poor outpatients who remained at home and took bed rest in their tenements, on the roof or balcony or in the yard. They were called on at home by a "friendly visitor," sometimes a nurse, who provided information and guidance to the patient and his family about bed rest, cleanliness, and nutrition, as well as encouragement over the long haul of a tuberculosis patient's treatment. The patients met weekly in small groups, first in Pratt's offices and later in the outpatient department of Massachusetts General Hospital, where Pratt provided medical supervision and inspected the record books personally kept by the patients. These meetings spawned many of the practices now utilized in Alcoholics Anonymous and Weight Watchers, such as weigh-ins (in this case, rewards were given for gaining weight), sharing of information about successful coping strategies, testimonials from patients who were progressing, and visits from former members who had "graduated" and were now working. The financing of this work was provided by the Emmanuel Church of Boston, which also developed a social service department that found employment for the recovered patients (Pratt, 1907, 1908). Elliott Joslin, a contemporary of Pratt in Boston, adapted the class method to teach diabetic patients about the management of their condition (Proger, 1937).

Two aspects of Pratt's methods stimulated major health system changes. First, his use of the "friendly visitor" influenced Richard Cabot to establish the first formal hospital social service department at Massachusetts General Hospital (Proger, 1937). Second, his provision of health information by group instruction influenced William R. P. Emerson to initiate health education classes in schools for malnourished children and their mothers that were conducted by pediatricians and internists. Out of Emerson's activities there developed many of the school health programs of the modern era (Emerson, 1910, 1922; Pratt, 1922). In these pioneer programs we find a partnership and division of labor among patients, families, medical care providers, and community institutions. In chronic illnesses, this partnership is of crucial importance. The bedrock of this partnership is the recognition that the experts in the meaning of illness for the organization and quality of life are the sufferers and their families. They have experiential knowledge gained through struggle with their problems and, often, expertise gained through successful coping with their predicaments (Borkman, 1976).

Descriptions of recent innovative uses of social support systems in community mental health practice have been provided by Shapiro (1969, 1971) on communities of the alone in single-room-occupancy hotels; by Fairweather, Sanders, and Maynard (1969) on the Lodge model, a residential program for the mentally ill; by Curtis (1973) on new roles for mental health workers; by Caplan (1974) and Caplan and Killilea (1976) on support systems and mutual help, including descriptions of the Harvard Laboratory of Community Psychiatry's development and testing of models—for example, Weiss's Seminars for the Separated and Caplan's work in organizing support systems in the community in a time of war; by Collins and Pancoast (1976) on natural helping networks and prevention; by Hansell and

Willis (1977) on screening-linking-planning conferences in the outpatient treatment of schizophrenia; by Gartner and Riessman (1977), Katz and Bender (1976), Lieberman, Borman, and Associates (1979), and Silverman (1976, 1978, 1980) on self-help groups; by Turner and Ten Hoor (1978) on the National Institute of Mental Health Community Support Program for the chronically mentally ill; by Froland and others (1981) on informal helping networks and human services; and by Vallé and Mendoza (1978) and Vallé and Vega (1980) on Hispanic natural helping networks and linkages to formal resources.

The report of the President's Commission on Mental Health (1978) took cognizance of these developments and began its recommendations with a call to acknowledge the contributions of the natural networks to which people belong and on which they depend, as well as with a call for research on the nature and functions of social support. The commission's *Task Panel Report on Community Support Systems* was probably the first systematic presentation of current research findings on social support, with programmatic examples utilizing social and community support systems concepts, across many disciplines and fields. Most recently, Veroff, Douvan, and Kulka (1981; Veroff, Kulka, and Douvan, 1981) in a follow-up to the earlier study, *Americans View Their Mental Health* (Gurin, Veroff, and Feld, 1960), found a general shift between 1957 and 1976 in the adaptation styles of people across the life cycle. They noted a profound change in the degree to which people seek and use informal help—family, friends, mutual help groups, and "alternative" services—to deal with everyday problems of worry and periods of unhappiness. They speculate on whether these informal networks will be able to serve people well. This can only be determined after a variety of well-designed studies are completed.

Convergence of Crisis Theory and Social Support Theory

Explicit in crisis theory were many of the elements now considered integral to social support theory and practice. These elements include the individual's signaling of distress in order to mobilize help from significant others; the individual's expectation that he or she will receive comfort, support, consensual validation, advice, and concrete aid with tasks; the individual's suggestible state and accessibility to intervention by informal as well as formal caregivers during a crisis; the role played by learned skills, competencies, and cognitive coping strategies; and an outcome that can be either positive and growth promoting or fraught with negative consequences.

In the crisis theory model, then, the focus is on the individual and his family, on short-term events, and on current influences. The support systems model enlarges this framework to include social aggregates, continuing socioenvironmental relationships, and communication patterns. Both models explicitly focus on coping and mastery.

Based upon present knowledge, the conceptual boundaries of crisis theory have been extended to the more inclusive framework of social support systems theory (see Figure 1). This expanded conceptual model has many implications for program strategies to be initiated by professionals, including the following:

1. *"Working through others"*; for example, working through family, significant others, and social networks; veterans of the experience or predicament (Silverman, 1966); natural helpers who are not role related (Collins, 1973); role-related informal caregivers; and community institutions, both traditional and unconventional.
2. *"Helping the helpers to help"* (Caplan, 1972); for example, helping through mental health consultation; mental health collaboration (Caplan, 1980; Caplan and others, 1981); and "burden sharing" between professionals and informal caregivers (Sainsbury and Grad, 1962).
3. *"Supporting the supporters"* (Caplan, 1976b); for example, offering backup to informal helpers; convening informal helpers for sharing of coping mechanisms; linking of similar peers—person-to-person and family-to-family; sharing information about community resources; and providing technical assistance.
4. *"Models of articulation"* (President's Commission on Mental Health, 1978); for example, recognizing and respecting

Figure 1. Significant Parameters of Expanded Model

Crisis Model	*Social Support Systems Model*
• Crisis period in social context	• Stressful life event and its contextual meaning
• Individual, with significant others, especially family	• Individual and family in networks of social relationships
• Personality factors and individual and family values and norms	• Network orientation and individual, family, and social network patterns of help seeking and help receiving
• Coping strategies, individual and family, including signaling of distress	• Coping strategies, individual, family, and social network, including ways of mobilizing social resources
• Informal role-related caregivers	• Natural helpers who are not role related and community resource brokers
• Settings: home, agency	• Settings: home, neighborhood, church, workplace
• Community volunteers	• Mutual help groups, person-to-person and family-to-family networks] fellow sufferers and veterans of the experience
• Formal community institutions	• Informal community resources
• Crisis intervention: brief involvement; professional and not professional	• Social and community support systems programming: brief and long-term involvement; professional and not professional

boundaries; developing coordinate relationships; facilitating bidirectional referrals between formal and informal resources; dividing labor between formal and informal caregivers based on different sources of knowledge and competence; carrying out community planning for services development by using informal caregivers as key informants, as interviewers in community surveys, and on agency advisory boards; linking formal and informal resources.

5. *Evaluative intervention models*; for example, models for providing adjuncts to clinical practice—at point of acute crisis, during management of transitions, and during aftercare in chronic illness; facilitating behavior change and adherence to medical regimens (Hansell, 1976); conducting preventive trials (Gruenberg, 1980) in situations of acute

stress; programming of social and community support systems for management of chronic illness; catalyzing development of mutual aid groups and networks in communities; strengthening intraorganizational support systems in, for example, the workplace, schools, and religious denominations; diffusing information through natural helpers who employ their usual patterns of communication (Salber, Beery, and Jackson, 1976); empowering communities by transfer of knowledge and skills; and engaging in advocacy and public policy formulation.

Directions for Future Research

The preceding review of crisis theory, coping, and social support theory points to the fact that several streams of research and clinical practice are now converging: (1) basic biological research on responses to stress; (2) basic social science research on stressful life events and their contexts; (3) basic social science research on the structures, processes, and functions of social support; and (4) experimentation with models for management of crises, transitions, and chronic deficit situations —models that involve professionals, families, and both informal and formal social and community support systems.

In the development of crisis theory, conceptual principles emerged from clinical practice; research always trailed far behind. Crisis intervention programming always moved very far ahead of both theory and research. In the social support systems field, theory has emerged slowly and, for the most part, it has emerged from the social and biological sciences; multidisciplinary basic research had been keeping pace with practice. However, in a manner analogous to the development of crisis intervention programs, we are now beginning to see both theory and research overtaken by the growth of social support systems programming—programming for health promotion and health education activities, as well as for the clinical management of illnesses. This is occurring for various reasons. First, there is the rising pandemic of chronic illnesses, along with greater longevity due to successful medical treatment (Gruenberg, 1977; Kramer,

1980). Second, there have been increased transfer of responsibility from professionals and formal institutions to individuals and families for health promotion (emphasizing self-care and life-style modification) and increased emphasis on the care of the chronically ill at home and in the community. Third, there has been questioning and sometimes even rejection by individuals and families of the use of high technology in the treatment and management of illness, with new definitions of the quality of life. Fourth, the term *expert* has been redefined to include those who are not professionals—for example, veterans of the experience or predicament—with a resultant redistribution of labor. Fifth, there has been increased awareness by professionals of the nature and characteristics of social support and of research findings on the functions of social support as protective of health. Finally, government is assuming less responsibility for providing health and human services, and there has been a consequent reduction of public resources.

Given these factors, continuing multidisciplinary basic research on the nature of social support is essential. Cross sectional, longitudinal, case control, epidemiological, and anthropological research methodologies should be utilized as appropriate. Evaluation of social support systems interventions and analyses of models of articulation between formal and informal care systems are also needed. Findings in these areas would provide a firm knowledge base for the decisions that must be made about deployment of scarce professional and public resources.

A number of research strategies consistent with this framework already have been suggested. Gore (1981), in an appraisal and clarification of research models on the stress-buffering functions of social supports, calls for a redirection of studies from those that presume support effects to those that document the nature of support mechanisms. This implies a closer examination of the links between particular stressors and social supports through analyses of process issues and structural questions, as well as a move in the direction of both descriptive and explanatory goals. As Figure 2 illustrates, Dohrenwend and Dohrenwend (1981) consider the relationship between stress and illness to be explorable within six hypotheses: (1) victimi-

Figure 2. Six Hypotheses About the Life Stress Process

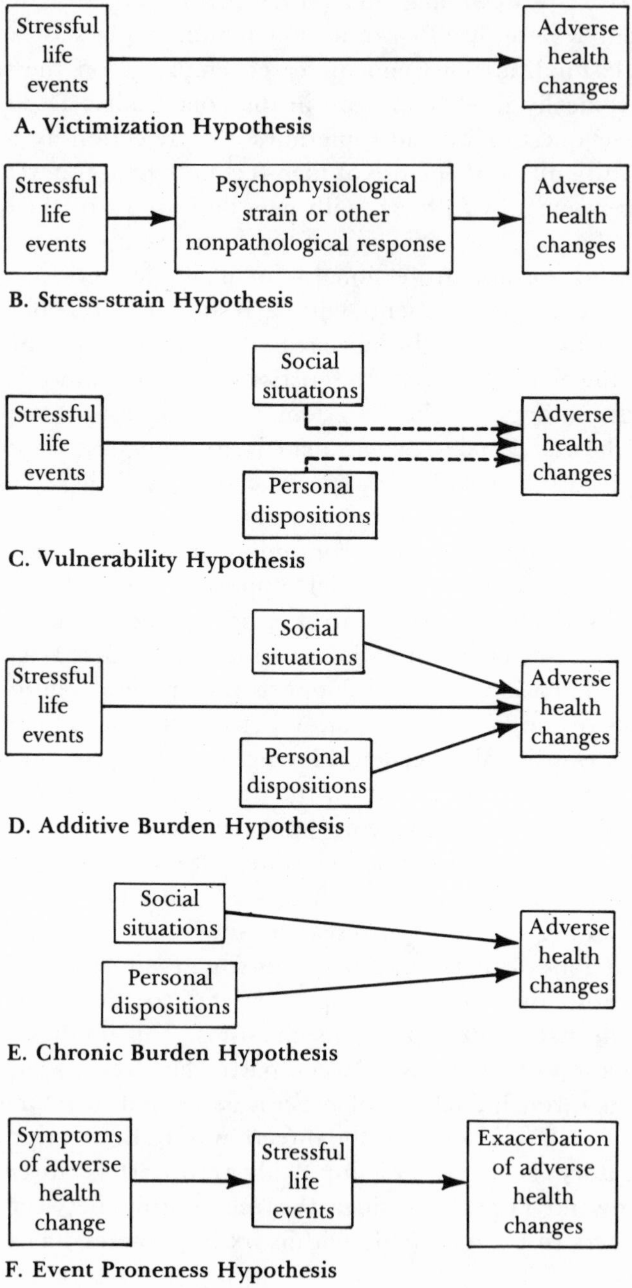

Source: Dohrenwend and Dohrenwend (1981).

zation, (2) stress-strain, (3) vulnerability, (4) additive burden, (5) chronic burden, and (6) event proneness. Golden and Dohrenwend (1981) outline a path analytic method for testing causal hypotheses about the life stress process that takes into account life events, personal dispositions, and social environmental situations.

As was noted earlier, although social support's true utility still requires elucidation, it already is being incorporated into the design of intervention strategies. Kornberg and Caplan (1980) present a model of primary prevention that emphasizes two sets of variables: (1) the biopsychosocial risk factors associated with an increase in psychopathology, and (2) a set of intervening variables that determine whether an individual becomes sick or not—personality factors, problem-solving skills, and behavior under stress in interaction with the social support network. This model is being utilized in Caplan's current work on risk factors and preventive intervention in child psychotherapy. On the other hand, Gruenberg (1980) suggests the development and testing of preventive trials—analogous to clinical trials—to lower disease prevalence. In a preventive trial, the investigator, in a population that is not ill, introduces an intervention to one part of the sample and withholds it from the rest in order to study the differential risk of developing the disease. The assumptions are that the interventions are harmless, socially acceptable, and not frightening to the subjects and that they can be expected, on some reasonable basis, to prevent a disorder. Gruenberg states that a preventive trial could be useful in documenting the effects of such social support program models as Widow-to-Widow in ameliorating the effects of loss of spouse. Bloom in Chapter Four of the present volume suggests a broad-based approach that would focus on identifying critical events in our environments that precipitate stress and on developing interventions to help in the mastery of these stresses, including strengthened sources of social support and improved social competencies. Each of these models permits the formulation of researchable hypotheses.

Based on the general research literature on social support theory and reviews of the literature on serious illness and social support (DiMatteo and Hays, 1981), I would like to suggest an evaluative intervention model for programming social and community support systems in the management of chronic illness. By definition, chronic illness places the person and his or her social system under everyday strain, with episodes of acute illness and other stressful life events occurring periodically. Strauss (1975) outlined the following problems of an individual living with chronic illness: (1) controlling symptoms; (2) carrying out prescribed regimens; (3) preventing medical crises and managing them when they occur; (4) preventing social isolation and normalizing life-style—redesign of social environment; (5) adjusting to changes in course of disease—periodic redefinitions of normality; (6) changing assumptive world and personal identity—coming to terms; (7) coping with drain on financial resources, including the results of, perhaps, partial or full unemployment.

Managing these problems successfully requires strategies that involve both personal and community social systems. On the assumption that these systems exist or can be established, Figure 3 presents a framework for testing numerous hypotheses

Figure 3. Social and Community Support Systems Intervention Model in Management of Chronic Illness

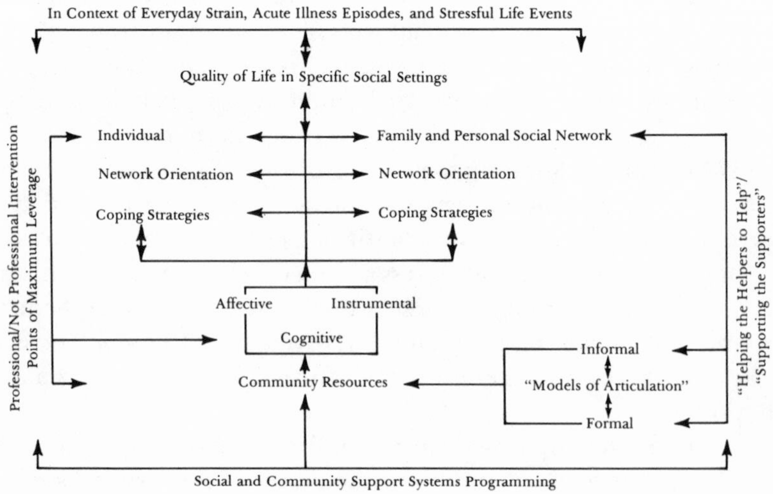

in a series of action-research, evaluative intervention studies. One or more parameters and their interactions could be investigated in a context of everyday strain or acute stress, including sociodemographic factors, personality factors, types of coping strategies, the effects of expectations of helpfulness or non-helpfulness from the personal social network on help seeking and help receiving, the types of community resources and the ways they are mobilized and by whom, and their availability and how and by whom delivered, both professional and not professional; effects of social support, positive and negative, on the individual and on his or her family and social network in terms of outcome criteria relevant to the quality of life in specific social settings. This latter assessment could include the effects of objective and subjective burden on the social network (Sainsbury and Grad, 1962; Cartwright, Hockey, and Anderson, 1973; Gruenberg and Sluss, 1980), as well as the explanatory power of changing health status, in the direction of severity and deterioration, over other explanations to account for changes in the quality of life for individuals with chronic illness and their families.

This intervention model obviously is complex, but it would generate various research designs and methodologies that could focus on the structure, processes, and/or functions of social support; on how individuals in situations of everyday strain and in periods of acute upset signal distress and elicit help from the social environment; and on which are the most effective pathways for improving the quality of life for the affected individual and his or her family. It could also explore how community resources can be matched with the usual coping strategies and network orientations of individuals and families—along the affective, cognitive, and instrumental dimensions of both—and how informal and formal care systems may be differentially utilized, with an appropriate division of labor. The intervention model could also focus on ways to "help the helpers to help" and to "support the supporters," as well as on the effects of strategies to improve the social competencies of individuals and their families in dealing with stress and strain and of strategies to strengthen or provide external social and community resources on the manifestations and course of the illness. In deficit situations such as chronic illness, this paradigm hypothesizes that the cognitive resources of the individual and his or her family, along with the cognitive and instrumental resources of the community, will be more powerful than affective support in increasing the quality of life along specified dimensions. The findings of such studies would give us enormously valuable information about what Schutz (1954) calls the biographically determined situation or circumstances, that is, the social reality of people attempting to manage their lives in chronic illness. These findings would also have crucial implications for public policy formulation in the planning of health and mental health services.

References

Ames, A. "Visual Perception and the Rotating Trapezoidal Window." *Psychological Monographs,* No. 324, 1951, *65* (entire issue).

Andrews, G., and others. "Life Event Stress, Social Support, Coping Style, and Risk of Psychological Impairment." *Journal of Nervous and Mental Disease,* 1978, *166,* 307-316.

Barker, R. G. *Ecological Psychology: Concepts and Methods for Studying the Environment of Human Behavior.* Stanford, Calif.: Stanford University Press, 1968.

Barnes, J. A. "Class and Committees in a Norwegian Island Parish." *Human Relations,* 1954, *7,* 39-58.

Becker, H. A. *A Social Psychological Study of Bereavement.* Unpublished doctoral dissertation, Department of Sociology, Northwestern University, 1927.

Belle, D. (Ed.). *Lives in Stress: Women and Depression.* Beverly Hills, Calif.: Sage, 1982.

Berkman, L. F., and Syme, S. L. "Social Networks, Host Resistance, and Mortality: A Nine-Year Follow-Up Study of Alameda County Residents." *American Journal of Epidemiology,* 1979, *109,* 186-204.

Bordow, S., and Porritt, D. "An Experimental Evaluation of Crisis Intervention." *Social Science and Medicine,* 1979, *13A,* 251-256.

Borkman, T. "Experiential Knowledge: A New Concept for the Analysis of Self-Help Groups." *Social Service Review,* 1976, *50,* 445-456.

Bott, E. *Family and Social Networks: Roles, Norms, and External Relationships in Ordinary Urban Families.* London: Tavistock, 1957 (revised edition, 1971).

Bowlby, J. *Maternal Care and Mental Health.* Geneva: World Health Organization, 1952.

Bowlby, J. *Attachment and Loss.* Vol. 1: *Attachment.* New York: Basic Books, 1969.

Bowlby, J. *Attachment and Loss.* Vol. 2: *Separation.* New York: Basic Books, 1973.

Bowlby, J. "The Making and Breaking of Affectional Bonds, Part I." *British Journal of Psychiatry,* 1977a, *130,* 201-210.

Bowlby, J. "The Making and Breaking of Affectional Bonds, Part II." *British Journal of Psychiatry,* 1977b, *130,* 421-431.

Bronfenbrenner, U. "Toward an Experimental Ecology of Human Development." *American Psychologist,* 1977, *32,* 513-531.

Brown, G. W. "Contextual Measures of Life Events." In B. S. Dohrenwend and B. P. Dohrenwend (Eds.), *Stressful Life Events and Their Contexts.* New York: Prodist, 1981.

Brown, G. W., Bhrolchain, M. A., and Harris, T. O. "Social Class and Psychiatric Disturbance Among Women in an Urban Population." *Sociology,* 1975, *9,* 225-231.

Brown, G. W., and Harris, T. O. *Social Origins of Depression: A Study of Psychiatric Disorder in Women.* London: Tavistock, 1978.

Bruhn, J. G., and others. "Social Aspects of Coronary Heart Disease in Two Adjacent Ethnically Different Communities." *American Journal of Public Health,* 1966, *56,* 1493-1506.

Budson, R. D. *The Psychiatric Halfway House: A Handbook of Theory and Practice.* Pittsburgh: University of Pittsburgh Press, 1978.

Cannon, W. B. *Bodily Changes in Pain, Hunger, Fear, and Rage.* New York: Appleton-Century-Crofts, 1929.

Cannon, W. B. "Stresses and Strains of Homeostasis." *American Journal of Medical Science,* 1935, *189,* 1-14.

Cantril, H. *The "Why" of Man's Experience.* New York: Macmillan, 1950.

Capildeo, R., Court, C., and Rose, F. C. "Social Network Diagram." *British Medical Journal,* 1976, *1,* 143-144.

Caplan, G. "Patterns of Parental Response to the Crisis of Premature Birth: A Preliminary Approach to Modifying Mental Health Outcome." *Psychiatry,* 1960, *23,* 365-374.

Caplan, G. "Emotional Crises." In A. Deutsch and H. Fishbein (Eds.), *Encyclopedia of Mental Health.* Vol. 2. New York: Franklin Watts, 1963.

Caplan, G. *Principles of Preventive Psychiatry.* New York: Basic Books, 1964.

Caplan, G. *The Theory and Practice of Mental Health Consultation.* New York: Basic Books, 1970.

Caplan, G. *Support Systems and Community Mental Health: Lectures on Concept Development.* New York: Behavioral Publications, 1974.

Caplan, G. "The Family as Support System." In G. Caplan and M. Killilea (Eds.), *Support Systems and Mutual Help.* New York: Grune & Stratton, 1976a.

Caplan, G. "Organization of Support Systems for Civilian Populations." In G. Caplan and M. Killilea (Eds.), *Support Systems and Mutual Help.* New York: Grune & Stratton, 1976b.

Caplan, G. "An Approach to Preventive Intervention in Child Psychiatry." *Canadian Journal of Psychiatry,* 1980, *25,* 671-682.

Caplan, G. "Mastery of Stress: Psychosocial Aspects." *American Journal of Psychiatry,* 1981, *138,* 413-419.

Caplan, G., and Cadden, V. "Adjusting Overseas: A Message to Each Peace Corps Trainee." In G. Caplan, *Principles of Preventive Psychiatry.* New York: Basic Books, 1964.

Caplan, G., and Killilea, M. (Eds.). *Support Systems and Mutual Help: Multidisciplinary Explorations.* New York: Grune & Stratton, 1976.

Caplan, G., Mason, E. A., and Kaplan, D. M. "Four Studies of Crisis in Parents of Prematures." *Community Mental Health Journal,* 1965, *1,* 140-162.

Caplan, G., and others. "Patterns of Cooperation of Child Psychiatry with Other Departments in Hospitals." *Journal of Prevention,* 1981, *2,* 40-49.

Caplan, R. B., in collaboration with G. Caplan, D. E. Richards, and A. P. Stokes, Jr. *Helping the Helpers to Help: The Development and Evaluation of Mental Health Consultation to Aid Clergymen in Pastoral Work.* New York: Seabury Press, 1972.

Cartwright, A., Hockey, L., and Anderson, J. L. *Life Before Death.* London: Routledge & Kegan Paul, 1973.

Cassel, J. C. "Psychiatric Epidemiology." In G. Caplan (Ed.), *American Handbook of Psychiatry.* Vol. 2. New York: Basic Books, 1974a.

Cassel, J. C. "Psychosocial Processes and 'Stress': Theoretical Formulation." *International Journal of Health Services,* 1974b, *4,* 471-482.

Cassel, J. C. "The Contribution of the Social Environment to Host Resistance: The Fourth Wade Hampton Frost Lecture." *American Journal of Epidemiology,* 1976, *104,* 107-123.

Cobb, S. "Social Support as a Moderator of Life Stress." *Psychosomatic Medicine,* 1976, *38,* 300-314.

Cochran, M. M., and Brassard, J. A. "Child Development and Personal Social Networks." *Child Development,* 1979, *50,* 601-616.

Coleman, J. V. "Psychiatric Consultation in Casework Agencies." *American Journal of Orthopsychiatry,* 1947, *27,* 533-539.

Coleman, J. V. "The Contributions of the Psychiatrist to the Social Worker and to the Client." *Mental Hygiene,* 1953, *37,* 249-258.

Coleman, J. V. "Mental Health Consultation to Agencies Protecting Family Life." In *The Elements of a Community Mental Health Program.* New York: Milbank Memorial Fund, 1956.

Colletta, N. C. "Support Systems After Divorce: Incidence and Impact." *Journal of Marriage and Family,* 1979, *41,* 837-846.

Colletta, N. C., and Gregg, C. H. "Adolescent Mothers' Vulnerability to Stress." *Journal of Nervous and Mental Disease,* 1981, *169,* 50-54.

Collins, A. H. "Natural Delivery Systems: Accessible Sources of Power for Mental Health." *American Journal of Orthopsychiatry,* 1973, *43,* 46-52.

Collins, A. H., and Pancoast, D. L. *Natural Helping Networks: A Strategy for Prevention.* New York: National Association of Social Workers, 1976.

Crogg, S. H., Lipson, A., and Levine, S. "Help Patterns in Severe Illness: The Roles of Kin Network, Non-Family Resources, and Institutions." *Journal of Marriage and Family,* 1972, *34,* 32-41.

Curle, A. "Transitional Communities and Social Reconnection." Part I. *Human Relations,* 1947, *1,* 42-68.

Curle, A., and Trist, E. L. "Transitional Communities and Social Reconnection." Part II. *Human Relations,* 1947, *1,* 240-288.

Curtis, W. R. "Community Human Service Networks: New Roles for Mental Health Workers." *Psychiatric Annals,* 1973, *3,* 23-42.

Dean, A., and Lin, N. "The Stress-Buffering Role of Social Support: Problems and Prospects for Systematic Investigation." *Journal of Nervous and Mental Disease,* 1977, *165,* 403-417.

de Araujo, G., and others. "Life Change, Coping Ability, and Chronic Intrinsic Asthma." *Journal of Psychosomatic Research,* 1973, *17,* 359-363.

DiMatteo, M. R., and Hays, R. "Social Support and Serious Illness." In B. H. Gottlieb (Ed.), *Social Networks and Social Support.* Beverly Hills, Calif.: Sage, 1981.

Dohrenwend, B. S., and Dohrenwend, B. P. (Eds.). *Stressful Life Events: Their Nature and Effects.* New York: Wiley, 1974.

Dohrenwend, B. S., and Dohrenwend, B. P. "Life Stress and Illness: Formulation of the Issues." In B. S. Dohrenwend and B. P. Dohrenwend (Eds.), *Stressful Life Events and Their Contexts.* New York: Prodist, 1981.

Eaton, W. "Life Events, Social Supports, and Psychiatric Symptoms: A Reanalysis of the New Haven Data." *Journal of Health and Social Behavior,* 1978, *19,* 230-234.

Eckenrode, J., and Gore, S. "Stressful Events and Social Supports: The Significance of Context." In B. H. Gottlieb (Ed.), *Social Networks and Social Support.* Beverly Hills, Calif.: Sage, 1981.

Egbert, L. D., and others. "Reduction of Post-Operative Pain by Encouragement and Instruction of Patients." *New England Journal of Medicine,* 1964, *270,* 825-827.

Eliot, T. D. "The Adjustive Behavior of Bereaved Families: A New Field for Research." *Social Forces,* 1930, *8,* 543-549.

Eliot, T. D. "The Bereaved Family." *Annals of American Academy of Political and Social Science,* 1932, *160,* 184-190.

Emerson, W. R. P. "The Hygienic and Dietetic Treatment of Delicate Children by the Class Method." *Boston Medical and Surgical Journal,* 1910, *163,* 326.

Emerson, W. R. P. *Nutrition and Growth in Children.* New York: Appleton-Century-Crofts, 1922.

Engel, G. L. "A Life Setting Inducive to Illness: The Giving Up, Given Up Complex." *Annals of Internal Medicine,* 1968, *69,* 293-300.

English, J. T., and Colmen, J. G. "Psychological Adjustment Patterns of Peace Corps Volunteers." *Psychiatric Opinion,* 1966, *3,* 29-35.

Erickson, G. D. "The Concept of Personal Network in Clinical Practice." *Family Process,* 1975, *14,* 487-498.

Erikson, E. H. *Childhood and Society.* New York: Norton, 1950.

Erikson, E. H. "Growth and Crises of the Healthy Personality." In *Identity and the Life Cycle.* Psychological Issues Monograph 1. New York: International Universities Press, 1959.

Fairweather, G. W., Sanders, D. H., and Maynard, H. *Community Life for the Mentally Ill: An Alternative to Institutional Care.* Hawthorne, N.Y.: Aldine, 1969.

Fine, P. "Family Networks and Child Psychiatry in a Community Health Project." *Journal of the American Academy of Child Psychiatry,* 1973, *12,* 675-689.

Finlayson, A. "Social Networks as Coping Resources: Lay Help and Consultation Patterns Used by Women in Husband's Post-Infarction Career." *Social Science and Medicine,* 1976, *10,* 97-103.

Fischer, C. S., and others. *Networks and Places: Social Relations in the Urban Setting.* New York: Free Press, 1977.

Folkman, S., and Lazarus, R. S. "An Analysis of Coping in a Middle-Aged Community Sample." *Journal of Health and Social Behavior,* 1980, *21,* 219-239.

Freidson, E. "Client Control and Medical Practice." *American Journal of Sociology,* 1960, *65,* 374-382.

Freidson, E. *Patients' Views of Medical Practice.* New York: Russell Sage Foundation, 1961.

French, J. R. P., Jr. "Person-Role Fit." *Occupational Mental Health,* 1973, *3,* 15-20.

French, J. R. P., Jr., and Kahn, R. L. "A Programmatic Approach to Studying the Industrial Environment and Mental Health." *Journal of Social Issues,* 1962, *18,* 1-47.

French, J. R. P., Jr., Rodgers, W., and Cobb, S. "Adjustments as Person-Environment Fit." In G. V. Coelho, D. A. Hamburg, and J. E. Adams (Eds.), *Coping and Adaptation: Interdisciplinary Perspectives.* New York: Basic Books, 1974.

Freud, S. "Mourning and Melancholia." In J. Strachey (Ed.), *The Complete Psychological Works of Sigmund Freud.* Vol. 14. London: Hogarth Press, 1957. (Originally published 1915.)

Froland, C., and others. *Helping Networks and Human Services.* Beverly Hills, Calif.: Sage, 1981.

Frydman, M. I. "Social Support, Life Events, and Psychiatric Symptoms: A Study of Direct, Conditional, and Interaction Effects." *Social Psychiatry,* 1981, *16,* 69-78.

Garrison, J., Kulp, C., and Rosen, S. "Community Mental Health Nursing: A Social Network Approach." *Journal of Psychiatric Nursing,* 1977, *15,* 32-36.

Garrison, V. "Support Systems of Schizophrenic and Non-Schizophrenic Puerto Rican Migrant Women in New York City." *Schizophrenia Bulletin,* 1978, *4,* 561-596.

Gartner, A., and Riessman, F. *Self-Help in the Human Services.* San Francisco: Jossey-Bass, 1977.

Gennep, A. van. *Rites of Passage.* (M. B. Vizedon and G. L. Caffee, Trans.) Chicago: University of Chicago Press, 1961. (Originally published 1908.)

Gerstel, N., and Riessman, C. K. "Social Networks in a Vulnerable Population: The Separated and Divorced." Paper presented at annual meeting of the American Public Health Association, Los Angeles, Nov. 1981.

Glass, A. J. "Lessons Learned." In Medical Department of the U.S. Army, *Neuropsychiatry in World War II.* Vol. 2. Washington, D.C.: U.S. Government Printing Office, 1971.

Goldberg, E. "Social Networks as a Factor in the Health of Older Married Women." Paper presented at annual meeting of the American Public Health Association, Los Angeles, Nov. 1981.

Golden, R. R., and Dohrenwend, B. S. "A Path Analytic Method for Testing Causal Hypotheses About the Life Stress Process." In B. S. Dohrenwend and B. P. Dohrenwend (Eds.), *Stressful Life Events and Their Contexts.* New York: Prodist, 1981.

Gore, S. "Stress-Buffering Functions of Social Supports: An Appraisal and Clarification of Research Models." In B. S. Dohrenwend and B. P. Dohrenwend (Eds.), *Stressful Life Events and Their Contexts.* New York: Prodist, 1981.

Gottlieb, B. H. "The Contribution of Natural Support Systems of Primary Prevention Among Four Subgroups of Adolescent Males." *Adolescence,* 1975, *10,* 207-220.

Gottlieb, B. H. "Lay Influences on the Utilization and Provision of Health Services: A Review." *Canadian Psychological Review,* 1976, *17,* 126-136.

Gottlieb, B. H. "Preventive Interventions Involving Social Networks and Social Support." In B. H. Gottlieb (Ed.), *Social Networks and Social Support.* Beverly Hills, Calif.: Sage, 1981a.

Gottlieb, B. H. (Ed.). *Social Networks and Social Support.* Beverly Hills, Calif.: Sage, 1981b.

Granovetter, M. S. "The Strength of Weak Ties." *American Journal of Sociology,* 1973, *78,* 1360-1380.

Gruenberg, E. M. "The Social Breakdown Syndrome: Some Origins." *American Journal of Psychiatry,* 1967, *123,* 1481-1489.

Gruenberg, E. M. "The Failures of Success." *Milbank Memorial Fund Quarterly,* 1977, *55,* 3-24.

Gruenberg, E. M. "Epidemiology." In H. Kaplan and others

(Eds.), *Comprehensive Textbook of Psychiatry.* (3rd ed.) Vol. 3. Baltimore, Md.: Williams and Wilkins, 1980.

Gruenberg, E. M., and Archer, J. "Abandonment of Responsibility for the Seriously Mentally Ill." *Milbank Memorial Fund Quarterly,* 1979, *57,* 485-506.

Gruenberg, E. M., and Sluss, T. K. "Role of Informal Helpers in the Care of the Elderly." Research project, Eastern Baltimore Mental Health Survey (National Institute of Mental Health–Epidemiology Catchment Area Program). Baltimore, Md.: School of Hygiene and Public Health, Johns Hopkins University, 1980.

Gurin, G., Veroff, J., and Feld, S. *Americans View Their Mental Health.* New York: Basic Books, 1960.

Gussow, Z., and Tracy, G. S. "The Role of Self-Help Clubs in Adaptation to Chronic Illness and Disability." *Social Science and Medicine,* 1976, *10,* 407-414.

Hamburg, B. A. "Early Adolescence: A Specific and Stressful Stage of the Life Cycle." In G. V. Coelho, D. A. Hamburg, and J. E. Adams (Eds.), *Coping and Adaptation.* New York: Basic Books, 1974.

Hamburg, B. A., and Killilea, M. "Relation of Social Support, Stress, Illness, and Use of Health Services." In the Surgeon General's Report on Health Promotion and Disease Prevention, *Healthy People: Background Papers.* Vol. 2. Washington, D.C.: U.S. Government Printing Office, 1979.

Hamburg, D. A. "A Life Span Perspective on Adaptation and Health." In B. Kaplan and M. Ibrahim (Eds.), *Family Medicine and Supportive Interventions: An Epidemiological Approach.* Chapel Hill: Institute of Research in Social Sciences, University of North Carolina, 1981.

Hamburg, D. A., and Adams, J. E. "A Perspective on Coping Behavior: Seeking and Utilizing Information in Major Transitions." *Archives of General Psychiatry,* 1967, *17,* 277-284.

Hamburg, D. A., Adams, J. E., and Brodie, H. K. H. "Coping Behavior in Stressful Circumstances: Some Implications for Social Psychiatry." In B. H. Kaplan, R. N. Wilson, and A. H. Leighton (Eds.), *Further Explorations in Social Psychiatry.* New York: Basic Books, 1976.

Hamburg, D. A., Hamburg, B. A., and de Goza, S. "Adaptive Problems and Mechanisms in Severely Burned Patients." *Psychiatry,* 1953, *16,* 1-20.

Hammer, M. "Social Supports, Social Networks, and Schizophrenia." Paper presented at National Institute of Mental Health Conference on Stress, Social Support, and Schizophrenia, Burlington, Vt., Sept. 1979.

Hammer, M., Makiesky-Barrow, S., and Gutwirth, L. "Social Networks and Schizophrenia." *Schizophrenia Bulletin,* 1978, *4,* 522-545.

Hansell, N. *The Person-in-Distress: On the Biosocial Dynamics of Adaptation.* New York: Behavioral Publications, 1976.

Hansell, N., and Willis, G. L. "Outpatient Treatment of Schizophrenia." *American Journal of Psychiatry,* 1977, *134,* 1082-1086.

Hatfield, A. B. "Help-Seeking Behavior in Families of Schizophrenics." *American Journal of Community Psychology,* 1979, *7,* 563-569.

Henderson, A. S. "The Social Network, Support, and Neurosis: The Function of Attachment in Adult Life." *British Journal of Psychiatry,* 1977, *131,* 185-191.

Henderson, A. S., with Byrne, D. G., and Duncan-Jones, P. *Neurosis and the Social Environment.* Sydney, Australia: Academic Press, 1981.

Henderson, A. S., and others. "The Patient's Primary Group." *British Journal of Psychiatry,* 1978, *132,* 74-86.

Hill, R. (Ed.). *Families Under Stress.* New York: Harper & Row, 1949.

Holmes, T., and Rahe, R. "The Social Readjustment Rating Scale." *Journal of Psychosomatic Research,* 1967, *11,* 213-218.

Ittleson, W. H., and Cantril, H. *Perception: A Transactional Approach.* New York: Doubleday, 1954.

Jacobson, G. F. "Programs and Techniques of Crisis Intervention." In G. Caplan (Ed.), *American Handbook of Psychiatry.* (2nd ed.) Vol. 2. New York: Basic Books, 1974.

James, D. (Ed.). *Outward Bound.* London: Routledge & Kegan Paul, 1957.

James, S., and Kleinbaum, D. G. "Socioecologic Stress and Hypertension: Related Mortality Rates in North Carolina." *American Journal of Public Health,* 1976, *66,* 354-358.

Janis, I. *Air War and Emotional Stress: Psychological Studies of Bombing and Civilian Defense.* New York: McGraw-Hill, 1951.

Janis, I. *Psychological Stress.* New York: Wiley, 1958.

Jones, M. *The Therapeutic Community: A New Treatment Method in Psychiatry.* New York: Basic Books, 1953.

Kahn, R. L. "Aging and Social Support." In M. W. Riley (Ed.), *Aging From Birth to Death: Interdisciplinary Perspectives.* American Association for the Advancement of Science Symposia Series. Boulder, Colo.: Westview Press, 1979.

Kahn, R. L., and Quinn, R. P. "Role Stress: A Framework for Analysis." In A. McLean (Ed.), *Mental Health and Work Organizations.* Chicago: Rand McNally, 1970.

Kahn, R. L., and others. *Organizational Stress.* New York: Wiley, 1964.

Kaplan, B. H., Cassel, J. C., and Gore, S. "Social Support and Health." *Medical Care,* 1977, *15* (supplement), 47-58.

Kaplan, D. M., and Mason, E. A. "Maternal Reactions to Premature Birth Viewed as an Acute Emotional Disorder." *American Journal of Orthopsychiatry,* 1960, *30,* 539-552.

Katz, A. H. "Application of Self-Help Concepts in Current Social Welfare." *Social Work,* 1965, *10,* 68-74.

Katz, A. H. "Self-Help Organizations and Volunteer Participation in Social Welfare." *Social Work,* 1970, *15,* 51-60.

Katz, A. H., and Bender, E. I. (Eds.). *The Strength in Us: Self-Help Groups in the Modern World.* New York: Franklin Watts, 1976.

Killilea, M. "Mutual Help Organizations: Interpretations in the Literature." In G. Caplan and M. Killilea (Eds.), *Support Systems and Mutual Help.* New York: Grune & Stratton, 1976.

Klein, D. C., and Lindemann, E. "Preventive Intervention in Individual and Family Crisis Situations." In G. Caplan (Ed.), *Prevention of Mental Disorders in Children.* New York: Basic Books, 1961.

Koos, E. L. *Families in Trouble.* Morningside Heights, N.Y.: King's Crown Press, 1946.

Kornberg, M., and Caplan, G. "Risk Factors and Preventive Intervention in Child Psychopathology: A Review." *Journal of Prevention,* 1980, *1,* 71-133.

Kramer, M. "The Rising Pandemic of Mental Disorders and Associated Chronic Diseases and Disabilities." In "Epidemiological Research as a Basis for the Organization of Extramural Psychiatry." *Acta Psychiatrica Scandinavica,* 1980, *62* (Supplement 285), 382-397.

Langsley, D. G., and Kaplan, D. *The Treatment of Families in Crisis.* New York: Grune & Stratton, 1968.

LaRocco, J. M., House, J. S., and French, J. R. P., Jr. "Social Support, Occupational Stress, and Health." *Journal of Health and Social Behavior,* 1980, *21,* 202-218.

Lazarus, R. S. *Psychological Stress and the Coping Process.* New York: McGraw-Hill, 1966.

Lazarus, R. S. "The Costs and Benefits of Denial." In B. S. Dohrenwend and B. P. Dohrenwend (Eds.), *Stressful Life Events and Their Contexts.* New York: Prodist, 1981.

Lazarus, R. S., Averill, J. R., and Opton, E. M. "The Psychology of Coping: Issues of Research and Assessment." In G. V. Coelho, D. A. Hamburg, and J. E. Adams (Eds.), *Coping and Adaptation.* New York: Basic Books, 1974.

Leutz, W. N. "The Informal Community Caregiver: A Link Between the Health Care System and Local Residents." *American Journal of Orthopsychiatry,* 1977, *46,* 678-688.

Levin, L. S., Katz, A. H., and Holst, E. *Self-Care: Lay Initiatives in Health.* New York: Prodist, 1976.

Lévi-Strauss, C. *Structural Anthropology.* (C. Jacobsen and B. G. Shoepf, Trans.) New York: Basic Books, 1963.

Lévi-Strauss, C. *The Elementary Structures of Kinship.* (J. H. Bell, J. R. von Sturmer, R. Needham, Trans. and Eds.) (Rev. ed.) Boston: Beacon Press, 1969.

Levy, L. "Self-Help Groups: Types and Psychological Processes." *Journal of Applied Behavioral Sciences,* 1976, *12,* 310-322.

Lewin, K. *A Dynamic Theory of Personality.* New York: McGraw-Hill, 1935.

Lewin, K. *Field Theory in Social Science: Selected Theoretical Papers.* New York: Harper & Row, 1951.

Liberman, R. "Personal Influence in the Use of Mental Health Resources." *Human Organization,* 1965, *24,* 231-235.

Lieberman, M. A., and Borman, L. D., and Associates. *Self-Help Groups for Coping With Crisis: Origins, Members, Processes, and Impact.* San Francisco: Jossey-Bass, 1979.

Lin, N., Dean, A., and Ensel, W. "Constructing Social Support Scales: A Methodological Note." Paper presented at National Institute of Mental Health Conference on Stress, Social Support, and Schizophrenia, Burlington, Vt., Sept. 1979.

Lin, N., and others. "Social Support, Stressful Life Events, and Illness: A Model and Empirical Test." *Journal of Health and Social Behavior,* 1979, *20,* 108-119.

Lindemann, E. "The Symptomatology and Management of Acute Grief." *American Journal of Psychiatry,* 1944, *101,* 141-148.

Litwak, E., and Szelenyi, I. "Primary Group Structures and Their Functions: Kin, Neighbors, and Friends." *American Sociological Review,* 1969, *34,* 465-481.

McKinlay, J. B. "Social Networks, Lay Consultation, and Help-Seeking Behavior." *Social Forces,* 1973, *51,* 275-292.

MacMillan, D. "Hospital-Community Relationships." *Mental Hospitals,* 1957, *8,* 29-50.

McQueen, D. V., and Celentano, D. "The Role of Social Support System and Problem Drinking Among Women." Paper presented at annual meeting of the American Public Health Association, Los Angeles, Nov. 1981.

Maddison, D. C., and Walker, W. L. "Factors Affecting the Outcome of Conjugal Bereavement." *British Journal of Psychiatry,* 1967, *113,* 1057-1067.

Mannheim, K. *Diagnosis of Our Time.* London: Routledge & Kegan Paul, 1943.

Menninger, W. W., and English, J. T. "Psychiatric Casualties from Overseas Peace Corps Service." *Bulletin of the Menninger Clinic,* 1965, *29,* 148-158.

Merton, R. *Social Theory and Social Structure: Toward the Codification of Theory and Research.* New York: Free Press, 1949.

Meyer, A. "The Life Chart and the Obligation of Specifying

Positive Data in Psychopathological Diagnosis." In E. E. Winters (Ed.), *The Collected Papers of Adolph Meyer.* Vol. 3: *Medical Teaching.* Baltimore, Md.: Johns Hopkins University Press, 1951.

Meyers, J. K., Lindenthal, J. J., and Pepper, M. P. "Life Events, Social Integration, and Psychiatric Symptomatology." *Journal of Health and Social Behavior,* 1975, *16,* 421-427.

Milbank Memorial Fund. *An Approach to the Prevention of Disability From Chronic Psychoses: Part I. The Open Mental Hospital Within the Community.* New York: Milbank Memorial Fund, 1958.

Mitchell, J. C. "The Concept and Use of Social Networks." In J. C. Mitchell (Ed.), *Social Networks in Urban Situations.* Manchester, England: Manchester University Press, 1969.

Moos, R. H. "Systems for the Assessment and Classification of Human Environments: An Overview." In R. H. Moos and P. M. Insel (Eds.), *Issues in Social Ecology.* Palo Alto, Calif.: National Press Books, 1974.

Moreno, J. L. "Foundations of Sociometry." *Sociometry,* 1941, *4,* 15-35.

Mueller, D. P. "Social Networks: A Promising Direction for Research on the Relationship of the Social Environment to Psychiatric Disorder." *Social Science and Medicine,* 1980, *14A,* 147-161.

Murray, H. A. *Explorations in Personality.* New York: Oxford University Press, 1938.

Nesser, W., Tyroler, H., and Cassel, J. C. "Social Disorganization and Stroke Mortality in the Black Population of North Carolina." *American Journal of Epidemiology,* 1972, *95,* 431-441.

Nuckolls, K. B., Cassel, J. C., and Kaplan, B. H. "Psychosocial Assets, Life Crisis, and the Prognosis of Pregnancy." *American Journal of Epidemiology,* 1972, *95,* 431-441.

Oxford English Dictionary: The Compact Edition. New York: Oxford University Press, 1971.

Parad, H., and Caplan, G. "A Framework for Studying Families in Crisis." *Journal of Social Work,* 1960, *5,* 3-15.

Park, R. E. "Human Migration and the Marginal Man." *American Journal of Sociology,* 1928, *33,* 881-893.

Parkes, C. M. "Psychosocial Transitions: A Field for Study." *Social Science and Medicine,* 1971, *5,* 101-115.

Pattison, E. M. "Clinical Social Systems Interventions." *Psychiatry Digest,* April 1977, *38,* 25-33.

Pattison, E. M., and others. "Social Network Mediation of Anxiety." *Psychiatric Annals,* 1979, *9,* 56-67.

Paykel, E. S., and others. "Life Events and Depression: A Controlled Study." *Archives of General Psychiatry,* 1969, *21,* 753-760.

Paykel, E. S., and others. "Life Events and Social Support in Puerperal Depression." *British Journal of Psychiatry,* 1980, *136,* 339-346.

Pearlin, L. I., and Schooler, C. "The Structure of Coping." *Journal of Health and Social Behavior,* 1978, *19,* 2-21.

Pearlin, L. I., and Schooler, C. "Some Extensions of 'The Structure of Coping.'" *Journal of Health and Social Behavior,* 1979, *20,* 202-204.

Platt, S., and others. "The Social Behavior Assessment Schedule (SBAS): Rationale, Contents, Scoring, and Reliability of a New Interview Schedule." *Social Psychiatry,* 1980, *15,* 43-55.

Porritt, D. "Social Support in Crisis: Quantity or Quality." *Social Science and Medicine,* 1979, *13A,* 715-721.

Pratt, J. H. "The Class Method of Treating Consumption in the Homes of the Poor." *Journal of the American Medical Association,* 1907, *49,* 755-759.

Pratt, J. H. "Results Obtained in the Treatment of Pulmonary Tuberculosis by the Class Method." *British Medical Journal,* 1908, *2,* 1070-1071.

Pratt, J. H. "The Principles of Class Treatment and Their Application to Various Chronic Diseases." *Hospital Social Service,* 1922, *6,* 401-411.

President's Commission on Mental Health. *Task Panel Report on Community Support Systems.* Vol. 2. Washington, D.C.: U.S. Government Printing Office, 1978.

Proger, S. H. "Joseph H. Pratt: A Biographical Sketch." In *Scientific Contributions in Honor of Joseph Hersey Pratt on His 65th Birthday by His Friends.* Lancaster, Pa: Lancaster Press, 1937.

Rabkin, J. G., and Struening, E. L. "Life Events, Stress, and Illness." *Science,* 1976, *194,* 1013-1020.

Rapoport, L. "Working with Families in Crisis: An Exploration in Preventive Intervention." *Social Work,* 1962, *7,* 48-56.

Rapoport, R. V. "Normal Crisis, Family Structure, and Mental Health." *Family Process,* 1963, *2,* 68-80.

Rapoport, R. V. "The Transition from Engagement to Marriage." *Acta Sociologica,* 1964, *8,* 36-55.

Riessman, F. "The Helper Therapy Principle." *Social Work,* 1965, *10,* 27-32.

Rosenfeld, J. M., and Caplan, G. "Techniques of Staff Consultation in an Immigrant Children's Organization in Israel." *American Journal of Orthopsychiatry,* 1954, *24,* 42-62.

Sainsbury, P., and Grad, J. "Evaluation of Treatment and Services." In Nuffield Provincial Hospitals Trust, *The Burden in the Community.* London: Oxford University Press, 1962.

Salber, E. J., Beery, W. L., and Jackson, E. J. R. "The Role of the Health Facilitator in Community Health Education." *Journal of Community Health,* 1976, *2,* 5-20.

Salmon, T., and others. In Medical Department of the U.S. Army, *Neuropsychiatry in the World War.* Vol. 10. Washington, D.C.: U.S. Government Printing Office, 1929.

Sanders, D. H. "Innovative Environments in the Community: A Life for the Chronic Patients." *Schizophrenia Bulletin,* 1972, *6,* 49-59.

Schutz, A. "Concept and Theory Formation in the Social Sciences." *Journal of Philosophy,* 1954, *51,* 257-273.

Selye, H. "The General Adaptation Syndrome and Diseases of Adaptation." *Journal of Clinical Endocrinology,* 1946, *6,* 117-230.

Shapiro, J. "Dominant Leaders Among Slum Hotel Residents." *American Journal of Orthopsychiatry,* 1969, *39,* 644-650.

Shapiro, J. H. *Communities of The Alone.* New York: Association Press, 1971.

Silverman, P. R. "Services for the Widowed During the Period of Bereavement." In *Social Work Practice.* New York: Columbia University Press, 1966.

Silverman, P. R. "Services to the Widowed: First Steps in a Program of Preventive Intervention." *Community Mental Health Journal,* 1967, *1,* 37-44.

Silverman, P. R. "The Widow as a Caregiver in a Program of Preventive Intervention with Other Widows." *Mental Hygiene,* 1970, *54,* 540-545.

Silverman, P. R. *If You Will Lift The Load, I Will Lift It Too: A Guide To Developing Widow-to-Widow Programs.* New York: Jewish Funeral Directors of America, 1976.

Silverman, P. R. *Mutual Help Groups: A Guide for Mental Health Workers.* Rockville, Md.: National Institute of Mental Health, 1978.

Silverman, P. R. *Mutual Help Groups: Organization and Development.* Beverly Hills, Calif.: Sage, 1980.

Speck, R., and Attneave, C. *Family Networks: Retribalization and Healing.* New York: Pantheon, 1973.

Stout, C., and others. "Unusually Low Incidence of Death from Myocardial Infarction." *Journal of the American Medical Association,* 1964, *188,* 845-855.

Strauss, A. L. *Chronic Illness and the Quality of Life.* St. Louis, Mo.: Mosby, 1975.

Talbott, J. A. "Community Psychiatry in the Army: History, Practice, and Applications to Civilian Psychiatry." *Journal of the American Medical Association,* 1969, *210,* 1233-1237.

Test, M. A., and Stein, L. I. "Training in Community Living: A Follow-Up Look at a Gold-Award Program." *Hospital and Community Psychiatry,* 1976a, *27,* 193-194.

Test, M. A., and Stein, L. I. "Practical Guidelines for the Community Treatment of Markedly Impaired Patients." *Community Mental Health Journal,* 1976b, *12,* 72-82.

Thomas, W. I. *Source Book for Social Origins.* Boston: Richard G. Badger, 1909.

Tolsdorf, C. C. "Social Networks, Support, and Coping: An Explanatory Study." *Family Process,* 1976, *15,* 407-417.

Turner, J., and Ten Hoor, W. "The NIMH Community Support Program: Pilot Approach to a Needed Social Reform." *Schizophrenia Bulletin,* 1978, *4,* 319-348.

Tyhurst, J. S. "The Role of Transition States—Including Disasters—in Mental Illness." In *Symposium on Social and Preven-*

tive Psychiatry. Washington, D.C.: Walter Reed Army Institute of Research, 1957.

Vallé, R., and Mendoza, L. *The Elder Latino*. San Diego, Calif.: Campanile Press, 1978.

Vallé, R., and Vega, W. (Eds.). *Hispanic Natural Networks: Mental Health Promotion Perspectives*. Sacramento: State of California, 1980.

Veroff, J., Douvan, E., and Kulka, R. A. *The Inner American: A Self-Portrait from 1957 to 1976*. New York: Basic Books, 1981.

Veroff, J., Kulka, R. A., and Douvan, E. *Mental Health in America: Patterns of Help-Seeking from 1977 to 1976*. New York: Basic Books, 1981.

Visotsky, H. M., and others. "Coping Behavior Under Extreme Stress." *Archives of General Psychiatry*, 1961, *5*, 423-448.

Walker, K. N., MacBride, A., and Vachon, M. L. S. "Social Support Networks and the Crisis of Bereavement." *Social Science and Medicine*, 1977, *11*, 35-42.

Wallace, A. F. C. "Stress and Rapid Personality Changes." *International Record of Medicine and General Practice Clinics*, 1956, *169*, 761-774.

Warren, D. I. *Helping Networks: How People Cope with Problems in the Urban Community*. Notre Dame: University of Indiana Press, 1981.

Weiss, R. S. "The Fund of Sociability." *Transactions*, 1969, *6*, 36-43.

Weiss, R. S. "The Provisions of Social Relationships." In Z. Rubin (Ed.), *Doing Unto Others*. Englewood Cliffs, N.J.: Prentice-Hall, 1974.

Weiss, R. S. *Marital Separation*. New York: Basic Books, 1975.

Weiss, R. S. "Transition States and Other Stressful Situations: Their Nature and Programs for Their Management." In G. Caplan and M. Killilea (Eds.), *Support Systems and Mutual Help*. New York: Grune & Stratton, 1976.

Weiss, R. S. *Going It Alone: The Family Life and Social Situation of The Single Parent*. New York: Basic Books, 1979.

Wellman, B., and Leighton, B. "Networks, Neighborhoods, and Communities." *Urban Affairs Quarterly*, 1979, *15*, 363-390.

White, R. W. "Strategies of Adaptation: An Attempt at Systematic Description." In G. V. Coelho, D. A. Hamburg, and J. E. Adams (Eds.), *Coping and Adaptation.* New York: Basic Books, 1974.

Wolff, H. G. "Life Stress and Bodily Disease: A Formulation." In *Proceedings of the Association for Research in Nervous and Mental Disease.* Vol. 29: *Life Stress and Bodily Disease.* Baltimore, Md.: Williams and Wilkins, 1950.

Chapter 7

Role of Support Systems in Loss and Psychosocial Transitions

Colin Murray Parkes

The life situations and events that are regarded as potentially damaging to mental health have been variously designated as *stresses, crises,* or *losses.* Although each of these words has its value, none of them is sufficiently precise. All tend to be defined in terms of their negative consequences, and we easily get caught in circular argument when we try to prove that a given stress is stressful or that a given loss is a cause of grief. Moreover, to define such situations independently of their meaning to the individual is to create a fresh set of problems. An event that is seen as a disaster by one person may be viewed as an unqualified blessing by another, and what may be a crisis in one man's life can be taken in stride by the man next door. Hence it is no surprise to find a wide variety of responses to particular events—even to events that seem, at first glance, to be relatively unambiguous.

Marris (1974) has attempted to clarify the issue by referring to significant losses as those that require an individual to revise his "context of meaning," but his fascinating book never quite succeeds in explaining the meaning of meaning. What is this elusive factor that decides how we evaluate the world we meet?

We assess events and situations in terms of our own assumed needs or goals. Thus it is reasonable to assume that the newborn babe has been preprogrammed to perceive and respond to a limited range of internal and external stimuli in ways that enable these needs to be met. At this stage it is reasonable to assume that a sensory stimulus has "meaning" only if it triggers one of these preprogrammed responses or instinctual response patterns. From the moment of birth, however, and possibly before birth, the child begins to learn and to improve its ability to act and to perceive in ever-more sophisticated ways to achieve its ends. The range of stimuli to which the child will respond and the complexity of the chains of responses increase enormously until it begins to be possible to speak of behavioral *plans.* The development of plans and the recognition of complex perceptions require the development of an internal world or "world model." Derived from our memories of previous experience, the "world model" enables us to explore in imagination possible events in the world around us and possible consequences of our own behavior. These vary from the essential thought processes by which we recognize and respond to the real world, to fantasies of gain and loss. Three types of world models can be distinguished: (1) the assumptive world (the world that we assume to exist on the basis of our previous experience of the world), (2) dreaded worlds (extrapolations of possible undesired consequences), and (3) hoped-for worlds (extrapolations of desired consequences). It is the first of these that is responsible for our ability to test reality. When a percept is found to accord with the internal schemata of the assumptive world, it has meaning for us and can be treated as familiar. Even our exploration of the unfamiliar or novel aspects of the world we meet has the object of discovering the underlying characteristics that "make sense" of these phenomena and enable us to incorporate them within the assumptive world. And as time passes, each person's assumptive world becomes more extensive, more complex, and more accurate as his experience of life extends and increases his awareness of his place in the world.

Psychosocial Transitions

But there are times when a person may discover a major discrepancy between the world he meets and the assumptions that, up to now, have guided his thoughts and behavior. Things that he had "taken for granted" prove fallacious, his world is "turned upside down," and for a while "nothing makes sense any more"; in short, "the world has lost its meaning." Situations of this kind are likely to arise whenever there is a major change inside or outside a person—sudden blindness, the loss of a limb, being unexpectedly made redundant at work, imprisonment, or the untimely death of one's spouse. Anything that requires a person, over a relatively short space of time, to abandon one view of the world and to develop another gives rise to a situation that, for convenience, I have termed a *psychosocial transition* (Parkes, 1971).

Psychosocial transitions are, by their nature, situations of danger. The person can no longer rely upon his Assumptive World to guide him, and it is no wonder that he feels frightened, bewildered, and upset. Even the recognition that such a change is imminent may be sufficient to cause severe anxiety, and it is not surprising to find that most of the "life events" that have been identified by Brown and Harris (1978), by Paykel (1974), and by Rahe (1969, 1975) as precipitants of a wide range of psychiatric and psychosomatic disorders are psychosocial transitions or threats of such transitions.

Paykel's work is of particular interest as it shows that life events that are negatively evaluated and changes that constitute "exits" from the environment are more traumatic than positive events and "entrances." In other words, losses are more traumatic than gains. Why should this be when both gains and losses may require major revision of the assumptive world and change the "context of meaning"? I suspect that two factors play a part. First, the identification of given situations as positive or negative (gain or loss) may be made with hindsight; hence those changes that lead to distress are more likely to be seen as losses than as gains. In addition, people are more inclined to anticipate and plan for a change that they hope for than a change that they dread. The possession of a realistic world model of an emergent change is one of the factors that mitigates the stress of transition. This was clearly demonstrated in the studies of unexpected and untimely bereavement that were carried out at the Laboratory of Community Psychiatry (Parkes, 1974), in studies of preparation for major surgery (Egbert and others, 1964; Lazarus and Hagens, 1968), and in studies of release from prison (Sinclair, Shaw, and Troop, 1974). In each of these cases it was those people who were unprepared for the psychosocial transition who subsequently got into difficulties.

Losses characteristically give rise to grief, and an important component of grief is the attempt to resist change and to retain or regain as much as possible of the world that has been lost. Thus we find newly blinded people refusing to learn necessary new skills and to accept the permanence of their blindness (Fitzgerald, 1970) and newly bereaved people searching for a means of contacting the person who has died (Parkes, 1970).

Anticipatory Guidance

It follows from these observations that anything that helps a person to anticipate a psychosocial transition by reducing the fear that causes resistance to confrontation or by providing information that will help the person to cope with the changes that are to come will reduce the risk of pathology. Hence there are good theoretical and practical reasons for including anticipatory guidance as a part of preventive psychiatry.

Perhaps because they are more easily anticipated, maturational changes and the other changes that constitute the milestones of life—leaving school, marriage, the birth of the first baby, retirement, and so on—are probably less damaging than accidental changes. But even these events are turning points for good or bad adjustment, crises when a little help may go a long way. Caplan (1981) and others have drawn attention to the opportunities that exist to identify people who are at special risk at times of crisis, but the need remains for systematic research to develop and evaluate the best methods of anticipatory guidance for people approaching a psychosocial transition. Many questions need to be answered: What are the relative merits of individual as opposed to group methods? Should education or counseling be given? Should it be conducted by highly trained professionals, lay volunteers, or veterans (people who have themselves come through the transition and can speak from their own experience)? Should it take place in the client's home, in the counselor's office, or over the telephone? Is it more effective if paid for by the client, by the state, or by some other body? How important is it to offer help to a few people who are at special risk as opposed to entire populations or subsections of the population?

Each of these alternatives has its adherents, and much ink has been spilled in recent years in defense of particular points of view. But in the last analysis it is systematic research that will provide the answers, and all involved with the development of services have a responsibility to evaluate their work, using the best scientific methods at their disposal. At a minimum these methods must involve the random allocation of clients to alternative methods of guidance and the assessment of outcome in all groups, using outcome measures of proven sensitivity and relevance. Caplan's Laboratory of Community Psychiatry played an important part in the development of such instruments in the 1960s and 1970s.

Whatever the arguments for anticipatory guidance, there are some events that are hard to prepare for. In fact there is strong psychological resistance to the anticipation of disasters. We recognize, for instance, that most married women will one day be widows, but nobody would dare to start a "school for widowhood." In psychological terms to plan for an event is to bring it about; conversely, by refusing to anticipate disaster, we attempt to ward it off. The good general does not admit the possibility of defeat any more than the good wife admits the possibility of widowhood. The surgeon who sets out to remove a breast lump reassures his patient that it is "probably benign," and when this prediction proves wrong he is at pains to explain that the cancer has been removed and that the ensuing radiotherapy is "only a precaution." Likewise the patient who has had his third coronary incident will seldom find anyone who is prepared to discuss the possibility that his next one may well be fatal.

While therapeutic optimism has some value in maintaining the morale of people under stress, it is sometimes taken to absurd lengths, and much of the undoubted success of the "hospice" approach to terminal care arises from the recognition of this fact. By providing an environment in which, as one patient put it, "It is safe to die," the staff recognize that, for many people, life can be lived more richly if patients and family members can be helped to anticipate the fact that they may not have very much longer together.

To reduce avoidance we must reduce fear, and we are obviously expecting a lot of doctors and nurses if we expect them to reduce their patients' fear of death when they are themselves afraid of dying. Yet it does not take very much imagination to realize that the fear of death is not a simple thing—it includes a package of fears. Analysis of the fears reported by dying patients (Parkes, 1973) reveals that these include:

1. Fears of Dying:
   a. Fear of pain or "death agony."
   b. Fear of physical mutilation as the illness gets worse.
   c. Fear of loss of control of physical powers and organs.
   d. Fear of not achieving life aims.
2. Fears of Being Dead:
   a. Fear of judgment or punishment.
   b. Fear of the unknown—death a step into the dark.
   c. Fear for one's dependents—what will become of them?
3. Reflected Fears:
   a. Fears picked up from the behavior of close family and friends.
   b. Fears picked up from the behavior of doctors, nurses, and other caregivers.

It is at once apparent that some of these fears are unnecessary, that some can be remedied, and that all can be reduced if the patient and his family are given the opportunity to share their feelings, are provided with information about their prospects when they are ready for it, and are permitted to express appropriate grief for the various losses that they must face. It is not possible in the space available to do justice to this important topic (see Saunders, 1978, for a more detailed exposition). Suffice it to say that several studies have demonstrated the effectiveness of hospice care in reducing anxiety or depression in patients and relatives (Hinton, 1979; Parkes, 1979). Terminal care, however, does not end with the death of the patient; the family continues and may have great need of continued support. Similarly, there are many bereavements for which family members may have had no opportunity to prepare themselves and many other transitions that give no warning of their coming. In these cases support may not be possible until after the change has begun.

Shneidman (1976) has coined the term *post-ventive guidance* for the counseling that begins after the onset of a transition to distinguish it from the *pre-ventive guidance* that anticipates that event. But these terms are confusing since "post-ventive guidance" is obviously a kind of "pre-vention" of the disorders that will arise if it is not carried out. The situation is further complicated by the fact that many transitions do not occur at a particular moment of time but are spread out over a longer period. Thus the occurrence of a progressively disabling illness, the deterioration of a marital relationship, or the occurrence of other circumstances whose outcome is, for a time, uncertain, require a different kind of help from that which is appropriate when the transition is instantaneous and the outcome clear cut.

The terms *midtransition* and *post transition guidance* may be more appropriate ways of designating help given during and after the period of external change, and it is interesting to note that the turning point (the moment at which the change finally becomes established in external reality) is often marked by some form of ritual. Thus, the person whose health has deteriorated is finally registered as "disabled" or the person whose marriage has crumbled obtains a divorce.

Midtransition Guidance

Midtransition guidance is often made difficult by the indeterminacy of the final outcome. Having no reasonable basis for prediction, it is hard for a person to know what plans to make and for his counselor to help him test reality. Both "wished-for" and "dreaded" models of the future may have to be rehearsed, and there may be a long period during which the client must live in a state of uncertainty. Continued high levels of tension and psychological preparedness will drain the physical and psychological resources of both client and counselor. Support systems must take this into account. Moreover, the client in such a situation may be "disabled by hope." For example, it is well recognized that partial blindness is more disabling than total blindness because it is so hard to persuade the client to accept as permanent the implications of his limited vision. Similarly, the woman whose husband has had an episode of coronary ischaemia may have no means of knowing whether she should prepare for his death, his full recovery, or for a lasting period of disablement.

The counselor must clarify the situation wherever this is possible, help the client to understand and prepare for the probable end results, mobilize familial and other social supports, and remain close enough to give further guidance when it is needed but not so close that he takes away from the client his ability to function autonomously. In view of the draining effects of continuing stresses of this kind, periods of escape (for example, holidays) may be needed, but these should be clearly seen for what they are rather than offered as permanent solutions to intolerable problems.

There is much need for further development and evaluation of methods of midtransition guidance. One successful example, however, is Rahe, O'Neil, and Arthur's evaluation of group support to patients with coronary artery disease—a condition whose outcome is notoriously unpredictable (Rahe, O'Neil, and Arthur, 1975). Rahe showed that those patients who received group support through the period of recovery from a coronary infarction were found to have better adjustment and health eighteen months later than patients who had not been supported in this way.

Posttransition Guidance

The type of help that is needed during the posttransition period depends upon the stage of psychological adjustment or grief that has been reached. Various classifications have been suggested for these phases or patterns of internal change, but the wide variation of response from one person to another must cause us to avoid too rigid an interpretation of these sequences. The progress of adjustment can probably best be viewed as a slowly resolving conflict between conserving and exploring tendencies. In the early stage the tendency to retain old models of the world and to resist change will predominate; later the old models tend to be abandoned and new ones sought for. The conflict is never completely resolved, and it is always possible for a person to swing back and forth between attempts at conservation and attempts at exploration.

The "guidance" literature can be divided into those papers that pay attention to grief and emphasize the importance of helping the client to review his old assumptions about the world (the "grief work") and those that focus on rehabilitation and emphasize the importance of providing information and training to acclimate the client to the new world that he is now entering. Lindemann's approach to bereavement counseling (1944) is a good example of the former. He recognized the importance of facilitating the expression of grief, examining with the client the world that he has lost, and encouraging him to allow appropriate feelings of pining, rage, guilt, and so on to emerge. Once this was done, it was expected that the person would be freed from ties to the past and would find new directions in his life without the need for further help. Lindemann's approach was taken up with enthusiasm by counselors in the mental health field.

Meanwhile, many of those concerned with the rehabilitation of the physically disabled have continued to emphasize gain rather than loss and to point to the obvious benefits of their courses of retraining. Their assumption is that common sense will prevail over intemperate grief and that a person would have to be blind not to take advantage of the offer of a guide dog (or other guidance)! Those who decline such offers of help are dismissed as "too old," "too rigid," or simply "uncooperative" and abandoned to the limbo of rehabilitation failures. Similarly those who emerge from a period of bereavement counseling without abandoning their grief are seen as "dependent" or intractable. The truth would seem to be that both approaches have their place in posttransition guidance. People need permission to grieve *and* permission to stop grieving. They need help in discovering what they have lost *and* in discovering what remains.

Van Gennep in his classic account of the rites of passage ([1909], 1960) pointed out that social rituals often mark both induction into a life change and the formal ending of the transition. The period in between is the time of internal change or the "liminal period." Thus, in the case of bereavement, the "liminal period" is the period of formal mourning and the induction ritual is the funeral. Rosenblatt, Walsh, and Jackson's (1976) comparative anthropological study of seventy-eight representative human societies shows that in 75 percent of them there is a second ritual to mark the end of mourning. In many societies the spirits of the dead are assumed to remain earthbound during the "liminal period," and it is only at the time of the second ritual that they depart for their final resting place. During the period of mourning the survivors are treated as, in some sense, "sick." That is to say, they are relieved of certain obligations and responsibilities and expected to express grief. Others treat them with gentleness and respect and protect them from competition and conflict. At the second ritual, however, they are released from the obligation to mourn and are expected to reassume more normal roles and responsibilities.

It is reasonable to suppose that these systems of belief and behavior foster healthy grieving. When these rituals or other support systems for the bereaved are absent, two kinds of problem may result. Absence of induction rituals can be expected to predispose to the avoidance of mourning; absence of ending rituals can be expected to foster the abnormal persistence of mourning. In Western societies both these problems arise and are commonly associated with distinctive forms of pathological grief (Parkes, 1965). On the one hand, we find people whose grief is delayed or inhibited, with all the resulting psychosomatic and psychological complications of repression or avoidance. On the other hand are those who suffer chronic grief and who may find it hard to give up the role of mourner.

Other psychosocial transitions also have their rites of passage. Thus, physically damaged people are attended by ritual specialists (doctors), who are authorized by society to admit individuals to the liminal status of those requiring rehabilitation. It is worth making a distinction between a "sick" person and a "disabled" one. The former implies that a person is in midtransition and the outcome uncertain, the latter that the outcome is now clear and that long-term changes have occurred for which "rehabilitation" is necessary. The rituals of rehabilitation, like the rituals of mourning, have the aim of inducing changes in a person's view of himself and his world—changes that will enable him to reenter society. But just as the bereaved person may avoid the role of "mourner" or may cling to it for longer than he should, so the disabled person may deny his disability or may cling to the role of "patient" when others think he should assume a new identity. I am not suggesting that the absence of effective social rituals is the sole cause of these pathological reactions but simply that abnormal grief will be less likely to arise or to persist in societies in which social rituals and other supports are present.

In the case of avoided grief it is reasonable to expect that any therapy that facilitates the expression of grief will be helpful. This is the basis of Volkan's use of "linking objects" (1972), Ramsay's "flooding" techniques (1977), and Mawson and others' "guided mourning" (1980). But these forms of therapy may do more harm than good when used to treat chronic grief. In this instance the person in transition may need permission to stop grieving rather than encouragement to express grief. Painful though perpetual grief may be, there are some who cling to it, either because of the secondary gains that arise from it or out of some supposed need to punish themselves for having survived. Thus they are doomed to make restitution to the dead by mourning them forever. In this instance the aim of therapy must be to help the bereaved to understand the self-defeating nature of their reactions and to discover new and more appropriate ways of behaving. Anger turned against the self can become creative if it is redirected against more appropriate objects. Thus a mother who is punishing herself for the death of her child may choose to devote her energies in support of an organization that aims to combat the disease responsible for the child's death.

The chronic griever and the hypochondriac may both be clinging to social roles that protect them from imagined dangers in the world around them. Others who can reassure them of their own abilities and help them discover a new place in the world will increase their chances of "recovery." Persons who have themselves come through a similar experience can often act as guides to those who are withdrawing from society. The doctor may play an important role by conducting the social ritual of a medical examination and issuing a declaration of health.

Scientific evidence is now accumulating that indicates that posttransition guidance to the bereaved can prevent deterioration in physical and mental health (see Parkes, 1980). Well-conducted random allocation studies seem to indicate that guidance is most likely to succeed when it is offered to bereaved individuals who are socially isolated or, for other reasons, at special risk and who are supported in their homes soon after the bereavement by properly trained professionals or by selected volunteers backed by professionals. Mutual help groups for the bereaved, although a logical and interesting development, have not, to my knowledge, been subjected to the test of scientific evaluation.

The success of posttransition guidance to the bereaved has obvious implications for those who are undergoing other psychosocial transitions and particularly for disabled people who require physical rehabilitation. Instances vary from the obvious example of the amputee to the less obvious example of the childless marriage. In this last case a couple may require both midtransition guidance during the period of uncertainty and posttransition guidance once it is established that their sterility is irreversible.

We live in a century that has seen the piecemeal disintegration of the social support system of the extended family in many parts of the world. The rate of cultural change has been so great that the beliefs and social rituals once hallowed by tradition have lost conviction. Thanks to the success of modern medicine in relieving physical distress, the casualties of change turn to doctors rather than priests as a source of help. But grief cannot be cut out or suppressed with drugs, and the medical profession, which tends to rely on such methods, is perplexed and embarrassed by the demands that are made upon it. Now that some methods of counseling have been shown to be effective, we can expect that others will emerge and help us to mitigate the effects of other types of loss. These should be employed by doctors and by other members of the caregiving professions, by clergy, by members of voluntary organizations, and by the many caring persons who are to be found in every community.

References

Brown, G. W., and Harris, T. O. *Social Origins of Depression: A Study of Psychiatric Disorder in Women.* London: Tavistock, 1978.

Caplan, G. "Mastery of Stress: Psychosocial Aspects." *American Journal of Psychiatry,* 1981, *138,* 413-419.

Egbert, L. D., and others. "Reduction of Postoperative Pain by Encouragement and Instruction of Patients: A Study of Doctor-Patient Rapport." *New England Journal of Medicine,* 1964, *270,* 825.

Fitzgerald,R. "Reaction to Blindness: An Exploratory Study of Adults with Recent Loss of Sight." *Archives of General Psychiatry,* 1970, *22,* 270.

Gennep, A. van. *The Rite of Passage.* (M. B. Vizedon and G. L. Caffee, Trans.) Chicago: University of Chicago Press, 1961. (Originally published 1909.)

Hinton, J. "Comparison of Places and Policies for Terminal Care." *Lancet,* 1979, *1,* 29-32.

Lazarus, H. R., and Hagens, J. H. "Prevention of Psychosis Following Open Heart Surgery." *American Journal of Psychiatry,* 1968, *124,* 1190.

Lindemann, E. "The Symptomatology and Management of Acute Grief." *American Journal of Psychiatry,* 1944, *101,* 141.

Marris, P. *Loss and Change.* London: Routledge & Kegan Paul, 1974.

Mawson, D., and others. "Guided Mourning for Morbid Grief: A Controlled Study." Unpublished manuscript, 1980.

Parkes, C. M. "Bereavement and Mental Illness: Pt. I. A Clinical Study of the Grief of Bereaved Psychiatric Patients. Pt. II. A Classification of Bereavement Reactions." *British Journal of Medical Psychology,* 1965, *38,* 1-26.

Parkes, C. M. " 'Seeking' and 'Finding' a Lost Object: Evidence from Recent Studies of the Reaction to Bereavement." *Social Science and Medicine,* 1970, *4,* 187-201.

Parkes, C. M. "Psychosocial Transitions: A Field for Study." *Social Science and Medicine,* 1971, *5,* 101-115.

Parkes, C. M. "Attachment and Autonomy at the End of Life." In R. Gosling (Ed.), *Support, Innovation, and Autonomy.* London: Tavistock, 1973.

Parkes, C. M. "Unexpected and Untimely Bereavement: A Statistical Study of Young Boston Widows and Widowers." In B. Schoenberg and others (Eds.), *Bereavement: Its Psychosocial Aspects.* New York: Columbia University Press, 1974.

Parkes, C. M. "Terminal Care: Evaluation of Inpatient Service at St. Christopher's Hospice. Pt. I. Views of Surviving Spouses on the Effects of the Service on the Patient. Part II. Self-Assessment of Effects of the Service on Surviving Spouse." *Postgraduate Medical Journal,* 1979, *55,* 5-7.

Parkes, C. M. "Bereavement Counseling: Does it Work?" *British Medical Journal,* 1980, *281,* 3-6.

Paykel, E. S. "Life Stress and Psychiatric Disorder: Applications of the Clinical Approach." In B. S. Dohrenwend and B. P. Dohrenwend (Eds.), *Stressful Life Events: Their Nature and Effects.* New York: Wiley, 1974.

Rahe, R. H. "Life Crisis and Health Change." In P. R. A. May and J. R. Wittenborn (Eds.), *Psychotropic Drug Response: Advances in Prediction.* Springfield, Ill.: Thomas, 1969.

Rahe, R. H. "Epidemiological Studies of Life Change and Illness." *International Journal of Psychiatry in Medicine,* 1975, *6,* 133-146.

Rahe, R. H., O'Neil, T., and Arthur, R. J. "Brief Group Therapy Following Myocardial Infarction: Eighteen-Month Follow-Up of a Controlled Trial." *International Journal of Psychiatry in Medicine,* 1975, *6,* 349-358.

Ramsay, R. W. "Bereavement: A Behavioral Treatment of Pathological Grief." *Behavioral Research and Therapy,* 1977, *15,* 131-135.

Rosenblatt, P. C., Walsh, R. P., and Jackson, D. A. *Grief and Mourning in Cross-Cultural Perspective.* New Haven, Conn.: Human Relations Area File Press, 1976.

Saunders, C. M. (Ed.). *The Management of Terminal Disease.* London: Edward Arnold, 1978.

Shneidman, E. S. "Introduction: Current Overview of Suicide." In E. S. Schneidman (Ed.) *Suicidology: Contemporary Developments.* New York: Grune & Stratton, 1976.

Sinclair, I. A. C., Shaw, M. S., and Troop, J. "The Relationship Between Introversion and Response to Casework in a Prison Setting." *British Journal of Social and Clinical Psychology,* 1974, *13,* 51-60.

Volkan, V. "The 'Linking Objects' of Pathological Mourners." *Archives of General Psychiatry,* 1972, *27,* 215-221.

Chapter 8

Impact of Public Policy on Mental Health Services

Dwight Harshbarger
Harold W. Demone, Jr.

Nearly a decade ago we wrote and edited the material that would later become *A Handbook of Human Service Organizations* (Demone and Harshbarger, 1974). It seems appropriate to reflect now on developments in the human services over the past ten years and to consider issues likely to confront community mental health administrators and service providers during the 1980s.

In reviewing our earlier work, we became keenly aware of the extent to which any analysis of community mental health services must rest on certain assumptions about the environment within which these systems function. It is of more than historical interest that in examining the environment of the early 1970s, we made the following assumptions:

1. The Vietnam War would end in two to four years.
2. The Republican party would hold the presidency through 1976.

3. The federal government would continue to fund Department of Health, Education, and Welfare programs at levels necessary to at least maintain and probably expand them. As the budget of this department continued its growth rate, it would soon exceed that of the Department of Defense.
4. The Republicans would decentralize authority to regional offices of the Department of Health, Education, and Welfare and to state governments.
5. Block grants for state and county government through revenue sharing and similar programs would become more common.
6. Legal considerations related to the rights of clients to secure services would increase in importance.
7. In the field of mental health:
    a. Deinstitutionalization would effectively reduce community reliance upon state hospitals.
    b. Funding for community mental health programs would continue to expand.
    c. State, local, and third-party funds would replace federal funds as the latter's support for community mental health centers (CHMCs) ended.
    d. The network model of service delivery would expand. We envisioned community mental health programs rather than centers.
8. In the field of social welfare:
    a. There would be an increasing emphasis upon the chronically dependent client.
    b. The multiproblem client and family would receive increasing priority.
    c. Multipurpose human service organizations and programs would be given high priority in funding and system design.
9. Planning would receive high priority, and planning organizations would be given increased authority to control costs and more effectively allocate limited resources.
10. Administrators would realize that there are limits to rationality in planning.
11. Planning would be greatly enhanced by client information

systems and data on program outcomes, thus enabling managers to more effectively determine resource utilization.

12. Program budgets and cost-benefit accounting would evolve into helpful tools for managers.
13. Neo-Keynesian economics would continue to characterize the American economy, which would enjoy steady growth and relatively low rates of inflation.
14. The principal resources for improving the quality of life for the poor would continue to emanate from the public sector.

Although the Vietnam War did end and the Republicans did hold the White House through 1976, we did not expect the heightened turbulence brought about by Vietnam and the Watergate disclosures or the adverse effects that these developments would have for community mental health programs. The war dramatically escalated in cost, feeding inflationary pressures and reducing the resources available for domestic problems. And the protests that were generated in part by the unfairness of the Selective Service System helped turn policy makers' attention toward issues of equity for disadvantaged Americans.

These pressures meshed with and helped intensify an unprecedented concern by newly formed public interest legal organizations for the basic constitutional rights of disabled Americans. As a result, the rights of mental patients began to be defined through major court decisions rather than by clinicians and public policy makers. When this trend was joined with the already powerful effort to secure equal opportunities for blacks and women, the product was a massive and new civil rights movement affecting every organization receiving federal monies. Affirmative action programs were mandated for all CMHCs receiving federal funds, architectural barriers for the physically handicapped began to be removed, maternity leave was granted male employees, and so on. Taken together, these societal pressures markedly changed the work environment of CMHC organizations.

Our assumptions about the continued expansion of funding for human service organizations proved correct up until the time that the 1981 budget of the Reagan administration was passed. Prior to that, these were relatively easy assumptions to make, simply because programs for better meeting the health, education, and welfare needs of communities were unlikely to be funded by state and county tax dollars. We did not anticipate what now appears to be the end of Keynesian economics, as a result of the sharp inflationary rise in prices and wages that was brought about by the pricing behavior of OPEC, the world's most powerful oil cartel. It is not that we did not anticipate so-called Reaganomics. For if Vietnam and Watergate had not interfered, Nixon would have headed in a similar direction durhis second term. What was not anticipated was the rate and speed with which conservative economic proposals were enacted in the Reagan administration.

The effects of these political and economic events upon community mental health systems have been profound. First, rising costs have reduced the available resources. Although levels of community need and demand have changed little, the funding available to combat the complex health, social service, and educational problems confronting community mental health clients has diminished. Even in those organizations that have been fortunate enough to withstand actual budget reductions, double-digit inflation has reduced the real value of available funds.

A second consequence of the funding constraint has been to require mental health administrators to closely analyze the services and outcomes produced by existing patterns of resource utilization. Client information systems, which were still being resisted in the mid 1970s, are now quite commonplace. Administrators now accept the challenge from funding sources to produce positive and demonstrable changes in client functioning. Although these are healthy developments, the more immediate danger is that inadequate evaluation technology will produce erroneous conclusions about service effectiveness. Human service organizations deal with highly complex problems, and they seldom, if ever, can control the major variables at which treatment is directed. Until a technology of outcome measurement is fully developed and refined, administrators would do well to sharpen their political skills and compete for budget dollars in the political rather than scientific arena.

Our substantive assumptions regarding mental health programs have remained intact on the whole, and events in this field appear likely to continue in the directions of the past decade. Resource problems will continue to vex policy makers. The chronically dependent and multiproblem client and family continue to be of major concern; but, except for adopting a "cash" or voucher system that allows the client to purchase services in the open market, there have been no major changes in the methods of meeting the needs of this disadvantaged group. The present categorical structure of human service programs and their administrative and accounting systems continues to be inordinately expensive, and ensuring that monies are used in the ways intended by legislation and regulations continues to escalate costs. While efforts to conceptualize and use natural support systems in community life as vehicles for treatment have begun to mature, very few mental health professionals are trained to utilize support networks. Perhaps the next decade will bring innovation in systems that support client purchase of services, and perhaps these systems will stimulate more imaginative entrepreneurial behavior among human service organizations. We doubt that such an approach would result in more waste than is already produced by present regulatory requirements.

It is unlikely that mental health organizations will voluntarily reform themselves, since jobs and power are at stake. Their environment must change, and we think that client control of the service dollar would be a powerful impetus to such change. An example of the impact of client choice can be found in the rapid decline of inpatient services experienced by public general hospitals (usually municipal) in the late 1960s and early 1970s when low-income clients were given the power by Medicaid to choose their own medical care. Many city hospitals found their inpatient censuses reduced by two thirds because their former clients chose to use voluntary general hospitals. One cautionary note in this regard is that the Department of Health and Human Services has concluded that the supply and demand characteristics of the marketplace do not apply in the case of physicians. Each physician generates fixed costs regardless of the degree of competition. Therefore, it has been proposed, as a way of controlling costs, that the number of practicing physicians be limited.

The funding of community mental health organizations has continued to be supported by the federal government, with state and local governments, private funds, and third-party fees providing the matching dollars necessary for federal support. Although the federal CMHC staffing grants have been phased out, relatively few centers have been forced to close because of insufficient funding. Fiscal support from state governments usually has offset the lost federal funds, and CMHCs have continued to function. However, the nature of their services has changed significantly, with a shift toward the provision of more direct and fewer consultative or indirect services. Decreased reliance upon state hospitals has been made possible by the greater availability of local services, more general hospital psychiatric services, federal fiscal supplements to aid clients living in the community (for example, Supplemental Security Income [SSI] and food stamps), and growth of the nursing home industry. The availability of nursing homes in particular has enabled tens of thousands of elderly patients to be moved out of mental hospitals.

Now that mental health centers have begun to secure federal support monies for clients, chronically dependent persons have been able to return to community life. Whether their quality of life has been improved by such a move is debatable (see "Mental Health Issues and Trends," 1979). Nevertheless, having mental health services available close to home has reversed a long American tradition of expelling behaviorally deviant people from community life. This new approach has resulted in the provision of services for a large population of chronically disturbed and dependent clients by CMHCs, and it has absorbed ever larger amounts of center resources.

As these changes have occurred, the mental health environment in the private sector has undergone significant changes as well. Insurers of health services have legitimized payment for certain types of psychiatric and substance-abuse services, thus encouraging health organizations and private practitioners that serve largely employed and insured clients to provide mental health services and to compete with CMHCs for the third-party dollar. CMHCs encumbered with state and federal regulations and concomitantly high overhead costs have experienced difficulty competing under these circumstances, and the result has been a movement of blue- and white-collar workers away from CMHCs. The public image of CMHCs has thus come to resemble that of other public agencies and of state hospitals.

Our assumption that deinstitutionalization would be effective has proved to be tenuous for at least some patients (see Bassuk and Gerson, 1978). Although the average daily census in state hospitals decreased from 559,000 in 1955 to well below 200,000 in 1980, admission rates, except in more progressive states, have remained high. Sometimes they have even increased due to high readmission rates among former state hospital patients. Moreover, as we noted, serious questions have been raised about the quality of life for persons who, after many years of institutionally dependent living, are now forced to fend for themselves in often inhospitable community environments (Lamb and Goertzel, 1972).

In addition to the hostility exhibited by many communities, four other factors have contributed to the unhappy fate suffered by some chronically disturbed clients. First, funds have not adequately followed clients into the community. Unfortunately, some advocates of deinstitutionalization have promoted it as a means of reducing expenditures, and politicians have either trimmed appropriations or have not permitted them to keep up with inflation. Second, the strategy of phasing down institutions rather than selectively closing them down has produced only minor budget adjustments. The fixed to variable cost ratio of large institutions allowed for significant savings only with closings. Third, the models of monitoring and supporting the chronic patient in the community derived from classic treatment regimes of psychotherapy and medication were much too narrowly conceived. Only recently have case management and other modalities been added so as to accommodate the more extensive needs of chronic patients in the community. Fourth, both the ideology and the therapeutic skills of the community-based practitioner are often incongruent with the needs of the chronic client. Not only are the therapeutic tools of these practitioners better designed to deal with acute and neurotic clients but so are their interests, beliefs, values, and reward systems.

Planning as an enterprise devoted to the most efficient and effective use of public and private resources was markedly enhanced during the 1970s. Although our assumption about the growing legitimacy and power of planning organizations was accurate, we did not anticipate the rapid escalation of human service costs and the compensatory and intense pressure for lean, nonduplicative human service systems. Prior to the Reagan administration, health systems agencies had in many states become powerful planning organizations, sometimes challenging the authority of a governor and a state's department of health ("HSA Spends . . . ," 1980). (We note, for the record, that it is only the sanctions and authority that have grown in human service planning. The absolute number of planners remained essentially unchanged during the decade.) One of the more curious recommendations of the Reagan administration has been to eliminate health systems agencies. These organizations both forged effective planning and became major cost-control vehicles that were themselves controlled by citizens and providers, not the government. They also met two major Reagan administration objectives: reduced governmental control and reduced expenditures. However, consistency has never been a hallmark of the political world.

Finally, and perhaps most importantly, our assumption that the principal resources for improving the quality of life for the poor would continue to rest in the public sector may no longer be tenable. New Deal programs in the 1930s that, with some modifications, were later to become the foundation of the Great Society in the 1960s seem to have run their course. The very real limits to what can be accomplished by simply providing money and services to chronically disadvantaged people without simultaneously altering their life-styles and the natural ecology of community life has become increasingly apparent. The shrinking human service dollar, combined with our growing awareness that deleterious environments and life-styles impact upon health and life adjustment (Harshbarger and others, 1973;

Dohrenwend and Dohrenwend, 1974; Boulding, 1978), have heightened our recognition that there are constraints and limits to the efforts of human service programs.

It is very probable that in the 1980s fewer resources will be available for public human service programs to confront the difficult and intricate problems of community life. Inevitably, this will force a reappraisal of public policies regarding such allocations. A likely result is that many human service programs will become "last-resort" resources to be used only when all else fails. This will be a marked departure in mission for the many human service organizations, including CMHCs, that have viewed themselves as "first-resort" forces for major social changes. The work of human service professionals is likely, therefore, to become difficult and frustrating as they are required to function more defensively with minimal control over program priorities. New resources and more active efforts to alter the natural ecology of community life will have to become the responsibility of the private sector in America's economy. There are few recent parallels to characterize the demands that will be made upon business and industrial organizations in the 1980s to positively alter community life. Therefore, the ability of a quasi-free market economy to serve the interests of both its corporate members and the public at large will be severely tested.

Managers and planners repeatedly experience problems in organizing and structuring staff behavior to best serve both clients and the long-term interests of their organizations. Teaching new staff and socializing them into the organization's behavioral norms, preventing burnout and maintaining the interest of senior staff, promoting effective change, and orchestrating productive professional relationships are never-ending tasks in the constantly evolving environment of community mental health programs. However, the substantive nature of management problems changes as social and economic shifts occur in the center's community and in the larger culture. Issues confronting human service systems in the 1970s included the following:

1. The relative absence of women and blacks in upper-level management positions was gaining legitimacy as a major problem to be resolved.

2. The damage to clients' lives resulting from the labels assigned to them by human service professionals was becoming increasingly recognized.
3. State and federal government efforts to solve newly emerging social problems by creating and funding new service programs were recognized as responsive and politically safe means of "doing good" that would inevitably have to end. Most administrators hoped this would occur in the distant future so they could avoid the immediate turbulence of reorganizing their existing systems.
4. There was a growing awareness that well-intended attempts to improve the quality of life for certain clients, for example, programs to generate low-cost urban housing and programs of deinstitutionalization, were sometimes producing serious and long-term harm.
5. Struggles for the control of programs among professionals, community advocates, and consumer advocates were creating friction and divisiveness.
6. Program planners were struggling to achieve a meaningful and functional definition of the term *community*.
7. How to establish time-limited, short- and medium-range goals and objectives based upon a more data-oriented approach to management became an increasingly important question.
8. The measurement of service outcomes was receiving at least minor recognition as an organizational need.
9. There was considerable concern about finding a means to reallocate resources so that they could be used to address the needs of populations receiving inadequate care.
10. Computers were assuming an increasingly significant and widespread role in management and planning tasks. There was concern about how to best finance, use, and effectively control this new resource.

Issues in Managing Community Mental Health Programs in the 1980s

During the 1970s, the Department of Health, Education, and Welfare, firmly backed by Congress and the courts, successfully implemented affirmative action programs in organizations receiving federal financial assistance. This led to the hiring and promotion of women and minorities, groups that historically had been statistically underrepresented among some of the mental health professions. Similar legal processes were begun in the 1970s to prevent discrimination against persons who had been diagnosed and treated in psychiatric and substance-abuse facilities. Programs to protect the rights of the physically handicapped were also sanctioned.

Legal debates associated with the right to employment and the equitable management of personnel practices promise to continue well into the 1980s. A growing body of laws, regulations, and court decisions has targeted organizations receiving federal dollars as having special obligations to remedy past employment inequities. Human service organizations, which confront the personal and behavioral consequences of institutionalized discrimination in American life, will be expected to provide continuing leadership in solving these problems. It remains to be seen how well this can be accomplished while simultaneously maintaining a reasonable level of high-quality professional services in the face of budgets that have been reduced both by inflation and real cutbacks.

Problems in reorganizing the human service bureaucracies of federal, state, and local governments, discussed throughout the 1970s, will continue in the 1980s. This is already occurring in medical services, as health systems agencies make ever more difficult decisions to control and limit the expansion of health facilities and programs. In those sectors of the human service economy that are growing more slowly but that nevertheless are already mammoth in size (for example, social and rehabilitative services), difficult decisions will have to be made about combining, limiting, and perhaps even eliminating programs that were affordable in an expanding but less inflationary economy. Jobs, patronage, political clout, and individual and community needs will collide as planners, politicians, professionals, and consumers scan these alternatives.

An idea reinvented each decade cannot easily be ignored. During the 1960s (the Johnson administration), the 1970s (the

Nixon administration), and the 1980s (the Reagan administration) serious efforts were and are being made to reduce the number of categorical programs and to give state governments more authority over the distribution of federal funds through the use of block grants for social programs. There were other goals as well, but the two mentioned above were generally found acceptable by liberals and conservatives alike. For community mental health advocates, the block grant proposals characterized in bold relief some of their fundamental political dilemmas. It was not then, nor is it now, true that the categorical direct investment by the National Institute of Mental Health in CMHCs was economically significant nationwide; block grants themselves did not jeopardize CMHC survival. Rather, the placing of block grant decisions in the hands of state mental health authorities tilted the probable decision outcomes toward the outmoded institutions that continued to be strongly supported in many states. To complicate matters further, CMHC advocates now find themselves competing for resources and influence with both their general health colleagues and their human service colleagues.

Just as environmental impact statements are required of plans to alter the physical environment, so it may be necessary for social impact statements to be drafted for public- and private-sector innovations that affect the natural ecology of community life. It does little good to build housing projects that quickly become slums or to move elderly state mental health patients into lower-quality boarding and nursing care homes. As the nation intensifies its concerns with cost controls for nondefense expenditures, technical planning and forecasting the consequences of efforts to improve the quality of community life will need far greater attention in the 1980s than in the previous decade.

The search for a more functional definition of community, the problems of designing more effective mechanisms whereby resource allocations can match changes in client populations, and the power struggles among professionals, consumers, and the community at large will receive far less attention during the 1980s. This change is in part the result of a natural resolution of some of these issues, and in part reflects the new priority placed on the organization, efficiency, productivity, and effectiveness of human services. Managers now find themselves facing sharply increased demands by funding sources for valid measurement and evaluation procedures. Given the still-limited technology available for such purposes, program managers substitute process measures ("who, what, where, and when") for the more fundamental criteria of effectiveness. We do not criticize these developments if they are seen as first steps toward developing an effective monitoring system and not as ends in themselves. However, unless a technology of measurement that is affordable and valid becomes readily available, there is a very real risk that inappropriate process-oriented accounting procedures will form a structurally flawed foundation for management and planning.

Professional or guild-related problems were of less importance in the 1970s than they are in the present decade. Issues include the rapidly expanding numbers of newly trained professionals entering a limited job market, threats to traditional professional domains through the declassification of positions in government-operated systems, and a vigorous effort to upgrade paraprofessionals in such areas as alcoholism treatment. Added to these problems is the movement being made by many professional groups toward unionization and collective bargaining, a movement that in many states is already colliding with attempts to reorganize and streamline human service organizations. The continuing growth and use of psychotropic drugs in mental health treatment has led to an increasing reemphasis upon the pharmaceutical aspects of treatment, hence a remedicalizing of the therapeutic process. And, the self-help movement that gained momentum throughout the 1970s continues to divert the efforts of many human service systems and their professional staff, since they view self-help programs as competitive rather than complementary.

As we approached the end of the 1970s, the *Report to the President* (President's Commission on Mental Health, 1978) was issued. This one-year study of the nation's mental health services, the first comprehensive examination of America's mental health services since the Report of the Joint Commission on Mental Illness and Health (1961), made strong recommendations about needed changes in mental health services and systems. These recommendations included the allocation of resources for comprehensive and integrated systems of care, minimizing community reliance upon institutional care, the improvement of aftercare services and services to special and minority populations, coordinated planning and increased citizen participation in planning, and the strengthening of natural helping agents and self-help groups.

Although the report of the President's Commission on Mental Health will be a major influence in legislation and funding priorities in the 1980s, it is doubtful that it will have the impact of its predecessor, the Joint Commission report. In 1960 the problems of human degradation in our mental hospitals were visible and shocking. The need to develop alternative, community-based mental health services was obvious, though the particular organizational models that could best provide these services was uncertain. In the 1980s alternative and community-based mental health organizations are in place throughout much of the nation, and we are becoming aware of the limitations in the performance of these new service delivery organizations. The pressures for system change today have less to do with human degradation than with system inadequacy. It is a more complex problem, and the costs and the benefits of our programmatic and organizational alternatives are far more blurred than those of 1960.

To a small but significant percentage of Americans, community mental health programs represent the only available help in coping with the problems of daily life. These organizations comprise our collective national attempt to intervene therapeutically in the lives of clients and correct inadequacies in the natural ecology of community life. The problems of clients are also a window through which one can glimpse the inner and interlocking workings of community and family systems in America.

Shrinking resources, the lower value placed on human needs, and intensified concerns with the service yield per public dollar spent will bring strong and unyielding pressures to narrow the focus and constrain the types of mental health services to be supported in the 1980s. This will confront planners and policy shapers with incredibly difficult decisions. Are mental health programs more or less valuable than cancer detection programs or additional diet supplements to elderly people with low incomes? Should programs of primary prevention receive a higher priority than emergency care in budget planning? To make such decisions, it is necessary that we more fully develop bio-psychosocial models and analogues of human coping and community life. Through such complex but workable models of human systems, we can anticipate the impact of prevention and intervention programs on the health and welfare of individuals and communities. It is a major challenge but one that must be met if we are to advance the quality of life in the United States during the decade of the 1980s.

References

Bassuk, E. L., and Gerson, S. "Deinstitutionalization and Mental Health Services." *Scientific American,* 1978, *238,* 46-53.

Boulding, K. *Ecodynamics.* Beverly Hills, Calif.: Sage, 1978.

Demone, H. W. "The Limits of Rationality in Planning." In H. W. Demone and D. Harshbarger (Eds.), *A Handbook of Human Service Organizations.* New York: Behavioral Publications, 1974.

Demone, H. W., and Harshbarger, D. (Eds.). *A Handbook of Human Service Organizations.* New York: Behavioral Publications, 1974.

Dohrenwend, B. S., and Dohrenwend, B. P. (Eds.). *Stressful Life Events: Their Nature and Effects.* New York: Wiley, 1974.

Harshbarger, D., and others. *A Survey and Analysis of Human Ecosystems and Human Service Systems in Appalachia.* Morgantown: Appalachian Center, West Virginia University, 1973.

"HSA Spends $25,815 to Contest New Hospital." *Charleston Gazette* (Charleston, W.Va.), January 22, 1980.

Joint Commission on Mental Illness and Health. *Action for Mental Health.* New York: Basic Books, 1961.

Lamb, H. R., and Goertzel, V. "The Demise of the State Mental Hospital—A Premature Obituary?" *Archives of General Psychiatry,* 1972, *26,* 489-495.

"Mental Health Issues and Trends." New York: *New York Times* Information Service, 1979.

President's Commission on Mental Health. *Report to the President from the President's Commission on Mental Health.* 4 Vols. Washington, D.C.: U.S. Government Printing Office, 1978.

Chapter 9

Effects of Value Systems on Service Delivery

Frank Baker

The way in which society helps those encountering personal difficulties periodically changes. As Schulberg and Baker (1975a) have noted: "The types of assistance and manner in which they are provided reflect each period's social values, political ideologies, technological capability, economic level, organizational practices, and manpower availability" (pp. 1-2). There have been a series of "movements" in the mental health field that have more or less reflected major shifts in the "world view" or "paradigms" of its community of practitioners. In *The Structure of Scientific Revolutions,* Kuhn (1970) presents the idea of a *paradigm* as a set of theoretical assumptions that are developed to explain difficult-to-understand phenomena. If the paradigm fits the basic values and social structure in a given professional field, it gradually becomes accepted as reality itself and begins to redefine that area. The paradigm becomes the normal way of conceiving things, and it expands as necessary to incorporate "anomalies" or to deal with difficult questions. Kuhn describes scientific revolutions in terms of challenges to the dominant paradigm of the times.

Three decades before Kuhn's work, Zilboorg (1941) proposed in a history of medical psychology that the development of mental health services could be conceptualized as a series of revolutions. He suggested that the first such revolution occurred after the French Revolution when society's perception of the mentally disturbed changed from viewing them as evil to viewing them as ill. Reflecting changes in the intellectual and social concerns of that period, new theories were developed regarding the mentally disturbed. Mental health services changed, and treatment replaced punishment and confinement; this is well illustrated by the work of Phillipe Pinel and Samuel Tuke. This period is generally thought to have witnessed mental health's first revolution symbolized by Pinel's striking the chains off the mentally disturbed. Similarly, there is widespread agreement that the second revolution occurred at the end of the Victorian period with Sigmund Freud's development of psychoanalysis and his interpretation of the human as a psychosexual being.

During the 1960s, a number of authors suggested that a third revolution was occurring as a result of the development of community mental health programs. But as Hollander (1980) observes, although there is agreement that revolutionary change began during this period, there is still some disagreement as to its basic parameters. Hollander concluded that part of the difficulty lies in the impossibility of associating the third revolution with a single event or person, as had been the case with the earlier revolutions, despite Hobbs' (1964) suggestion that the third revolution might be identified through a number of "seemingly disparate innovations."

Rose (1979) has noted the irony in the fact that the first mental health revolution involved the establishment of the asylum or hospital, and that, over a century later, the community mental health revolution was stimulated by a desire to rectify the problems created by the first revolution. Rose further notes that the physician's view about sanity has changed very little from the pre-Civil War era, that is, insanity is still seen as a disease either of the brain or in the brain: "Essentially, the medical view of mental illness has gone unchanged, and the transformation that did take place was one of type rather than kind—one in which the same basic types of service would be delivered through a new community-based delivery system. Put another way, the nature of the change was to move predominantly old, medically defined, inpatient services to new outpatient facilities. The hospital came under attack as if it somehow existed independently of the profession that managed it, proclaimed its virtues, and supervised its decline, while always rationalizing its existence—a process that allowed for continued medical control" (pp. 436-437).

Bassuk and Gerson (1978) have observed what may be considered a further historical irony in that much of the initial motivation for developing state hospitals in the nineteenth century was economically inspired. The state hospitals were viewed as a cost-effective treatment setting to be preferred over the smaller, more numerous county institutions. In the 1970s, the opposite thinking prevailed. Rose (1979) has described the recent policy of deinstitutionalization as demonstrating "the power of reigning and socially stabilizing paradigms; organizational rearrangements are made in the name of humane social change, while, simultaneously, traditional orientations and practices are maintained in new settings" (p. 455). He noted the emergence of a further development in the community mental health movement: "The 'new' new era already on the horizon, with offices in NIMH and small-scale projects in a limited number of states, is that of Community Support Systems (CSS) programs. This new development is obviously an effort to recognize the failures of the old new era to anticipate and plan for concrete problems of daily life among those pushed out of hospitals and into deprived and exploitative living environments" (p. 456).

Ideological Changes

The various revolutions in mental health practice have been associated with changes in the basic ideologies of mental health practitioners. The ideological beliefs of caregivers have long been recognized as crucial variables affecting the type and quality of helping services offered to clients. Beliefs and attitudes are particularly important in areas where there is inadequate scientific evidence to serve as a basis for informed opinion. A belief system—that is, a set of interrelated, although not necessarily logically organized, ideas to which the members of a collectivity are strongly committed—can provide a common rationale for the behavior of the group's members. Mental health and other human service disciplines have developed new programs more often on the basis of belief than on the basis of empirical, well-supported clinical evidence. Faced with a variety of social and professional pressures for change, those charged with the design and operation of professional delivery systems are likely to proceed on the basis of what is believed to be good and right rather than what is likely to be effective.

Humanistic Ideologies of the 1950s. As mental health service delivery programs developed during the last three decades, a number of studies were made of the ideologies utilized by professionals in choosing and treating persons defined as needing help. The rebirth of humanism in the United States during the 1950s resulted in a redefinition of the mental hospital as a community of persons rather than a rigid institution of incarceration. The Custodial Mental Illness (CMI) Scale was developed by Gilbert and Levinson (1957) to measure custodialism and humanism as ideological orientations of mental hospital staff. Gilbert and Levinson found that hospital units having the most custodial policy consisted of personnel with the most custodial ideologies and the most authoritarian personalities.

An examination of therapeutic ideologies among psychiatric residents and senior medical staff undertaken by Sharaf and Levinson (1957) focused on the bipolar dimensions of a "psychotherapeutic" versus a "sociotherapeutic" treatment orientation. In their study of psychiatric services to New Haven residents, Hollingshead and Redlich (1958) similarly defined the practitioners as adhering to either of two orientations: directive-organic or analytic-psychotherapeutic. The attempt to clarify the ideological orientations of mental health workers was advanced by Strauss and others (1964) when they integrated the somatic dimension refined by Hollingshead and Redlich with the psychotherapeutic and sociotherapeutic dimension measures identified by Sharaf and Levinson.

Although Strauss and his colleagues hypothesized that each of these orientations represented a separate and distinct ideology, their data indicated that only "sociotherapeutic" was an independent dimension. The somatotherapeutic and psychotherapeutic orientations were strongly negatively correlated, suggesting the existence of a continuum of "psycho" versus "somato" ideology. Using data from a nationwide survey of hospital psychiatrists, Armor and Klerman (1968) found factor analytic support for the independent ideologies of somatotherapy and psychotherapy. Since only a small amount of the variance could be explained by each factor, these researchers saw the need for refined measures and predicted that sociotherapy might develop into full ideological status under the egis of community mental health.

Community Mental Health: Ideology of the 1960s and 1970s. In the second half of the 1960s, Baker and Schulberg (1967) postulated that a growing collectivity of mental health professionals was forming a new social movement in mental health and beginning to share a common ideology. Baker and Schulberg described this new ideological movement of community mental health as particularly concerned with such issues as professionals' assuming responsibility for an entire population rather than only the individual patient; primary prevention of mental illness through the amelioration of harmful environmental conditions; treating patients with the goal of social rehabilitation rather than personality reorganization; comprehensive continuity of care and concern for the mentally ill; and total involvement of both professional and nonprofessional helpers in caring for the mentally ill. Schulberg and Baker (1969) later described community mental health ideology as the mental health professional "belief system of the 1960s."

Through the development of a valid and reliable Community Mental Health Ideology (CMHI) Scale (Baker and Schulberg, 1967), it was possible to demonstrate that this new ideological orientation existed as a major belief system among nationwide samples of various professional disciplines. Degree of commitment to this ideology was significantly higher among those individuals who had received additional training in community mental health. Evidence of highly satisfactory psychometric properties for the CMHI Scale was obtained in the first study and in subsequent research by Langston (1970) and Breeskin, Wolff, and Witzke (1972). Gross (1972) found that mental health workers with high scores on the CMHI Scale were more likely to work in community settings than workers with low scores. In a nationwide study of graduate students in psychiatric nursing, Howard and Baker (1971) found that commitment to community mental health ideology was related to an acceptance of broader community-oriented role functions for the psychiatric nurse. Block (1974) administered the CMHI Scale to service directors, line staff, and student aides in a community mental health center and found that the psychiatrists had the greatest degree of variance in their responses and the lowest overall mean on the CMHI Scale. Examining service units, Block found considerable variation in overall identification with community mental health ideology; mental health workers had the weakest identification with it. Block also found CMHI Scale scores of service units to be related to the degree to which the units were involved in community activities.

Community mental health ideology has been empirically related to expanding roles for mental health professionals, but also with liberal versus conservative values among mental health professionals and citizens at large. For example, Baker and Schulberg (1969) found that attitudes strongly in favor of a community mental health approach were negatively correlated with dogmatism and political and economic conservatism. Hersch (1972) similarly related the community mental health movement and its underlying ideology to social and historical changes in the United States. He asserted that it was not accidental that the community mental health movement blossomed in this country during the decade of the 1960s, a period characterized by the spirit of social and political reform and an emphasis on a "revitalized humanistic concern for the disadvantaged, the oppressed, and the powerless" (p. 749). In an epilogue to Ruth Caplan's book tracing the recurring concern with environment in the prevention and treatment of mental disorder in nineteenth-century American psychiatry, Gerald Caplan (1969) similarly suggested that ideology might play an important role in the survival of community psychiatry once economic, social, and political forces changed again.

Human Service Ideology in the 1970s and 1980s. During the 1970s, still another ideology evolved among mental health professionals and other community caregivers who had come together from the community mental health, consumerism, and New Careers movements (Baker and Northman, 1978, 1981). Baker (1974) labeled this developing set of beliefs as "human service ideology" and suggested that it is characterized by five general themes:

1. *Systemic integration:* the belief that genuinely effective, comprehensive services can be provided only by linking the various caregiving agencies that provide a complex array of resources, technologies, and skills.
2. *Comprehensive accessibility:* the view that services should be inclusive and available to clients without geographic, administrative, or other barriers.
3. *Problems in living:* the belief that client problems should be defined and analyzed with regard to the fit between a person and his or her environment rather than through diagnostic labels focusing on individual deficiencies.
4. *Generic helping activities:* the assumption that a universal quality exists in the helping actions of caregivers that transcends disciplinary and professional barriers.
5. *Service provider accountability:* the view that service providers are responsible not only to themselves and their colleagues but, more importantly, to their clients and the public at large.

Baker and Baker (1981) developed the Human Service Ideology (HSI) Scale with psychometric procedures similar to those employed for the Community Mental Health Ideology Scale (Baker and Schulberg, 1967). An initial pool of items was constructed on the basis of five thematic categories derived from the relevant literature. These items were subjected to content validity review by a panel of expert judges, edited on the basis of the judges' ratings, assembled into a questionnaire containing other questions to be used in checking concurrent and construct validity, and then submitted to a large national sample of respondents. Respondents were selected from relevant groups "known" to have differing commitments to this particular ideological orientation.

Unlike the CMHI Scale, the HSI Scale is multidimensional. A factor analysis supported the existence of four of the five hypothesized subdimensions, namely, systemic integration, comprehensive accessibility, generic helping activities, and service provider accountability. The problems-in-living items did not stand out as a separate dimension, but rather they tended to blend with the systems integration items that focus on the whole person and his or her problems. Scale factor and total scores were related to self-reports of human service orientation. Scale reliability data, item-total correlations, and interfactor and factor-total correlations supported the general utility of the thirty-six-item total score as a measure of one's adherence to human service ideology. The HSI Scale also successfully distinguished between "known groups," thus giving further evidence of its validity.

Libertarian Mental Health Ideology of the 1980s. Nevid and Morrison (1980) have developed an attitude scale to measure another contemporary ideology, namely, the radical psychosocial or libertarian belief system. This ideology posits that "mental illness" is really a metaphor that has outlived its usefulness. Based on Szasz' (1974) assertion that mental illness is a reified metaphor and hence a myth, the libertarian ideology rejects "the medical model treatment of behavioral problems as epiphenomena of organic diseases, preferring to regard such deviant conduct in terms of psychosocial, communicative, cognitive, or existential antecedents" (Nevid and Morrison, 1980, p. 72).

Nevid and Morrison (1980) have successfully constructed the Libertarian Mental Health Ideology (LMHI) Scale to measure this radical view of the nature of mental illness and mental health practices. Their scale was refined by choosing items that distinguish between extreme scores on a dimension of strength of identification with a "Szaszian-libertarian" position. On the basis of a principal components factor analysis, four scale factors were defined:

1. *Mental illness mythology* deals with the belief that mental illness is a myth and that mental health problems relate not to medical considerations but rather to personal, social, and ethical ones.
2. *Antimedical model* deals with rejection of the belief that behavior disorders are the results of biochemical defects, that the thinking of schizophrenics is incomprehensible, or that schizophrenics lack free choice in their behavior.
3. *Social deviance control* describes the view that medical justification for controlling social deviance is provided by the institutional mental health system.
4. *Anticoercive treatment* is a view that coercive treatment should be prohibited since it is not justified by science.

In their earlier publications, Nevid and Morrison suggested that psychiatric patients change their self-concepts in response to the implicit ideology communicated by their therapists (Morrison and Nevid, 1976; Nevid and Morrison, 1976a; Nevid and Morrison, 1976b). More recently, Nevid and Morrison (1980) suggest that the LMHI Scale will be particularly useful for distinguishing therapists who do and do not have a commitment to the medical model of therapy. Since client behavior change often is affected by whether or not they perceive personal problems as the result of inherent disease, Nevid and Morrison suggest that the scale be used to select staff who will encourage behavioral solutions to clients' problems.

The Strain Toward "Newism." Schlosberg (1976), in describing progress in community psychiatry in European countries and the U.S., observed that Americans passionately search for whatever is new, be it something material, a scientific theory, or an ideology. While recognizing the positive aspects of such a quest, he notes that it has occasionally "resulted in a sometimes premature, uncritical, and too rapid adoption of new concepts—the kind of 'jumping on the bandwagon' mentality which produces an easy acceptance of popular enthusiasms whenever they may be fashionable—which leads to painful disillusionment and frustrations" (p. 123). He explained this phenomenon by suggesting that it "may be due to [the] supposedly typical American attitude of pragmatism, adopting a concept or method simply because it works" (p. 123).

The concept of "newism" appears to have first been described by Eaton (1962) in his portrayal of how group therapy techniques were introduced into the California prison system. A basic assumption of "newism" is that fresh developments or practices are superior to those preceding them. Austin (1978), applying this concept to the emergence of paraprofessionals, has noted that the concept of "newism" has the following qualities that may generally apply to the human service industry: It emphasizes innovation and belief, it relies on "newistic" validation, it offers an antidote to organizational ritualism, and it calls into play the self-fulfilling prophecy. Applying the elements of "newism" to the community mental health movement, it becomes apparent that beliefs contained in this ideology generated intense faith that services would greatly improve. These beliefs included the notion that primary prevention would successfully decrease the incidence of mental disorder and that community mental health centers would replace state hospitals. Belief in improved services was also congruent with society's cultural norms during the 1960s, which strongly favored experimental innovations.

The contribution of community mental health centers also received "newistic validation." For example, there were no empirical studies to show large-scale success for primary prevention activities or the successful impact of community mental health centers on state mental hospital populations, but such studies did not seem necessary. It was simply assumed that because such programs were new, they were effective. Eaton has emphasized that in climates of innovation, novelty per se provides validity, and it is presumed that currently existing activities should be evaluated negatively. Austin (1978) has also pointed out that innovative experiments are used to combat organizational ritualism. Thus, paraprofessional manpower was introduced as an antidote to organizational ritualism. Collectively, the experiments of the community mental health movement encouraged new organizational patterns and procedures.

A further aspect of "newism" described by Eaton (1962) and Austin (1978) involves the working out of self-fulfilling prophecies. As Austin has described it: "The introduction of paraprofessionals involved an ideology which encouraged change. The concept of self-fulfilling prophecy, on the other hand, postulates that if an ideology is espoused almost totally, its propositions will in fact become true, or manifest themselves in actuality" (pp. 43-44).

Since a high proportion of community mental health professionals and paraprofessionals firmly believed that new community mental health centers would substantially alleviate the problems of mental illness, it was expected that this prophecy would be fulfilled. However, reports by skeptics have seriously questioned the community mental health center movement and have threatened its continued viability (Chu and Trotter, 1974; Comptroller General of the United States, 1977).

This analysis of "newism" has implications for other ideological movements within mental health and other human services. Fresh beliefs develop quickly and are accepted because they are new. However, the seeds of their own self-destruction are inherent in their emphasis on faith rather than on science. Novel approaches to resolving difficult problems appear doomed and will be replaced by a succession of ideologies if they are not strongly committed to program evaluation and other accountability mechanisms (Schulberg and Baker, 1979; Cronbach and others, 1980). Of particular relevance, then, is the evidence that one of the newest ideologies, Human Services Ideology, contains a belief in the accountability of providers to consumers as one of its basic tenets (Baker, 1974; Baker and Baker, 1981). If this tenet is put into practice, perhaps this ideology's viability and survival possibilities will be enhanced.

Effect of Ideology on Service Delivery Behavior

It is necessary to consider the effects of staff ideology in conjunction with other sociopsychological variables and non-human resource variables in order to understand the effect of ideology on service delivery behavior. Although attitudes and related human response variables have been a central concern of social psychology since its inception, clear and direct relationships between the attitudes and behavior of individuals and groups have been difficult to document. In the last decade, however, investigations have abandoned attitudinal variables as the sole basis for predicting behavior, and attitude-behavior processes are now being studied as multivariate relationships. The view that attitudinal variables must be examined in the context of the numerous reality-based situational variables that shape behavior implies that individual response dispositions are simply one of the factors contributing to overt behavior decisions. Other relevant situational variables include the psychological, social, and cultural influences that combine in action situations to influence behavioral outcomes.

Acock and DeFleur (1972) describe the key to understanding behavior by means of attitudes as "discovering interrelated configurations of attitude and social or cultural variables that accurately predict action" (p. 715). Behavioral predictions can be improved by combining attitude and social situational variables in a linear model based upon the interaction between these variables. As an example of this strategy, Acock and DeFleur collected data from 202 subjects regarding their attitudes toward the legalization of marijuana, as well as data on the subjects' perception of the position of peers and family on this matter. At a later date, subjects were observed in an experimental situation in which they were asked to vote on the question of legalizing marijuana. Although a multiple-regression solution showed that the independent effects of these several variables did not clearly predict behavior, their additive effect did somewhat better, and the resulting configurations led to the clearest behavioral predictions. Thus, Acock and DeFleur's results suggest that a configurational approach emphasizing the interaction of attitudinal and social situational variables is an effective approach to examining the relationships of attitude and behavior.

The relevance of this multivariate conceptual approach to the study of ideological influences upon service delivery changes was anticipated by Strauss and others (1964). They identified three mechanisms that produce ideological differences among institutions or among their subsystems: (1) variations in policy and procedure for the recruitment of professional personnel; (2) organizational variables such as resources, prevailing local patterns of treatment, and institutional necessity; and (3) opportunities for and constraints upon the feedback of practice into the formulation of refined ideological positions. Strauss and others also observed that persons with diverse ideological positions functioning under similar institutional conditions select differing clinical priorities and then organize treatment programs accordingly. Thus, although specific organizational and situational variables certainly affect how ideology is translated into practice, ideology also influences the way in which professionals organize their working situations and treatment preferences.

The relationship of community mental health ideology to program development was analyzed by Schulberg and Baker (1975b) in their study of Boston State Hospital. They found that the differing community mental health orientation of two successive psychiatric directors of the hospital's outpatient clinic affected the type of treatment services that each sought to develop. Of particular relevance was the clinic directors' differing policies regarding such key community mental health concepts as population focus, treatment goals, and continuity of care. The executive's belief system is emphasized because in situations of "medical dominance" (Freidson, 1970), the psychiatric director's ideology is the predominant vector, even though staff beliefs may exert constraining influences.

Delgaudio and others (1976) investigated the relationship of community mental health ideology to psychotherapy practice. In their study, thirty-three therapists rated the case histories of eight psychiatric outpatients on the five dimensions of likability of the patients, comfort in dealing with them, interest in treating them, interest in friendship with them, and prognosis of the patients. Social class, diagnosis, and insight level were systematically varied within the case histories. Therapists scoring high on the CMHI Scale were found to like patients significantly more than other therapists did and to assign patients significantly more favorable prognostic ratings. Delgaudio and others suggest that professionals who score high on the CMHI Scale tend to believe in the "essential goodness and perfectibility of people," and that "the CMHI Scale may be, in part, measuring level of optimism about the prospects of helping those in distress" (p. 653). These researchers also reported that their therapists preferred middle-class, high-insight, less disturbed patients; therapists scoring high on the scale assigned equal likability ratings to all patients except for the lower-class, schizophrenic group to whom they assigned much lower ratings.

Role of Ideologies in Natural Support Systems

Ideology may influence mutual help and other natural support systems as well as professional service delivery. Antze (1976) has described the role played by ideologies in promoting therapeutic cognitive change in such natural support systems as Alcoholics Anonymous, Recovery, Inc., and Synanon. He notes that peer therapy organizations have five common structural characteristics:

1. They are fixed communities of belief. When one joins such a group, he or she is placed in close and lasting proximity to others having very definite ideas about the world.
2. The sharing of experience is a basic function of such groups. The storyteller's recasting of his personal experiences in a manner consistent with group beliefs both serves as an object lesson for members and reinforces the storyteller's own acceptance of the group's ideas.
3. When he or she offers advice to peers or explains the group's ideas to visitors, there is a deepening of the member's personal convictions.

4. Peer therapy groups bring together people who have something in common. Since newcomers perceive old-timers as similar to themselves, they are more likely to be influenced by "veterans" deemed to have achieved success.
5. These groups deal with extreme problems. Since new members enter with a high degree of despair, they are quite willing to adopt a new belief system that promises comfort or relief.

Antze believes that these characteristics permit peer psychotherapy groups to be very persuasive in changing their members' ideology. Since these groups are very highly specialized, their ideology functions as a "cognitive antidote" to the problems shared by members. For example, Alcoholics Anonymous teaches surrender to counter the inordinate assertiveness characteristic of alcoholics; Recovery, Inc., promotes will power to block the surrender tendencies of ex-mental patients; and Synanon emphasizes the expression of strong feelings in social engagements to reverse the addict's social and emotional detachment. Thus, argues Antze, "every affliction has its typical attitude or style of action, every therapy group its countervailing ideology" (p. 345).

Thus, ideology is affected by socially induced changes in service delivery patterns, but it in turn affects mental health practice by providing a justification and the impetus of faith.

This paper argues that mental health ideology has undergone a series of evolutions in the last three decades to reflect changes in social values, politics, and economics. Unfortunately, theoretical parsimony about ideology's role is not fully served by available evidence. Ideology does not appear to be simply and linearly linked to changes in service delivery patterns. Rather, ideology and service delivery are better conceived as interdependent variables systemically linked with each other as well as with other professional, personal, and environmental factors. Professional ideology seems to be related not only to attitudes and values but also to basic personality variables, giving support to Levinson's (1964) "postulate of receptivity." New ideologies emerge as earlier ideologies lose their novelty and are challenged by "scientific-minded" evidence. Mental health professionals are increasingly aware that personal beliefs influence their behavior. Just as evidence exists that particular therapeutic ideologies meet the needs of particular clients, so perhaps do ideologies help professionals resolve their problems as well. Recognition of ideology's influence on professional practice should immeasurably help those involved in changing service delivery systems.

References

Acock, A., and DeFleur, M. "A Configurational Approach to Contingent Consistency in the Attitude-Behavior Relationship." *American Sociological Review,* 1972, *37,* 714-726.

Antze, P. "The Role of Ideologies in Peer Psychotherapy Organizations: Some Theoretical Considerations and Three Case Studies." *Journal of Applied Behavioral Science,* 1976, *12,* 323-346.

Armor, D., and Klerman, G. "Psychiatric Treatment Orientations and Professional Ideology." *Journal of Health and Social Behavior,* 1968, *9,* 243-255.

Austin, M. J. *Professionals and Paraprofessionals.* New York: Human Sciences Press, 1978.

Baker, F. "From Community Mental Health to Human Service Ideology." *American Journal of Public Health,* 1974, *64,* 576-581.

Baker, F., and Baker, A. P. "Dimensions of Human Service Ideology." Unpublished manuscript, State University of New York at Buffalo, 1981.

Baker, F., and Northman, J. E. "The Ideology and Education of the Future Human Service Executive." In J. Chenault and F. Burnford (Eds.), *Human Services Professional Education.* New York: McGraw-Hill, 1978.

Baker, F., and Northman, J. E. *Helping: Human Services for the '80s.* St. Louis, Mo.: Mosby, 1981.

Baker, F., and Schulberg, H. "Development of a Community Mental Health Ideology Scale." *Community Mental Health Journal,* 1967, *3,* 216-225.

Baker, F., and Schulberg, H. "Community Mental Health Ideology, Dogmatism, and Political-Economic Conservatism." *Community Mental Health Journal,* 1969, *5,* 433-436.

Bassuk, E. L., and Gerson, S. "Deinstitutionalization and Mental Health Services." *Scientific American,* 1978, *238,* 46-53.

Block, W. E. "The Study of Attitudes About Mental Health in the Community Mental Health Center." *Community Mental Health Journal,* 1974, *10,* 216-220.

Breeskin, J., Wolff, S., and Witzke, D. "Community Mental Health Ideology in the Military." Paper presented at 19th annual conference of Air Force Behavioral Scientists, Jan. 1972.

Caplan, G. "Epilogue: Implications for Community Psychiatry: Personal Reflections." In R. B. Caplan and G. Caplan, *Psychiatry and the Community in Nineteenth-Century America.* New York: Basic Books, 1969.

Chu, F. D., and Trotter, S. *The Madness Establishment: Ralph Nader's Group Report on the National Institute of Mental Health.* New York: Grossman, 1974.

Comptroller General of the United States. *Returning the Mentally Disabled to the Community: Government Needs To Do More.* Washington, D.C.: U.S. Government Accounting Office, 1977.

Cronbach, L. J., and others. *Toward Reform of Program Evaluation: Aims, Methods, and Institutional Arrangements.* San Francisco: Jossey-Bass, 1980.

Delgaudio, A. C., and others. "Attitudes of Therapists Varying in Community Mental Health Ideology and Democratic Values." *Journal of Consulting and Clinical Psychology,* 1976, *44,* 646-655.

Eaton, J. W. *Stone Walls Do Not a Prison Make.* Springfield, Ill.: Thomas, 1962.

Freidson, E. *Professional Dominance: The Social Structure of Medical Care.* New York: Atherton Press, 1970.

Gilbert, D., and Levinson, D. "Custodialism and Humanism in Staff Ideology." In M. Greenblatt, D. Levinson, and R. Williams (Eds.), *The Patient and the Mental Hospital.* New York: Free Press, 1957.

Gross, H. W. "The Community Mental Health Ideology Scale:

Validation." Mimeographed paper, Buffer Hospital, Providence, R.I., 1972.

Hersch, C. "Social History, Mental Health, and Community Control." *American Psychologist,* 1972, *27,* 749-754.

Hobbs, N. "Mental Health's Third Revolution." *American Journal of Orthopsychiatry,* 1964, *34,* 822-833.

Hollander, R. "A New Service Ideology: The Third Mental Health Revolution." *Professional Psychology,* 1980, *11,* 561-566.

Hollingshead, A., and Redlich, F. *Social Class and Mental Illness.* New York: Wiley, 1958.

Howard, L. A., and Baker, F. "Ideology and Role Function of the Nurse in Community Mental Health." *Nursing Research,* 1971, *20,* 450-454.

Kuhn, T. *The Structure of Scientific Revolutions.* Chicago: University of Chicago Press, 1970.

Langston, R. D. "Community Mental Health Centers and Community Mental Health Ideology." *Community Mental Health Journal,* 1970, *6,* 387-392.

Levinson, D. "Idea Systems in the Individual and Society." In G. Zollschan and W. Hirsch (Eds.), *Explorations in Social Change.* Boston: Houghton Mifflin, 1964.

Morrison, J. K., and Nevid, J. S. "Demythologizing the Attitudes of Family Care Takers About 'Mental Illness.' " *Journal of Family Counseling,* 1976, *4,* 43-49.

Nevid, J. S., and Morrison, J. K. "Preventing Involuntary Hospitalization: A Family Contracting Approach." *Journal of Family Counseling,* 1976a, *4,* 27-31.

Nevid, J. S., and Morrison, J. K. "Humanistic Approaches in the Delivery of Community Mental Health Services." Paper presented at annual meeting of the American Psychological Association, Washington, D.C., September 1976b.

Nevid, J. S., and Morrison, J. "Attitudes Toward Mental Illness: The Construction of the Libertarian Mental Health Ideology Scale." *Journal of Humanistic Psychology,* 1980, *20,* 71-85.

Rose, S. M. "Deciphering Deinstitutionalization: Complexities in Policy and Program Analysis." *Health and Society,* 1979, *4,* 429-460.

Schlosberg, A. "Some Factors and Issues Concerning Community Psychiatry." *International Journal of Social Psychiatry,* 1976, *22,* 120-129.

Schulberg, H., and Baker, F. "Community Mental Health: Belief System of the 1960s." *Psychiatric Opinion,* 1969, *6,* 14-26.

Schulberg, H., and Baker, F. "Introduction: Social Values, Economic Influences, and Integrated Human Services." In H. Schulberg and F. Baker (Eds.), *Developments in Human Services.* Vol. 2. New York: Behavioral Publications, 1975a.

Schulberg, H., and Baker, F. *The Mental Hospital and Human Services.* New York: Behavioral Publications, 1975b.

Schulberg, H., and Baker, F. *Program Evaluation in the Health Fields.* Vol. 2. New York: Human Sciences Press, 1979.

Sharaf, M., and Levinson, D. "Patterns of Ideology and Role Differentiation Among Psychiatric Residents." In M. Greenblatt, D. Levinson, and R. Williams (Eds.), *The Patient and the Mental Hospital.* New York: Free Press, 1957.

Strauss, A., and others. *Psychiatric Ideologies and Institutions.* New York: Free Press, 1964.

Szasz, T. "The Myth of Mental Illness: Three Addenda." *Journal of Humanistic Psychology,* 1974, *14,* 11-19.

Zilboorg, G. A. *A History of Medical Psychology.* New York: Norton, 1941.

Chapter 10

Leading and Managing Mental Health Centers

Anthony Broskowski

After a brief period of optimism in the closing years of the last decade, we are now facing the certainty of dramatic, possibly traumatic, changes for community mental health services in the 1980s. The period of uncertainty regarding the federal government's role ended when Congress repealed the Mental Health Systems Act and created a single block grant for mental health, drug abuse, and alcohol abuse services. How each state will respond is still uncertain. Clearly, long-range planning will be at once more critical and more difficult. The purpose of this chapter is to speculate on some of the most likely future scenarios that will affect community mental health center (CMHC) management, with an emphasis on the role of the executive director in providing the necessary leadership and administrative skills for the future.

Along with the demise of a categorical mechanism for funding CMHCs, we can expect a continued decline in the relative contribution of federal dollars, especially when measured in terms of their true purchasing power. We are told to expect a decline in federal regulations, although many administrators, including state officials, doubt that greater flexibility will be forthcoming. Federal leadership, evidenced by advocacy, experimentation, and demonstrations of innovations, is more likely to decline than are federal regulations. Already many respected professionals at the National Institute of Mental Health (NIMH) have "jumped ship," and the NIMH may yet be subsumed into the larger health bureaucracy.

A more optimistic view would consider the possible benefits to be achieved by shifting responsibilities for funding and leadership to the state level. Many think that the past categorical system was unnecessarily costly and that it produced fragmentation and discontinuities for the ultimate service recipient (Attkisson and Broskowski, 1978). The existence of federal standards for comprehensiveness also made it difficult to develop local programs that were both responsive to local conditions and efficient in the total expenditure of resources.

The potential benefits to be achieved during this transitional period will depend heavily on how each state government responds. Theoretically, the block grant mechanism will allow states to consolidate services where appropriate, to improve coordination across categorical services (for example, linking general health and mental health services), and to be more responsive to variations in local need. Again, the cynics doubt that state government can be trusted to accomplish such goals, either due to the motivations of politicians or the lack of a sufficient pool of qualified personnel in the state bureaucracy. For example, states are likely to increase the number of state regulations affecting CMHCs, more than making up for the "loss" of federal regulations. It is the nature of government to have little confidence in those assigned program responsibility and to withhold necessary authority from them. At worst, there are fears that some states will retreat from the commitment to community mental health.

Part of the Reagan administration's rationale for a reduction in federal dollars is that monitoring and administrative costs will be reduced. There is also an implied promise to provide states a greater ability to generate tax revenue at the state level, allowing them to "make up" the loss of federal dollars through fewer bureaucratic regulations. Again, the cynics are doubtful that citizens will support increases in local or state taxes.

Although the funding and tax policies of the various states are still unclear, we can anticipate an increasing demand for mental health services, especially from those high-risk groups that are losing other federal entitlements or experiencing reductions in other services. In a very broad sense, the need and demand for mental health services will covary inversely with the general state of the economy. If Reagan's economic policy does lead to higher employment, a reduced rate of inflation, and lower taxes, then the need and demand for mental health services will show a relative decline. There will be a long lag period, however, and the demand curve is likely to continue to rise long before the benefits of a stronger economy can rescue CMHCs. But CMHCs are not passive entities, and there are important steps that can be taken in the years ahead to guarantee that services will be maintained. The balance of this chapter will review the major options open to centers. While these options involve board members, management, staff, clients, and other advocacy groups, this chapter will focus primarily on the role of the executive director and associated management personnel.

Long-Range Perspective

The quality of the CMHC's adaptation response will depend on the ability of the leader to clarify and, if necessary, redefine the center's long-range mission. The leader must think about the center as an institution, a permanent and enduring community resource. Planning for how that institution will look in 1991 will be critical for guiding decisions about how it will respond in 1982 or 1984 (Broskowski, O'Brien, and Prevost, in press). Crisis management, in an effort to maintain the status quo, can dissipate the energy needed for long-term survival. Furthermore, a long-range institutional perspective allows leadership to make difficult decisions by buffering it from immediate pressures to protect existing commitments to particular interest groups among staff and clients.

In the broadest sense, the CMHC has three major options as it faces a future of political and economic uncertainty. One, it can choose to accept a series of planned cutbacks, working out the transition as smoothly and ethically as possible. Two, it can attempt to maintain size or growth by expanding into new "markets." This can be done by providing traditional services to new clients (for example, industrial employee assistance programs), by providing new services to current or new client groups (for example, health promotion programs), or by developing the capacity to manage programs that have traditionally been outside the CMHC's interests (for example, starting nursing homes). A third option is to do both, that is, to make selective cutbacks and to attempt to grow in very well-targeted areas. Later we will address these options more fully, along with some of their associated strategies and tactics. At this point we must emphasize that it is likely to be the responsibility of one "leader" to set forth the options, assess the major opportunities and risks associated with such choices, and realign the center's existing personnel and material resources to move forward. The leader must develop a consensus in the midst of crisis, articulate the conflicting values inherent in making changes, and assume responsibility if the endeavor fails.

Leadership and Management. The temptation is great to develop a table that would contrast the critical difference between the roles of leadership and the tasks of management. For example, it has been said that "leadership inspires while management controls." Rather than emphasize such differences, however, we need to recognize that the effective CMHC director must be both a leader and a manager. The decade of the 1980s will demand a dynamic blend of attitudes, technical skills and knowledge, and vision from the mental health administrator. As with any blend, however, the relative balance of critical ingredients will change over time.

Although there is a voluminous literature on mental health administration (Feldman, Goldstein, and Offutt, 1980), we still cannot define with certainty the ingredients of successful CMHC leadership. The reasons why successful CMHC directors behave as they do remain a well-respected mystery (Howell, 1976, 1979; Macindoe and Houge, 1980). What works in one particular time and place is seldom transferable; hence, mental health administration is not a science or a profession. The use of such words as "planning," "evaluating," and "deciding" to describe executive actions does not really explain behavior but at best organizes and catalogues activities, and at worst disguises our ignorance about the management of CMHCs.

In his excellent review of "The Short and Glorious History of Organizational Theory," Perrow (1974) reaches five general conclusions; the fourth concerns leadership:

> The burning cry in all organizations is for "good leadership," but we have learned that beyond a threshold level of adequacy it is extremely difficult to know what good leadership is. The hundreds of scientific studies of this phenomenon come to one general conclusion: Leadership is highly variable or "contingent" upon a large variety of important variables such as nature of task, size of group, length of time the group has existed, type of personnel within the group and their relationships with each other, and amount of pressure the group is under. It does not seem likely that we'll be able to devise a way to select the best leader for a particular situation. Even if we could, that situation would probably change in a short time and thus would require a somewhat different type of leader.
>
> Furthermore, we are beginning to realize that leadership involves more than smoothing the paths of human interaction. What has rarely been studied in this area is the wisdom of even the technical adequacy of a leader's decision. A leader does more than lead people; he also makes decisions about the allocation of resources, type of technology to be used, the nature of the market, and so on. This aspect of leadership remains very obscure, but it is obviously crucial [p. 18].

Burns (1978) defines leaders as those with followers. Leaders have a capacity to convince others to subordinate individual goals in order to achieve larger collective goals. This capacity is based on the leader's ability to sort out the multiple goals and values of the individual followers, to understand the power and limitations of the technologies, skills, and attitudes of the followers, and to match these with a reasonably accurate vision of the future environment. The CMHC leader must do no less.

Based on a recent Delphi survey of forty-two distinguished and nationally recognized mental health professionals, representing a range of disciplines and settings, Noren and Peterson (1979) isolated 165 specific areas of knowledge (k), skills (s), and attitudes (a) that will be needed by mental health administrators of the future. These specific k/a/s areas were developed only after earlier iterations among the panelists identified the most important future mental health goals. For our purposes, it is important to note the *pattern* of priorities among these 165 items. Each k/a/s item was rated by each respondent on a scale of one to ten. Table 1 summarizes my retabulation of Noren and Peterson's original findings.

Table 1. Number of Knowledge, Attitude, and Skill Items at Each Level of Importance to Mental Health Administrators.

	Type of Item			
Level of Importance	*Knowledge*	*Attitude*	*Skills*	*Total*
Most important (Ranks 1-33)	7	13	13	33
Very important (Ranks 34-66)	11	11	11	33
Important (Ranks 67-99)	19	8	6	33
Less important (Ranks 100-132)	24	8	1	33
Least important (Ranks 133-165)	29	1	3	33
Totals	90	41	34	165

Note: Chi square = 43.73
d.f. = 8; $p < .001$

It is noteworthy that formal knowledge items (for example, "knowledge of components of a total system of mental health") are less frequently ranked as "most important" than attitude items ("respect for data that conflicts with one's own bias") and skill items ("confront and resolve conflict tactfully"). Given that there were only 34 skill items in the original pool of 165 items, and although knowledge items occur at all levels of importance, the overall pattern of findings would reinforce Mintzberg's (1973) view that managerial effectiveness requires more than the mastery of formal knowledge. Based on the systematic observation of what managers actually do with their time, Mintzberg (1973, 1975) attempted to separate management fact from folklore. His analysis is especially critical to mental health administrators because, in time of crisis, the tendency is to cling to established myths and deny the realities of change. If we are to reach an understanding of how to integrate leadership with management skills, we must begin to recognize the limitations inherent in the manager's job and the limits associated with management technologies.

Planning. The CMHC director is considered responsible for deliberative planning, based on reflective thought about the current and future state of affairs. In reality, Mintzberg (1973) found that managerial work is characterized by brevity, variety, and fragmentation and is carried out over long hours at an unrelenting pace. Continuity of thought or action seemed impossible for the chief executives observed by Mintzberg; thus, half their activities lasted less than nine minutes and only 10 percent exceeded one hour. Over a five-week period the average deskwork event lasted fifteen minutes, telephone calls averaged six minutes, and unscheduled meetings averaged eleven minutes. One major reason for this pace and work load is the "open-ended nature of the job" (Mintzberg, 1973, p. 30). Unlike specialists, the leader is responsible for the overall success of a complex operation, with few "tangible mileposts where he can stop and say, 'Now my job is finished' " (p. 30). If preoccupation and superficiality are inherent risks for the manager, then it is all the more important for the CMHC director to integrate, from time to time, the tremendous variety of events and issues crossing his or her path, sorting out the critical strategic issues from the trivial ones. Planning, therefore, requires information.

Information Processing. The demand for more and better information is a familiar one. Manual and computerized "management information systems" spring up like weeds on the organizational landscape. In the ideal world, the manager has ready access to well-organized information files, built on well-defined data elements, reliably recorded and collected by cooperative employees and clients, and based on internally and externally agreed-upon needs for information that seldom change over time (Broskowski and Attkisson, forthcoming). The real world, however, does not operate that way. Managers of businesses with elaborate, computerized information systems do not, in fact, spend much time using such formalized intelligence systems (Mintzberg, 1973; Cox and Osborne, 1980). Simon (1973) correctly points out that few managers lack sufficient information. Most suffer from information overload, and the really scarce resource is the time to attend to information on a selective basis.

While CMHC leadership should not overestimate the value of formalized information systems for accomplishing the strategic tasks of planning cutbacks or expansions, such systems are obviously necessary. A management information system has value because it contains information that is useful for planning and prediction in a stable environment. As environmental turbulence increases, however, the leader will be forced to shift to reliance on less formalized systems. Leaders have a strong need for current and future-oriented information, even information that is speculative and based on highly informal and interactive modes of communication. They may thrive on "rumors" about what is happening inside or outside the agency. Timeliness is commonly more important than precision. Leaders must continuously make decisions that will not wait, and they appear quite willing to accept a high degree of uncertainty in their information rather than wait for more or better "answers." A decision delayed is often a crisis invited (Kissinger, 1979).

The CMHC director's sources of information form a complex network of subordinates who report on a formal basis, close associates and peers, clients, competitors, politicians, and critics. As part of such a network, the director is continuously picking up information, evaluating its utility, and selectively storing that information or transmitting it to others in the network. Because of its emphasis on past events and aggregated details, a formalized management information system will seldom entirely serve the strategic planning needs of the contemporary

CMHC director. This statement is not an indictment of such formal systems, because they are truly useful for some specialized applications, such as financial accounting, billing, inventory control, scheduling, and statistical data processing (Broskowski, 1979). But with respect to the majority of the demands placed on him, the leader operates more in the manner of an information artist than an information technologist.

In their longitudinal study of a small sample of CMHC directors, Cox and Osborne (1980) attempted to relate the characteristics of problems (that is, familiarity, complexity, instability, ambiguity) to the decision processes used by the directors. They found that directors were generally satisfied with their available levels of information and were fairly confident of their ability to make adequate, even optimal decisions.

The directors were very clear about their objectives and the criteria they would use in selecting an acceptable solution. They "were readily able to identify key beliefs that defined and structured their problems (e.g., 'Professionals provide better quality care . . . , Agency X does not have any commitment to a mental heath program for adolescents. . . .')" (Cox and Osborne, 1980, p. 179). Such key beliefs served to simplify the problem-solving process by ruling out many decision alternatives from early consideration and by guiding the subsequent search for information. The directors responded to the instability of problems—"the degree to which criteria, goals, and constraints of the problem change during and after the decision" (Cox and Osborne, 1980, p, 179)—by being proactive in their attempts to change the characteristics of the decision environment, reduce the number or change the nature of the constraints, or modify the risks or probabilities of success associated with alternative solutions. Instability was viewed as an advantage in affecting the choice of a solution. The decision-making process was a highly interactive one; alternative solutions, and hence the need for information, evolved over time—and partly in response to the decision-maker's efforts to modify the decision environment.

Leaders commonly operate on the assumption that they presently know enough, perhaps because they have so little time to learn more. As Kissinger noted in his *White House Years*

(1979), new cabinet members are quickly "overwhelmed by the insistent demands of running their departments. On the whole, a period in high office consumes intellectual capital; it does not create it. Most high officials leave office with the perceptions and insights with which they entered; they learn how to make decisions but not what decisions to make" (p. 27). Center directors seldom have time to read and thus to learn new methods and approaches. Their information needs are not tolerant of long treatises on management, such as the one you are now reading. They come to depend on their network of associates and subordinate specialists to learn and implement new procedures. The leader's depth of knowledge of any new procedure or project is likely to be superficial, given the breadth of information that must be mastered. The costs of information overload and the dangers of superficiality must be continuously assessed as waves of new information enter the picture.

Limits on the Director's Control

CMHC staff may envy the director, who seems to have power to make final decisions, to initiate new projects, to reallocate existing resources. But how many CMHC executives truly feel that "sense of power"? The director more likely feels pressured to respond to multiple, incompatible, even conflictual demands from a host of constituencies: the board of directors and its individual members, middle managers, professional staff, unions, special-interest groups, associates in peer organizations, and numerous funding and regulatory agencies. The director's authority may be narrowly limited by board policies, professional standards, and government controls.

Kouzes and Mico (1979, 1980) describe three "domains" in the human service organization: the policy domain, the management domain, and the service domain. Each has its own members, as well as its characteristic principles, structures, success measures, and working modalities:

Policy Domain: *Members:* Board members.
Principle: Consent of the governed.

Success measure: Equity.
Structure: Representative and participative.
Work modes: Voting, bargaining, and negotiation.

Management Domain: *Members:* Top and middle managers.
Principles: Hierarchical control and coordination.
Success measures: Cost efficiency and effectiveness.
Structure: Bureaucratic.
Work modes: Use of linear techniques and tools.

Service Domain: *Members:* Service staff.
Principles: Autonomy and self-regulation.
Success measures: Quality of service and good standards.
Structure: Collegial.
Work modes: Client specific and problem solving.

Differences among these domains inevitably generate disagreements and conflicts. Many potential problems can be avoided, however, when the management domain serves as a buffer between the policy domain and the service domain. But each domain has its own powers and controls, and the CMHC is truly a system of checks and balances.

Is the CMHC director, thus, a puppet manipulated by others, or is he an orchestra conductor directing a composition written by others? Drucker (1954) says that the leader is composer *and* conductor. Mintzberg (1973) agrees: "The manager is challenged to gain control of his own time by turning obligations to his advantage and by turning those things he wishes to do into obligations" (1975, p. 60). We are all familiar with the CMHC leader who complains that he cannot get the job done because of unreasonable or conflicting demands. Failure is blamed on his numerous obligations. However, successful (or at least satisfied) directors appear to turn obligation into opportunity. A meeting is a chance to pick up more useful information, a speech is an opportunity to advance a new project, a site visit by a regulator is an opportunity to gain new feedback or obtain sanction for a change. Leaders also gain control by forcing or obligating themselves to perform unpleasant but important tasks—tasks that perhaps only the leader considers important. For example, writing a chapter on the problems and opportunities of management forces me to reflect on my personal progress. Furthermore, unpleasant tasks must be forced onto the director's schedule. "Hoping to leave some time open for contemplation or general planning is tantamount to hoping that the pressures of the job will go away" (Mintzberg, 1975, p. 61). Thus, the CMHC director's control over events is seldom as clear as his obligations and responsibilities are. The CMHC leader must force himself to concentrate on priorities and be willing to devote his time and energies to even the most unpleasant tasks.

Management of Cutbacks. Levine (1978) provides a range of options for leaders who are experiencing a decline in resources. He divides his tactics into those that are useful for resisting decline and those that are useful in planning a smooth decline. In a follow-up article, Levine (1979) argues that managing cutback is different in many respects from managing growth. First, an organization cannot be systematically dismantled in the same way as it was built. Second, many of the sophisticated and expensive technologies that were built in a time of growth, such as elaborate management information systems, tend to be jettisoned when cutbacks begin, making it even more difficult to solve problems as time continues. Levine (1979) notes that "the management science paradox means that when you have analytic capacity you do not need it; when you need it, you do not have it and cannot use it anyway" (p. 180).

Frequent or infrequent personnel turnover can also become a significant problem. Employees that perform the poorest generally hang on to their jobs because they have few better alternatives. However, many superior employees tend to leave the organization when it begins to experience decline; they can find better alternatives elsewhere. Another problem is the unrealistic optimism that tends to pervade the staff when cutbacks have just begun. Staff seem to believe that somewhere out of the sky will come a magical solution so that the cuts need be only temporary. The leader is faced with difficult trade-offs between equity and efficiency. Should cuts be made across the board so that all programs and employees experience the cuts equally or should the cuts be made on the basis of community priorities? Cutbacks on the basis of equity may be emotionally easier for the governing board to make, but such cuts are probably less useful for the overall organization.

Another problem is the so-called participation paradox. Although major changes generally require center-wide participation, an invitation to staff to participate in making cutback decisions can lead to self-protective behavior and a paralysis of action, since no one wants to cut his or her own program. This process can lead one back to such irrationality as making across-the-board cuts in order to avoid a collapse of morale. Cutbacks in productivity can cause further vulnerability. Improved productivity often requires the investment of new money for either equipment or staff training. Under conditions of stringency it is very difficult to find funds and justify their expenditure to improve the organization and offset further declines. Decline breeds decline.

A further problem is described by Levine (1979) as the "efficiency paradox." This dilemma is perhaps the most troublesome for a well-managed agency. Inefficiently run CMHCs have obvious areas of slack and waste that can be identified and cut in times of stringency. In contrast, an efficiently run CMHC will likely have enmeshed its slack resources into the core services and priorities of the agency. For example, it may have committed spare resources to long-term planning and capacity-building efforts. When forced to make cuts, this efficient agency must cut into its critical core operations; thus, efficient units of the organization may be cut as much as inefficient ones.

McTighe (1979) provides some useful suggestions for scaling down an organization. The first prescription is to critically review the organizational mission, including its legal mandates and its time-honored activities. The next step is to examine marginal investments, including financial unit costs, client volume, alternatives provided by other agencies, and the possibility that immediate cuts will stimulate even further revenue reductions or serious public reactions. He argues for "rational choice mechanisms" such as zero-based budgets to be installed. Unlike Levine, McTighe argues for employee participation, while stressing that personnel cutback decisions be carried out promptly, once made. Finally, he stresses that the agency maintain its "openness" by communicating its problems to clientele, political bodies, and the general public.

Management of Expansion and Diversification. Community mental health centers must also consider opportunities for program expansion and diversification. A well-managed CMHC may wish to consider starting new services that the community needs and is willing to pay for. Another alternative is to actively compete in areas where public services are being demanded but are poorly operated by existing public or private agencies. For example, delinquency programs, nursing homes, therapeutic nurseries for handicapped children, and primary health care represent significant human services where CMHC management experience can be applied. Leadership must carefully assess, however, the risks of such strategies. Will crises in the domain of mental health services be ignored or glossed over as a result of overly optimistic plans to take on new problems? Does the CMHC have its own middle-management and administrative support systems sufficiently organized to tackle such new ventures? Will energy be wasted fighting entrenched competition? Will the center lose its reputation for quality services?

In general, the choice to diversify must depend heavily on local community circumstances, the center's history and general community reputation, and the mix of board and staff leadership styles and skills. For example, fighting reductions by diversifying into new programs requires a reservoir of financial support, an entrepreneurial leadership style, and the requisite variety of staff skills and motivation. Funding for expansion and diversification will be problematic in any case. Nevertheless, many centers are beginning to be more aggressive in their fund-raising and marketing strategies, particularly in providing such services to industry and public agencies as employee assistance programs, health promotion and wellness programs, and consultation, training, and educational programs.

The Northside CMHC in Tampa found it useful to organize its strategies for resource development into several broad categories, each one associated with specific tactics and action steps, different time frames, risk factors, and implementation requirements. The general resource development strategies are: (1) securing more government grants and contracts, (2) securing private grants and contracts, (3) turning to private philanthropy, (4) charging higher fees, and (5) forming interorganizational linkages. These strategies are not totally independent. For example, forming interorganizational linkages may be a part of securing a government grant. Furthermore, simultaneous pursuit of all strategies will not be feasible for Northside CMHC. For example, the business office staff configuration that is ideal for collecting insurance fees is not the same one that is suitable for maintaining multiple grants and contracts. Also, the mix of professional specialists versus generalists will necessarily vary as the center pursues one or more of these strategies. Unless an organization is very large, it will have to selectively pursue only one or two strategies.

The choice of any given strategy for fund raising will affect and be affected by internal policies and procedures. For example, both stated personnel policies and unwritten personnel philosophies are critical factors in the choice of strategies for dealing with the environment. Policies that support seniority and encourage tenure without regard for productivity or the quality of work will make the organization less cost efficient over time. Employment practices based on inflexible written job descriptions will also make it more difficult to respond flexibly to new grant or contract opportunities. Staff must be able and willing to do a variety of new and different jobs if the center chooses to pursue a grants and contract strategy.

In order to keep salary rates within reasonable limits and tied to quality and quantity of effort, Northside CMHC is currently revising its own personnel philosophy to reflect the needs and interests of three different categories of employees: support staff, entry-level and mid-level professional staff, and "key personnel." Key personnel are those whose skills are very specialized and difficult to replace, or those who are good generalists, capable of assuming a wide range of different duties over time. Key personnel could occupy support positions or professional line positions at any level of the organization. They are not necessarily only top management staff, but they are identified by objective criteria and by demonstrated consistent performance. Incentives, salary increases, and other prerogatives will be extended to key personnel in order to retain them in the center. In contrast, a controlled rate of turnover will be expected and encouraged among the entry-level professional staff. Salaries for support staff, who generally are less career oriented, will be tied to the level of salaries prevailing for similar jobs in the community.

Following a process of successive approximation, the CMHC leader must continuously move from the inside to the outside, looking for feasible matches between internal capabilities and external demands. The process starts with knowing what the center presently does best, what it can afford to sacrifice, and what else it could do if sufficient interest and financial support were forthcoming. Furthermore, strategies to seek new levels and types of support cannot be clearly separated from the need to make simultaneous internal changes. In fact, the dichotomy between external demands and internal capabilities is primarily a fiction, useful for planning and delegation of responsibilities.

Corporate Configuring

Another step being taken by CMHCs to improve their chances of survival and to open up new growth opportunities has been called "corporate configuring" (Avery, Packard, and Vorwaller, 1980). Corporate configuring calls for the creation of one or more nonprofit corporations, each designed to take advantage of specific service or funding opportunities, to avoid regulatory disincentives, or to shelter the parent center from undue liability or risks. This strategy is analogous to internal reorganization or differentiation to match the constraints and/or opportunities of a complex but turbulent environment. It is also parallel to strategies used in the profit sector to diversify product lines and services or to disassociate high-risk/high-gain ventures from a more stable but less profitable line of activity. The most common options (and provisions in the Internal Revenue Service [IRS] code) regarding new corporate structures include:

- Starting one or more new 501 (c) 3 nonprofit corporations to offer new or existing services.
- Creating a new 501 (c) 2 subsidiary corporation to own and lease land, buildings, or equipment.
- Establishing a 501 (e) 1A subsidiary corporation to provide administrative services (for example, payroll, personnel, and billing) to one or more 501 (c) 3 corporations.
- Creating a 501 (c) 9 subsidiary corporation, or employee benefit trust, to provide more relevant and responsive fringe benefits to employees (for example, a self-insured health plan with health promotion incentives).

There are many legal and administrative considerations that must go into making the decision to pursue a strategy of corporate configuring. For example, there are federal and state laws governing the creation of nonprofit corporations and their contractual relationships with one another. To take one instance, the Internal Revenue Service requires an "arms-length" relationship between separate corporations. Furthermore, although one 501 (c) 3 corporation may donate its reserves to another, such arrangements may not be so designed that one is a "feeder corporation" for the other.

Another consideration involves the degree of control that the CMHC wishes to maintain over any additional 501 (c) 3 corporations. The new corporations must be sufficiently independent for legal purposes, but sufficiently related to the original CMHC so that they operate in concert, as a single service delivery *system,* to achieve the major missions of the CMHC. Furthermore, does the CMHC have the staff capability to provide the types of services that can potentially generate additional revenues? If so, are these best organized and delivered through a second corporation? Does the center have the administrative and support-staff talent needed to manage the legal and accounting complexities inherent in this approach? Will local or state funding bodies misinterpret the center's efforts to start a new corporation as only a means to avoid accountability? Are there sufficient markets, such as private industry, foundations, or the general public, in the community to support the revenue needs of an additional corporation?

To those who are interested in the administrative and legal technicalities of corporate configuring, we recommend two texts: *The Law of Tax-Exempt Organizations* (Hopkins, 1980) and *Tax-Exempt Charitable Organizations* (Treusch and Sugarman, 1979). The IRS provides numerous pamphlets, books, and other documents on regulations pertaining to nonprofit corporations. Legal and accounting advice is also warranted when undertaking such ventures. Because corporate diversification in profit-making organizations is well established, there are many legal and accounting experts in that area. However, corporate configuring in the nonprofit sector is still a novelty, and there are few "experts" to guide us. Consequently, any CMHC taking this approach is doing so at some risk and prudence is well advised.

Although there may be limitations imposed by local or state circumstances, several types of advantages may result from increasing a CMHC's corporate flexibility. First, funding sources that provide only deficit ("last-dollar") financing are not lost when the center is aggressive and successful in providing services to private organizations or individuals that can and will pay for services. Second, certain services are more easily promoted by a corporation that does not carry with it the stigma of "mental illness" or "mental health" in its corporate name. Third, more flexible and motivating personnel policies can be implemented in a corporation that is not hamstrung by federal or state restrictions on hiring and reimbursement systems. Fourth, competing priorities can be separated out. The success of a new corporation in serving the well-off, for example, does not have to be compromised, while its financial gains after costs can be used to benefit the original CMHC corporation that serves the poor. Similarly, board representation can be adjusted so that expertise and influence are maximized in one corporation while community representativeness is maintained in the other corporation. Fifth, administrative flexibility in start-up and ongoing program operation can be achieved because decisions to purchase or lease, borrow or not borrow, hire or contract can be made on a case-by-case basis, depending upon such factors as a project's funding sources and associated regulatory constraints. Cash reserves can be built, and the monetary positions of the various corporations can be adjusted through contracts to purchase or lease services from one another. Cost control and predictability are enhanced through the centralization of support services and the intercorporate agreements to lease or purchase equipment or services at controllable rates. Northside CMHC expects to save $12 to $15 thousand annually through self-insurance and to apply such savings to more benefits and incentives for healthy employees. Finally, staff development and morale are enhanced when employees can work in one corporation as employees and serve in another as consultants. Work diversity and financial incentives are then readily made available to the better employees of the center.

The Director as Integrator

Most CMHC directors will be faced with both cutbacks and opportunities for growth. To provide leadership and management for both may prove to be a schizophrenogenic experience. While cutting some services, the leader will be encouraging the board to start new corporations. While laying off some clinical staff, the leader will be arguing for merit increases to retain the most competent general managers. Certainly this process will tax the cognitive and emotional assets of everyone, but primarily the director's.

We urge CMHC directors to face this uncertain future with a clear structure and process to assist them. At Northside CMHC the board has established a long-range planning committee, staffed by the executive director and the manager of program planning and evaluation. This committee has undertaken to review existing services on the basis of multiple criteria (for example, community needs, cost-recovery potential, availability elsewhere, board's value commitment). The committee has explored the current funding mix and different financial scenarios for the future. Interorganizational linkages have been evaluated to determine if they need to be expanded or improved. A Delphi survey of other CMHCs has been undertaken to learn about their strategies and tactics for possible application. Recommendations are being made to the full board and its existing subcommittees to reexamine the board's own structure, to focus on state legislative issues, to establish a resource development committee, to review the center's current personnel policies (for example, the role of seniority in lay-offs, incentive systems, pay-grade systems, retention and retraining opportunities) and to reexamine policies and procedures for cost recovery through contracts and fees. For example, the staff has been directed to consider alternatives to the standard sliding fee scales (Shields, 1981) and to seek Joint Commission on Accreditation of Hospitals (JCAH) accreditation.

Growing out of this committee's work, the center will undertake steps to cut some programs, and will cooperate with other organizations to take on some services that they plan to drop while supporting their efforts to pick up some of ours. The center will also establish a new 501 (c) 3 corporation to provide health promotion and employee assistance programs, while generally trying to improve its internal structure and management strength (White and Broskowski, 1980). Although cutting some programs will cause the director stress and sorrow, the opportunity to redirect resources and strengthen the organization will undoubtedly provide him or her with an equal measure of enthusiasm and personal growth.

The current decade will present a severe test of our abilities to manage the delivery of mental health services within the community. The survival and success of the CMHC will undoubtedly depend on many factors outside the control of its executive director. Nevertheless, the odds of success for the director and the center can be greatly improved by attention to some general principles:

- Clarify and redefine the CMHC mission, maintaining a long-range, institutional perspective.
- Avoid making pronouncements about the limits of the current environment without at the same time speaking of future possibilities.
- Master the skills and processes of cutback management.
- Help "mourn the loss" of valued programs that cannot be sustained.
- Master skills in diversifying services and resources and instill renewed commitment among CMHC supporters.
- Continue to articulate and clarify the fundamental *values* of human concern that will motivate a drive for excellence, while accepting the pain of making some decisions that are alien to that value system.
- Maintain an emphasis on existing management technologies that allow for the most effective and efficient organization and use of limited resources.
- Consciously design and utilize formal and informal information networks. Avoid actions that would reduce feedback from internal and outside sources.
- Try to get out and around as much as possible rather than simply remaining within existing orbits; solutions to problems are generally found in the environment.
- Use multiple theories and models to guide analysis and decision making; maintain multiple managerial and organizational success measures; strive for *optimal* size, influence, growth rates, and diversity; blend and balance the symbolic and technological realms of action.
- Build and maintain multiple personal support systems, including those made up of friends, peers, and family.
- Avoid interagency competition for control over limited resources. Confront the challenges and benefits of cooperation and mutual support.
- Choose new personnel and commitments carefully; once chosen they are difficult to change.

- Remember that people are more important than procedures. Good people can make a poor system work, and poor people can foul up a good one. Rigid commitment to procedures usually disguises an inability to recruit, select, and motivate good people.
- Strive to be a generalist while developing a few specialties for purposes of personal reputation and future equity.
- Learn to tolerate ambiguity and uncertainty and to take risks on the basis of limited information.
- Try to be as clear as possible in your own mind about what goals are most important in the short and long runs.
- Do not waste time regretting inequities.

While not all CMHC directors will find it possible to adhere consistently to these general guidelines, we recommend that conscious attention be given to such concerns on a daily and weekly basis. The director's ability to make good decisions, under pressure, about how and where to cut resources may hinge on little else.

References

Attkisson, C. C., and Broskowski, A. "Evaluation and the Emerging Human Service Concept." In C. C. Attkisson and others (Eds.), *Evaluation of Human Service Programs.* New York: Academic Press, 1978.

Avery, B. J., Packard, R., and Vorwaller, C. J. *Corporate Configuring for Human Services.* Colorado Springs, Colo.: Pikes Peak Mental Health Center, 1980.

Broskowski, A. "Management Information Systems for Planning and Evaluation." In H. C. Schulberg and F. Baker (Eds.), *Program Evaluation in the Health Fields.* Vol. 2. New York: Human Sciences Press, 1979.

Broskowski, A., and Attkisson, C. C. *Information Systems for Health and Human Services.* New York: Academic Press, forthcoming.

Broskowski, A., O'Brien, G., and Prevost, J. "Interorganizational Strategies for Survival: Looking Ahead to 1990." *Administration in Mental Health,* in press.

Burns, J. M. *Leadership.* New York: Harper & Row, 1978.

Cox, G., and Osborne, P. "Problem Characteristics, Decision Processes, and Evaluation Activity: A Preliminary Study of Mental Health Center Directors." *Evaluation and Program Planning,* 1980, *3,* 175-183.

Drucker, P. F. *The Practice of Management.* New York: Harper & Row, 1954.

Feldman, S., Goldstein, C., and Offutt, J. *Mental Health Administration: An Annotated Bibliography.* Department of Health and Human Services Publication No. (ADM) 80-548. Washington, D.C.: U.S. Government Printing Office, 1980.

Hopkins, B. R. *The Law of Tax-Exempt Organizations.* (3rd ed.) New York: Wiley-Interscience, 1980.

Howell, J. "The Characteristics of Administrators and the Effectiveness of Community Mental Health Centers." *Administration in Mental Health,* 1976, *3,* 125-132.

Howell, J. "Leadership Behavior and Organizational Effectiveness." *Administration in Mental Health,* 1979, *7,* 120-132.

Kissinger, H. *White House Years.* Boston: Little, Brown, 1979.

Kouzes, J. M., and Mico, P. R. "Domain Theory: An Introduction to Organizational Behavior in Human Service Organizations." *Journal of Applied Behavioral Science,* 1979, *15* (4), 449-469.

Kouzes, J. M., and Mico, P. R. "How Can We Manage Divided Houses?" In S. L. White (Ed.), *New Directions for Mental Health Services: Middle Management in Mental Health,* no. 8. San Francisco: Jossey-Bass, 1980.

Levine, C. H. "Organizational Decline and Cutback Management." *Public Administration Review,* 1978, *38,* 316-323.

Levine, C. H. "More on Cutback Management: Hard Questions for Hard Times." *Public Administration Review,* 1979, *39,* 179-183.

Macindoe, I., and Houge, D. "The Impact of Roles on the Evaluation of Administrative Effectiveness." *Administration in Mental Health,* 1980, *8,* 71-82.

McTighe, J. "Management Strategies to Deal with Shrinking Resources." *Public Administration Review,* 1979, *39,* 88-90.

Mintzberg, H. *The Nature of Managerial Work.* New York: Harper & Row, 1973.

Mintzberg, H. "The Manager's Job: Folklore and Fact." *Harvard Business Review,* 1975, *53* (4), 49-61.

Noren, J., and Peterson, R. Personal communication, February 1979.

Perrow, C. "The Short and Glorious History of Organizational Theory." In H. L. Tosi and W. C. Hamner (Eds.), *Organizational Behavior and Management: A Contingency Approach.* Chicago: St. Clair Press, 1974.

Shields, P. "Public Pricing: One Answer to the Human Service Fiscal Dilemma." *New England Journal of Human Services,* 1981, *1,* 18-24.

Simon, H. A. "Applying Information Technology to Organization Design." *Public Administration Review,* 1973, *33,* 268-278.

Treusch, P. E., and Sugarman, N. A. *Tax-Exempt Charitable Organizations.* Philadelphia: American Law Institute, 1979.

White, S., and Broskowski, A. "Critical Management Tasks: The PERFORM Model." In S. L. White (Ed.), *New Directions for Mental Health Services: Middle Management in Mental Health,* no. 8. San Francisco: Jossey-Bass, 1980.

Chapter 11

Diagnosis and Intervention in Organizational Settings

Harry Levinson

As it becomes increasingly apparent that forces within organizations have significant effects on the mental health of the individuals who belong to them, it will become equally apparent that intervention into the organizational system is an advantageous way of preventing emotional distress and of fostering mental health. Many mental health professionals, therefore, will be moving toward a mental health consultation role in and with organizations. This is what Gerald Caplan has called consultee-centered administrative consultation (Caplan, 1970).

When such a role shift occurs, it requires a new model of practice, new methods of intervention, different conceptualizations, and certainly a significant difference in the way in which professional mental health workers go about their work. Mental health workers who seek to undertake organizational consultation will discover that there are three established ways of consulting with organizations. There is first of all the classical and historical mode of studying an organization or one or another of its major problems and of arriving at a series of recommendations that are then presented to organizational authorities as the preferred mode of behavior. Such studies may focus on engineering, finance, marketing, organizational structure, feasibility, and so on. They are characteristic in fields other than those having to do with human relations and usually do not take people significantly into account.

Much of human relations consultation takes one of two different orientations or involves a combination of them. Both of these orientations arise from the discipline loosely called organizational development. Organization development, as a consultation discipline, grew out of social psychology and the group dynamics movement. For a long time it concentrated heavily on the application of various kinds of group-based techniques to solve problems in organizations. That movement has been criticized for being technique oriented, sometimes for being little more than a series of techniques in search of a problem. Indeed, there is a pervasive tendency for the same techniques to be applied to a wide range of problems without careful analysis of particular organizations or of the specific problems that those organizations are experiencing. Another orientation arising from that movement is the survey feedback technique. Here a questionnaire is given to all the members of an organization. The results are then tabulated and reported either to these members or to the organization's management. Sometimes such questionnaires are modest in scope, sometimes they are extremely comprehensive. They are variously called morale studies, attitude surveys, climate surveys, or diagnostic studies. Sometimes the feedback process involves the use of group process orientations and group dynamics skills. More often it does not. In both cases the organizational participants define and describe the organization's problems, and the professional then works in varying ways with the organization to help resolve those problems. Most of the consultants who use such techniques have no theory of individual motivation or clinical experience in working with individuals, and therefore they have little sense of unconscious dynamics and forces.

The third method of consultation derives from a clinical

(psychological) orientation. Psychodynamics—especially concepts of unconscious motivation—and an understanding of the adaptive history of the organization, as well as of the contemporary forces operating on it, are the foundations for understanding the problems of the organization and the basis for subsequent intervention. It is this orientation that both Caplan and I bring to organizational consultation.

A clinical orientation requires a heavy emphasis on understanding and defining problems in terms of the organizational, environmental, and historical contexts in which they occur. With respect to mental health organizations, for example, Caplan advocates preparing a cumulative history of the economic, political, and sociocultural life of the community, with particular reference to problems in the health, education, corrections, and welfare fields and to the institutions and services that have been developed to deal with them (Caplan, 1970). He speaks of a series of maps and tables that should be developed indicating the main demographic and ecological indexes of the community. He notes further that cumulative statistics should be kept on the adaptive casualties of the population, not merely routine physical morbidity and mental disorder indexes, such as admissions and discharges to hospitals and outpatient clinics and visits to physicians, but also as much information as is available in the general public health, education, corrections, labor, and welfare fields. He advises developing a register of populations with special risk and that there be a cumulative register of those caregiving agencies and individuals who are potentially or usually most helpful to those high-risk populations. He notes that the consultant should focus on the problems of an organization, not of a client, and that he should present a plan for administrative action instead of recommendations in regard to case management.

As contrasted with the kind of consultation derived from the group dynamics tradition, in this mode a consultant is personally responsible for correctly assessing the problem and for giving a specific action recommendation or a range of options to be carried out by the consultees. Caplan (1970) notes that "it is therefore essential that the information upon which the consultant bases his recommendations be accurate and that he have the expert knowledge to deliver a wise plan. He does not in this regard have the leeway of the consultee-centered case consultant or administrative consultant whose contract calls for him only to improve the understanding and operational effectiveness of his consultees" (p. 223).

In this orientation the organizational consultant is expected to come into the organization, study its problems, assess the significance of the relevant factors, and then present a report containing his appraisal of the situation and his recommendations for dealing with it. Caplan (1970) recommends that a consultant make a study of the traditions, values, and customary practices of the organizations with which he consults. He speaks of the skill and techniques that mental health consultants need when collecting information and when communicating their plans in acceptable ways to those who have responsibility for the action outcomes. He reports how he (Caplan), by reading, prepares for a visit to the client system and how he gets a bird's-eye view of the problem and its ramifications by traveling around the setting. He points out that there is a need to obtain a view of the total organization in order to identify issues that are not brought to his attention by consultees. He therefore widens his range of data collection to achieve that view. Once he accepts responsibility for identifying and dealing with problems in the organizational structure beyond those brought to his immediate attention by his current informants, he confronts the question of how far to go in initiating action to achieve organizational change through his influence on consultees. Caplan contends that the consultant must therefore operate in three phases: (1) collecting information, (2) making a consultation plan, and (3) implementing the latter in his specific consultation intervention.

Caplan (1970) eschews the more common modes of mechanistic diagnosis:

> He [the consultant] should not be misled by the format of group discussions and the need for motivating staff to collaborate, through the utiliza-

> tion of group dynamics skills and knowledge of group process, into the belief that his role is to catalyze their collecting only the information they think relevant in working out their own solutions to their problems. He must usually go beyond this, both in fact finding and in problem solving, because he will be held responsible for the content of the assessment and of remedial recommendations, and these must be based on his own expert judgment and not restricted in any way by the limitations in knowledge, skill, and objectivity of the staff. Moreover, because program-centered administrative consultation is usually only a short process of a few days to a few weeks in duration, the consultant is operating under considerable time pressure, and he cannot afford to move at the slow speed that is likely to be comfortable for his staff, which is confused and is struggling with communications blocks or is relatively ineffective because of reduced morale associated with the problems that stimulated the request for consultation [p. 227].

Caplan makes little or no use of survey techniques and instead relies on a "clinical" approach that is based on data collected through personal interview or direct observation.

Case-Study Outline

In the same tradition, I have devised a systematic mode of organizational diagnosis (Levinson, 1972). This organizational diagnostic method is based on a highly detailed case-study outline. The outline calls for detailing the chief complaints or events leading to the consultation, the problems as stated by key figures, and the background of the organization in terms of its cycles of development as seen by both those inside and outside the organization and by the consultant. It asks also for a history of the major crises experienced by the organization, its product or service history, and the circumstances surrounding the diagnostic effort. It calls attention to and asks questions about the organization's formal structure, its plant and equipment, the distribution of its personnel, demographic variables and variables within the organization, its structure for handling personnel, its policies and procedures, and the time span and rhythm of the organization's operation. It also requires the consultant to follow the manner in which information is received by the organization, how it is processed as communication, and how it is responded to; this line of inquiry will give some sense of the adaptation processes of the organization.

Once the factual data are noted, the case-study outline asks the consultant to infer from those data and from data that he has collected by interview, questionnaire, observation, and examination of historical documents how the organization perceives stimuli, processes those stimuli, and acts on them. Thus, this is an ego psychology model that calls for the consultant to make judgments about the effectiveness of the organization's adaptation to its employees, markets, materials, as well as to its competitors, the economy, and the government.

The consultant is asked to ascertain how the organization acquires knowledge and what it does with that knowledge; to examine the organizational language as reflected in employee publications, in advertising, and in organizational ideology; to evaluate the emotional atmosphere of the organization; and to assess the organization's relationship with both its internal and external constituencies. The outline asks the consultant to consider the attitudes of the people in the organization toward the consultant and the consultant's attitude toward them. It asks also what kind of self-image people in the organization have and their feelings about that image. It calls attention to intraorganizational relationships among individuals and groups. Finally, it asks the consultant to review the organization's integration with its host community, as well as to note the special assets of the organization and its particular impairments.

On the basis of these inferences, the consultant is required to make a generalized cross sectional description of the organization in its environment at one point on the time spectrum—the present. This description is an integration and summary of the material discussed under the topics noted above. That integrative summary should capture the essence of the current situation in which the organization finds itself and the conclusions that the consultant has drawn. Such a statement will have a genetic orientation: It will explain the present status of the organization in terms of its entire life process, taking into account those significant events that have molded and influenced the organization.

The consultant is also asked to make a dynamic formulation, that is, he is asked to explain organizational behavior and the environmental response in terms of energy systems, defensive maneuvers, conscious and unconscious conflicts, and multiple causation and motivation. Such a formulation will also see the organization as moved by forces of which it is often unaware and as continually making compromises and adjustments in order to achieve the best level of functioning that it can. From these formulations the consultant is asked to prepare prognostic conclusions. Specifically, what kind of change is it reasonable to expect this organization to accomplish, given its resources and limits, its history, the level of intelligence and the personalities of its leadership, and the talents, skills, and limits of the consultant?

The diagnostic process is necessarily and simultaneously an intervention. The consultant engages with the organization and the organization with him. The consultant is asked to keep a diary of continuous contacts with the organization, to consider the nature of his impact on that organization, and to examine the expectations that both the consultant and organization members come to have of each other and the feelings that members of the organization generate in the consultant and vice versa.

This process calls for attention to the significance of the consultant in the organization. This means that consultants must use themselves as their most important diagnostic devices and learn to trust their psychological antennae. It also means that consultants must be able to justify their inferences by pointing out the relationships between the inferences they have drawn and the data from which they have drawn it. This is a critically important issue. As Lippitt (1969) puts it:

> It is not easy to overstate the importance of diagnosis in the renewal process, although in the same breath we must note that diagnosis generally does not stand as an end in itself and that in most cases it must be translated into a course of action for change. The history of planned change shows that most renewal stimulators approach each problem with a predetermined diagnostic orientation. Some of them always feel the basic problem is either a maldistribution of power, caused by faulty interchange of ideas, or the result of poor utilization of energy by the organization. It seems almost axiomatic among industrial consultants that poor intraorganizational communication lies at the root of low productivity. A renewal stimulator with a particular diagnostic orientation undoubtedly will find data to fit his preconception; this does not limit the usefulness of his diagnosis provided he changes in the face of contrary data [p. 158].

Having evolved and written a diagnostic case study, the consultant is then asked to prepare a formal report to be presented to the organization. Depending on the nature of the problem and why the consultant was invited into the organization, that report may be presented to top management or to management and all the employees in the organization. That report, which should be about twenty pages in length, has four components: (1) a description of how the consultant went about gathering his information, (2) the consultant's findings, (3) the consultant's understanding or interpretation of those findings, and (4) the consultant's recommendations based on those findings. Having presented this report and having helped the client or client system to examine it critically, the consultant is then prepared to leave the organization. By this I mean that the diagnostic phase is a comprehensive first step that, ideally, will set in motion the process of change. At this point the organization should be free to make its own decisions about whether it wants to continue working with that particular consultant, whether it wants to make use of his recommendations, or whether it prefers to take another direction. The consultant then either renegotiates his contract with the organization or brings the relationship to a close.

This comprehensive method, which at first seems overwhelming, nevertheless provides consultants with the assurance that they have looked at all the details of organizational functioning. In addition, it provides a logical base for amassing and distilling data and then focusing it in a way that specifies both the possibilities and the options available to the consultant and to the organization. Thus, consultants have the comfort of a detailed structure that compels them to make a logical analysis of the situation. This analysis will lead to conclusions that take into account critical elements in the organization, the psychological aspects of the leadership, and the limits of the knowledge and competence of the consultant. This model is adaptable not only to all kinds of organizations but also to communities. It is a systematic way of gathering, organizing, integrating, and interpreting information that will lead to the intervention of choice. In other words, it will specify what method or methods should be used in working with this organization, given its particular problems, its particular circumstances, and a particular consultant.

Such a diagnostic method provides a rationale for mental health professionals to take on a more aggressive and action-oriented role. But there is another important reason for having a comprehensive diagnostic method. Put simply, to operate without that kind of method, particularly with respect to complex social systems, is to "psychologize" or, more often, to "sociologize" organizational or community problems. Thus, we have a wide range of social problems defined in sociological terms and assessed by sociological means without careful analysis of the multiple forces operating in a given situation, the kinds of people involved, the nature of their resources, their modes of communication, their value systems, and so on. As a result, much public money has been thrown at problems ranging from education to rehabilitation of offenders to little avail.

For example, sociologists, with no knowledge of individual motivation (or even hostile to the whole concept) become criminologists and seek to apply normative solutions to problems that when examined at the individual level, turn out to have significant individual psychological dynamics that are neither recognized nor appreciated by the sociologist turned criminologist. This same kind of problem occurs when economists seek to deal with problems of absenteeism and labor turnover. It is not that these people are ignorant or narrow in their conceptual orientations. It is rather that people who deal with organizational problems are all too often not well informed psychologically, and do not take the trouble to systematically pursue, integrate, and analyze information that they can then use as a logical basis for recommending action.

Organizational consultation requires thorough knowledge of personality theory, together with an awareness of a wide range of fields—economics, anthropology, sociology, organizational theory, and so on. Caplan (1970) notes: "A mental health consultant cannot be expected to be equally expert in all these areas of psychology, psychiatry, small-group processes, sociology, anthropology, administration, and economics. He must, however, develop some generalist working competence in all these areas. He must also make a study of the traditions, values, and customary practices of the organizations in which he consults. His own expertise consists in his specialized knowledge of certain aspects of the field and his being able to help his consultees strengthen their mastery of those aspects in a balanced relation to other factors" (p. 281).

The consultant, then, must be both a generalist, capable of taking the broad view, and a specialist in diagnostic process. Like an internist the consultant must himself undertake the diagnostic study of the organization as a central part of his role. He may then refer the actual carrying out of his recommendations to other people or he may, as Caplan notes, do it himself. Most of the time such consultation does involve intervention by the consultant, although operations such as setting up a new method of handling finances or of reaching out to constituents, whether parishioners of a church or clients of a community mental health center, may require the expertise of others. Sometimes a problem may call for community analysis, and this might mean turning to a sociologist or political scientist.

A question of ethics also enters here. A consultant who is unaware of what he does not know, regardless of his discipline, cannot set his own limits, nor will he know to whom to refer a consultee when those limits have been reached. The clinical psychologist or psychiatrist must be able to know when he is dealing with a patient who may have a brain tumor or who may be suffering from toxic poisoning. Neither may ethically undertake to treat such a person, but each must know enough about the symptoms of such pathology to be able to refer the patient to someone who does have the training and experience to do so. The requirement for referrals is built into the codes of ethics of all professions. Certainly it must also be a part of the ethical code of people who would do organizational consultation. Thus, it is not merely that one should be knowledgeable, but rather that one cannot be responsible without being knowledgeable.

The diagnostic consultant must define for himself and for client systems the limits of his knowledge, skill, and expertise. Not all consultants, even in the same discipline, are equally expert in dealing with the total range of problems with which that particular discipline professes special competence. Prognosis is the handmaiden of diagnosis. The consultant who does not define for himself and for the organization what is reasonably possible in a given period of time, with the resources and limits at hand, including those of the consultant, usually tries to do too much or tries to cover all bases too quickly. This leads to disillusionment, often to frustration and failure. Every consultant must define for himself what he can reasonably expect to do with this problem, in this organization, under this set of circumstances. Only then can he go about doing what needs to be done in a rational way.

Applying Organizational Consultation

But how does all this work in practice? Here is one example: A consulting team agreed to take on the problems of a community mental health center. As with so many other community health centers, this one found itself confronted with increasingly complex constituencies in its host communities. There were more power centers in the various communities it served than there had been a generation ago, and each of these centers wielded both financial and psychological influence. There was more criticism from the public at large and from those who were being served. There was greater demand for more medically effective and cost-effective service. There was great, sometimes conflicting, pressure from the various disciplines in the mental health professions at the center. Each of these wanted greater autonomy, greater flexibility, higher pay, and less accountability to formal authority. Each also wanted to resist those forces outside the agency that were trying to influence its activities. These forces variously took the form of community boards, laws having to do with licensing, third-party payers, minority groups, persons with certain kinds of illnesses, those with problems unique to youth or old age, or workers in other community agencies who had to deal with the proliferation of demands for help in the absence of supportive resources either in the family or other aspects of the community.

The Wabash Mental Health Center served a population of 280,000 people in nine communities. It provided outpatient treatment, specialized assistance for retarded and emotionally handicapped children through a nursery school program, rehabilitation services for mentally retarded adolescents and adults, community consultation in mental health and community agencies, community education in mental health, advanced professional training for clinical students, and assistance in finding community health and retardation resources. Its staff members were strong in individual and group therapy processes. They had less interest in working with community agencies.

A new director was trying desperately to reorganize the center, which was still mourning the loss of his predecessor, a charismatic leader. Competition was rising in the form of other public and private service groups in the various communities. Communities supporting the center increasingly wanted its expenditures justified. There was increasing consumer dissatisfaction with the quality, kind, and frequency of services, as reflected in the concerns of school systems, police departments, and other community agencies. There was also internal conflict among staff members. New therapeutic "techniques," which promised rapid cures and required limited training, seemed to appeal to younger clinical students, who were reluctant to undergo the formal discipline required to attain the professional sophistication that the senior staff valued. The students and junior staff felt that the senior staff, particularly the administration, was authoritarian and rigid. Goals and objectives were in conflict—service versus training, clinical versus community service—and there was conflict among the professional disciplines.

There was also little quality control over consultation efforts. Some citizens and officials were angry because the center had not provided much assistance for a desperately needed drug treatment program. The various communities were demanding that the center expand both the breadth and depth of its services and become much more flexible and responsive to consumer needs. Despite numerous meetings, teams within the center had little sense of what was going on beyond their own work groups. The center was a fragmented assembly of autonomous subunits that operated according to various professional norms rather than on the basis of central policy. The administration had an impact only in terms of financial control; there was no formal overall planning.

There was little concern on the part of the staff about the adequacy and timeliness of the services that it delivered to the communities. The communities naturally wanted to know what they were getting from the center, but the center could not accurately measure its own output, costs, or results. The center was withdrawing from the communities it supposedly served, just as the staff was withdrawing from the center. This process was accelerated by the guilt and frustration generated by the staff's low self-esteem, resulting from the measurement of today's performance against yesterday's ego ideal.

The center was paralyzed by its internal divisions. It could not directly attack its internal problems, even though staff members expended a great deal of energy on them. The lack of staff confidence in the director was compounded by the staff members' professionally based belief that they should avoid conflict and control their personal feelings. The center was losing its reputation, its support, and the commitment of its staff, and, therefore, its effectiveness. The new leader was trying to reshape the organization into a structure better suited to its size and task without the managerial tools to do so or the support of his staff. This task was overwhelming and forced the director into regressive behavior patterns. The organization, in short, was in a crisis.

All this information arose out of the consulting team's interviews with members of community agencies and with members of the center's board and staff, as well as from a review of the history of the organization, its finances, management, and internal processes. The consulting team then made clear to the staff the difference between its historic ego ideal (good, individual therapeutic effort) and the operations now demanded of it. The team recommended that the staff upgrade its present program so that both the needs of the environment and the expectations of staff members could be more fully met. The staff, it said, should revise and clarify its present ego ideal by discussions with one of the members of the consulting team. The team also recommended that the organization be differentiated and decentralized according to task groups to increase each group's investment in both the center and the environment. The head of each task group would be a member of an eight-person team that would clarify the roles, purposes, and goals of the center, specifically stating what the center could and could not do and how much it would do in each area.

The organization's strategy was based on this work, which was used in published statements by the center. The strategy included formally setting priorities for various activities and programs and establishing broad guidelines for the allocation of man-hours to these programs and activities. The task group leaders thus came to constitute a policy-making body. Department (discipline) heads were made responsible for teaching, training, evaluation, and personnel matters.

Each task group leader and department head was asked to

become a full-time staff member. Each was also asked to become involved in the negotiation for funds from the communities that he served, and this required him to maintain personal contacts with the various service recipients and service-purchasing groups. That also required him to provide information to them. Each task unit had to develop its own time budget to show how the time of its members would be allocated over the coming year and to update that budget quarterly, when it would be reviewed by the policy committee. That committee was also asked to develop a method of quality control to check service, follow-up, and termination.

These and other recommendations and the supportive help that went with them were gratefully received by the staff, which arrived for the first time at a clear picture of the complex morass in which it had become embedded. The recommendations gave the staff a chance to debate and discuss both the findings and the consultant's proposed solutions for the problems, as well as to modify the recommendations in keeping with what they felt they could reasonably expect to do. The diagnostic process, therefore, did not limit itself to the center's staff alone. In essence, it was almost a community diagnosis in that it discovered and integrated information that members of the center's staff did not themselves have and could not perceive on their own. Note also that the consulting team dealt with the agency as an agency rather than with people in an agency.

Furthermore, the diagnostic model held out for the staff members the possibility of their working with their community agencies in the same way. One-to-one relationships with professional peers, while important, do not have much effect on the formal structure of an agency or organization, even though that structure affects how a given professional or group of professionals may do his or their work. It is one thing to consult with a teacher about a pupil, with a pastor about his consultees, or with a policeman about juveniles, but quite another to examine the school as an organizational system, the church as an institution, or the police department as a quasi-military organization, along with the pressures and demands of each one of those institutional forms as an institution. Increasingly, services are rendered by institutions of which individual professional persons, often transient, are merely agents. The hospital renders a caring service, but many different nurses may be the caretakers at different times. So it is with many social service agencies. How effectively, reasonably, and accountably the members of an institution are able to perform will hinge significantly on how that institution—as an institution—is able to perform.

Importance of Leadership

Mental health centers, like other organizations, are becoming more complex. Service is rendered by these organizations as *organizations* rather than by individual providers. (For example, persons seeking help become clients of the center and are assigned a therapist by the center.) Therefore, the issue of leadership of the organization becomes crucial. The leader of any organization is its core, and he or she must set its standards. The leader defines external reality and is a main figure in dealing with it. He or she frequently allocates roles and resources, entertains hostility and tries to deflect it into problem solving, and, in the last analysis, is responsible to a board or to the community for the functioning of the agency or organization as a whole. Leaders must deal with increasingly higher levels of complexity and abstraction for reasons noted above and, in addition, must be capable of resolving interprofessional conflicts, as well as evolving complementary professional roles to meet the demands of the community for service. This was a critical issue in the case of the mental health center discussed earlier.

Leadership is not easily come by in social service and community mental health organizations, or for that matter in educational or religious institutions. People who enter the serving or helping professions do so in order to practice a professional skill rather than to take charge of an institution and to exercise leadership. There is often role conflict when people who pride themselves on their excellent professional skills are asked to give up those skills to assume managerial roles with which they usually are not familiar. Their ambivalence about the leadership role that they must carry out will reflect itself in the kind of uncertain functioning characteristic of many such organizations. Thus, leadership demands a great deal of support from those outside the organization, especially consultants, because leaders often cannot talk with their subordinates about some of the problems with which they are confronted and often need outside objective observers who can help them cope with the issues of management.

In his discussion of organizational consultation, Caplan gives considerable attention to the psychological dynamics of the leaders with whom he worked. He speaks of the manner in which he had to work with them in order to accomplish the goals of the consultation. Caplan clearly arrived at a professional understanding of the psychodynamics of those leaders and the modes of behavior required of him if he were to avoid becoming entrapped and defeated by the characteristic behavior of the leaders. Leaders of organizations in a consultative relationship may well act toward the consultant as patients in one-to-one therapy sometimes act toward the therapist. Individuals always have ambivalent feelings about seeking help, and this brings into play transference phenomena. The consultant must be psychologically sophisticated enough to understand this and to work with the leadership in ways that will enable that leadership to assume a more responsible and psychologically sound role with respect to the organization and its problems. Diagnostic effort therefore requires as fundamental preparation a sophisticated understanding of psychotherapeutic techniques.

Role Strain

It is imperative to note that when one undertakes to deal with community institutions and with the problems of formally constituted groups, such consultation involves a more aggressive mode of action than client- or consultee-centered consultation does. I make a point of this because, in other forms of consultation, the consultant's task is to stay out of the way and to help the consultee formulate and focus on the problem himself. The consultant's is a more passive, nonresponsible role, as Caplan has indicated. For that matter, an aggressive personality style is not congenial in the mental health field. Indeed, mental health workers tend to be poor administrators because in most cases they cannot comfortably take charge of situations and express their aggression constructively by giving appropriate direction to the institutions that they head. More often they handle aggression by reaction formation and then rationalize that behavior as serving others. By permitting others to depend on them, they serve their own dependency needs. Too often, then, theirs is a depressive orientation. This same orientation may inhibit them in making diagnostic formulations and recommendations in organizations. How many people would feel comfortable taking charge of a consultation as Caplan did when he walked in on a meeting of a government agency division chief and his staff and redirected the meeting to his consultation needs (Caplan, 1970, pp. 229-230)?

This problem makes it even more imperative to have a method that *requires* consultants to gather data and removes from them the onus of penetrating the system of their own accord, a form of behavior that they may perceive to be inappropriately aggressive. Such a diagnostic framework or outline demands of diagnosticians that they actively pursue the information. It therefore serves as a rationale to appease the sense of unconscious guilt that people often feel when they are "digging out" information or examining organizational phenomena that they believe to be none of their business.

An example of a consultation in which the team had to make such a vigorous effort follows. In still another consultation, the consulting team interviewed nearly 150 persons within a community mental health center system and its environment. This center included inpatient and outpatient facilities, as well as a wide range of supportive activities. In addition to interviewing employees from all levels of the organization, professional and nonprofessional, and sampling the ethnic and gender composition of the hospital, the consulting team attended meetings and spent a good deal of time in informal conversation in the coffee shop with employees. The team also talked with long-time employees, read other studies that had been done at the center, reviewed its annual reports, and put together a history of the organization. The team also examined the external organizations that impinged on the hospital, including various governing and appropriation bodies, to determine the kinds of relationships they had with the center and their perceptions of it.

Few members of the center's staff appreciated the history of the organization before the consulting team detailed it. The team presented a history, tradition, and values of which that institution could be proud. Its innovations had had significant impact on the practices of all professional disciplines. But the center had been compelled to shift its focus as a result of legislation from long-term individual psychotherapy to briefer, community-oriented services. The new director was called upon to protect his organization from unpredictable fluctuations in funding and had delegated many of the internal operations of the center to subordinates. One consequence was the feeling that the director was detached and not as involved in the center as his predecessor was thought to have been. Government budgeting processes and rigid civil service requirements further inhibited the flexibility of the center. Its major building was obsolete. Its programs and services had expanded, but its patient population had changed as a result of changes in its catchment area; the staff enjoyed fewer of the satisfactions associated with treating well-educated, neurotic patients and felt more of the frustrations that working with chronically ill patients entails.

Despite the efforts of the director, there was a general lack of communication. Staff members felt a sense of cohesion within their respective departments but felt little relationship to other departments; outlying clinics were isolated from the main part of the center. Few had been oriented to the center and what it did. Rules and guidelines seemed to be nonexistent. Performance feedback was either highly structured or totally lacking. There was perceived competition between departments for the same limited resources, and this increased the distance between them. The administrative structure was not clear. In some cases employees reported to two or even three superiors. The psychiatrists felt that their schedules were too hectic and heavily overloaded. The other members of the staff complained about the complexity of doing even simple tasks because of the need to share resources. Memorandums sometimes seemed not to reach their destinations.

To cope with all this, employees sometimes went directly to key figures in the hierarchy—therefore bypassing the usual administrative channels—and demanded results. As a result, half the people responding to the questionnaire and interviews used in the consultation said that the center was not very interested in their welfare. Nevertheless, people did want to work in that center and were dedicated to excellence of patient care. There was a strong indication of interpersonal cohesion despite low pay, poor working conditions, and relative isolation from fellow workers.

When staff members were asked to describe the organization as though it were a person, this composite view emerged: The center was like a middle-aged person, somewhat frumpy, disheveled, and depressed; someone no longer young, but still with a lot of energy and "clout"; a person lacking direction but still, with a limping gait, searching for it; someone not in the best of health because of internal problems of some complexity, possibly even schizophrenic in that there was no acknowledgment of reality and various internal units seemed to operate independently of each other. Typically the image was of a person in conflict with himself or herself, a leaky ship with no connection from the steering mechanism to the water.

The director and other top managers felt as unappreciated as the staff did; they also thought that employees were unaware of the extent to which they had been working to improve conditions at the center. As a result there was a pervasive lack of common purpose or sense of belonging to the center. In addition, the organization was being pulled in several directions at once. Some staff members tended to identify upward with top management and long-term goals and ideals, others with patients and nonprofessionals. Nonclinical employees felt alienated and excluded from the mainstream. There was a conflict between inpatient work and community population work. Longitudinally, the center was torn between members who idealized the good old days and those who could hardly wait for the future to arrive.

There was insufficient delegation of authority to middle managers, and in fact there were too few people designated as middle managers. As a result, senior people were continually entangled in operations-level problems and lacked the help of intermediate-level subordinates, who in turn felt bitter about being bypassed. Consequently, top managers spent a lot of time troubleshooting and reacting to crises. They were both too busy and too exhausted to support the efforts and emotional needs of subordinates who were also overwhelmed. As part of a state system, the center was also plagued with financial and political problems. Unknown to many of the staff, decisions were often imposed from above, and this led them to feel that decisions were made arbitrarily.

The consulting team recommended that the center formulate a unified ideal and that its director increase his personal contacts, improve promotion opportunities, develop an orientation program, and more clearly define middle-management responsibilities. The director was dismayed at these findings because of his already intensive efforts to cope with the many problems of the center and his sense that he was fighting a difficult uphill battle. However, his continuing discussions with the consulting team relieved some of his anger and anxiety and led him to take steps to implement the recommendations. A slide orientation program was developed for new employees. He and his top staff people evolved a new organizational structure with the help of an outside consultant.

With that same assistance, the director then held an all-day meeting of his professional staff in which he presented his new structural plan for open discussion. The staff was next divided into small groups that were made up of people from different units of the center and with different professional disciplines so that they could discuss his proposals from the point of view of their identification with the center as a whole. Delegates from each of the groups then reported the discussion of that group. The luncheon speaker, the director of a major professional association, brought the staff up-to-date on current developments in the field of community mental health. There followed two other discussion groups. In the first, staff members met as members of a discipline—social work, psychology, nursing, and so on. Persons chosen from each of these groups then reported to the larger plenary session. The second discussion group was composed of all the staff of each of the subsidiary units; the same reporting procedure was used. This was followed by a summary of the experience of the day and its high points by the outside consultant, followed in turn by a farewell from the director.

During the following year, two other one-day meetings were held to review how things were going and what problems needed more focused attention. The staff reported increased satisfaction with the center as a result of these efforts and increased identification with its myriad and complex problems, as well as with its leadership.

Systematic comprehensive diagnosis is fundamental to community mental health efforts. As both of the cases discussed in this chapter illustrate, that diagnostic process may involve assessment of community forces, assessment of leadership, and assessment of the internal structure and processes of the organization. An intervention of choice must then be worked out. That is, it must be determined what recommendations this organization will be able to make use of, given its level of knowledge and sophistication, its history and leadership, as well as its resources and the state of its morale. Special sensitivities are required in understanding and dealing with the leadership, which sometimes itself is the core problem in the organization.

Diagnosis involves constructing a clear picture of the reality the organization faces, of the demands being placed on it, and of how those both inside and outside the organization perceive it. The highly detailed outline for undertaking this complex task is the core of *organizational diagnosis.* It provides a structure that the consultant can use to organize, interpret, and summarize his findings, which then can become a solid basis for recommendations. The model is useful with all kinds of organizations and even communities. It can be used for self-study and is particularly helpful in teaching students the techniques of organizational consultation.

References

Caplan, G. *The Theory and Practice of Mental Health Consultation.* New York: Basic Books, 1970.

Levinson, H. *Organizational Diagnosis.* Cambridge, Mass.: Harvard University Press, 1972.

Lippitt, G. L. *Organization Renewal.* New York: Appleton-Century-Crofts, 1969.

Chapter 12

Consultation to Organizations in Transition

Ralph G. Hirschowitz

Critical changes in the workplace provide the mental health consultant with rare opportunities for the promotion of healthy organizational adaptation. In helping leaders cope with the disruption of organizational change, the consultant draws upon his schooling in diagnostic analysis, public health practice, personality, group, and social systems dynamics, and the application of systems and crisis theories. Given the value placed by the mental health consultant on primary prevention, investment of his time produces its most gratifying return when his help is sought early rather than late in the course of organizational crisis. Unfortunately, organizations tend to seek help in their first encounters with dramatic change only when system dysfunction is advanced. Lacking prior experience with significant change, their leaders are usually slow to identify indicators of adaptive distress. Even when these have been identified, help is often sought from the wrong consultants. Initial entry into such organizations is therefore likely to be late rather than early, compelling the consultant to practice tertiary and/or secondary prevention. As organizations become more comfortable with consultants, interventions occur earlier so that primary prevention goals are ultimately attainable. This occurs in ideal form when consultation is sought in anticipation of change. The case examples that follow, while drawn from three different organizations, illustrate stages of this evolutionary process. They are therefore offered as examples of late, earlier, and early intervention. Each represents different facets of prevention.

Case 1: Late Intervention

In this case, which is detailed in a previous publication (Hirschowitz, 1979), a plant manager sought help for prolonged employee absenteeism. Over three and a half years, three of which preceded his tenure, absenteeism had risen from 2 to 20 percent. The latter rate had been sustained for some months. Almost all the employees had been absent with orthopedic complaints. In the three and a half years, this very stable manufacturing plant had been buffeted by winds of change, emanating from many directions. Cutbacks, "speedups," departures of leaders, and capricious divisional staff interventions had generated endemic fear and anxiety. Assumptions of organizational predictability and dependability were shattered as long-established "psychological contracts" (Levinson and others, 1962) were violated. The situation worsened when the paternalistic manager, who had maintained the stability of the traditional regime, was prematurely retired. Employees mourned his loss. The new, younger manager's "professional" style did not mesh with theirs. He was perceived as distant and had yet to be sanctioned as successor. Many other factors conspired to produce the eventual absenteeism. Some are captured in the following excerpts from the consultant's report to the plant manager:

> The past three years have been punctuated by unusual changes and demands. These all placed heavy pressure on workers who were already working hard and conscientiously. The expectation that they work still harder must have generated profound feelings of "felt unfairness." Since the typical worker is a loyal, obedient person unaccustomed to expressing feelings of resentment directly

to superiors, her unexpressed feelings would therefore have been repressed and internalized. This tendency to internalize resentment would have caused workers to become "wound up" and "uptight." When emotional stress reached threshold levels, this unconscious tightening would then have been consciously registered as muscle discomfort, eventually to be reported as symptoms. Symptoms would have been more likely in the most conscientious workers, since they would have been less likely to take time out to unwind and restore tired muscles. Fatigue, as in the stress familiar to engineers, would then have caused loss of elasticity in muscles and joints. This would have impaired the workers' capacities to "roll with the punches," so that some would have sustained small muscular injuries from which they were normally protected.

The changes of the past three years must have been particularly stressful for this group of workers because they had experienced so little change prior to this. Their work lives and the composition of the work force were unusually stable. Compared with other plants in the division, they appeared to have been insulated and protected from change. . . .

Loss was experienced in many ways by the workers during these three years and must have been a source of particular upset. Loss was precipitated particularly by the cutback and then the successive retirements of your predecessor and the personnel and cafeteria managers. . . . In addition to such obvious losses, the workers have experienced the loss of control associated with the dissolution of a familiar, predictable regime—and have not yet accepted the new one. Losses have therefore been both actual and symbolic, direct and indirect, real and feared.

These losses would have triggered such emotions as aggrievement, anger, and protest. As suggested earlier, your typical worker is unaccustomed

> to expressing—and, for some, even consciously acknowledging—feelings of anger toward authority. Feelings were, however, communicated indirectly as "soreness" or "complaints." . . .
>
> Why did the condition assume epidemic proportions? When the first workers with orthopedic complaints were rewarded by attention, paid leave, and, sometimes, less demanding jobs when they returned, other workers probably paid attention to signals from their muscles and joints that they might previously have ignored. Signals of "soreness" that had been switched off were now amplified. For similar reasons, discomfort that might previously have been resolved by a night's rest now became the subject of lingering preoccupation and eventual ground for "complaint." The spread was also assisted by the phenomenon described as "group psychological contagion." Individuals who were highly suggestible would have been particularly susceptible to these psychological group pressures.

As the report demonstrates, consultation provided the new manager with an authoritative analysis of previously inexplicable "complaints." This provided the rationale for a number of corrective recommendations. The manager subsequently increased his visibility on the shop floor, interacted frequently with workers, and established grievance committees and procedures to legitimize the expression of grief and provide forums for review of the past years' traumas. He instituted "state-of-the-plant" meetings and made his personal posture and values clear. He listened carefully, acknowledged past suffering, responded to legitimate grievances, and negotiated mutual expectations. Work was redesigned for workers with residual disabilities, and "speedup" pressures were reduced. A sensitive personnel manager who won the confidence of the workers was recruited to become an advocate for their needs. As complaints were aired and redressed and the manager's concern was repeatedly demonstrated, the orthopedic complaints subsided.

Case 2: Earlier Intervention

In this case, intervention occurred earlier because a corporate medical officer sought consultation for a rising incidence of psychophysiological problems in a corporate division. He convened a meeting between the consultant and the division's general and personnel managers. Consultation and education followed.

The division, an entrepreneurial component of an apparel and sporting goods enterprise, had been instituted to implement a corporate business strategy requiring penetration of a growing winter sports market. To lead the division, an aggressive committed leader was recruited who was able, in turn, to attract competent, ambitious young managers to his team. During the first two years of the division's embryonic life, it was given the seed financing needed to position itself for market entry. Those two years, 1978 and 1979, proceeded smoothly; planned objectives were realized, and few unpleasant surprises were encountered. In planning for 1980, the group had reason to project its first profitable year. However, the fiscal year ended with the division seriously in the red. This outcome was determined by two unpredicted (and substantially unpredictable) events: Little snow fell in the northeastern states to which the division's marketing thrust had been directed, and bank interest rates soared to unprecedentedly high levels. Sales declined and accounts went unpaid. Many customers hovered on the brink of bankruptcy so that additional pressures could not be placed upon them.

The psychological response of many members of the management team to this predicament was to resort to denial and reaction formation. Pollyannaish schemes were elaborated and busily pursued. Sales managers' travel and communication expenses mounted as they attempted unsuccessfully to sell their products in unfamiliar national and international markets. Cancellations were ignored and inventories were permitted to soar. Interminable meetings were held in pursuit of strategies by which to snatch victory from the jaws of imminent defeat. The divisional president, oppressed by his fear of "failure," collaborated in this desperate search for solutions.

Denial, reaction formation, and wishful thinking thus fused with the "busyness" triggered by the threat of loss to direct energies away from realistic cutting of losses and toward unrealistic attempts at undoing. Despite pessimistic marketing news, group denial of failure continued to abet impulsive plans to "turn things around." As evidence of their failing battle began to mount, the managers became irritable and fatigued, blaming themselves or others for their predicament. At that point, some managers developed the psychophysiological symptoms that attracted the attention of the corporate physician. Consultation with the personnel manager confirmed his diagnosis of divisional stress. By that time, the divisional president had also become uneasily aware that his and his team's extraordinary efforts were proving fruitless, so that he was ready to "cut losses." In initial consultation, he acknowledged that overwork was "getting to them" (the managers) in the form of marital and drinking problems as well as medical ones. He welcomed consultation.

The consultant met with the members of the management team, conducted group interviews with their subordinates, and then submitted a brief written report upon which an extensive discussion was based. In meetings, the events of the previous months were retraced, and the devastating impact of threatened loss upon personal and group pride was discussed. The various attempts to buttress self-esteem were analyzed. Meetings were supplemented by seminars that illuminated the dynamics of the group's denial and undoing behavior. A three-day retreat with the management team followed. It was conducted in a setting conducive to sorely needed reflection and restoration. An initial formal seminar provided concepts and language with which to examine the behavior of the previous months and to place recent loss events in perspective. In so doing, grief was acknowledged and assuaged. Renewed hopes and aspirations for the future could then be asserted. With reality acknowledged, feelings brought to the surface, and fatigue remedied, psychophysiological symptoms abated. No recurrence was observed in the course of ongoing consultation.

Case 3: Early Intervention

In this case, consultation was provided in anticipation of change. The leaders had been sensitized to the merits of preventive intervention by previous programs of consultation and education. They had learned "the hard way" that adaptive casualties were easier to prevent than repair.

Consultation was requested because significant resistance to an impending reorganization was predicted. The production division of an oil company was to be split into entirely independent oil and gas companies, entailing geographical and personal dislocations for hundreds of people. It was expected that identification with the change would be compromised for other reasons. The rationale for change, rooted in long-range strategic considerations, was likely to be obscure since the existing organization was very profitable and displayed no obvious evidence of need for transformation. Further, the contemplated reorganization ran counter to the conventional wisdom of other oil companies. This wisdom decreed the fusion of oil and gas operations because oil and gas were often extracted from the same wells. The many geologists, geophysicists, and petroleum engineers who were crucial to the organization's continuing operations were members of professional reference groups in which the reorganization was certain to be debated. These professionals would therefore need to be persuaded of the reorganization's strategic rationale. Yet another source of expressed concern was the likelihood of "winners and losers" reactions to reorganization assignments. People assigned to the future oil company would experience more restricted career mobility than in the embryonic gas company.

Given the complexity and magnitude of change, a task force was therefore charged with planning the transition. Consultation was provided to the task force, to existing leaders, and to the leaders of the new company. An early decision was made to extend the time between the announced reorganization and its eventual implementation. Thirteen months were to be devoted to communication, personal counseling, planning, and preparation for the impending change. A variety of vehicles were devised to ensure that people would *understand* the change, *appreciate* its rationale, and *identify* with its leaders. Also, processes were installed to ensure that people would be helped to make personal decisions, come to terms with their consequences, and eventually *accept* the change. Avenues for *contracting,* that is, the negotiation of need, were also constructed. (The rationale for this sequential approach to managing change is developed at the conclusion of this chapter.)

Multiple structures were designed to help people deal with the impact of the reorganization on their personal and professional lives. Transition managers were selected and schooled to provide the transitional supports described by Levinson (Personal communication, 1981) as "psychological scaffolding." In addition to planned meetings, a special newspaper was created to provide an additional forum for information exchange and debate. The task force elaborated principles and guidelines for communication, including the following:

1. Decisions about the disposition of material assets and human resources were to be made only after consultation with the persons who knew most about them.
2. People were to be informed about the decision alternatives available to them as soon as these were agreed upon.
3. Decisions were to be communicated in face-to-face meetings. Written communications could follow, but were not to precede, such meetings.
4. All requests for information, general or specific, were to be dealt with openly and candidly.
5. Everyone was to receive adequate time and counsel to make choices and negotiate special needs.
6. All leaders and their representatives were to be visible and accessible throughout the transition.
7. Managers were not to make decisions for people; they were cautioned against indulging in salesmanship. People in conflict were to receive counseling.
8. After the initial announcement, meetings were to be held in all regions and at all levels. Initial meetings were designed to clarify the reorganization; later meetings were designed

for interactive discussion. At regional levels, meetings were to be conducted by regional managers with the visible assistance of central office leaders.

Policy about "transition supports" was refined. Adequate financial, emotional, and counseling support was to be given to employees and their families. This was to be provided irrespective of decisions to accept proferred positions or leave the company. Every employee was to be assured in writing that he would be offered a position in the new organization. The relocation policy included adequate compensation for homes that could not be profitably sold, reimbursement for house-hunting trips, and professional help with house selection.

After the reorganization was announced, transition managers met frequently to inform employees, invite questions from them, listen to their problems, and clarify company policies. The meetings that ensued were often highly critical of the reorganization, and derogatory, sometimes paranoid interpretations of it were common. The reorganization's content, intent, and rationale required repeated clarification before most employees moved from incredulity and protest to some acceptance of the decision. During the thirteen months' delay of execution, interactive exchanges in large and small meetings, as well as through the special newspaper, made a considerable measure of anticipatory grief work possible. Leave-taking ceremonies were conducted, new relationships and assignments explored, and needs for orientation and training met. Stress arousal was thus maintained within a range where realization and acceptance could be promoted.

Eventually, the reorganization was ceremonially launched in a workshop for the managers who were to direct the new companies. Spouses were invited to attend and to participate in the seminar component of the workshop. The seminar reviewed the experience of transition and its effective management. It emphasized the leaders' roles in providing information, general support, and the modeling of mature coping. The corporation's chief executive and senior officers attended to participate in a ceremonial dissolution of pre-existing organization. Fears about the future were aired and hopes projected. Spouses were given the opportunity to voice their concerns. The workshop concluded with a period of recuperation punctuated by informal interaction.

The preceding description does poor justice to the patient, exhaustive, and exhausting interactions sustained by the transition managers over many months. Human resource professionals were often overextended by the need to inform and counsel employees over and over. They had to absorb considerable fear and ambivalence. Also, these human resource professionals supported and counseled the transition managers. Consequently, a useful role played by the external consultant was to provide support and consultation to these internal consultants.

Information for evaluation of this program of preventive intervention was provided by attitude surveys conducted for the transition's newspaper. In the first months of change, most responses to questions about the reorganization were "strongly disapprove." Later, most respondents answered "approve," with a few in the "neither approve nor disapprove" camp. When initially asked, "Do you approve of the way in which the change is being managed?", most respondents were strongly negative; at implementation, the overwhelming majority "strongly approved" of the way in which the change was managed. Public health indicators were monitored and reflected a low incidence of health problems before and after implementation. Evidence for the organization's "holding power" was particularly striking. To the considerable surprise of the transition managers, very few people decided to leave. Large emigrations had been predicted because geographical relocation would involve considerable disruption for most people. Since oil company professionals were in high demand, the transition managers had projected the resignation of some 100 professionals. The eventual figure was 9. This holding power reflects the high level of organizational coherence and cohesion attained during the transition.

Case Discussion: From Practice to Principles

In Case 1, a substantial number of workers became ill or disabled while a residual population remained at risk. Intervention was designed to contain existing disability, heal dysfunction, and maintain health in the unimpaired population. Measurable tertiary, secondary, and primary prevention results were achieved. In Case 2, managers had symptoms but no chronicity had occurred. Earlier intervention therefore confidently pursued secondary and primary prevention goals. In Case 3, the consultant helped to design and implement a primary prevention program for an employee population acknowledged by its leaders to be at risk. Despite differences in populations, targets, and tactics, similar principles informed consultant practice in all three cases. These principles were anchored in the following concepts:

1. Loss, change, and the tasks of transition.
2. Defense, resistance, and mastery.
3. Requisite supplies.
4. Requisite leadership processes: the model for modulation of change.

Concept 1: Loss, Change, and the Tasks of Transition. The cases illustrate one of change's axioms—that all change involves loss. This axiom has been developed psychologically by Levinson and others (1962) and sociologically by Marris (1970). The related psychological tasks have been conceptualized by Janis (1958).

In unraveling the meaning of human behavior in transition, the consultant recognizes that organizational change compels people to relinquish attachments to familiar people, as well as to familiar places, habits, identities, functions, and/or roles. The problems caused by this may be compounded when self-esteem is fractured by the temporary loss of habitual mastery or effective role performance. When change is massive, as in Case 3, or cumulative, as in Case 1, grief may emerge in such varied ways as aggrievement, outrage, physiological disturbance, emotional distress, and/or irritability. The depth of grief and worry experienced is greatest when change produces a transformation in organizations previously protected from change. Distress, hurt, and outrage are intensified when change is sudden, unanticipated, and imposed.

News of impending organizational change sets in motion a search for information. The primary search is for information about the likely impact of the announced organizational change upon the individual. Often, this information must await the translation of strategies for change into tactical decisions. Emotional responses are then further aggravated by the need to endure sustained ambiguity and uncertainty.

As information about an imminent change becomes clear, individuals confront the twin tasks of psychological demolition and reconstruction. The intensity of these tasks varies with the degree of cumulative impact upon relationships, roles, identities, and attachments. With multiple changes, the pace of grief work is perforce slow. The more devastating the perception of actual or anticipated loss, the greater is the likelihood that those affected will resort to individual and group psychological defenses to reduce emotional intensity. The consultant's initial diagnostic forays are therefore designed to assess the meaning of news about a coming change to people in the organization. He seeks to establish the magnitude of felt loss and change. In his search he is primarily concerned with people's perceptions and secondarily with the content and sources of the information from which perception derives.

This analysis of people's perceived loss and concern assigns weight to grief and worry work. When perceptions stem from misinformation, the need for corrective information flow is also defined. With weight assigned to the tasks of transition, people's behavior can be interpreted and cast within a normative frame. The normative frame for construing behavior during organizational change is anchored in the second salient concept: defense, resistance, and mastery.

Concept 2: Defense, Resistance, and Mastery. Announcements of transforming organizational change produce levels of emotional arousal that only the most mature persons can consciously sustain, curb, and constructively channel. When arousal levels exceed personal stress thresholds, emotional flooding is averted by resort to such initial emergency defenses as numbness, dissociation, and incredulity. This is common when change is heavily freighted with massive and multiple losses, whether actual, threatened, or imagined. These initial shock responses then surrender to psychological security operations that seek to deny or attenuate the more painful aspects of news about impending change. (Denial provided the basis for the reaction formation and undoing behavior exhibited by managers in Case 2.) With the passage of time, psychobiological rage and contact-seeking responses are activated. When the rage response of grief-stricken employees is repressed, it may be displaced, projected, or, as Case 1 attests, expressed somatically. Rage may be directed toward others in the form of paranoia or toward the self as guilt or depression.

Contact-seeking responses are often evident in the form of peer huddling: interdependent exchanges between peers. When leaders are invisible, such huddling may fortify paranoid social system defenses against the grief, worry, and anxiety of change (Jaques, 1955; Menzies, 1967). The consultant deciphers observed behavior in change so that his report can move from description to reasoned analysis, diagnosis, prognosis, and prescription. Behavior is encoded by working with the constructs of defense, resistance, and mastery. These have been fashioned as working constructs from the formulations of White (1974) and Vaillant (1977).

White emphasizes that *defense* pursues immediate biological ends: survival, safety, and protection. When life is not in jeopardy, defensive maneuvers contain anxiety. When news of a coming change suffuses an organization with threat, uncertainty, and ambiguity, defense protects people from excessive arousal of fight-or-flight responses and the reckless, impulsive action that might otherwise ensue. Defense "buys time" for future mastery. By this definition, defensive behavior early in organizational change is inevitable, necessary—and normal. With the passage of time—and incremental doses of valid information from reliable sources—reality-attenuating defenses should diminish, and tentative attempts at problem mastery should begin.

Defense yields to *mastery* as retreat and avoidance surrender to the increasingly realistic information seeking, information processing, and planning that precedes movement toward resolution of the tasks of transition. Mastery vanquishes reality while defense avoids it.

When defensive avoidance becomes excessively prolonged by exclusive reliance on the primitive defenses described by Vaillant (1977) as "immature," then defense shades into resistance. Resistance represents the "freezing" of immature defenses prolonged over considerable periods of time. It is profoundly regressive, attempting to deny reality by "digging in." Resistance attempts to conserve and "hold on" to the familiar while mastery "lets go." Resistance is exhibited in overt or covert, passive or active forms. Passive forms are passive-retreatist or passive-aggressive; active aggression is more overtly oppositional and is "rationalized" on the basis of paranoid formulations. However, resistance as here discussed refers to behavior substantially mediated by unconscious psychological mechanisms. It does not refer to the active opposition of employees who choose consciously to mobilize against change. This kind of resistance requires a different analysis, along with firm, directive responses from leaders. The topic is important but falls outside the scope of this chapter.

When the consultant has identified and categorized behavior in change as defense, resistance, and/or mastery, he can guide leaders toward appropriate interventions. Since the implications of early defense are benign, leaders are taught the virtue of selective inattention. In populations where defense lingers, mastery is promoted by graduated doses of reality abundantly punctuated by human contacts that produce comfort. For countering resistance, application of the model for modulation of change (discussed later) is aggressively pursued. Meetings are structured to promote understanding, dissolve paranoia, and negotiate legitimate needs. Residual resistance after these interventions, which provided information to counter paranoia, is addressed on a case-by-case basis. Where effective mastery is evident, efforts are recognized. Selective attention provides reward, reinforcement, and support.

In sum, the application of Concept 1 in a changing organization defines the meaning of change events to people and weighs the tasks of transition confronting them. Application of Concept 2 categorizes manifest behavior as defense, resistance, and/or mastery: This provides the basis for differentiated leadership action.

When consultation is provided prior to change, the concepts are applied in order to project need, predict behavioral responses, and mobilize supplies. The consultant can do this in language congenial to executives by engaging in "psychological cost accounting" (Hirschowitz, 1973). Whether counseling before or after change, the consultant assesses the supplies and processes needed to ease transition and makes specific recommendations for their introduction. The prescription of *supplies* is derived from the third salient concept: requisite supplies.

Concept 3: Requisite Supplies. The supplies required to promote mastery of the tasks of transition reflect people's ministration, mastery, and modeling needs (Levinson, 1968). Ministration supplies meet dependency needs by providing direct relief for the psychophysiological pain, emotional distress, and existential agony of people burdened by the tasks of transition. Representative supplies in this category are care and affection; reassurance and encouragement; hope, faith and confidence; and worth and esteem. These are the primary constituents of social support. The vehicle for delivery of these supplies is contact comfort. Ministration needs are delivered by the creation of opportunities for interpersonal contacts.

Mastery supplies *follow* the delivery of ministration supplies and are advanced through the alliances forged by demonstrated concern and regard. Ministration fortifies hope and confidence, raising stress thresholds so that mature defenses can be mobilized and mastery efforts promoted. Mastery is induced by reality-focused problem solving. The leader paces the process of realization in such a way that his people can maintain adaptive equilibrium while responding to the multiple demands that converge upon them in transition. Psychological balance is maintained by nourishing self-esteem and meeting dependency needs while channeling aggressive energies toward mastery. The consultant therefore helps leaders to expect—and accept—people's inevitable oscillation between approach and avoidance, attention and inattention, impulse gratification and overcontrol, overdependent searches for reassurance and counterdependent rejections of help.

Modeling supplies are tendered as ministration supplies

are provided. The leader "lends ego" in the course of lending his presence. Because followers are dependent and suggestible during change, the leader can utilize this to their and his adaptive advantage by modeling coping behavior. By offering himself as a role model for mature coping, he invites imitation and identification. He simultaneously models mature coping mechanisms (such as humor) for the reduction of distress and extends people's intelligence activities by the modeling of problem solving. He also provides a model for the maintenance of self-esteem by the communication of reasonable expectations of self and followers. He makes clear that he expects eventual, not immediate, competence in responding to the demands of change.

When modeling need dictates, leaders are candid about personal fears and concerns while continuing to project visions of reasoned optimism. On the one hand, many ministration and modeling supplies are delivered nonverbally; some are, indeed, ineffable. On the other hand, mastery supplies require verbal exchanges. Because of the dialectic oscillation between reality comprehension and flight from it, mastery is profoundly dependent upon verbal interaction in which information must often be repetitively and redundantly communicated. News about a coming change must be repeated because initial doses of information often elicit more apprehension than comprehension. The proper sequencing of news can prove elusive without the guidance of an explicit model for leadership processes to modulate the pace of transition. Such a model has been elaborated elsewhere (Hirschowitz, 1977) and is presented here in condensed form.

Concept 4: Requisite Leadership Processes: The Model for Modulation of Change. This model for modulation of change formulates the sequential interactive steps required to breach defenses, disarm resistance, and promote mastery of the tasks of transition. Because news of significant impending change is inherently disorienting, time is required to recognize and work through the losses and transitions demanded by change. Comprehension is eased and the working through of transition's tasks facilitated when information is supplied incrementally and at a slow pace. Comprehension ceases when news floods psychobiological or social systems with rage, fear, or anxiety. The leader "doses" information so that unsteadying reality-focused dialogue is counterbalanced by steadying ministration.

Because the leader's presence both comforts and lends ego support, it is possible for him to alternate between the presentation of information that arouses distress and the support that alleviates the distress. He does so by demonstrations of active listening, concern, and regard; this reduces distress and defensiveness to levels that permit the assimilation of additional doses of news about the change at hand. However, not all difficulty in realizing and accepting information about a change stems from stress arousal. Many difficulties stem from people's use of differing cognitive maps. Information processing may require numerous interactions because of differences in people's appreciative systems. The concept of appreciative systems, that is, the integration of percepts, cognitions, values, and judgments into coherent frames of meaning, is developed by Vickers (1968).

The unraveling and sifting of change information are regulated by cognitive maps. When such information is profoundly unsettling, calling the organization's and/or individual's mission, integrity, or identity into serious question, personal value frames—ontological maps—may color or distort further information processing. The use of different cognitive and ontological maps causes people to interpret the same information in very different ways: much confusion is generated in change by the failure to comprehend consequent differences in meaning attribution. The model for the modulation of change recognizes that cognitive dissonance occurs early, frequently, and repetitively in response to change news. Frequent clarification is needed to guard against the misapprehensions that distort information processing. The model requires that the leader communicate interactively through four sequential stages, the immediate, intermediate, ultimate, and end outcomes of which are: *understanding, appreciation, acceptance,* and *commitment.* The stages represent an inexorable sequence: When any one step is omitted, adaptive distress will blunt problem solving and retracing of steps will be required.

The interactions required to achieve these sequential outcomes are:

1. *Exchanges of facts.* Initial meetings are held to communicate *what* has been decided. The purpose of these meetings is to orient and clarify. The desired outcome is that news about the impending change be *understood.*
2. *Answering "Why . . . ?"* Because these interactions are challenging, emotionally intense, and sometimes hostile, they are often avoided or mismanaged by too rapid closure or overcontrol. Frequent meetings are needed to ensure that the intent, rationale, and criteria for decisions are adequately challenged and tested. In this phase, both substantive and process outcomes are pursued. The phase ideally concludes with *appreciation* for the rationale for change and identification with its purpose. Also, the leader's tolerance for challenging questions should give legitimacy to the right to question (and experience or express the underlying emotions). An ideal intermediate outcome, therefore, is identification with the leader's style; that is, appreciation for his active listening and realistic, nondefensive interaction. By the end of this phase there should be appreciation for *what* has been communicated and *how* it has been communicated.
3. *Exchange of meanings.* With change appreciated, the grief process can move toward acceptance. This is assisted in the leader's interactive meetings by exchanges of meaning. Reviewing what change *means* to people allows grief to be expressed and worry work to be consolidated. Condolence, consolation, and mutual support are generated. The desired outcome of *psychological acceptance* is achieved as people are helped to come to terms with change.
4. *Reciprocation exchanges.* In this phase, expectations are clarified, roles negotiated, interdependencies consolidated, and psychological contracts negotiated. The ideal end outcome is renewal and *commitment.*

In a final emphasis, this model defines the iterative, redundant, and interactive processes required of leaders. It combats the action-oriented tendencies of leaders by clarifying the step-by-step pattern of advance and retreat by which eventual commitment to change is achieved. The model emphasizes that statements such as "I can understand it but cannot appreciate it" or "I can appreciate it but it is difficult for me to accept it" epitomize the need for leadership processes that follow an orderly sequence.

The Consultant's Role

When an organization is in transition, the consultant supplies comprehensive diagnoses and provides leaders with authoritative guidance on requisite leadership processes. When the consultant discovers that the relevant information flow has been restricted or distorted, he encourages interactive engagement so that people can make sense of change and begin to exercise control over their changing lives.

During the stress of imminent or actual transition, the consultant operates from multiple vantage points to sharpen awareness of the need for injection of requisite supplies and leadership processes. Where change has caused organizational continuity to be severed or coherence to be paralyzed, the consultant helps leaders to explore repressed psychological meanings, to legitimate grief, and to restore continuity. This is often necessary after massive organizational transformation, when emotional distress evokes "all is lost" responses. The leader can then be helped to distinguish for his people between changes in structural form and issues of spirit and essence. People welcome reassurance about continuity of cherished values and images.

When reorganization has been introduced in too summary a fashion, the consultant often fashions strategic retreats. In these retreat structures, the decision steps of leaders are retraced: Information is given about the reasons for reorganization and appreciation is sought. Negotiations of need are encouraged so that people are assured of specific supplies to ease transitional distress. The consultant plays a teaching role in such retreats by introducing the objective aspects of the situation —and the lexicon by which to maintain it. The consultant applies this model for the modulation of change both diagnostically and reparatively: He not only diagnoses the leadership processes that have been neglected in reorganization but also guides the repair of errors of omission or commission. When change is in prospect, as in Case 3, he helps leaders anticipate and rehearse the necessary modulating steps. In modulating change, the consultant deploys himself flexibly. He builds new relationships and strengthens existing ones; he provides support wherever he can. As he becomes organically involved in a changing enterprise, he may extend his availability.

Throughout, the consultant supports leaders in supporting their people. He prescribes the specific supplies needed by people to surmount the adaptive tasks of transition. He affirms the universality of need for ministration, modeling, and mastery supplies and stimulates the leadership processes required to provide them. In addition to his diagnostic and prescriptive functions, the consultant functions as teacher, preceptor, coach, and counselor. He often plays an invaluable role in rehearsing the leader for interactions that are likely to be hostile or testing. Rehearsal helps the leader anticipate what the likely responses of his people will be so that he can regulate the emotional climate of potentially tense meetings. When leaders have intuitive appreciation of the requisite processes, the consultant supplies authoritative assurance.

Consultation in the throes of transition is demanding, intense, and emotionally wearying. The consultant absorbs the pain of those who trust him and must counter the paranoid hostility of those who do not. When consultation to an organization in distress occurs late in the process, the consultant must also counter pressures for "quick fixes" from leaders. The maintenance of relationships and sanctions then compels frequent interactions. His reserves will be further eroded as he encounters the distrust and suspicion often endemic in organizations where change has been mismanaged. Ambivalence, negative transference, and testing are often more dramatic in consultation than in clinical work. Distrust and hostility may be at catastrophic levels when paranoia has become the entrenched social system defense.

Enmeshed in such a context, the consultant may have to struggle to maintain balance, reserves, objectivity, and confidence. When objectivity is lost, his ability to inspire confidence suffers and consultation may fail. The consultant entering such an organization therefore needs to know what to expect (derived from appropriate experience and learning) and how to maintain adequate reserves and supports. He draws strength from his support systems but may need collegiate consultation to sustain objectivity and maintain cognitive control. He is further sustained by the certainty of realizable objectives and the durability of anchoring values. In turbulent organizations, cognitive mastery and value anchors provide the consultant with protection against drift. He can then maintain behavioral consistency with some certitude. Congruence between concepts, values, and behavior communicates integrity and inspires confidence. Research studies by Tichy (1974) attest to the positive correlation between this kind of congruence and consultant effectiveness.

This chapter has affirmed the mental health value of the consultant to changing organizations and has introduced concepts and cases to illustrate behavioral congruence. The principles that flow from these concepts are neither inclusive nor exclusive; when their application proves fruitless, the consultant, like the failed experimenter, must refine existing models and generate new ones. Finally, no consultant can hope to survive frequent immersion in changing organizations without dependable internal and external supports. Representative internal supports are intellectual curiosity, appreciation for the absurd, and a sense of humor. Of external supports, those provided by family, friends, and professional reference groups are invaluable.

References

Hirschowitz, R. G. "Psychological Cost Accounting." *Management Practice,* Fall 1973, pp. 1-5.

Hirschowitz, R. G. "Consultation to Complex Organizations in Transition." In S. C. Plog and P. I. Ahmed (Eds.), *Principles and Techniques of Mental Health Consultation.* New York: Plenum, 1977.

Hirschowitz, R. G. "An Epidemic of Orthopedic Complaints in Industry." *Psychiatric Opinion,* 1979, *16* (3), 33-39.

Janis, I. L. *Psychological Stress.* New York: Wiley, 1958.

Jaques, E. "Social Systems as a Defense Against Persecutory and Depressive Anxiety." In M. Klein, P. Hermann, and R. E. Money-Kryle (Eds.), *New Directions in Psychoanalysis.* London: Tavistock Institute, 1955.

Levinson, H. *The Exceptional Executive.* Cambridge, Mass.: Harvard University Press, 1968.

Levinson, H. Personal communication. Cambridge, Mass.: Levinson Institute, 1981.

Levinson, H., and others. *Men, Management, and Mental Health.* Cambridge, Mass.: Harvard University Press, 1962.

Marris, P. *Loss and Change.* New York: Pantheon, 1970.

Menzies, I. E. P. "The Functioning of Social Systems as a Defense Against Anxiety: A Report on the Study of Nursing Services of a General Hospital." Tavistock Pamphlet, No. 3. London: Tavistock Institute, 1967.

Tichy, N. M. "Agents of Planned Social Change: Congruence of Values, Cognitions, and Actions." *Administrative Science Quarterly,* 1974, *19* (2), 168-182.

Vaillant, G. E. *Adaptation to Life.* Boston: Little, Brown, 1977.

Vickers, G. *Value Systems and Social Process.* London: Tavistock Institute, 1968.

White, R. W. "Strategies of Adaptation: An Attempt at Systematic Description." In G. V. Coelho, D. A. Hamburg and J. E. Adams (Eds.), *Coping and Adaptation.* New York: Basic Books, 1974.

Chapter 13

Providing Services to the Elderly

Robert D. Patterson
Ruby B. Abrahams

The mental health needs of the elderly are particularly amenable to population-focused interventions. First, the aged are more sensitive than younger persons to environmental changes —more vulnerable to poor environments but also more able to benefit from positive ones. Second, there are many formal and informal sources of help for the elderly, such as government programs and families. These support systems offer many opportunities for creative input from community mental health practitioners. In this chapter we will examine the characteristics of the elderly population, formulate a theoretical approach to their mental health needs that is not isolated from their medical and other needs, and describe some pioneering mental health programs for the elderly.

The elderly are generally defined as persons over age sixty-five. It should be stated at the outset that this is a heterogeneous group of people, showing a wide range of differences in health status, functioning ability, and need for services and supports. Studies of the community elderly (for example, Shanas, 1971) have shown that the majority of elderly persons function independently, or with some help from family and friends, and that the majority rate themselves as in good health, physically and mentally, in spite of the chronic illnesses experienced by many. Fragility tends to increase with age, and it is mainly in the group over age seventy-five that supports and helping services are needed, both by the elderly person and by the caregiving family. Nevertheless there are many instances of healthy, active eighty-year-olds, and stories abound of these independent characters.

The elderly are the fastest growing segment of the U.S. population. In 1900, one person in twenty-five was aged sixty-five or over; by 1950 the ratio had grown to one in twelve, and by the year 2030, if the present low birthrate and declining death rates hold steady, one in every six Americans will be over sixty-five (17 percent of the population). According to 1976 Census Bureau estimates, the sixty-five and over population numbers about 22.9 million, or 10.6 percent of the population. At the turn of the century the average life expectancy was 47.3 years, now it is 72.8 years. A woman reaching sixty-five today can expect to live an additional 17.5 years, while a man of sixty-five can expect another 13.4 years. Moreover, the percentage of the seventy-five plus age group is projected to increase at about twice the rate of the over sixty-five group as a whole.

One characteristic of the current elderly population that is not likely to change is the greater number of elderly women than men. The 1970 U.S. census showed that among those over sixty-five, 55 percent were women. The sex ratio increases with increasing age. Most men over sixty-five are married; only one out of seven is widowed and only one out of seven lives alone. By contrast, more than half the women in this age group are widowed, and more than one third of the women live alone. Hence, greater attention needs to be directed to helping older women with problems of widowhood, living arrangements, and isolation.

Contrary to some popular opinion, the vast majority of older people in the United States live in family settings. Only 5 percent of the elderly are in institutions, and over 80 percent of those are seventy-five or over. Of the 95 percent noninstitutionalized elderly, 83 percent of men and 60 percent of women are living as married couples or with relatives, mainly children; 17 percent of men and 40 percent of women live alone or with nonrelatives (National Clearing House on Aging, 1975). Elderly persons living with children are more likely to be older and sicker, while those living alone are usually younger and in better health. At any rate, the idea that families in the United States no longer care for their elderly relatives is a myth.

Health Status of the Elderly Population

The National Health Survey has shown that 80 percent of persons over sixty-five have some chronic illness. But a more useful measure of health status in the elderly is the degree to which their functional capacity is impaired. A recent Census Bureau report shows that 38 percent of older persons had some limitation of their major activity (work or housekeeping), as compared to only 7 percent of younger persons. The major chronic conditions resulting in limited activity were: heart conditions (21 percent), arthritis/rheumatism (21 percent), visual impairments (7 percent), hypertension without heart involvement (6 percent), mental/nervous conditions (3 percent), and all other (42 percent). If we focus on that proportion of the community elderly that is truly in need of support services due to physical incapacity, a major epidemiological study of disability (Nagi, 1976) indicates that 5.2 percent are severely impaired, requiring assistance in personal care (that is, assistance in clothing, feeding, bathing, and toileting) and 11.5 percent require assistance in mobility, both in- and outside of the home, and need help with housekeeping and shopping. Therefore, a total of 16.7 percent of the community elderly in this study need help to perform the tasks of daily living.

In spite of a negative image of aging projected in Western cultures, a recent survey (Harris and Associates, 1974) showed that one third of persons over sixty-five described their lives as better than expected and only 11 percent called it worse than expected. The Human Aging Study sponsored by the National Institute of Mental Health (Birren and others, 1963) found that very healthy elderly men reported many favorable changes in their social and emotional lives as they aged. Examples were relative freedom from competitive pressures and greater freedom to pursue their interests.

Estimates of psychological impairment among community elderly have varied depending on the definition used (see Eisdorfer and Cohen, 1978; Juel-Nielsen, 1975). A rate of 15 to 17 percent was consistently found in community studies that defined psychological impairment as that which impacted severely on daily functioning and indicated a need for mental health services (see Lowenthal, Berkman, and Associates, 1967; Berg and others, 1970; Abrahams and Patterson, 1978).

Most people with psychiatric symptoms in old age have experienced similar problems earlier in their lives. Schizophrenia probably always makes its appearance before old age, and manic-depressive diseases usually do so. Major depression more frequently appears anew, however. Neurotic and characterological problems may become greater sources of distress in the later years, but they also may become less troublesome or disappear altogether. Alcoholism, which affects 2 to 10 percent of the elderly, typically has begun in the person's forties rather than young adulthood (Schuckit, 1977). The incidence of psychosis in persons over sixty-five is estimated at 8 percent. More than two thirds of these cases are organic brain syndromes (Roth, 1976).

Depression is the most common mental health symptom among the elderly. This is reflected in suicide rates, which increase with each succeeding decade of life in elderly men. In women, the peak rate is in the sixth decade with a decreasing but still substantial rate in old age. One quarter of all suicides in the United States are among the elderly—predominantly among persons who had never been suicidal at earlier ages (Miller, 1979). Anxiety or agitation is often a concomitant of depression, but it may occur as an isolated symptom. For example, elderly people often develop an incapacitating fear of falling after once falling and injuring themselves. Hypochondriacal symptoms are also frequent in the elderly. Paranoia is more common in the elderly than in younger age groups. It is especially common in people with hearing defects or other organic difficulties in processing information about their environments.

Chronic organic brain syndrome is especially important

from a public health standpoint because persons suffering from it require a large amount of family and institutional care. Organic brain syndrome is a major cause of many of the behavioral problems seen in the elderly, such as wandering, hoarding, neglecting their homes or personal hygiene, or unnecessarily calling police or fire departments. Acute organic brain syndrome, which is frequently totally reversible, may be caused by many medical illnesses and by toxic levels of prescribed or unprescribed drugs. Symptoms alone frequently do not dictate a treatment program. It is the interaction between the symptomatic person and the environment that determines what is needed.

In the United States, as in most Western countries, the movement to deinstitutionalize long-term care in the mental health system has resulted in dramatic changes in the delivery of mental health services to the elderly. Along with other groups, there has been a decline in the rate of admission of the elderly to state and county hospitals. At the same time, however, there has been a substantial increase in admissions to acute care hospitals—with mental disorders as primary diagnoses—and in the number of persons with mental disorders admitted to nursing homes. Nursing home use has increased rapidly, and this trend has resulted in a current capacity of over 1.2 million beds, 90 percent of which are used by the elderly. Levine and Willner (1976) estimate that expenditures for patients with primarily mental health problems in nursing homes exceeded $4.2 billion in 1974. At the same time outpatient psychiatric clinics typically provided only 2 percent of their services to the elderly.

An Ecological Perspective

In this section we will explore the application of an ecological systems model to meet the mental health needs of the elderly. An ecological model sees a person and his environment as reciprocally interacting components. A person's behavior is influenced by his current and his past environment, and his behavior in turn influences the environment (Holahan and others, 1979).

The ecological perspective is based on epidemiological studies that show that if there is a good fit between an individual and the environment, the individual will usually flourish. But if the person-environment fit is not good, the likelihood of physical and emotional problems is greatly increased. Epidemiological research supports the notion that disease incidence is influenced by the quality of social relationships, by the social position of the individual, and by the amount of preparation the individual has for the adaptive challenges presented (Cassel, 1974). It is usually not possible to predict which particular kind of problem will develop. Similar stresses increase the incidence of hypertension, cancer, depression, and so on. Thus, prevention models based on simple cause-effect relations are not very useful to program designers.

The ecological perspective takes a macroscopic view of the person and his environment or, better, of groups of people and their environments. Elements of the environment that have traditionally been peripheral to the concerns of mental health professionals gain new importance. These include income, housing, personal safety, and transportation facilities, as well as work, recreation, and social support opportunities. An approach that limits itself to concern with intrapsychic conflicts is seen as too narrow.

As a general rule, aging reduces the individual's capacity to adapt to environmental changes. From a systems point of view, this is the essence of aging. With advanced age, difficulty in maintaining homeostasis becomes evident in many organ systems, including the nervous system. In the biological sphere examples are less capacity to cope with toxins such as excess salt or with infectious organisms that can cause pneumonia. This dependence on the environment in the elderly makes the ecological perspective especially appropriate for this group. Lawton and Simon (1968) concluded that as the competence of the individual decreases, the proportion of behavior attributable to environmental rather than personal characteristics increases. Comparisons of elders who adapted well to institutional settings with those who did not have demonstrated the great importance of the environment (Lieberman, 1969; Brody, 1977).

In youth and middle age, individuals frequently are very actively attempting to change their environments. With advancing age, however, individuals become more absorbed in maintaining their equilibrium in the face of destabilizing environmental forces. A practitioner with a community mental health orientation will aim to use his special skills to reduce destabilizing forces. This effort will likely have an effect on the incidence of both mental and physical illness; it will help to create a sense of well-being among the population, and it may serve to increase longevity.

Physical and social changes in old age sometimes make adaptive behaviors that served throughout earlier adulthood no longer suitable. For example, opportunity for activities that maintain self-esteem may be lost upon retirement or when the person can no longer take part in physically demanding activities. Our rapidly changing social values challenge old people to change principles they lived by for decades or risk disapproval and isolation because they are "out of step." Often psychotherapy is recommended to help people adapt better to their environments. But there are many additional ways to facilitate adaptation in the elderly. For example, when elderly people get together, they can share information about how to adapt. Some people have many of these opportunities and learn quickly while others have few such interchanges or cannot incorporate others' experiences in order to help themselves.

Support System Needs of the Elderly. Caplan (1974) defined social support systems as "continuing social aggregates that provide individuals with opportunities for feedback about themselves and for validations of their expectations about others, which may offset deficiencies in these communications within the larger community context" (p. 4). For the very old or for the elderly who are physically frail, such support systems also provide many practical services such as meal preparation and transportation.

Families are the major support system of the elderly. However, people who do not have families must use formal support systems, and as a result they may be institutionalized too often. Even with a family, after just a brief absence, the elderly person may find that his family or other informal support system has deteriorated, thus closing the door to his return.

The death of family members and friends often depletes the social support systems of old people. Simultaneously, social and physical changes make it harder to establish new supportive relationships. To get support beyond the immediately available family and friends, people need to know about other helping resources, both formal and informal. Yet the complexity of our human services system makes this quite difficult for even the most sophisticated consumer.

Major life changes such as retiring from work, becoming a widow, changing residence, or developing an illness that limits mobility frequently seriously disrupts peoples' informal support systems. It is true that, as old age advances, there is typically a gradual "social disengagement" (Cumming and Henry, 1961). Thus most people in their eighties want more quiet time for personal chores, contemplation, or napping. But this change in the quantity of social interaction as distinguished from social supports does not mean that social supports are less essential for maintaining mental health in advanced age.

The value of social supports for the elderly must not be misinterpreted as meaning that more service always makes for better service. Blenker and others (1971) showed that a program of intensive social service led to more institutionalization of the experimental group (mostly in nursing homes) than of the control group. More deaths also occurred among the institutionalized, high-service group. It appears that the social and physical disruption of moving to a nursing home caused the excess deaths.

Physical Support Systems. The relatively healthy elderly have some physical needs common to their age. They need a physical environment that will compensate for their greater tendency to fall and their reduced physical stamina. Ocular changes often lead to the need for glasses. Hearing defects increase. The elderly have less tolerance for cold weather. Their slower reaction times require both social and physical adaptations; for example, old persons may need long walklights at intersections to allow them to cross slowly. The elderly who have major chronic illnesses often require special equipment such as wheelchairs, braces, and walkers. Persons with organic brain syndrome need so many physical modifications to protect and aid them that the term *prosthetic environment* has been coined.

Applying the Ecological Model

The needs of the elderly population cover a broad spectrum, ranging from the need for life enrichment opportunities for the active elderly, so that their coping skills can continue to grow, to the need for supports that will help the frail elderly to reach medical, psychiatric, and social services. Caregiving for the elderly requires multidisciplinary responses from many sources, professional and nonprofessional. Various services need to be coordinated so that an older person can move in and out of a continuum of services as needs change. It is extremely important that natural informal support networks of the older person be strengthened. Caplan (1974) identifies three helping elements provided by the natural network of family, friends, neighborhood, and community. First, the individual is helped by significant others in the network to mobilize his psychological resources. Second, he shares his tasks with them. Third, they provide him with extra resources to handle the situation (for example, money, feedback, skills, and cognitive guidance).

Mental health professionals should have involvement in many programs that support the elderly (for example, adult education, self-awareness groups, housing, congregate meal and drop-in centers, adult day centers, home care programs, nursing homes, hospices, and respite care facilities). They should be involved in two ways. First, by showing community planners how these programs support community mental health aims, they can help increase support for them. Second, they should provide consultation and coordination services. The staffs of these agencies frequently have client problems with which mental health experts can assist. Too often, such agencies have very little contact with mental health professionals and have only minimal knowledge of what services they might obtain from them. Although frequent regular consultation may not be practical with all these organizations, they at least need to have a working relationship with one or more mental health professionals whom they feel comfortable to call on for consultation, crisis assistance, or referral. Participation in the in-service education of these organizations can be very valuable. Unfortunately, even federally assisted community mental health centers have barely scratched the surface in providing these services.

When a comprehensive range of services for the elderly is planned, the whole spectrum of needs must be considered. Resources should be made available to enrich the later years and encourage development of coping skills to prepare for the stresses of aging. Such preparation should begin in middle life or earlier. Neugarten (1968, 1978) has identified the "young-old" as a meaningful division of the life cycle. This group, drawn mainly from those aged fifty-five to seventy-five, is distinguished from the middle-aged by retirement and from the "old-old" by continued vigor and active social involvement.

In recent decades there has been a downward trend in retirement age, so that there is now a sizable group of active retired people with high potential for useful roles in society, especially if opportunities are provided for continuing education, training for new, appropriate job skills, part-time work, volunteer work, and leisure time enrichment activities. This group is increasingly becoming politically active through such organizations as the Gray Panthers, the American Association of Retired Persons (AARP), and the National Council of Senior Citizens. In addition, the federal volunteer agency called ACTION administers the Foster Grandparent Program and the Retired Senior Volunteer Program. Through such programs, senior citizens can find opportunities to help others—both children and adults. Organizations like Mature Temps find paid work for older persons and have been increasingly successful in highlighting the many skills of older workers. Action for Independent Retirement is a division of AARP that helps people between the ages of fifty and sixty-five to plan their retirement; it provides guidance and information on finances and the pros and cons of moving, as well as information on retirement communities and leisure and recreational options.

Self-Care, Self-Help. In the health area, the growing movement for self-care has considerable potential for stimulating preventive action among the elderly (Butler and others, 1979). There are many support and self-help groups that focus on such areas as nutrition, diet, exercise, smoking cessation, and alcohol abuse. There are also a growing number of multi-disciplinary agencies dedicated to a holistic approach to health care; these agencies have medical and mental health personnel who counsel and teach clients to understand their own bodies, as well as the relationship between physical symptoms and psychological stress. One self-care program described by Sehnert (1977) was the "Health Activation Course," in which Medicare participants were taught to check their own respiration and blood pressure. A self-help medical guide outlined home procedures during illnesses and danger signals requiring a physician's attention. Participants learned to be realistic about what to expect from a doctor and were given lessons in "speaking the doctor's language." An interesting outgrowth of this course was the formation by the elderly of their own health clubs, which meet monthly and feature talks by medical experts and discussion of self-care practices. Such clubs could become effective mutual help groups by allowing members to share knowledge and reinforce each other in pursuing healthier life-styles. To change behavior, in fact, such reinforcement through mutual help groups is often required.

One of the more comprehensive self-help groups for the elderly is Senior Actualization and Growth Exploration (SAGE). Started by a psychologist in 1974 in California, it has spread to fifteen states. Described as "a growth center for people over sixty-five," it is based on the premise that "old age can and should be a rich creative culmination, involving as much growth as early childhood" (Fields, 1978). SAGE-sponsored groups, some in nursing homes, meet weekly, and their activities include deep breathing exercises, massage, limbering exercises to music, biofeedback, and counseling. Similarly the Institute for Creative Aging in Los Angeles stresses psychosocial well-being. Gordon (1978) reports that in a mutually supportive group setting, old people have the opportunity to share with one another and to learn to use nonpharmacological self-help techniques to alleviate pain and increase function. Participation in self-care and self-help groups is particularly relevant to the elderly who suffer from attrition and role loss. The Administration on Aging has recently made grants to develop curricula for government agencies to use in building self-help groups. These include food cooperatives for elderly person, programs to maintain homes and neighborhoods, self-protection programs, urban gardening, and consumer education. In these enterprises it is reported that older helpers benefit as much as those they help, develop self-esteem, and become actively involved in their communities (Citizens Committee for New York City, Inc., 1978).

Formal and Informal Helpers. For the elderly who are less able to act on their own behalf, the ecological model of helping identifies informal and formal caregivers who may also need support networks to reinforce their helping skills. Families are the natural caregivers to the elderly and the first line of defense when the older person becomes ill or disabled. Too often this family support system breaks down under the prolonged stress of caring for a severely impaired elder. With adequate supports, however, many families could continue to care for their elderly relatives, so that early and inappropriate institutionalization could be prevented.

Eisdorfer (1979) has assisted in the formation of a mutual support group for families of persons with chronic organic brain syndrome. Considering the emotional stress that this condition places upon families and the enthusiasm of the current group members, this organization seems likely to grow (Eisdorfer and Cohen, 1981). Hausman (1979) describes a series of short-term counseling groups for persons with elderly parents. Common problems, fears, and goals were shared. The major goals of all the groups were (1) to find a balance between responsibility to oneself, one's nuclear family, and one's parents; (2) to make specific decisions about the extent and limits of the members' duties and obligations to their parents; and (3) to learn to deal with one's parents in a mature way, leaving behind the conflicts, rebellions, and unresolved issues from childhood and adolescence. Support groups for families of chronically ill elderly patients could be organized through the social service departments of hospitals, nursing homes, adult daycare centers, and other such agencies. Respite care is needed to provide relief to the family caring for a disabled elderly person.

There is a minority of fragile elderly who are lacking a family support network. When a medical or psychiatric emergency occurs, they have little to rely upon except hospital care. These elderly have longer stays in hospital and then are more likely to be transferred to a nursing home. Without a family as advocate, they are in danger of neglect and repeated transfers between hospitals and nursing homes. Multiple environmental changes are likely to lead to regressive and antisocial behavior that can further compound the person's problems. These elderly need above all an advocate for guidance through the system.

Coordinated, Comprehensive Programs. The present health care system is not designed to take care of chronic illness. Medical care, psychiatric care, and social services are fragmented by separate jurisdictions, regulations, and funding. Few mechanisms exist to integrate the range of psychiatric, medical, and social services that a chronically ill elderly person may need at any one time. Two programs that have attempted to achieve comprehensive coordinated care for the fragile elderly are the Chicago Council for the Jewish Elderly and the East Boston/Dorchester program (Masters and others, 1980) for inner-city elderly.

The Chicago Council for the Jewish Elderly is operating a multifaceted program that is a fine example of a program designed from an ecological perspective (Glasscote and others, 1977; Weinberg, 1979). The program is located in the East Rodgers Park section, which has about 7,000 Jewish elderly. The following is an abbreviated list of the services provided: numerous drop-in centers and an extensive outreach program; casework services and limited psychiatric services; home health and housekeeping services; home-delivered and congregate meals; transportation; residential facilities (temporary shelter, group residence, and well elderly housing); and daycare programs.

The overall aim of this array of services is to assist aged

individuals—especially those who are mentally confused—to remain in the community as independent functioning persons making maximum use of their resources and strengths. The services are designed to be a generic helping program. They also fulfill the requirements of a community mental health program. The drop-in centers (neighborhood services centers) are places for socialization and recreation and points of access for counseling and other services. Since there has been a tendency for people to see the centers as only for recreation, the staff has been working to make people aware of the additional functions. A portion of the center's staffing is provided by a "senior service corps" of elderly paid local residents. Professionally trained caseworkers are frequently available at the centers to provide consultation, counseling, and evaluation. The caseworkers' presence in the informal and nonstigmatizing atmosphere of the centers makes it easier for the elderly to avail themselves of help. There is a medical unit that acts primarily as an advocate to help people get better care from local physicians. The psychiatrist attached to the medical unit also gives high priority to helping people get services from nearby mental health programs.

The residences—two apartment buildings, a complex of six town houses, and an eleven-bed temporary shelter—are designed to provide housing to meet the needs of the frail elderly who frequently have some organic mental impairment that is not so severe as to require total institutional care. The temporary shelter also provides respite care when relatives need a vacation or break from caregiving. It also accommodates persons who are moving into or out of hospitals, nursing homes, or other residences. Unfortunately, the unique character of these residences has made them unable to fit the categories for which state and federal support is provided.

The East Boston/Dorchester program is a more modest attempt to coordinate existing resources in an inner-city area. Promoted by a group of physicians, it has brought together several neighborhood health centers, a teaching hospital, nursing homes, and several home health agencies in a coordinated system of care. The role of primary provider and advocate for the elderly person is assumed by trained nurse practitioners and physician assistants, backed by physicians. These nurse practitioners and physician assistants visit patients at home and are aided by visiting nurses, home health aides, physical and occupational therapists, and social workers. The home health aides are recruited from the local community whenever possible and are in a position to reinforce family and neighbor support networks. Health care, including physical and mental health services, is provided at the local neighborhood health center or at home for the homebound. When hospital care is needed, the patient is admitted under the care of his own physician, not by house staff or a doctor on call. If admission to a nursing home is required, the patient is followed there by his own nurse practitioner and then brought back into the home care program as soon as possible. Hospice care is delivered through the home care program for the terminally ill. Skilled medical and psychological counseling is provided to support both patient and family in the process of dying.

To initiate the East Boston/Dorchester program it was necessary to bend the existing system in a number of ways. A special waiver of Medicaid regulations was required to permit nurse practitioners to deliver care in nursing homes. Special arrangements with the teaching hospital were made to admit these welfare-assisted program participants as private patients.

Most clinical mental health services for the elderly can be provided along with those for other adults. Psychiatric hospitals frequently have separate units for elderly patients. This has some advantages in that their special needs can be met but also a disadvantage in that institutional discrimination against the elderly is made easier. In all service programs, overcoming prejudices and undue pessimism against the elderly must be a matter of concern. Therapy groups exclusively for the elderly are uncommon, yet they have been successful. Age integration group therapy involving members of all age groups from teen-agers to the elderly have been described by Lewis and Butler (1974). The interaction that was promoted between the differing generations proved therapeutic. Psychiatric day hospital programs can accommodate many elderly patients. However, frail and confused elderly persons need separate day programs. These had been rare in the United States (though common in England) until recently when Medicaid funds became available to support them. They provide a valuable alternative to full-time institutionalization.

Making Dying a Part of Life. The final task of the life cycle is the process of dying and death. Since Kubler-Ross's (1969) work in the late sixties, much attention has been focused on the psychological needs of the terminally ill. It has been well documented that the death denying attitudes of Western societies create severe problems for the terminal patient and his caregivers (Becker, 1974; Feifel, 1963; Toynbee, 1968; Weisman, 1977). Kastenbaum and Costa (1977) found that many of those who relate to the dying person (physicians, nurses, and others) are in distress themselves and resort to various evasive and self-protective maneuvers. Increasingly in recent decades, people have been going to hospitals to die, but hospitals are not organized around dying; they are organized around curing. For a hospital, death is a failure and a cause of anxiety for the staff. Dying patients therefore are often either the targets of superhuman efforts at resuscitation, or they are emotionally ignored. Death then occurs in isolation and loneliness.

Before the age of high-technology medicine, death was not such an isolating crisis. In a study of death scenes in eighteenth-century literature, Caplan (1976) has described death at that time as "the culmination of a social role, a moment within the continuum of life . . . in which the community finally evaluated and benefited from the moral worth of the dying member" (p. 155). Deaths were a major social occasion requiring the presence of family and community. Achieving a peaceful end and dying with dignity were expected of the virtuous person. His performance while dying set an example for those who watched and, if well done, could bring to them some acceptance of the contemplation of their own end. The final role of the dying person was to educate the living.

Death rituals in many societies are designed to include the living in the act of dying. The hospice movement in Western societies is an attempt to reintroduce the notion that dying is a family and community event. Like other important life cycle events—births, weddings, anniversaries, and retirements—dying should be shared as an event meaningful not only to the dying person but to others in the community. It is in response to the inhumane death situations that occur within medically oriented institutions that the hospice movement has grown both in Europe and the United States and has sought to establish special terminal care facilities where people who cannot recover from illnesses may die comfortably and meaningfully.

St. Christopher's Hospice in London, founded in 1949, has been the model for hospices in the United States. The facility is homelike and open to the community. Not only family but neighbors and children are encouraged to spend time there. Patients, family, staff, and neighbors share in the caregiving process. Patients provide other patients with inspiration and encouragement, giving them a sense of service in their last days. Considerable skill has been developed in the use of drugs as pain-killers, without oversedation. Hospice patients are described as appearing more alert and less sedated, as well as more cheerful and less depressed, than patients with similar conditions being cared for in hospitals (Stoddard, 1978). In the United States the hospice movement is comparatively recent. But over fifty hospice groups have already been established, mostly operating through home care programs but sometimes affiliated with terminal care departments in hospitals. However, there are currently less than twenty American general hospitals that have terminal care departments.

Human Services in Other Countries. The experience of European countries in developing human services for the elderly is instructive. Comparative studies (Kamerman, 1976; Wershow, 1979) found that their social policy objectives were very similar to ours, although the means to achieve them varied, especially in emphasis. Some countries rely heavily on a system of providing cash to meet needs, while other countries provide the needed services directly, with or sometimes without a means test. Generally the European countries provide a higher level of financial and social service support to their elderly populations than does the United States. Recently, however, even European countries with progressive social programs have experienced a leveling off of growth in these services as competition for funds among government programs grows.

The United Kingdom has the most extensive array of services: Health care is universally provided, as are regional geriatric mental health facilities; geriatric daycare or day hospital programs are frequent; homemakers are available in about ten times the quantity as they are in the United States; 6 percent of the elderly use meals programs (compared to 1 percent for the United States); 3 percent of the elderly reside in long-term care facilities (compared to 5 percent in the United States). The United States is unique in having long-term care facilities that are mostly proprietary while European countries have predominantly publicly owned or nonprofit facilities. Difficulty in coordinating medical, social, and housing services is a major problem for most of the countries.

Health Care Costs and the Older Patient

The elderly comprise only 10 percent of the population but account for 30 percent of all health costs in the United States. They are admitted to general hospitals at two to five times the rate of admission for younger adults. Before Medicare and Medicaid went into operation in the mid 1960s, public funds paid for only 30 percent of health care costs for the elderly (U.S. Senate Special Committee on Aging, 1977). By 1978, that share had grown to 63 percent. However, since 1970 direct out-of-pocket expenses for health care have been increasing. Direct expenses for physicians' services rose from $84 per capita in 1971 to $96 per capita in 1978. In 1978 about 52 percent of nursing home care was financed out of pocket; the per capita cost for such care rose from $109 in 1970 to $271 in 1978. By 1978 persons aged 65 and over paid an average of $698 for health related items out of pocket, which represented 12 percent of their $5900 average income (Fisher, 1980). Though more recent figures that are comparable are not available, it is likely that these trends have continued and probably accelerated. High out-of-pocket expenses tend to inhibit patients from seeking needed care at an early stage, and they often wait until illness has reached acute or emergency proportions before seeking help.

Medicare and, to a lesser extent, Medicaid are based on the medical model. Both provide some coverage for home health care, but these services must be dictated by "medical" need. Medicare-certified home health agencies are medical agencies. They provide nursing care, physical and occupational therapy, home health aide services, speech therapy, and medical social services. The services are prescribed by physicians and must follow a period of hospitalization. If a person needs help only with household tasks, shopping, home repairs, or transportation, Medicare will not pay the bill. Medicaid will provide home health services without a prior period of hospitalization, but again these services have to be certified by a physician and are oriented toward medical benefits.

Most lacking in the medical model, which is basically designed to care for episodes of acute illness, is the capacity to deliver a flexible range of services in a continuum of care and so to accommodate the constantly shifting needs of the older patient with chronic illness. Chronic illness requires a form of organization suitable for repeated interaction over months and years between patient and health workers. The medical, psychological, and social needs of these patients fluctuate and require the interaction of many different disciplines and agencies to effect proper management both of the patient and his environment. The financing of services, the benefits covered, and the methods of payment shape the delivery system and its utilization. Services that do not receive third-party reimbursement will remain peripheral, while reimbursed services will tend to grow. Thus, many elderly patients, who might remain at home if adequate support services were available, are admitted to institutions because this care is paid for.

There has been much discussion recently on the issue of extending benefits for social support services and broadening eligibility for home health benefits. It is sometimes argued that dollars might be saved by providing home care and thereby preventing institutionalization. However, concerns are expressed that by expanding benefits for home care, other populations would be picked up that are now managing independently. Most disabled Americans, who are at home, manage with their families and are not dependent on government funding. There is an ambiguity in trying to maintain peoples' independence based on family support, on the one hand, and trying to expand entitlements that might undermine family responsibility, on the other. The charge that health costs increased rapidly after the introduction of Medicare and Medicaid has not been answered. The influx of such funds, in a cost-based reimbursement system, can indeed be highly inflationary. Some experimentation in cost control has been made, but so far no cure has been found for the inflationary growth of hospital and nursing home costs.

These are complex issues, and frustrating to providers of care for the elderly. Current licensure and reimbursement practices tend to emphasize institutional care, to require licensed professionals, and to prefer use of the most highly skilled and expensive personnel. Many of the support services needed to build strength in the home and family environment could be provided by trained paraprofessionals or nonprofessionals who at present cannot be reimbursed under third-party mechanisms. Monitoring services and setting standards for them are difficult in these areas. It is easier to regulate large institutions such as hospitals than a myriad of small agencies that provide social and support services. Managing home health payment programs, fixing payments at fair levels, assessing need, and measuring outcomes and quality of care are extremely difficult. Until innovative changes are made, so that more resources can flow from medical care institutions to preventive, primary care, and support services, it will be difficult to develop the appropriate array of supportive services to maintain the optimum functioning and independence of the elderly.

In recent years the Federal government has initiated a number of demonstration projects that attempt to coordinate long-term care and support services for the elderly. The government has also encouraged enrolling more elderly in Health Maintenance Organizations (HMOs), which deliver coordinated medical care, and most recently is supporting a Social/HMO demonstration project that combines medical and long-term care services in a prepaid, coordinated delivery system (Callahan and Wallack, 1981). These experiments offer promising approaches to solving some of the problems of uncoordinated, fragmented, costly, and often poor quality care found in the current system.

The elderly are a growing proportion of our population, but this proportion will stabilize in future decades. Their mental health and medical needs are great compared to other age groups. There is a substantial body of epidemiological and experimental data upon which to build an ecological approach to meet their mental health needs. Population-focused mental health efforts should be integrated with acute and long-term medical care as well as with recreational and educational programs. Support of caregiving families and of enlightened self-care and self-help groups deserves high priority. Creative programs are being tried, and we expect activity in this direction to increase. Nevertheless, poorly designed benefit packages in Medicare and Medicaid can potentially inhibit delivery of mental health care and sometimes tend to destroy the social and emotional networks that are extremely important for mental health.

References

Abrahams, R. B., and Patterson, R. D. "Psychological Distress Among the Community Elderly: Prevalence, Characteristics, and Implications for Service." *International Journal of Aging and Human Development,* 1978, *9,* 1-17.

Becker, E. *The Denial of Death.* New York: Free Press, 1974.

Berg, R. L., and others. "Assessing the Health Care Needs of the Aged." *Health Services Research,* 1970, *5,* 36-59.

Birren, J. E., and others. *Human Aging: A Biological and Behavioral Study.* Washington, D.C.: U.S. Government Printing Office, 1963.

Blenker, M., Bloom, M., and Neilsen, M. "A Research and Demonstration Project of Protective Services." *Social Casework,* 1971, *52,* 483-499.

Brody, E. M. "Environmental Factors in Dependency." In A. N. Exton-Smith and J. G. Evans (Eds.), *Care of the Elderly: Meeting the Challenge of Dependency.* New York: Grune & Stratton, 1977.

Butler, R. N., and others. "Self-Care, Self-Help, and the Elderly." *International Journal of Aging and Human Development,* 1979, *10,* 95-114.

Callahan, J., and Wallack, S. (Eds.). *Reforming the Long-Term Care System.* Lexington, Mass.: Lexington Books, 1981.

Caplan, G. *Support Systems and Community Mental Health.* New York: Behavioral Publications, 1974.

Caplan, R. B. "Deathbed Scenes and Graveyard Poetry: Death in Eighteenth-Century Literature." In G. Caplan and M. Killilea (Eds.), *Support Systems and Mental Health.* New York: Grune & Stratton, 1976.

Cassel, J. C. "Psychiatric Epidemiology." In G. Caplan (Ed.), *American Handbook of Psychiatry.* Vol. 2. New York: Basic Books, 1974.

Citizens Committee for New York City, Inc. *The Older Persons Handbook and New York Self-Help Handbook.* New York: Citizens Committee for New York City, Inc., 1978.

Cumming, E., and Henry, W. E. *Growing Old: The Process of Disengagement.* New York: Basic Books, 1961.

Eisdorfer, C. "Developments in Dementia: Clinical Implications." Paper presented at McLean Hospital, Belmont, Mass., Dec. 1979.

Eisdorfer, C., and Cohen, D. "The Cognitively Impaired Elderly: Differential Diagnosis." In M. Storandt, I. C. Siegler, and M. F. Elias (Eds.), *The Clinical Psychology of Aging.* New York: Plenum, 1978.

Eisdorfer, C., and Cohen, D. "Management of the Patient and Family Coping with Dementing Illness." *Journal of Family Practice,* 1981, *12,* 831-837.

Feifel, H. "The Taboo on Death." *American Behavioral Scientist,* 1963, *6* (9), 66-67.

Fields, S. "Senior Actualization and Growth Exploration (SAGE)." In R. Gross, B. Gross, and S. Seidman (Eds.), *The New Old: Struggling for Decent Aging.* New York: Doubleday, 1978.

Fisher, C. "Differences by Age Groups in Health Care Spending." *Health Care Financing Review,* 1980, *1* (4).

Glasscote, R. M., Gudeman, J. E., and Miles, D. G. *Creative*

Mental Health Services for the Elderly. Washington, D.C.: Joint Information Service, 1977.

Gordon, J. S. *Final Report to the President's Commission on Mental Health: Special Study on Alternative Mental Health Services.* Unpublished report. Washington, D.C., 1978.

Harris, L., and Associates. *The Myth and Reality of Aging in America.* Washington, D.C.: National Council on Aging, 1974.

Hausman, C. P. "Short-Term Counseling Groups for People with Elderly Parents." *Gerontologist,* 1979, *19,* 102-107.

Holahan, C. J., and others. "The Ecological Perspective in Community Mental Health." *Community Mental Health Review,* 1979, *4* (2), 2-7.

Juel-Nielsen, N. "Epidemiology." In J. G. Howells (Ed.), *Modern Perspectives in the Psychiatry of Old Age.* New York: Brunner/Mazel, 1975.

Kamerman, S. B. "Community Services for the Aged: The View from Eight Countries." *Gerontologist,* 1976, *16,* 529-537.

Kastenbaum, R., and Costa, P. T. "Psychological Perspectives on Death." *Annual Review of Psychology,* 1977, *28,* 225-249.

Kubler-Ross, E. *On Death and Dying.* New York: Macmillan, 1969.

Lawton, M. P., and Simon, B. B. "The Ecology of Social Relationships and Housing for the Elderly." *Gerontologist,* 1968, *8,* 108-115.

Levine, D. S., and Willner, S. G. "The Cost of Mental Illness in 1974." Mental Health Statistical Note No. 125, Department of Health, Education, and Welfare Publication No. (ADM) 76-158, 1976.

Lewis, M. I., and Butler, R. N. "Life Review: Putting Memories to Work in Individual and Group Psychotherapy." *Geriatrics,* 1974, *29,* 165-173.

Lieberman, M. A. "Institutionalization of the Aged: Effects on Behavior." *Journal of Gerontology,* 1969, *24,* 330-340.

Lowenthal, M. F., Berkman, P. L., and Associates. *Aging and Mental Disorder in San Francisco: A Social Psychiatric Study.* San Francisco: Jossey-Bass, 1967.

Masters, R. J., and others. "Creating a Continuum of Care for the Inner City." Boston: Urban Medical Group, Inc., 1980.

Miller, M. *Suicide After 60: The Final Alternative.* New York: Springer, 1979.

Nagi, S. "An Epidemiology of Disability Among Adults in the United States." *Health and Society,* 1976, *54,* 439-467.

Neugarten, B. L. *Middle Age and Aging.* Chicago: University of Chicago Press, 1968.

Neugarten, B. L. "The Rising of the Young Old." In R. Gross, B. Gross, and S. Seidman (Eds.), *The New Old: Struggling for Decent Aging.* New York: Doubleday, 1978.

Roth, M. "Psychiatric Disorders of Later Life." *Psychiatric Annals,* 1976, *6,* 57-101.

Schuckit, M. A. "Geriatric Alcoholism and Drug Abuse." *Gerontologist,* 1977, *17,* 168-174.

Sehnert, K. W. "A Course for Activated Patients." *Social Policy,* 1977, *8,* 40-46.

Shanas, E. "Measuring the Home Health Needs of the Aged in Five Countries." *Journal of Gerontology,* 1971, *26,* 37-40.

Stoddard, S. *The Hospice Movement.* New York: Stein and Day, 1978.

Toynbee, A. *Man's Concern with Death.* New York: McGraw-Hill, 1968.

U.S. Senate Special Committee on Aging. "Health Costs and Problems in Medicaid and Medicare." In *Developments in Aging.* Washington, D.C., 1977.

Weinberg, J. "Community Programs for the Elderly: Alternatives to Institutionalization." In *Issues in Mental Health and Aging.* Vol. 3: *Services.* Department of Health, Education, and Welfare Publication No. (ADM) 79-665. Washington, D.C.: National Institute of Mental Health, 1979.

Weisman, A. D. *On Death and Denying.* New York: Behavioral Publications, 1977.

Wershow, H. J. "The Outer Limits of the Welfare State: Discrimination, Racism, and Their Effect on Human Services." *International Journal of Aging and Human Development,* 1979, *10,* 63-75.

Chapter 14

Serving the Chronically Mentally Ill

Norris Hansell

The impaired social connectedness of the chronically mentally ill presents special problems in designing effective service. Much of the difficulty with these groups flows from the long shadow that any impairment in the biological underpinnings of bonding or adaptation can cast both on ordinary life and on the narrower activities of being a patient. For the foreseeable future it will remain necessary for some patients to receive assistance in bonding and adaptation and in forming links with mutual support groups in addition to technical service relating to presumably altered central nervous systems.

The basic difficulty in schizophrenia and schizophreniform conditions appears to involve the foundation of chemical systems that produce and remove such synaptic neurotransmitters as dopamine, serotonin, gamma-aminobutyric acid, and neuropeptides. Damage to these systems sits so close to the genetically transmitted, basic cellular systems as to be likely to resist any downstream remedies. The condition in some patients constitutes a lifelong disorder, detectable at birth and thereafter never fully absent. Schizophrenia radically interferes with the bonding process, yielding the solitary and fragilely bonded individuals who are so difficult at times to assist through narrow, technical services.

Chronic affective disorders also periodically disrupt the bonding and adaptive work of persons carrying these defects and present the need for stretched services—services that extend beyond traditional clinical services. Affective disorders as well appear to involve basic cellular chemical systems, including, for example, the sodium-efflux pump on the cell membrane, as well as the apparatus for making and recycling such neurotransmitters as serotonin and norepinephrine. Substance abuse and other nonheritable damage to neural tissue also can interfere with the neural systems that underlie bonding and adaptive change. Many of the chemicals people employ to modify mood and experience exert their effects in ways that persistently alter the kinetics of neurotransmitters and so can ablate a set of critical experiences that underlie bonding and adaptation. Damage to the brain also can yield massive or subtle alterations in the work of bonding or adapting and create the same need for a pattern of services that includes linking and other assistance with bonding.

The range of services that chronically mentally ill persons may at times need is as large as the scope of activities within a human settlement, but it certainly includes medication, affiliation, adaptation, housing, and financial subsidy. The recent President's Commission on Mental Health (1978) has attempted to enumerate the scope by referring to the need for a network of specialized services; for small, local residences; for services to manage or integrate an individual within this array; for broad medical insurance; for advocacy and guardianship; but most of all for assistance to the kith and kin and other natural groupings that can provide a supportive connectedness. The American Psychiatric Association (1979) has also enumerated the scope of needed services, including public financing, persisting medical care, enlarged social supports within local group residences, legal remedies for discrimination against ill persons, and a focus on the importance of assistance to the patient in bonding and adapting. When the defect is as general as a lack of bonding and adaptation, the range of remedies will be long and variously enumerated, sometimes to the point of dismay or exhaustion. Caplan (1981) has repeatedly returned the attention of clinicians and planners to the simplicity of purpose within this range—to assess and support bonding and adaptation.

Medication to Assist Adaptation

Current concepts of the treatment of schizophrenia, affective disorders, substance abuse, and brain damage typically include the use of medication within a relationship, an educative clinical approach, and efforts to link the patient with support systems and mutual help groups. In order to prevent some acute episodes and reduce chronic dysfunction, it is often helpful to use medication for extended intervals. Neuroleptics, lithium, and tricyclics are the principle materials used, and each has significant long-term hazards. Indications for use of medications over prolonged periods are narrow. The conditions of efficacy, necessity, medical observation, cooperation of the patient, and arrangements for emergency need to be met. When possible, there should be efforts to educate patients regarding recognition and reduction of hazards. A body of information is developing that persons with schizophrenia and affective disorders may use in the same way as diabetics use information on nutrition and insulin.

Neuroleptic medications have a demonstrated value in the management of acute and chronic schizophrenia. However, not all chronic schizophrenics benefit from them, and the problems of tardive dyskinesia and neuroleptic-induced dysphorias occasionally can be serious. Because neuroleptics can dramatically control symptoms and prevent job loss, school failure, and suicide, we have the classic clinical situation of a high-gain, high-risk decision. The risks can be reduced by stretching services so as to include a component of education.

The clinical indications for placing a presumed schizophrenic individual into a program of continuous or semicontinuous neuroleptic use are narrow. The diagnosis of schizophrenia should be secure; that is, it should be based on criteria such as thought disorder, affect reduction, delusions, hallucinations, all in the absence of gross brain disease, intoxicated state, or broad affect, and showing a duration of more than six months. It is particularly important to distinguish between single-episode forms of schizophrenia and chronic remitting or chronic unremitting forms. In the case of a young individual with no previous episodes, use of the neuroleptic may be gradually reduced toward a trial of discontinuance, while the patient is kept under observation for at least one year. The physician should see a reduction of symptoms that is dose related and improves the patient's quality of life. Because chronic schizophrenia may comprise a heterogeneous group of biological aberrations, some of which may not require or benefit from neuroleptics, it is essential that the clinical impact of use and nonuse be assessed for each patient during a prolonged interval of outpatient observation. If an individual does not appear to require neuroleptics but is otherwise presumed to exhibit symptoms of chronic schizophrenia, an extended program of service and surveillance can proceed with continuing openness to the later necessity of prescribing neuroleptics.

The safety and reliability of prolonged medication programs for schizophrenics have increased in recent years through the use of a strategy that combines a low-dosage pattern of maintenance with rapid increases in dose at the time of any episodic reappearance of symptoms. This plan offers the prospect of lower side effects and smaller cumulative lifetime doses but requires instruction and a degree of cooperation from patients. Not all schizophrenics can make use of such instruction, particularly when their histories include mental retardation or prolonged tumbling in psychosis. Typical instruction focuses on analogies to chronic metabolic diseases like diabetes. Patients can be counseled that their disease may be lifelong but that it is often substantially modifiable with chemical and psychotherapeutic regulation.

The development in the patient of an attitude of personal responsibility for making changes from a base-line dose in relation to criterion observations underlines the successful use of the low-dose strategy. In order to avoid the episodic reappearance of symptoms usually seen with a low-dose pattern, the patient is instructed to increase temporarily the usual dose for the duration of each episode, using as guidepost observations the reappearance of a sleeping disturbance, difficulty concentrating, preoccupation with a narrow range of topics, anhedonia, and floating affects. The term *floating affects* comprises the experiences of sadness, panic, suspicion, anger, and perplexity when they rise to high levels and last for hours or days. These observations constitute an early warning system because typically they appear in advance of psychotic symptoms and offer a signal to increase the dose of medication promptly. At the first appearance of such symptoms, patients are to double their daily maintenance dose, wait three days, then assess the effect. They may repeat this maneuver several times. The low-dose approach employs as a base-line dose the least amount that will control the sleeping disorders and floating affects between episodes. The method for lowering the dose is similar. Patients are instructed that feeling "slowed down," sleepy, or separated from their experience indicates that the dose is too high. At the first appearance of such signs they are to reduce the dose by one third and wait three days to assess the effect. They may also repeat this maneuver several times.

The didactic component in this model of service is of major importance. Some patients can best learn about their disease and its control in group formats. Snyder's book, *Madness and the Brain* (1974), can serve as a practical tool for such instructional meetings. Groups of this kind can combine beginners with those more experienced in self-regulation. Some schizophrenics use such groups only briefly, some for months or years. The usefulness of a group lies in the context it may provide for a novice to learn what he needs to know when deciding whether or not to use medications and makes it possible for the more skilled to teach the less skilled in self-regulation. Participants learn through hearing reports from one another about how well target symptoms are being controlled. They also hear reports on side effects and receive help in setting the next objectives for improving self-regulation. A useful feature of such groups is their potential for converting reluctant or careless medication users into skilled self-regulators and for raising the average level of self-regulation to near the best level represented in the group. Many of these groups form the beginnings as well of mutual help groups. The availability of such a cooperative format and support system allows a major improvement in the patient's ability to learn and to adapt within the constraints of the disease.

The availability of continuing medical care throughout the career in service of a chronic schizophrenic offers the patient an ally in the struggle against disability, and it also allows the essential element of surveillance. Many patients will consider a prolonged program of medication only if it is part of a treatment relationship that they recognize as a broadly responsive one. Moreover, the didactic component so important in using the low-dose strategy and for achieving reliability over decades can conveniently commence as part of the physician's general therapeutic relationship to the patient. Continuing access to crisis services is central to any condition marked by an episodic course. Activity during such crises includes counseling, placement into a pattern of closer supervision than pertains ordinarily, and possible entry into inpatient care. Counseling enables many schizophrenics to move through episodes in a more orderly fashion. They are better able to enter counseling promptly at the onset of an episode if the groundwork has been laid earlier.

A similar approach to the treatment of chronic affective disorders employs medication within a relationship that includes didactic and affiliational assistance. Again, a focus on bonding and adaptation guides the process. The risks of school and job loss, family disruption, and suicide are substantial for persons with repeating affective disorders. A program of continuous or semicontinuous medication offers demonstrated value in reducing the frequency and severity of episodes and the degree of accumulating disability. But such a program carries risks and does not benefit all persons with affective disorders. Again, the conditions of efficacy, necessity, surveillance, cooperation, and emergency arrangements need to be met. The tricyclics and lithium in particular require a close watch on the patient's physical status, including laboratory monitoring.

The clinical indications for placing an individual with an affective disturbance into a program of continuous or semicontinuous prophylactic use of a tricyclic, lithium, or monoamine-oxidase inhibitor are narrow. Most physicians would want to see at least two hospitalizations or an otherwise serious episode benefited distinctly by medication. A suicide attempt or a strong family history of mental illness are additional markers of severity. Efforts to diagnose the type of affective disorder are significant because lithium generally is reserved for bipolar disorders that have included at least one serious manic episode. Tricyclics may be more desirable when effective because, although they have a serious overdose hazard and several largely reversible side effects, they do not appear to possess a serious cumulative hazard other than weight gain. Lithium in prolonged use may carry a risk of renal changes, which have an as yet undefined clinical significance. It is sometimes feasible to use tricyclics within a pattern of close regulation for bipolar patients as long as manic attacks are not provoked. In this connection, the manic components of a bipolar illness can appear in several forms besides a typical hyperactive euphoria–including catatonic, paranoid, dysphoric, and episodic aggressive forms. An attempt should be made to lower the dose or to withdraw the tricyclic periodically in order to reassess the necessity for its use. In the case of lithium, many physicians would make an evaluation of discontinuation after a period of several years in which there had been no recurrence. Individuals using lithium on a continuing basis can receive a periodic review of their health status with particular attention to the possibilities of hypothyroidism and altered renal function.

The safety and reliability of tricyclic antidepressant use can be increased by using an instructional effort similar to that employed in connection with neuroleptics. A low-dose strategy is combined with rapid increases from a base-line dose at the beginning of any episode. The low-dose strategy offers advantages in safety and reliability because the patient experiences fewer side effects and is less likely to discontinue the medication than if he were taking large doses. The method requires the patient to cooperate, adapt, and learn new skills. When such cooperation cannot be achieved, the low-dose strategy does not succeed. This strategy is not used with lithium, which is ordinarily employed at a steady level.

In order to suppress an incipient depressive episode, the increase in dosage must be early and quick. Patients are instructed to watch for changes in the sleeping-waking cycle, loss of social interest, loss of pleasure, decreased work energy, and preoccupation with a few, repeating topics of thought as early markers of a beginning depressive episode. Early hypomanic signs include feelings of speed and urgency and major deviations from a prior daily schedule. Typically these markers appear days or weeks before the major signs of the episode and, with a medication response, allow its control. When such markers appear, depressed patients may double the base-line dose, wait three days, and assess the effect. Manic patients halve the dose or reintroduce a base-line level of neuroleptic. They may repeat these maneuvers several times.

Counseling and Assistance with Bonding

Counseling can assist the patient's efforts to start, stop, pace, and focus the current adaptive work. Regulating the pace of efforts to get rest, food, water, and relaxation during a period of challenge reduces the risk of exhaustion. Patients can be encouraged to keep in regular reporting contact with their helpers, particularly throughout each episode within a chronic illness. After an episode is resolved, counseling can shift to a less frequent, less intense pattern and be held in readiness for the future.

At the beginning of an adaptational episode, patients can change their dose of medication in the manner reviewed and watch the sleeping-waking and resting-working rhythms as markers of the precision of their regulation. They can be encouraged to feel for a comfortable pace while entering and moving through the situation and to regulate the working-resting cycle during the period of challenge, remembering that the problem-solving effort can extend over many weeks. They can be asked to define the current problem and its relation to their aims for the future. They can be encouraged to name their helpers and to keep in regular reporting contact with them. The regulation of adaptive work seems to proceed best when all parties in the process have an opportunity to form a task group. Above all, patients can be counseled to avoid getting exhausted or becoming isolated. They are assisted with bonding and adaptation so as to remain linked to others, to a path, and to a pace.

The importance of assistance with linkage and bonding is derived from the effect that such supports offer during adaptive intervals, as, for example, during an episode of illness. An individual's signals of distress and displays of affect ordinarily have the effect of convening around him a task group who help him (see Caplan, 1981; Hansell, 1976a, 1976b). But these basic systems are defective in many chronically mentally ill persons. For example, the schizophrenic's chaotic signaling and his proclivity under stress to isolate himself may deprive him of the presence of a group that otherwise might assist him. Many have regarded the schizophrenic person's sometimes solitary condition as central to the disability that then begins to accumulate. Schizophrenic individuals who receive help in maintaining social contacts do distinctly better than those who receive only medication. Many clinicians have observed that schizophrenics who maintain or acquire affiliations appear more capable of problem solving during episodes. This relationship is likely part of the basis for the effectiveness of residential programs of the Lodge-type and of contemporary foster communities in the tradition of Gheel. It is helpful during episodes to convene the schizophrenic person's often fragmentary networks—family, friends, work associates—so as to provide bonding opportunities during the adaptive process. Also useful are linkages to mutual help groups such as First Friends and Recovery, Inc.

Convening key people of the patient's social network can greatly increase its innovative power. Bringing together persons who have bonds or key daily roles with the patient makes more visible and more unitary the operating social field. Persons in turbulent, stressing degrees of trouble may be using alienating or visibly incompetent patterns of behavior. Persons convened in crisis may experience a strong renewal of attachment feelings.

The individuals in a patient's network, when convened, may develop a dramatic new awareness of their conjoint impact. Constructive changes in their behavior often result from this.

Facilitating Other Support Systems

Services that assist in the forming of new bonds are a radically helpful service for individuals found not to have convenable kith or kin. Some patients may not have been recently strongly bonded members of groups. In this situation, it can be useful to establish a support group, for example, a spin-off group. Spin-off groups have ten or so members and learn within the first eight or ten meetings such roles as "the convener," "the arbiter," "the social chairman," "the recorder," and so on. The format of the group is designed to allow it to function without continuing professional direction. Such groups can provide a means for persons previously without a group support system to meet and help one another. The group can serve as an extended family and offer social support to its members. Typically, it begins under the direction of a professional who proceeds to teach the group a set of conventions, roles, and exercises that members can employ to form new social bonds. Roles in the group are distributed so that each person has one or two. Each individual knows the roles of the others; therefore, alternate roles can be assumed in case a member is absent or unable to function. The professional operates from the premise that the convened individuals would probably experience a reduction in distress if they became able to form bonds within a group. He expects them to carry out their roles and provides structure and instruction during the early meetings. During these meetings he also tries to make preparations that will signal that an interesting, possibly enduring group is assembling. He then demonstrates a set of roles, conventions, and exercises. But he expects others to gradually take over these functions and transforms his own role from that of member to that of facilitator.

Service for chronically mentally ill persons is not likely to be continuingly effective in maintaining noninstitutional status unless an individual without a convenable network is given a means to become to some degree a bonded member of a network. Arranging for such a social context, whether temporary or long term, appears to place in operation a set of semiautomatic actions that have the regulatory effect of advancing an individual's adaptive work. These regulatory functions may be conducted by several types of small clusters of people. The cluster may be comprised of relatives, of friends, or of persons with a religious or situational affiliation. It may be an ad hoc mutual help group or, quite often, a set of persons who happen to be in service at the same time. Professionals have sometimes provided themselves as a bonding point to assist with adaptation. However, although very serious limitations lie in the path of individuals trying to conduct problem-solving work while in social isolation, equally serious risks lurk in the service approach that tries to correct such isolation by arranging bonds with professionals. The resulting adaptive work may continue to depend on contact with professionals. And problem-solving work regulated mainly by professionals results in constrictive bonds between patients and professionals. The patient becomes disablingly attached. The service resources can become dysfunctionally encumbered. Consequently, many workers employ practices that convene and enable rather than supply and replace.

Observations of the effectiveness of such convening activities suggest that they are emerging as a major component of services. Convening is made possible by significant although temporary increases in the potential for realignments that are often seen in family and friends at times of crisis. Convening previously isolated persons while they are in service also makes use of such increases in bonding potential as are present during crises. Newly formed groups of otherwise isolated persons can gain affiliations that are not dependent on continuing contact with service personnel. Some of the resulting groups last only for weeks whereas others persist for years. The value to isolated persons of even temporary bonding resides in the more effective variety of the adaptive work conducted as well as in the availability of bridges to more persisting affiliations.

Assistance with bonding can proceed within many varieties of settings—residential, daycare, outpatient care, and shelter-care homes and lodges. Little about the setting seems to interfere with bonding as long as the group members can exercise a measure of control over the use of a space during the time that they employ it. Assistance with bonding can be joined smoothly with many other components of service, for instance, instruction concerning use of medication, counseling, or job training.

A focus on the simple issues of bonding and adaptation also shows in the efforts of many practitioners to manage the majority of acute episodes within a chronic illness by prescribing hospital stays that are as short as feasible. Short hospitalizations appear more likely to preserve affiliations and to yield lower rates of subsequent rehospitalization. Those individuals who remain in contact with a familiar social context between episodes of acute illness seem to experience fewer episodes. Individuals who participate in outpatient counseling or in mutual help groups show more ability to maintain their family affiliations than do persons relying only on the family.

Some mutual assistance groups develop a pattern of regular meetings in a particular place. These groups differ in that some also reside in the building where they meet, while others do not. It is too early to make a judgment on the relative merit of residence clustered in one place—for example, a lodge versus residence spread throughout the community with individuals meeting together in social centers or clubs. Many observers conclude that the separated-domicile lodge holds a remarkable potential to widen, rather than narrow, the social reach of its members. This design may emerge as a useful way to provide long-lasting affiliations without turning the lodges into asylums.

Mutual help groups can be set up with or without a building or major property, with or without a shared domicile, and with or without professional assistance. They have in common a method for recruiting, bonding, regulating, and giving dignity to their members. Because they can be both effective and inexpensive, such groups appear likely to play a continuing role in the service system. Activities such as the convening of people around a person-in-distress and pacing or focusing his problem solving show themselves everywhere in the life of these groups.

Support groups act to start, pace, focus, and stop adaptive efforts in an atmosphere that brings out an individual's identity and enhances his dignity. These groups appear to constitute the radical center of the stretching effort to broaden services for the chronically mentally ill.

Stretched Format of Services

What has been learned about the chronically mentally ill, particularly about the need to rearrange services to include the elements of long-term management, self-regulation, and assistance with bonding and adaptation, may foreshadow a whole set of advances in services. On the one hand, attempts to use hospital services more briefly and to use local services whenever possible appear clinically sound. On the other hand, the concern for promoting early discharge from long-term service in the community will fade in the face of experience in providing such services. The continuing vitality of mutual help groups and other community support systems appears assured and likely to enlarge as medical services become more effective.

The interest in preventive efforts will continue, but with respect to the chronically mentally ill, the earlier, somewhat mischievous dalliance with broad social programming may be supplanted by more solid measures of prevention that are possible with an early and continuous pattern of service. Some of the most reliable preventive work possible today pertains to what may be done in preventing school and job failure, hospitalization, and suicide for persons who can remain functional if they receive services specific to their condition. Schizophrenia and affective disorders may now offer the most solid domain for preventive efforts since preventions were first recognized for neurosyphilis and pellagra.

The large instructional component required for effective services for life-cycle-length disorders may portend the advent of a major set of classroomlike activities. An individual can learn what he needs to know about his disorder and its management in a variety of settings (individual and group) and formats (books, tapes, and clubs). The majority of observers conclude that the most desirable case manager is an individual managing himself, within a supporting system to which he is vitally connected, and employing a personal understanding of his situation, illness, treatment, and goals. We may have only scratched the surface of what may be attempted in teaching people how to regulate their circumstances so as to realize a fuller potential within a chronic mental illness. Throughout a wide range of services for the chronically mentally ill—for example, medication, counseling, instruction, linkage, and surveillance—there should be a centering on bonding and adaptation. The more that basic biology is altered in a persisting way, the more will assistance with bonding and adaptation be needed.

References

American Psychiatric Association. "Position Statement on the Chronic Mental Patient." *American Journal of Psychiatry,* 1979, *136,* 748-753.

Caplan, G. "Mastery of Stress: Psychosocial Aspects." *American Journal of Psychiatry,* 1981, *138,* 413-420.

Hansell, N. "Enhancing Adaptational Work During Service." In R. G. Hirschowitz and B. Levy (Eds.), *The Changing Mental Health Scene.* New York: Spectrum, 1976a.

Hansell, N. *The Person-in-Distress: On the Biosocial Dynamics of Adaptation.* New York: Behavioral Publications, 1976b.

President's Commission on Mental Health. *Report to the President.* Vol. 1. Washington, D.C.: U.S. Government Printing Office, 1978.

Snyder, S. H. *Madness and the Brain.* New York: McGraw-Hill, 1974.

Chapter 15

Working with the Mentally Retarded and Developmentally Disabled

Lewis B. Klebanoff

Mental retardation has had a long and, until recently, not particularly illustrious history. Heaven's curse, God's chosen, freaks of nature, bad seed, and bad family were among the explanatory concepts. In the past, severely or profoundly retarded persons seldom lived long enough to be noticed by neighbors. The more severe the retardation, the more likely were physical anomalies. Recent medical advances, however, have sometimes kept alive many quite impaired persons who require extensive, continuing, and expensive care. Unlike milder forms of mental retardation, which tend to appear in the more economically and socially deprived segments of the population, the more severe forms occur in all social strata. Along with a slowly emerging scientific interest in the manifold issues of mental retardation, it was the middle-class parents of more impaired children who, about the mid 1950s, sparked a demand for social attention and services for persons affected by this complex and distressing problem, with all its social, psychological, medical, educational, vocational, economic, and religious implications. So successful were they that parents of children with somewhat similar, and often overlapping, disabilities organized on behalf of their own children's disabilities and helped to generate federal acceptance and support for the umbrella concept of "developmental disabilities."

In considering how to present recent developments and issues in the area of mental retardation, I found it difficult to separate and recombine the issues to tell a coherent story. Thus, I decided to launch a discussion of modern developments with an example with which I am quite familiar, namely, the community clinical nursery schools (CCNS). Further justification for using this example is that these schools were profoundly influenced by community mental health principles (Caplan, 1959, 1961, 1970).

Before turning to the CCNS movement, however, we might note that intense debates have occurred as to the prevalence of mental retardation. The figure used most widely is 3 percent of the population. But it is generally agreed that most of the persons in that group would, with the ideal combination of social and educational interventions, disappear into the working world after leaving the schools that tested them and identified them as retarded. As widespread as moderate to severe mental retardation is, its prevalence does not approach the six million figure generally used. Ironically, this confusion is beneficial to organized parent groups because it allows for a strong impact on the public consciousness.

Epidemiological studies offer diverse findings, due in no small part to their differing assumptions and methods and to the fact that they study different populations. Conley (1973), in reviewing many of these studies, concludes that although there were an estimated 5.6 million retarded persons under age sixty-five in the United States in 1970 who had IQs under 70—almost exactly 3 percent of the population—most were mildly retarded; 88.2 percent had IQs between 50 and 70, 8.3 percent had IQs between 25 and 50, and 3.5 percent had IQs below 25. The overall estimate of the prevalence of mental retardation is almost identical to what would be predicted if intelligence were normally distributed with a mean of 100 and a standard deviation of 16. Conley emphasizes, however, that a closer inspection of the demographic composition of retarded persons destroys the apparent resemblance of this total population to the normal distribution curve. Among children, the prevalence of mental retardation is slightly greater and among adults slightly less than would be predicted by the normal curve. Among whites, the true prevalence is slightly over half of what would be predicted; among nonwhites the prevalence is four times the predicted rate. Unless carefully analyzed, the combined data would give the overall appearance of congruence with expected frequencies. These data also have to be considered in light of changing definitions of mental retardation. Intellectual level is no longer the overriding criterion. Adaptive behavior is fundamental to the definition promulgated by the American Association on Mental Deficiency, and this criterion is widely accepted in the United States and elsewhere.

Community Clinical Nursery Schools

Until the late 1950s, except for some special education programs in the public schools and a few private facilities, organized investment in mental retardation in the United States was primarily in large public institutions that provided little more than custodial care. One of the more famous institutions, the Walter E. Fernald State School in Massachusetts, had begun as a training school for mild and moderately impaired students. It was so successful that a greater number of students than could be served—including some with serious impairments—were placed there. Without sufficient professional staff for the new tasks, the school slowly deteriorated into an institution for chronic patients. With funding from a recent consent decree and operating under new management, it is struggling to regain its leadership position or at least to provide first-class habilitative services in a decent living environment and to return as many clients as possible to functional lives in the community. In most states, chronic mental facilities were developed for clients whose problems had, or were thought to have, something to do with the brain. Such facilities tended to be part of state mental hospitals or were placed under departments of mental health. Attitudes of professionals were generally pessimistic, and chronic institutional care for mentally retarded persons was the modal pattern. In the late 1950s, however, professional and parental attitudes began to change in more positive directions, and, although sometimes in conflict, they generally stimulated and challenged each other toward greater progress. Whereas mental retardation facilities had usually been directed by superintendents who were, in their way, as institutionalized as the clients, the infusion of community ideas began to produce an aura of hope for the future.

Massachusetts was among the first states in which a parent movement developed in a setting of receptive professionals. The first new programs developed in this state were community clinical nursery schools (CCNS), and they exemplified the many problems in linking the fields of mental health and mental retardation (Bindman and Klebanoff, 1959). Operating on the strong belief that integrated services are to be preferred over separate departments and programs of mental health and mental retardation, we made every effort to integrate the nursery schools into the local guidance clinics or the fledgling mental health centers (Klebanoff, 1964). The chief rationale for this was that families of young children with chronic disabilities are themselves at high risk for emotional difficulties. It should be noted that we did not subscribe to the then popular notion that all parents of retarded children are emotionally disturbed but rather that they are at risk. It was expected that the mental health clinics would provide support and counseling groups for the parents as part of a broader program, including three to five mornings per week of nursery school, to accelerate and maximize the development of children who might otherwise have remained at home with no program, leading to a frequent family expectancy of institutional placement. When parents were given facts about mental retardation, along with higher expectancies for their children, their abilities to cope were strengthened and the risk of emotional disturbance was lessened. A number of years were spent trying to build a community mental health program that would also serve this population of retarded children and their families (Bindman and Klebanoff, 1960; Klebanoff and Bindman, 1962).

Positive expectation was a major concept of the CCNS program. Heretofore, a great many retarded children developed slowly and learned little. It was believed that they had little or no developmental potential, and their treatment resulted in behavior that seemed to confirm this hypothesis. It was decided that the major criteria for selecting teachers for the CCNS program would be familiarity with young children and the expectation of positive responses, even if slow and uneven, from them. The teachers could be taught what they had to know about mental retardation. This manifestation of what was more thoroughly developed in Scandinavian countries as "normalization" endeavored to maximize the developmental potential of the enrolled children, give hope and encouragement to their families, and avoid the then prevalent notion that institutionalization was the child's inevitable fate.

The program grew over the years and came to include more than 100 nursery schools. The clinical services, alas, did not grow apace. They developed by fits and starts, and in only a minority of communities did they fulfill the high hopes held out for them. Mental retardation was not a priority for many mental health personnel. Even after acknowledging the "at risk" concept, they were reluctant to provide clinical services. But several senior psychiatrists, who were also clinical directors, accepted the responsibility cheerfully, developed good services, and even proselytized among their more reluctant colleagues. In the early years of the CCNS program, however, the prevailing national pattern was one of mental health agencies neglecting mentally retarded persons and even exploiting resources earmarked for them. Funds appropriated for mental retardation services never seemed to arrive intact but were diverted and used for mental health purposes. Programs for retarded children were filled with emotionally disturbed children. In many states, parental resentment at this discrimination produced periodic efforts to emulate states such as Connecticut and New Jersey that had established independent mental retardation agencies. While this effort succeeded in only a few states, parents had at least begun to organize themselves.

As the years went by, it became clear that services for the age range of three to seven were not adequate to meet the needs of children and families in the communities. Daycare programs were developed for "graduates" of school age for whom the public schools offered no place. CCNS classes were held for only a half day so that, during the remainder of the day, teachers and their clinical colleagues could hold diagnostic nursery schools for younger children or children with multiple impairments. Special nursery school groups were developed for some of these children, and the teachers increasingly began to visit residences of younger and younger children to encourage the parents to keep their children at home and stimulate their development through materials and techniques suitable for home use. This later developed into a broad effort of home-based programming.

Role of the Federal Government

In 1965, the federal government became significantly involved in mental retardation by providing funds for supplementary services under P.L. 89-313 (Federal Assistance to State-Operated and Supported Schools for Handicapped [Amendment to the Elementary and Secondary Education Act]). A special education, early childhood grant program was developed in the U.S. Office of Education, the purpose of which was to encourage program development throughout the country. While these federal efforts had many positive aspects, they also had two major and related flaws. First was the desire to scatter programs as widely as possible. Second was an often naive emphasis on "innovation"—a problem that has plagued other social programs as well. But why did these apparently reasonable goals turn out to be mistaken ones? In the interest of program proliferation, many small, tenuous organizations—community and church groups—were funded. Most of them could not survive when federal funding ceased. It was also unreasonable to expect much innovation of the kind that could be documented and disseminated from such groups. If the goal was a rapid increase of services, a more productive approach would have been to offer a choice of several tested and packaged models to agencies, preferably public ones. This would have provided some assurance that services would continue even when federal funding stopped, but such admonitions did not fit the populist tenor of the times. Thus, the money and services were scattered and generally ran out together at the end of the grant periods.

It should be noted, however, that the federal program continued and expanded under the Education of the Handicapped Act, P.L. 91-239 Title VI, Part C, 20 U.S.C. 1423, as amended by P.L. 95-49. In the budget for fiscal year 1979, $22 million was allocated to provide "therapeutic service" for an estimated 22,000 children from birth to eight years of age. The initial program has been modified, and its goals are now to serve a wider age range to support experimental demonstration, outreach and state implementation of preschool and early childhood projects for handicapped children. One of the lamentable aspects of the growing concern and increased funding for services to persons with disabilities ("handicapped individuals" in government parlance) is the failure to integrate insights derived from university and highly funded special-project research into the real-world services of public and private agencies. Project Head Start, perhaps more than most others, has bridged much of that gap.

It would be difficult to overstate the federal role in developing new approaches and comprehensive services to persons with mental retardation. In 1961, President Kennedy delivered a message on mental retardation that came from a deep personal and family concern and surprised even the National Association for Retarded Children (now the National Association for Retarded Citizens). President Kennedy established a Panel on Mental Retardation, and armed with data from its inquiries and the 1961 reports of the Joint Commission on Mental Illness and Health, he issued, on February 5, 1963, a "Message from the President of the United States Relative to Mental Illness and Mental Retardation" (Kennedy, 1963). His message led the 88th Congress to pass P.L. 88-156 (the Maternal and Child Health and Mental Retardation Planning Amendments of 1963). This legislation provided grants to each state to develop statewide plans for the mentally retarded.

In P.L. 88-164, passed in October 1963, Congress authorized the construction of "university-affiliated facilities." These were to be associated with a college or university; aid in demonstrating specialized services for the diagnosis, treatment, care, education, and training of mentally retarded persons; and conduct interdisciplinary training of physicians and other specialized personnel needed for the activities named above. The U.A.F. program, as it came to be known, grew quickly and developed a number of facilities, most of them medically centered. This legislation, section 1 of P.L. 88-164, was known as the Mental Retardation Facilities and Community Mental Health Centers Construction Act of 1963. In 1967 it was amended to include other neurologically handicapping conditions. Although the legislation was entitled the Mental Retardation Amendments of 1967, Congress was already edging toward the concept of developmental disabilities.

By executive order, President Johnson established the President's Committee on Mental Retardation in May 1966 (Boggs, 1972). President Kennedy had a special adviser, but the Johnson executive order formalized a group to "provide such advice and assistance in the area of mental retardation as the president may from time to time request," including coordination, evaluation, and information gathering and dissemination. As so often happens with such efforts, the results were mixed. On the one hand, the strategy of having a president's committee was positive; it attracted more attention to the issues than might otherwise have been the case, and the committee pursued many issues that later led to needed legislation. On the other hand, appointments to the committee were often political and did not always represent the field of mental retardation very broadly.

Sections of P.L. 88-164 and its later amendments provided for demonstration and training grants for states to develop and implement a comprehensive and continuing plan for meeting the needs of persons with developmental disabilities. The concept of developmental disabilities, which was translated into legislation before it was subjected to very full public discussion or professional acceptance, seemed to emanate from two major sources. The first source included certain professionals who recognized the similarity of many developmental conditions associated with the nervous system; they saw, for example, that these conditions manifested some similar behaviors, particularly difficulty in learning, and often were at least partially responsive to similar interventions. Related to this was the habit of some professionals to assign whatever diagnostic labels would entitle children to more and/or better services. The second major source included parents who saw that major progress had been made in public recognition of and provision of services for persons with mental retardation. Although prejudice and discrimination existed among families whose children had different disabilities, the gradual destigmatization of all diagnoses (still far from complete), along with the desire to obtain help and services, prevailed over these feelings. A striking example of this phenomenon is the contrast between parents who hoped their child was autistic or schizophrenic despite certain implications of their role in the etiology because there was hope for treatment, and parents who hoped their child was mentally retarded which, despite its irreversibility, was organic, and therefore not their fault but God's will. Thus autism, cerebral palsy, epilepsy, and learning disabilities joined mental retardation as the developmental disabilities. The possibilities for coalitions to lobby and obtain support for the needs of all persons with these disabilities made the umbrella concept of developmental disabilities attractive to many. The problems, however, were not minor. As was stated earlier, legislation preceded the concept's refinement. Furthermore, the organizational base for this legislation was in the federal Bureau of Developmental Disabilities. But since no comparable administrative base existed in most of the states with services for mental retardation, epilepsy, cerebral palsy, and autism, federal money went to state developmental disability councils that, for the most part, were and still are totally independent of and isolated from service delivery systems.

Parent Power, Rights, and Advocacy

One of the phenomena reflected in these expanding definitions of populations to be served is that of *parent power.* The strong advocacy manifested by so many other societal groups was adopted by the parents of children with developmental disabilities. Overcoming shame, guilt, and embarrassment, they slowly came to recognize that there was much need for mutual effort. The membership of these parent groups consists largely of middle-class workers, businesspersons, professionals, that is, of persons who tend to vote. The largest and strongest parent group remains the National Association for Retarded Citizens (NARC), although it has never reached its full membership potential. One of the major reasons for that is that it has a largely middle-class membership. The milder the degree of mental retardation, the more likely it is to be related to lower sociocultural status. But since families in the lower end of the socioeconomic scale are less likely to join parent organizations, the initial issues pursued by parent organizations related to the needs of moderately to severely retarded children and of those with organic involvement.

Largely as an outgrowth of the parent movement but also related to the women's movement, the black pride and power movements, and the welfare rights and gay rights movements, the concept of rights and advocacy for the mentally handicapped has become a dominant one with many manifestations. The battle for legal rights and entitlements is waged on many fronts: legislative, administrative, and judicial. A major effort was to legislate entitlement to a free public education. For example, Massachusetts in 1972 passed a law that was to serve as a model for the 1975 Federal Education for All Handicapped Act, P.L. 94-142, which followed a series of amendments to the Elementary and Secondary Education Act (Gettings and Mersh, 1980). The Education of the Handicapped Act provides states with basic grants to cover a percentage of the costs of providing special education and related services (defined as "transportation, developmental, corrective, and other supportive services to assist a handicapped child to benefit from special education, including speech pathology and audiology, psychological services, physical and occupational therapy, recreation, medical and counseling services [for evaluation purposes], and early identification and assessment of handicapped conditions in children"). Funds are allocated on a formula basis to state educational agencies, and they are required to pass on 75 percent of them to local educational agencies. The act included preschool incentive grants to encourage the states to provide special education and related services to preschool handicapped children aged three to five, as well as continuation of the preschool project grants mentioned earlier in this chapter. The original act provided almost $10 million for regional resource centers that would give advice and technical assistance to educators. Among the act's other features were services for deaf-blind children, innovative programs for severely handicapped children, regional postsecondary programs, research and demonstration programs, teacher training and recruitment, information and referral services, and instructional media and captioned films.

The amendments to the Elementary and Secondary Education Act had included the important provision requiring a maintenance of effort; that is, states could not use federal funds to replace state and local money but only to expand services. The Education for All Handicapped Act went much farther than that. To avoid colliding with state laws that established age restrictions, it indicated that federal funds were conditional on the state's agreeing to establish a goal of serving all handicapped children between the ages of three and eighteen by September 1, 1978, and between three and twenty-one by September 1, 1980. Those states where mandatory services were inconsistent with state law or a binding court order were offered an entitlement of $300 for each handicapped child between the ages of three and five.

The aforementioned Massachusetts legislation had made heavy service demands upon the local systems without providing adequate state funding. In fact, the initial regulations provided more generous benefits than did the legislation itself. As the years passed and more services, including such costly ones as intensive clinical care, legal appeals, repeat evaluations, and private residential treatment and education, were added, public objections mounted. The fact that "children with special needs" had long been deprived of the right to a free public education was never adequately impressed on the public, and far too much of an adversary tone developed. These problems have surfaced in many states that implemented P.L. 94-142. And, as tax crises arose in 1980 and 1981, these special education services became a ready target in Massachusetts and many other states.

The federal legislation, P.L. 94-142, specified that an individualized educational plan be developed for each child, gave first priority to unserved children and second to severely handicapped children who were not receiving adequate services, continued the maintenance of effort provision, described procedures for evaluating program effectiveness, established advisory panels to state education officials, and established record and accounting procedures. The due process safeguards that had appeared in P.L. 93-380 in 1974 were continued and enlarged. The additional rights enabled parents or guardians to examine all records pertaining to identification, evaluation, and placement of their children; to receive written notice of these events in the parents' language; and to obtain an impartial due process hearing at which the parents could be represented by counsel, present evidence, and cross examine and compel witnesses to attend. Parents were also given the right to receive a statement of facts, findings, and decisions. Although this was a great step forward, some families could not cope with all these complicated, even incomprehensible rights, and others were intimidated by schools into keeping silent. Since public schools, with some exceptions, had a sorry record of discrimination and neglect of children with special needs, a new breed of "helper" appeared in response to the confusion. Often untrained in anything relevant to assessment and services, these new "helpers" frequently condemned the schools, indeed all of organized society, as oppressors and wrongdoers deserving punishment. Their confrontation tactics often made it very difficult for parents and decent, concerned school professionals to work together with a shared concern for the child.

In the early 1970s, the notion of "advocacy" burst into flower and became the latest vogue. It had two main manifestations, although each had many variations. One major theme, and the more valuable one, was advocacy by those who became friends of mentally retarded persons, spent time with them, took them places, and taught them to negotiate the complex worlds of travel, shopping, and community life in general. Sometimes these advocates represented the retarded person before various agencies. The other major type of advocate was the self-proclaimed champion who asserted that society did not care about retarded persons and would not treat them fairly without the advocate's intervention. There were, of course, many sincerely concerned advocates who were motivated by the most compassionate of ideals. However, the spotlight was preempted by the strident and the arrogant. It is true that many clinicians and educators were unwilling to serve mentally retarded persons. Many others, however, considered advocacy part of their professional role and thought that they could well and caringly represent their clients' best interests. These issues are not yet fully resolved even though much money was spent employing untrained, inexperienced people who were attuned primarily to the antiprofessional temper of the times.

Parents and Service Delivery

To understand the role of parents in service delivery, it is necessary to be aware of the history of the mental retardation parent movement. The quality of parent leadership at the national level has generally been quite high, if somewhat more variable at the state and local levels. A problem that often confronted citizen leaders, however, was the conflict between organizational goals and the service needs of their own children. Thus, the key early leaders in Massachusetts who had preschool children fostered a large preschool program with few other services available except special classes and state institutions. In Pennsylvania, by contrast, a similar situation with parents of older children produced a large sheltered workshop program but little else.

In many states, parents gained growing access to political and opinion leaders. They engaged in fund raising and, partly because of the general public perception of retarded persons as children, helped to change public attitudes in directions supportive of their interests. Progress was somewhat slowed, however, by several peculiar twists. One was that many officers of parent associations were, for the first time, hobnobbing with governors, legislators, and mayors. This newfound prominence was so beguiling that the officers were successfully sidetracked from pursuing needed organizational goals. The officers were reluctant to risk "friendships" with powerful persons by challenging them with the fact that, although meetings were often pleasant and the officials publicly praised their groups, real progress was agonizingly slow.

Another conflict involved a refusal on the local level to accept the national policy to "obtain, not provide" services. Many of the first projects undertaken by newly organized parent groups were direct service projects intended to compensate for the lack of needed community programs. Their operation required various combinations of dues, fees, fund-raising efforts, and perhaps some public money. There was often a strong feeling that no other agency knew how to provide for their children as well as the parent groups. The more farsighted leadership understood, however, that for the vast array of services required by retarded persons over their lifetime, the concept of their right to care, education, treatment, and public funding was vital. Nevertheless, the immediate gratification earned by many local committee chairpersons operating direct services was so rewarding that they were reluctant to give up their fiefdoms and sometimes refused to implement available public programs or delayed in doing so.

At the national level, the National Association of Retarded Citizens (NARC) exemplified how several small, local parent efforts could grow into a large, effective, respected national advocacy organization in a relatively few years. This movement has not been without problems, however. State chapters have retained considerable autonomy, and national policies have not been uniformly followed. The provision of direct services at the local level never completely disappeared. In fact, with the growth of government's purchase of services from local agencies in the late 1970s, this trend accelerated again. In many communities, there were few local vendors who could bid for the contracts or, indeed, were even motivated to try to do so. The parent organizations were available, they had corporate structures and staffs, and they wanted to have services provided. Once they became contract vendors, moreover, they often delivered quality services.

At the same time, however, new problems arose. First, staff members developed a vested interest in their jobs and in keeping NARC in the provider business. Second, the advocate organizations were now vendors with a financial stake in governmental action, and it is becoming increasingly questionable whether an advocacy group receiving large amounts of public money can have the same standing in public discourse as a group without that kind of financial conflict. It is also likely that some parent groups were lured into providing direct services by public officials deliberately seeking to co-opt some of their strongest critics. Third, there is now the risk that as the parent movement achieves growing success in obtaining or providing services and as the needs of retarded persons are increasingly met, the motivation for parents to join or remain active in parent organizations will fade. Since no social issue remains forever in the limelight of public concern and support, it will be vital to have strong organizations guarding the gains of the mental retardation movement, if not seeking new victories. Concerned families and friends must understand this concept if the movement is not to disintegrate.

Quality of Services

The American Association on Mental Deficiency (AAMD), starting in 1952, began to consider standards for public institutions. This led in 1966 to formation of the National Planning Committee on Accreditation of Residential Centers for the Retarded, which was composed of representatives of several national organizations. This National Planning Committee developed the structure for an accrediting agency and in 1969, looking for an experienced organizational base, became the first of several accreditation councils in the Joint Commission on Accreditation of Hospitals (JCAH). In the early years of this affiliation, the council, called the Accreditation Council for the Mentally Retarded, grew in numbers of corporate members, in scope of standards, and in methods of assessing compliance with those standards. Within the benign constraints of a "gentlemen's agreement" under which the JCAH commissioners would either approve the council's recommendations or remand the issue to council for further work and negotiation, council activities progressed and the relationship with JCAH was relatively satisfactory. New standards were developed through truly extensive and intensive consultation with all relevant professions and citizens. The resulting set of standards, as much of a national consensus as is likely to be achieved, covered residential and community services and followed a broad developmental model. However, because this model was at variance with the medical model followed by JCAH, tensions began to develop. In 1979, JCAH reorganized its administrative structure, and agreements with accreditation councils were terminated. They were replaced by professional and technical advisory committees for programs now to be accredited directly by the JCAH. Efforts at negotiation failed and after careful consideration, member organizations of the Accreditation Council for Services for Mentally Retarded and Other Developmentally Disabled Persons voted to withdraw from JCAH (as did several other councils) and to establish an independent accreditation program in order to:

1. Preserve consumer participation in the accreditation process;
2. Maintain the developmental model, the principle of normalization, and the interdisciplinary approach as bases for providing services; and
3. Assure that decisions regarding standards and accreditation for developmental disability services are made by persons having the requisite knowledge and concern (Accreditation Council for Mental Retardation and Developmental Disabilities [AC MRDD], 1980).

Most of the corporate members of the council (with the exception of the American Academy of Pediatrics, the American Nurses Association, and the American Psychiatric Association) joined the new group. The current sponsoring organizations are the American Association on Mental Deficiency, the

American Occupational Therapy Association, the American Psychological Association, the Council for Exceptional Children, the Epilepsy Foundation of America, the National Association for Retarded Citizens, the National Association of Private Residential Facilities for the Mentally Retarded, the National Association of Social Workers, the National Society for Autistic Children, and United Cerebral Palsy Associations, Inc. Each organization has two representatives on the board of directors. Although the medical organizations did not rejoin, three distinguished physicians represent three of the current member organizations on the board.

The council still faces many major problems. It is supported in large measure by a federal grant that reflects enlightened government operation at its best. For a relatively small (in federal terms) amount of money, the government supports a major interdisciplinary and citizen-backed quality assurance program and also makes it possible for the fee structure for applicant agencies to be much more modest than that of the JCAH. This differential is particularly important because the council has not yet been granted "deemed status." A facility accredited by JCAH is deemed in compliance with federal standards and can receive federal reimbursement for its services. However, a facility accredited by AC MRDD still requires a governmental evaluation. (Ironically, the government standards were taken directly from an earlier version of the AC MRDD standards.)

The AC MRDD standards have recently been updated and the residential and community service components combined. The major thrust of this accreditation process, in fact its distinguishing feature, is less concern with physical structure and whether there is dust over the doorways (although life-safety codes and state and local fire and safety code compliance are mandated), and greater concern with whether there is a comprehensive program plan for each individual client and whether it is being implemented. "Program audits" are conducted on a representative sample of clients served by the agency in order to assess the agency's compliance with standards directly related to appropriate and adequate services to individuals. Whether this uniquely conceived service can survive governmental budget slashing and the implacable hostility of the well-entrenched and influential JCAH, which would like to continue in the developmental disability accreditation business provided that such programs and facilities are regarded as medical or health enterprises, remains to be seen. If the council does not survive, American society will be deprived of a broadly endorsed service that seeks to ensure that public and private funds are used to purchase only high-quality care.

Medical and Developmental Models

The so-called medical model has generated controversy in the mental retardation field for many years. It is often invoked as an incantation by those who have little understanding of its meaning or history. The controversy appears especially puzzling to well-trained, competent physicians who have only recently become involved with mental retardation programs and often find themselves facing considerable hostility and suspicion. The problem has two main sources that, although related, can be best analyzed separately.

The first is the now widely held commitment to a developmental model of understanding mental retardation: "The most useful way to view mental retardation and other developmental disabilities is within the context of a developmental model that acknowledges each individual's capacity for learning, growing, and developing, regardless of how severely disabled he or she may be. Services must be provided to meet the developmental needs of the disabled individual throughout his or her life-span, so as to maximize the individual's human qualities, increase the complexity of the individual's behavior, and enhance the individual's ability to cope with his or her environment. Services must be provided in accordance with the principle of normalization, defined as the use of means that are as culturally normative as possible to elicit and maintain behavior that is as culturally normative as possible" (AC MRDD, 1980, p. vi). Under this conception, and almost no matter how impaired the person, medical services are to be ancillary to and supportive of the person's growth. For the vast majority of retarded persons, this model holds, medical care is required only for intercurrent illness and should not become the central focus of their lives. Medical care, diagnosis, and monitoring are needed to help the individual carry on with living, learning, and working; the individual does not exist to receive medical care.

The second source of the conflict is rooted in the history of mental retardation services. For many years, the major focus of attention and expenditures was on public institutions. Whether called hospitals or state schools, they tended to be medical feudal baronies. Although there were exceptions, far too many incompetent, unmotivated, unlicensed, and non-English-speaking physicians controlled the institutions. Their salaries were low, but their perquisites were often high. The physicians controlled patients and other staff, and only they could make decisions about who was "good" enough to go home for the weekend, who could go to school, who should live where, and so on. The rituals developed in some institutions were so stifling that young professionals, training in nonmedical disciplines, were affronted by the hierarchical structure. They reported back to their universities, and a general attitude of hostility was engendered to physician control of service facilities. Partly as a result of the antiestablishment tenor of the late 1960s and partly as a result of revelations in court suits about misuse of psychotropic drugs as chemical restraints, not to mention the use of mentally retarded clients as research subjects, a "throw the rascals out" philosophy began to prevail and, unfortunately, turned into a strong antimedical bias.

This attitude has, perhaps, begun to run its course; increasingly, major medical centers and skilled physicians have become involved in the care of retarded persons. These physicians speak the language of the staff and the clients and concentrate on their specialties. Consequently, the other disciplines and program managers are coming to recognize that the mentally retarded need good medical evaluations and appropriate treatment.

Several related health issues illustrate the complex interplay of scientific advances and political factors in the care of mentally retarded persons. The first is in the realm of prevention, particularly of the biomedical kind that saves relatively few lives but does so dramatically. Prevention has been strongly pushed through research programs, as well as through screening and intervention programs. This occasionally leads to a paradox. In the case of phenylketonuria, a metabolic disorder, a particularly prominent family wanted to emphasize that this form of retardation might well be prevented and that a test and treatment for it were available. The family lobbied for legislation in several states to implement this test, even though it had not yet received thorough scientific documentation. Thus, several states mandated blood screening of all newborn infants and established different levels of blood phenylalanine as indicating the disorder. Some children died on the prescribed special diets until it was recognized that the special substance that prevented phenylketonuria had to be balanced with many other dietary components. It was a dramatic example of politics distorting science.

A second health issue of special interest involves the prenatal tests for determining genetic disorders that also allow for termination of pregnancy. This use of amniocentesis continues to provoke considerable controversy as the abortion issue generates increasingly intense political conflict. Paralleling these developments in prevention of mental retardation is the general progress in obstetrics, neonatology, and general medical care. One ironic consequence is that many infants who previously would not have survived are now kept alive and face a future of severe or profound disability.

Role of the Courts

Although they could easily fill a chapter of their own, issues pertaining to court appeals, usually federal, for the redress of grievances of the mentally retarded will be addressed in the remainder of this one. This role of the courts has been a major phenomenon of recent years and, despite the fact that decisions have been generally favorable to mentally retarded and other developmentally disabled persons, this development raises profound policy questions. Is it good public practice for a single appointed judge to override the decisions of hundreds of elected officials? Does this principle of judicial decision making, applauded today, carry the seeds of great future harm to our system of government? Finally, if judicial decisions should begin to go against advocates of the handicapped, will they unwittingly have provided ammunition for legislators to also refuse to redress grievances?

One of the first major court victories for the mentally retarded occurred in the U.S. District Court for the Eastern District of Pennsylvania in the case of *Bowman et al.* v. *Commonwealth of Pennsylvania*. The orders that issued from this suit in 1971 specified that no child can be denied admission to school or have his or her educational status changed without notice and that parents have a right to a hearing, to an independent evaluation of the child, to swift justice, and to the best alternative (not the cheapest or most convenient) for the child (The Exceptional Parent, 1971-1972). This suit, as did many later ones, produced consent decrees in which the states and their relevant constituent agencies stipulated to the accuracy of many of the allegations and consented to at least some of the demanded remedies. These agreements by plaintiffs and defendants were ordered by the courts with full force of law and were usually overseen by a court-appointed monitor. But governors and legislators, required to provide necessary funds, sometimes resisted doing so, and the plaintiffs often had to request that judges prod the defendants into fulfilling fiscal commitments.

Major suits concerning state institutions were launched in Massachusetts, at Willowbrook in New York, at Pennhurst in Pennsylvania, in Alabama, and in New Hampshire. Because most resulted in smashing victories for the plaintiffs, expenditures for services then rose sharply. In Massachusetts, for example, mental retardation programs had long been poor stepchildren in the state's Department of Mental Health. Presently, the mental retardation division still lacks funds for vital services, particularly for persons not residing in institutions and therefore not parties to class action suits. Nevertheless, retardation is better funded now than mental health services, which have gone into a relative decline in terms of funding and public support. It is also noteworthy that because the judge did not trust Massachusetts to deliver on its promises, he mandated that certain state institutions be rebuilt, even though their residents were expected to be in community placements by the projected completion time. The cost of this capital program has continued to bedevil legislators and governors.

The judicial case currently causing the most consternation is the Pennhurst State School suit, which was based on provisions of the Federal Developmentally Disabled Assistance and Bill of Rights Act. This statute provides federal grants to help states care for and treat the developmentally disabled. The act's "bill of rights" provision states that mentally retarded persons "have a right to appropriate treatment services and habilitation" in "the setting that is least restrictive of personal liberty." In 1974 a resident of Pennhurst brought a class action suit on behalf of herself and others in which she alleged, among other things, that since conditions at Pennhurst were unsanitary, inhumane, and dangerous, class members were being denied various constitutional and statutory rights. The plaintiffs suggested that Pennhurst be closed and community living arrangements provided for its residents. The U.S. District Court found certain of the rights violated and granted relief. The U.S. Court of Appeals substantially concurred but based its agreement on the Developmentally Disabled Assistance and Bill of Rights Act rather than on constitutional claims.

The case was appealed to the U.S. Supreme Court, which in April 1981 reversed the decision of the Court of Appeals and remanded the case for further proceedings. The Supreme Court held that section 6010 of the act does not create any substantive rights to "appropriate treatment" in the "least restrictive" environment. The thrust of the justices' decision was that Congress meant to encourage and help states to improve services but not to impose a mandatory and massive financial obligation on them. Any state could have refused to participate under the act and merely caused itself to forfeit relevant federal funds; it was encouraged but not obligated to accept the money or the service mandate. The Supreme Court also questioned whether the legislation can be interpreted to have gone as far as the original plaintiff maintained. Thus, the court affirmed the District Court's holding that Pennhurst residents have a state statutory right to adequate habilitation. The case has been remanded to the U.S. District Court for relief that does not include the closing of Pennhurst or guaranteeing the least restrictive environment ("Supreme Court Opinions," 1981).

Congress will have to speak much more clearly than it is likely to in the near future if full guarantees of these desirable rights to habilitation and least restrictive environment are to be obtained. The Pennhurst case has created much consternation among families of mentally retarded persons, professionals, and concerned citizens. Several decades of enormous progress had been capped by the original Pennhurst decision. Not only is that now to be limited in its scope, but other courts are also likely to retreat from what they have granted mentally retarded persons.* Many justifiably fear that administrative and legislative officials who have heretofore expended large sums of money to support consent decrees, perhaps in some cases to avoid court action, will in the light of this Supreme Court decision and pressing financial problems not only bring progress to a halt but may even undo some of the gains of recent years.

The moving finger writes. In just three decades, we have seen a social revolution of very real dimensions better the lot of countless persons at the unfavored end of our social scale. It can perhaps be said that the United States has, in that time, made more progress than has any other country, but we must also face the grim fact that few places in the world have had facilities for mentally retarded persons as appalling as those in Amer-

*In 1982, the U.S. Supreme Court ruled in *Youngberg* v. *Romeo* that mentally retarded people in institutions have the constitutional rights to "personal security" and "freedom from bodily restraint." The Supreme Court also found that these persons have the right to such training as would ensure their security and facilitate their freedom. The standard by which infringement of these rights is to be ascertained is delimited to whether professional judgment in fact was exercised.

ica. During these three decades we have witnessed complaints, controversy, vast funding increases, scientific progress, program advances, new definitions, and changed social attitudes. The field has often been a pressure cooker, and although many competent people have entered it, others have left in frustration, often because of the unrealistic but relentless demands by certain advocates for ideological purity. Perhaps in a situation of such enormous social change that kind of conflict is inevitable.

In this chapter, I have highlighted some of the undersides to the bright clouds of progress, because these issues seldom, if ever, appear in print and they may help us to understand changes that will occur in the future. For the first time in several decades, there is outright opposition to the cause of mental retardation and other developmental disabilities. The twin forces of a troubled economic system and a conservative Supreme Court may not only slow progress but even produce regression. Whatever the eccentricities of the retardation field and some of its prominent personalities, and however difficult it is to meet all the needs of troubled families, the developmentally disabled nevertheless have the right to those opportunities that will allow them to develop to their fullest potentialities. History will measure our society not by how many rockets we produce but by how we care for the disabled, the elderly, and the poor. If we fail them, we fail ourselves. But if we can use our scientific and technical intelligence to solve human problems, we may move into the next century as a civilized society.

References

Accreditation Council for Mental Retardation and Developmental Disabilities (AC MRDD), "Standards for Services for Developmentally Disabled Individuals." Washington, D.C.: Accreditation Council for Services for Mentally Retarded and Other Developmentally Disabled Persons, 1980.

Bindman, A. J., and Klebanoff, L. B. "A Nursery Center Program for Preschool Mentally Retarded Children." *American Journal of Mental Deficiency,* 1959, *64,* (3), 561-573.

Bindman, A. J., and Klebanoff, L. B. "Administrative Problems in Establishing a Community Mental Health Program." *American Journal of Orthopsychiatry,* 1960, *30* (4), 696-711.

Boggs, E. M. "Federal Legislation 1966-1971." In J. Wortis (Ed.), *Mental Retardation.* Vol. 4. New York: Grune & Stratton, 1972.

Caplan, G. *Concepts of Mental Health and Consultation: Their Application in Public Health Social Work.* Washington, D.C.: U.S. Department of Health, Education, and Welfare, Social Security Administration, Children's Bureau, 1959.

Caplan, G. *An Approach to Community Mental Health.* New York: Grune & Stratton, 1961.

Caplan, G. *The Theory and Practice of Mental Health Consultation.* New York: Basic Books, 1970.

Conley, R. W. *The Economics of Mental Retardation.* Baltimore, Md.: Johns Hopkins University Press, 1973.

Gettings, R. M., and Mersh, S. *Summary of Existing Legislation Relating to the Handicapped.* Publication No. E-80-22014. Washington, D.C.: U.S. Department of Education, 1980.

"Justices Plan to Define the Rights of Retarded Held in Institutions." *New York Times,* May 19, 1981.

Kennedy, J. F. "Message from the President of the United States Relative to Mental Illness and Mental Retardation." Washington, D.C.: House of Representatives, Document No. 58, 1963.

Klebanoff, L. B. "Facilities for the Mentally Retarded: Integrated or Separate but Equal." *American Journal of Public Health,* 1964, *54* (2), 244-248.

Klebanoff, L. B., and Bindman, A. J. "The Organization and Development of a Community Mental Health Program for Children: A Case Study." *American Journal of Orthopsychiatry,* 1962, *32* (1), 119-132.

"Supreme Court Opinions." *United States Law Week,* 1981, *49* (41), 4363-4377.

The Exceptional Parent. *The Pennsylvania Court Orders.* Boston: Psy-Ed Corporation, 1971/1972, *1* (4), 8-12.

Chapter 16

Intervening with Disaster Victims

Raquel E. Cohen

Intervention programs designed to assist victims of natural disasters are beginning to emerge in the United States. Models are being developed to plan these programs and to structure mental health intervention assistance in collaboration with other disaster relief efforts. Professionals who are trained in community mental health practice are particularly cognizant of the necessity, as well as the multiplicity of opportunities, for service to disaster-affected populations in order to prevent pathological or maladaptive consequences. Congress has recognized and legitimated mental health intervention activities as part of federal disaster relief programs in the Disaster Relief Act (1974). The act reads in part as follows: "The president is authorized through the National Institute of Mental Health to provide professional counseling service, including financial assistance to state or local agencies or private mental health organizations to provide such service or training of disaster workers to provide such service, to victims of major disasters in order to relieve mental health problems aggravated by such major disaster or its aftermath."

This chapter defines postdisaster crisis counseling as a mental health intervention technique that seeks to restore the capacity of individuals to cope with the stressful situations in which they find themselves and to provide assistance for these individuals to reorder and reorganize their worlds. Education about and interpretation of the overwhelming feelings produced by postdisaster stresses are offered to help strengthen their sense of capability and hopefulness. Postdisaster intervention programs offer a unique model for including mental health activities, for broadening the perspective of community caregivers, and for offering the possibility of a resolution to crisis reactions for victims. To be effective, however, the mental health component of the intervention program must prove continuously useful to both the victim *and* the community caregivers. Mental health intervention activities in disaster work that are based on a reconceptualization of traditional clinical roles and on the adaptation of therapeutic procedures described by others in the general clinical literature, as well as on skills and methods introduced and refined by the author as a result of her own experiences, will be documented in this chapter.

It is, of course, a monumental task to sort out the concrete and psychological needs of a disaster-stricken population. The success with which it is done depends largely on the concerted efforts and logistical coordination of many individuals from a wide variety of professional disciplines. The approach to establishing and maintaining cooperative relationships must be fluid, spontaneous, and, above all, sensitive and compassionate. A number of conditions will influence how the mental health professionals will participate in work at the disaster site. A key issue will be the service priorities selected by governmental and voluntary agencies as they organize themselves to assist. Generally, providing for the physical comfort of victims and caring for physical injuries are first priorities. Another issue concerns the kind of knowledge that mental health professionals bring to the situation and whether or not this knowledge is sufficient to guide them through multiple types of postdisaster intervention activities. One major consideration will be the particular skills they bring to or can mobilize in the community to evaluate the traumatic psychological symptomatology exhibited by the population.

Two main areas of community mental health theory and

practice can be helpful in addressing these issues. The first concerns knowledge of loss and mourning theories, that is, knowledge about reactions to overwhelming losses of limb, of familiar physical surroundings, and of significant others. Understanding the progression of crisis reactions and phases of resolution will assist mental health professionals to cope with the inherent stresses of the situation and will facilitate their conceptualization and categorization of the phenomena present at the disaster scene.

The second valuable body of knowledge is that which can be obtained from the practices of community mental health. The techniques of crisis resolution, short-term therapy, and counseling and support to couples, families, and groups will form part of the mental health worker's repertoire of expertise (Lindemann, 1944, 1979; Caplan, 1974, 1976). Mental health workers in previous disasters have defined and documented the phases of psychological reaction that follow a disaster as (1) impact, (2) recoil, and (3) reorganization. The experiences of these workers offer examples of how to organize and mobilize professional resources within a community to assist disaster victims in the various phases of reaction to the event (Tyhurst, 1951, 1957; Cohen and Ahearn, 1980).

Key authors who have contributed to basic and applied knowledge helpful in disaster assistance work are Lindemann (1944), who documented the bereavement reactions of individuals after the Coconut Grove fire in Boston; Lifton (1967), who developed a theory of postdisaster behavior based on his studies of victims at Hiroshima; Fritz and Williams (1967), who addressed issues of reactive behavior according to intensity and scope of psychological impact; Titchener and Kapp (1976), who participated in many recovery program activities following the Buffalo Creek flood in Appalachia; Erikson (1976a, 1976b), who was able to contrast behavior before and after the Buffalo Creek flood; Caplan (1976), who described the organization of support systems for civilian populations in time of war; Ahearn and Castellon (1978), who researched emotional responses to the Managua, Nicaragua earthquake and found that admissions to the only psychiatric hospital in the country increased by 27 percent after the catastrophe; and Frederick (1981), who compared the effects of natural versus human-induced violence upon victims.

Conceptual Framework

The conceptual framework for postdisaster mental health intervention presented here incorporates information from community mental health theory and practice:

1. *Effects of Loss and Bereavement.* The consequences of a disaster can affect an individual by producing loss of "world view" of his environment, loss of symbolic meaning to his life, loss of independent economic status, symptoms of transitory or longer-lasting mental disorder, and loss of life (Lindemann, 1944, 1979).
2. *Reactions to Crisis.* The individual's feelings, attitudes, perceptions, and behavior are affected by and in turn affect social systems disorganized by the disaster (Tyhurst, 1951, 1957).
3. *Strategies of Adaptation.* Each individual has unique coping defenses and mastery mechanisms to deal with stress (Dohrenwend and Dohrenwend, 1974).
4. *Support Systems.* Social and community support systems can be variously effective in supplying physiological, psychological, social, and economic assistance to the individual in the aftermath of disaster (Caplan, 1974, 1976).

Each individual involved in a natural disaster can be characterized by the following: (1) demographic factors (age, sex, ethnicity, and so on); (2) personality traits, developmental stage, marital status, occupation, and level of economic independence; (3) previous life experiences; (4) effectiveness in the past of usual coping mechanisms; (5) type and intensity of impact of the disaster on the individual; (6) adaptive behavior as an indication of the reactive responses of the individual; and (7) support systems availability and "fit"; how the individual utilizes them. Information gathered from each of these categories will provide a profile of the individual, his psychosocial reactions to the disaster, and his stage of crisis resolution. This information will also suggest his current vulnerabilities and thus indicate what he needs and requires to regain functional equilibrium. The mental health worker can then incorporate these psychological and sociocultural factors into an intervention strategy to assist the victim of the disaster.

Many interlocking factors influence the outcome of the crisis for the disaster victim, including the economic and political characteristics of the community in which the disaster occurs. Any conceptual framework for developing a postdisaster mental health intervention model must also take into account the level of community disorganization following the disaster and the corresponding availability of relief resources.

Intervention Model

It is the contention of this intervention model for the resolution of crises following the impact of a natural disaster that a mental health team must mobilize quickly and gain rapid entry into the federal, state, and local disaster-assistance systems in order to be effective.

Initial Basic Information Gathering. There are two basic sets of information that must be acquired prior to entering the disaster area and initiating participation. First, the mental health team must obtain descriptions of the circumstances of the catastrophic event and descriptions of the populations affected:

- Was the impact immediate and without warning, or was the population prepared?
- Was the public kept informed of the situation, as in a storm or hurricane; or was there a sudden, violent upheaval, as in an earthquake?
- Was the site of the disaster an urban setting where the congestion of buildings added to the destructive impact of the event, or was it on the edge of a city with little structural loss?

- What were the salient population characteristics (for example, age and ethnicity) before the event?
- How has the population sustained the impact of the disaster?

The tornado that slammed through Windsor Locks in Connecticut in 1979 caused $179 million worth of damage in three communities. Ninety-five homes and thirty-eight businesses were destroyed, two individuals died, and more than 500 were injured. All this happened in a matter of minutes when the wind ripped through a suburban area one mile wide and three miles long.

The Appalachian population affected in the Buffalo Creek disaster of February 1972, in which many children were lost, lived in a community that highly valued family bonds (Erikson, 1976a, 1976b). Families living in isolated conclaves provided the major support systems for dealing with everyday life. The family was a structural entity from which every member could draw some resources and to which every member gave of himself or herself unquestioningly and spontaneously. Livelihood revolved around coal mining. The torrential rain caused overloading of the capacity of the mining dam, and, when the dam broke, it sent millions of gallons of water roaring down the valley. The effects of the rain became the center of the controversial investigation and litigation about the cause of the disaster. The impact of the disaster and its aftermath seriously disrupted normal family, work, and community networks of relationships and patterns of assistance.

Second, the mental health team must obtain descriptions of political and organizational responses to the disaster:

- What were the immediate, official governmental measures taken to develop human support systems to parallel financial emergency assistance programs?
- What groups were mobilized to provide the survival needs of the individual—for food, shelter, and assistance for physical injury?
- What was done to counter the effects of the disarray of social organizations?

After a severe earthquake struck Managua, Nicaragua in 1972, senior members of the government took over leadership of the relief agencies and organized them along military lines. Ministers and all other heads of programs gathered in the president's house, which became the headquarters for daily centralized planning. Meetings were held continuously, and orders were given for relay of food and housing resources. Medical supplies and vehicles shuttled continually in and out of the compound. The clergy was also a strong influence working to reconstruct the social organizations of the country.

The flood that ripped through the city of Corning, New York in June 1972, crippled trade and industry to an extent that caused a serious unemployment problem (Kliman, 1976). The Corning Glass Works geared itself to meet the short- and long-term problems subsequent to the flood. Exhibiting leadership and concern, a group of representatives from the industry organized services to seek out and assist individuals in need. The introduction and support of a crisis team under the sponsorship of the Corning Glass Works and the Family Service Agency, both of them integral to the community, made the team more acceptable than a group of outsiders would have been.

Initial Action Plan. Three modes of action for the mental health team take priority (Cohen, 1976):

1. Enter the specific geographic area where disaster assistance is being organized, whether it is a shelter, a displaced population camp, or a congregation of tents on a safe level of the terrain. Link into the network of assisting individuals, guided by the knowledge obtained during investigatory activities.
2. Conduct a rapid needs assessment to ascertain the ethnic, cultural, and economic characteristics of the displaced and traumatized population. For example, was this a population whose members had many needs before the disaster and may now have insufficient resources to reconstruct their lives? This kind of information will help to determine the extent of needed assistance, both physical and psycho-

logical. Whether the needs are minimal, moderate, or severe, some accommodation for mental health procedures must be incorporated into the disaster operation activities.

3. Establish and develop collaborative procedures with governmental units and voluntary agencies. These may include state government agencies, Civil Defense, the Red Cross, and/or the various community agencies working in the relief operation. The leader of the mental health team must introduce, describe, and explain the services that mental health professionals can offer to help these agencies in their recovery assistance tasks.

The actions listed above become a means for the mental health team to learn and help at the same time. They must be carried out as soon as the team enters the disaster area so as to hasten the process of mobilizing the resources that the mental health team will need in doing its specific work.

Guidelines for Intervention. All activities must be directed at developing useful procedures that will be of immediate value. First, because the number of mental health workers in disaster work is generally small in relation to the need, it is important to begin with *triage.* Traditional clinical procedures must be streamlined and simplified to a first-aid approach, especially in the first hours or days. In the aftermath of one disaster, for example, several individuals were referred to the mental health team in a shelter. Among them was a young woman in her fourth month of pregnancy. She was anxious, agitated, and fearful that she would have a miscarriage because the corner of a roof had fallen on her during an earthquake. She needed reassurance and education about her fearful reactions; she was given these after a quick physical exam by the physician on the team revealed no signs of an imminent miscarriage.

Second, rapid mobilization of mental health teams must occur in a unified rhythm of activity with the other crisis caregivers. In another example, a Red Cross worker asked for assistance from the mental health team with a thirty-year-old white woman who appeared tense and was speaking angrily. She was complaining about "being pushed around." The mental health worker elicited the following story: The woman had lost her apartment because of severe flooding and now had to find a new place to live. She felt weak and helpless about finding a place at a rent that she could afford. She also felt entitled to government help but wasn't getting it. Because of her psychological distress, this woman was unable to articulate her needs. The mental health worker helped her to ventilate her anger and disappointment at her loss, and the Red Cross worker guided her through the bureaucratic system to get some rental assistance.

Third, as opportunities arise, mental health workers should participate in the postdisaster services provided by the community's usual health, education, and welfare institutions. Take the case of a forty-five-year-old woman who became depressed and anxious while her husband was going through an episode of alcohol withdrawal. He refused to be examined and was hostile and aggressive with the physician while his wife tried unsuccessfully to calm him—she was too upset herself to exert any influence on him. When he finally agreed to accept help, a mental health professional joined the medical team to assist the wife. The mental health worker was able to elicit a story of long suffering and difficulties in the marital situation before the disaster. There was a deep dependent need to control each other's behavior. The wife revealed the depth of her depression in expressing her reactions to her husband's behavior in the shelter. She insisted on going with him to the hospital to which he was transferred. The mental health worker talked on the phone with the hospital staff and prepared them for the couple's arrival, sharing with them his understanding of their behavior within the crisis context of the disaster.

Fourth, mental health workers should not only strive to offer direct help to individuals traumatized by the disaster but should also seek opportunities to offer indirect services, such as consultation and education, to the other caregivers. The leader of one crisis-counseling team, for example, developed a plan to meet all the senior personnel in one of the federal relocation centers set up to deal with a particular disaster. She walked over to their assigned areas, introduced herself, and explained the role of the crisis counselors. She also provided a schedule of the hours and names of the mental health workers. As time allowed, she would "visit" to share the information about people and their expectable reactions to crisis that she had gained through her own mental health intervention activities in this and previous disaster-assistance programs.

Fifth, as the organization of the disaster aid network develops and more knowledge of the prevailing situation and available services begins to emerge, psychological procedures can become more elaborate, and areas of responsibility for the mental health team will begin to broaden. To give one example, a black married man, thirty five years old, whose house had been destroyed by a storm, related that his wife had been hospitalized with severe back pain the day after the disaster. His daughter, eighteen years old, was now staying with a neighbor because the father could not find temporary housing for the whole family. A son was living with two young men whom the father didn't approve of or like. The father had found an apartment in an adjoining town. As he spoke of the problems of his family, it became evident that their relationships previously had been ambivalent. Subsequent to the disaster the family ties appeared even more strained. The mental health worker supported and helped the man to acknowledge his pain, encouraging him to express anger and disappointment. He then was assisted to develop a plan of action to put together all the disparate pieces of his scattered world.

Sixth, postdisaster psychological reactions and resolutions occur in phases over an extended period of time. Mental health intervention activities must be developed and sustained within the community to provide phase-appropriate help in collaboration with other community efforts. Finally, data and documents relating to mental health activities should be accumulated, organized, and analyzed so that they can be shared, as appropriate, with other workers and key sanctioning groups. These individual data are useful for collaborative efforts in the immediate disaster relief activities, and aggregated data are useful for long-range community planning to prepare for future disasters.

The following example will illustrate and clarify some of the concepts and guidelines for action of the intervention model presented. This example is taken from the activities of a mental health team that intervened in the aftermath of the blizzard and tidal surge of February 16, 1978, in a community near Boston, Massachusetts.

Case Example: The Boston Blizzard, 1978

Basic Information. The storm set state records for snow accumulation in a twenty-four-hour period and for the most snow from one storm; it was also catalogued as the tenth worst disaster in United States history. The storm lasted thirty-three hours, with wind gusts of sixty-nine miles per hour inland and ninety-two miles per hour on Cape Cod. There was a violent, swirling northeast wind. Together with high tides, this wind resulted in major flooding that severely damaged many of the state's coastal communities. Twenty-eight persons died, over 2,250 were injured, and 450 were hospitalized during the blizzard. It was reported that 2,133 homes were destroyed, 9,000 homes were seriously damaged, and over 25,000 other homes were hurt to some degree by the flood. More than 30,000 people had to be evacuated from their homes, and many individuals were trapped in their cars for up to thirty-six hours.

Initial Action Plan. On the second day following the blizzard, a mental health team composed of professionals from different disciplines set about to coordinate its activities with personnel from other state and voluntary agencies. Initially, the mental health team's activities took place in emergency shelters that were organized for displaced persons. The mental health team's first objective, as soon as it entered the system of disaster assistance, was to establish links to the ongoing governmental group that had assembled the day before their arrival. It must be noted here that *entering a disaster assistance system necessitates crucial linkage activities.* This becomes the responsibility of one of the members of the group; a particular individual must take on the leadership role at this juncture and negotiate the conditions of collaborative efforts.

The blizzard and storm destroyed several neighborhoods

in the catchment area where I was the mental health director. Assuming the role as head of mental health operations in the disaster assistance program, I took full responsibility for organizing the mental health staff and linking it to other activities as they unfolded throughout the period covered by the postdisaster relief program. At the same time, I worked with staff and administrators in the state's Department of Mental Health to set up a small, rapid-decision-making mental health group, under state auspices, directly focused on the disaster response effort. In this case, the entrance of the mental health team into the disaster assistance system was facilitated by the fact that the mental health professionals had previously been practicing in the affected community. They were already linked to the Community Neighborhood Health Center, which was operating emergency and first-aid units in the shelter. They were also able to quickly establish a collegial relationship with the Red Cross workers, who welcomed their assistance. I introduced myself to the Red Cross senior staff and explained how the mental health professionals could be of assistance.

From this beginning, relationships were extended to include the official community representatives in the disaster area. These consisted of a representative of the mayor, a senior civil defense staff person, and representatives of state and federal disaster assistance agencies and various state human services agencies. The mental health professionals and these other individuals collaborated with and assisted one another in conducting a rapid needs assessment of community and individuals' problems.

A logistics plan for mental health intervention activities was developed and implemented in the first days following the disaster. It delineated the number of mental health professionals required, the shifts that would be covered, the location of the team, and the administrative procedures that would be followed. Means of communicating information and methods of decision making were agreed on by all the team members. Objectives were conceptualized and defined; collaborative mental health, general health, and social services first-aid assistance techniques were agreed upon. These were immediately communicated to the health team and Red Cross staff.

Early Intervention Activities. The mental health workers quickly developed a system of instruction, covering some of the characteristic mental disorder syndromes to be expected, for the staff of the health team and the Red Cross, since disaster victims were already being interviewed and assisted by these two groups. The members of the health team and the Red Cross would gather for sessions lasting fifteen to thirty minutes. Anxiety syndromes, depressive symptoms, and reactions of uncontrollable anger were explained to these professionals so that they could understand them as part of the expectable effects of disaster trauma. They were also told that they could manage individuals themselves or ask for assistance from the mental health professional.

In one instance, a mental health professional met with the senior members of the health unit and the Red Cross team in one of the small areas assigned to them in the shelter. They identified their areas of need for assistance. For example, one victim was identified as being a problem to the health officer. She was a forty-five-year old white, single female who kept coming to the health unit to ask for sleeping pills. She had lost all her belongings in the storm. She was at times incoherent and tearful and constantly paced around her cot. She could be calmed down for a few hours, but she would later return to the health unit in the same condition. The mental health worker used this opportunity to explain the symptoms and describe the process of crisis intervention. He established a procedure with the other workers on how to refer a person with this type of problem to the mental health team.

The mental health team also participated in direct, face-to-face therapeutic intervention with disaster victims outside the referral system. Members offered their time and energy to help individual victims who were exhibiting such critical symptoms as uncontrollable epileptic attacks, threatened miscarriages, drug and alcohol withdrawal, somatic equivalents of tension, acute anxiety states, and depressive syndromes.

During the first days, the triage model was used to divide needs into general health and mental health needs, physical problems, and housing needs. Professionals from the three units —mental and physical health, Red Cross, and housing allocation

—worked closely and interchangeably with the people who had congregated in the shelters, and they collaborated and kept the flow of needy people moving to the appropriate teams. If, for example, after talking with staff attending to housing needs, someone seemed to need psychological services, he would then be taken to the mental health team. Many rapid mental health interventions were given with a team member sitting next to an individual on a cot or sitting with a group of persons on the shelter floor. Mental health professionals would approach individuals who appeared upset, despondent, or anxious, offer to hear what they were "going through," and make a determination if any further help should be offered. If the individual needed a brief diagnostic intervention and he agreed to it, he would then be escorted to an area where a team member was on duty. This small area consisted of a corner of one room where a modicum of quiet and privacy made it possible to offer psychological diagnosis and time-limited counseling.

Phases of Reactions to Disasters and Sustaining Intervention Responses. There are three phases of postdisaster psychological and social reaction. Each phase lasts several days or weeks depending on the severity of trauma and loss.

Phase I: Three types of population needed the most immediate help during the first phase: ex-mental patients who didn't have their medication; drug and alcohol users unable to obtain their usual amounts of stimulants; and individuals who had no previous history of mental illness but who were decompensating under the intense stress. Mild sedatives and antidepressant medications were prescribed. Supportive therapy, ventilation, clarification, and guidance were the main psychological interventive processes used in the emergency shelters. For example, a married couple and the wife's brother asked to see the mental health worker. They were asking for help to rehospitalize the brother, who was an ex-patient discharged on medication several months ago. They felt they could not take care of him in their present situation, since their home had been partially demolished and they could not handle the patient anymore. They were given assistance and support to share and ventilate their feelings. It was suggested to them that if the wife's brother were closely monitored with his medication, and if a member of the team met with them daily while they were in the shelter, they might reconsider. They accepted this advice and, a few days later, decided to keep the ex-patient with them.

Phase II: The next two weeks presented opportunities to ascertain the degree and variety of postdisaster problems. Families were followed as they moved back to their damaged homes or into relocation housing. Emotional reactions multiplied, and new modalities of intervention were offered. Team members were deployed in the disaster relief centers throughout the city, so that they could continue their relationships with troubled individuals and the staffs of relief-assisting agencies. One difficult case involved a forty-nine-year-old man and a forty-seven-year-old woman who were the parents of fourteen children, ten of whom still lived in the house. The mother walked into the disaster relief center "to find out if I am going crazy." She felt as if her personality were changing, as if she were not the same, and she had heard that people were getting help in the center. She reported crying for hours and feeling depressed and said that she was not motivated to do anything and was unable to follow through with the normal operation of the home. Her social drinking had increased, and she was beginning to worry about it. She found herself drinking throughout the day and would occasionally resort to drinking when she had trouble sleeping.

The basement and first floor of the family's home had been severely damaged. She had rearranged the first floor in order to flood proof it; however, this had not been enough. Most of her complaints and expression of her difficulties centered on a husband who, five years ago, had had a stroke that resulted in his partial paralysis and difficulty with speech. Despite his disability, he wanted to control all the house repairs and the assistance money that they were getting from agencies. She felt that this was unrealistic, but she did not seem to know how to handle the situation. She was ambivalent about keeping him at home and began talking seriously about finding a nursing home for him. Her marital situation, already shaky, had become worse and she felt trapped. In the past, she had been able to function with strong realistic defenses and with support from her children. Now, everything seemed to be falling apart.

Crisis intervention helped this woman to reassess and re-evaluate her situation. By getting some relief through verbal expression of her feelings and then seeing the disaster relief agency respond appropriately by helping her to arrange for the repair of her home, she gained better control of her alcohol intake. She also recognized that it was her own internal feelings that were troubling her, and she started to work with the mental health worker to regain her ability to manage her daily life. She began to feel more positive about her ability to deal with her family. The mental health worker supported her in her difficult reality situation and was appreciative of her numerous skills. She became more assertive and more effective in dealing with her husband and her children.

Phase III: After the activities of the first three weeks of the postblizzard intervention came to an end, plans for the next six months had to be operationalized. The mental health team delineated a new interventive model for the follow-up period. Thus, teams of mental health professionals would be attached to various human services agencies in each community where disaster victims lived or had relocated and would have direct links to clinics of the Department of Mental Health. The teams would provide mental health crisis intervention services and would link people to the federal and local disaster relief agencies. Outreach and advocacy programs to assist individuals traumatized by their postdisaster living situations would be instituted. Longer-term psychological counseling would be mobilized to aid those in continuing difficulties.

One such case involved a fifty-six-year-old widow who had always lived in the beach area of the town. Five years ago, her husband had died, but she continued living alone in their home. Some weeks after the blizzard, she came into a local social agency. She was seen wringing her hands, she reported losing fifteen pounds in weight, and she looked agitated and cried very easily. She talked uninterruptedly for several hours. She was obsessed with the government's delay in processing her claim and with not being able to make choices or to get reimbursement for the repair workers assigned to her by the government agency to fix her house. Her stress symptoms seemed to parallel very much her dissatisfaction with the way the government officials were responding to her letters and phone calls. She complained that she had great difficulties in functioning and dealing with the relief agencies "because I don't have a man."

It was clear that the woman's dependency needs had overwhelmed her. Her defenses had been shaken by the stressors of the disaster and its aftermath, and she was still having episodes of mourning. She had a rather rigid and obsessive personality structure that did not allow her to deal with her rage and her anger. She felt that she did not know how to deal with a masculine world. The mental health worker was able to guide her through all the intricacies of dealing with the various assistance agencies to try to get more appropriate help. The worker also helped her to get back in touch with the good support system that she had, namely, a large local family and many close friends. The worker helped her recall the times when she and her husband were able to handle difficulties and thus rekindled her awareness of her own skills.

After six or seven visits, the woman appeared much better. But then she called the agency again, and, when she was visited at home, she looked exhausted and was agitated with pressure of speech. One of her problems was that "I have not paid my bills and people are expecting their money which I don't have." It appeared that her assistance check had been lost and some of the repair payments were delayed. The worker began to deal with the replacement of her assistance check and told her, "If you have not heard in two days, call me." The woman called a day or two later saying, "I could not wait any longer." She then walked to the agency and was able to begin to handle the problem in a realistic way. When she did receive her money a week later, she returned to her normal behavior.

A couple with a newborn baby made contact with the author at the local mental health center, asking mainly for concrete things. Although they were seen as rather manipulative, it became evident that they were unable to deal with all the intricacies of getting assistance. They were showing a flat affect, confusion, and depression. They asked for help with a family grant, a loan to repair their house, and some assistance from the

Catholic charities. They needed much help in clarification of the issues in order to plan their budget, to get assistance from the welfare department, and to use daycare for a child from the husband's first marriage. The young wife also needed help with baby care and with sibling issues. This family was able to use intervention and guidance. Mental health workers assisted them in linking with the appropriate community supports and agencies to get the help they needed.

An airline stewardess who walked into the disaster relief office was agitated, very bitter and angry, and asking for emotional support. She showed pressure of speech, inability to sit quietly and listen, constant tearing, and anxiety. The content of her speech was a preoccupation with the amount of damage done to her home. She had almost lost her life as she was being rescued; however, she denied many feelings about and memories of the experience. She felt that the insurance company was not moving fast enough and that her whole life was interfered with and disorganized. She wanted to ask for a leave of absence from her job because she was unable to deal with her emotions. She asked the mental health worker for a letter of recommendation for this leave because she was frightened to face her employer. She feared that she was going to break up with her boyfriend because she was exploding in such rage. She vacillated between feeling pressured and crying.

Even though the mental health worker made a schedule of appointments, the woman broke many of them and would come only when she was in a crisis or when her emotions were uncontrollable. Little by little, she seemed to calm down, but she was unable to use brief psychological help. The worker linked her to the services of a community mental health clinic.

As these plans for Phase III were translated into operations, it was essential that the community perceive the mental health workers as part of an overall effort to support, guide, and assist victims in recovering their former coping abilities. It was also important that the mental health workers assist community caregivers to find ways to approach the individual who was having trouble coping not as if he were sick—which might simply encourage him to adopt the role of "patient"—but as a person having expectable problems in a difficult situation. This view necessitated the adoption of a consistent educational approach in working with community caregivers, who tended to stereotype mental health workers as professionals who dealt only with illness and psychopathology. Mental health professionals must be skilled in establishing and value these community relationships in order to be accepted as collaborators by members of the other disaster assistance groups. Unless this professional link is well developed and functional, requests for mental health intervention assistance will diminish as the months elapse. Disaster victims will use the opportunities available for needed longer-term mental health services only if the services offered are made accessible to them and in settings without organizational or professional barriers.

Many variables need to be considered, within a coherent conceptual framework, to plan a crisis resolution strategy. The intervention model for postdisaster mental health services outlined in this chapter has aimed at systematic presentation of both direct and indirect procedures.

An individual first relies on his own familiar coping mechanisms following a disaster. If he is unable to master his stress reactions, he reaches out and tries to link to a source of community support. Hansell (1970) has described how an individual calls attention to his desperate needs; he will attempt to take advantage of all available resources, simultaneously and in a complementary manner.

Therapeutic intervention that gives immediate support and guidance offers the best potential resource for the disaster victim. A rapid evaluation has to be completed to ascertain the level of functioning of the individual, the length of time he has been in a postdisaster traumatic situation, and his most pressing needs. Then the mental health professional determines what resources are available to meet those immediate needs. During the later postdisaster recovery stages, different needs will emerge. In these stages, mental health professionals will require the knowledge and skills needed to assess the situation within a developmental frame of reference, so that they can match the problem with the appropriate resources. Coordination of different types of assistance—both concrete and psychological—characterizes this kind of crisis intervention. Although psychological assistance is under the direct control of the mental health professional, he participates indirectly in all the other types of postdisaster assistance through collaboration with other disaster relief agencies, both federal and local.

Continuation of needed mental health services requires certain outreach efforts on the part of mental health professionals, as well as long-term planning for these activities. Their crisis-oriented work continues as the affected population begins to deal again with daily life. It is essential to systematize the link between the postdisaster mental health teams and the formal mental health services system. This linkage will ensure continuing community mental health services for disaster victims suffering from severe emotional dysfunction. Finally, it is important to note that postdisaster crisis counseling cannot be practiced in the same way as therapy offered in a clinic or private office setting. The mental health professional must help disaster victims deal with their immediate physical and psychological problems and must quickly sort out the complicated life circumstances in which he finds the victims and assist them in planning to reconstruct their lives. Moreover, he must perform these tasks within the complex network of services deployed by governmental and voluntary agencies to aid these individuals. This is what makes the experience of disaster work a unique frontier and a unique challenge for mental health workers.

References

Ahearn, F. L., and Castellon, R. S. "Problemas de Salud Mental Despues de Una Situacion de Desastre." *Boletin,* 1978, *85,* 1-15.

Caplan, G. *Support Systems and Community Mental Health.* New York: Behavioral Publications, 1974.

Caplan, G. "Support Systems for Civilian Populations." In G. Caplan and M. Killilea (Eds.), *Support Systems and Mutual Help: Multidisciplinary Explorations.* New York: Grune & Stratton, 1976.

Cohen, R. E. "Postdisaster Mobilization of a Crisis Intervention Team: The Managua Experience." In H. J. Parad, H. L. P. Resnick, and L. G. Parad (Eds.), *Emergency and Disaster Management: A Mental Health Source Book.* Bowie, Md.: Charles Press, 1976.

Cohen, R. E., and Ahearn, F., Jr. *The Handbook for Mental Health Care of Disaster Victims.* Baltimore, Md.: Johns Hopkins University Press, 1980.

Disaster Relief Act, P.L. 93-288 (93rd Congress), 1974.

Dohrenwend, B. S., and Dohrenwend, B. P. *Stressful Life Events: Their Nature and Effects.* New York: Wiley, 1974.

Erikson, K. T. *Everything in Its Path.* New York: Simon & Schuster, 1976a.

Erikson, K. T. "Loss of Commonality at Buffalo Creek." *American Journal of Psychiatry,* 1976b, *133,* 302-304.

Frederick, C. J. "Violence and Disasters: Immediate and Long-Term Consequences." Paper presented at a working group conference on the psychosocial consequences of violence, sponsored by The Netherlands and the World Health Organization, April 1981.

Fritz, C. E., and Williams, H. B. "The Human Being in Disaster." *The Annals,* 1957, *309,* 42-51.

Hansell, N. "Decision Counseling Method: Expanding Coping at Crisis-in-Transit." *Archives of General Psychiatry,* 1970, *22,* 462-467.

Kliman, A. S. "The Corning Flood Project: Psychological First Aid Following a Natural Disaster." In H. J. Parad, H. L. P. Resnick, and L. G. Parad (Eds.), *Emergency and Disaster Management: A Mental Health Source Book.* Bowie, Md.: Charles Press, 1976.

Lifton, R. J. *Death in Life: Survivors of Hiroshima.* Los Angeles: S and S Enterprises, 1967.

Lindemann, E. "The Symptomatology and Management of Acute Grief." *American Journal of Psychiatry,* 1944, *101,* 141-148.

Lindemann, E. *Beyond Grief: Studies in Crisis Intervention.* (E. Lindemann, Ed.) New York: Jason Aronson, 1979.

Titchener, J. L., and Kapp, F. T. "Family and Character Change at Buffalo Creek." *American Journal of Psychiatry,* 1976, *133,* 295-299.

Tyhurst, J. S. "Individual Reactions to Community Disaster: The Natural History of Psychiatric Phenomena." *American Journal of Psychiatry,* 1951, *107,* 23-27.

Tyhurst, J. S. "The Role of Transition States–Including Disasters–in Mental Illness." In National Research Council (Ed.), *Symposium on Preventive and Social Psychiatry*. Washington, D.C.: U.S. Government Printing Office, 1957.

Chapter 17

Brief Family Crisis Therapy

Howard J. Parad

Crisis intervention, an important part of virtually all community mental health programs, is mistakenly regarded by some as a dangerous fad and by others as a panacea for the mental health problems of mankind. Still others, including myself, regard crisis intervention as just beginning to be systematically investigated as a promising approach toward helping individuals, families, small groups, and communities to cope with and master a wide variety of disequilibrating stresses (Parad, Resnik, and Parad, 1976; Brown, 1980).

This chapter provides an overview of selected aspects of theory and practice relating to an eclectic approach to brief family crisis intervention. My approach draws upon and updates certain features of the pioneering work that I carried out with Gerald Caplan and other colleagues at the Family Guidance Center of the Harvard School of Public Health in the early 1950s when both crisis intervention and family therapy were just getting underway (Parad and Caplan, 1965). In these early attempts, we had two general goals: (1) to reduce the impact of stress by immediate emotional and environmental first aid and (2) to strengthen the family in its adaptive and integrative efforts by what Redl (1959) has described as "clinical exploitation of life events" through on-the-spot interpretations and clarifications. Subsequent experience in crisis intervention interviews with families that were reacting to severe stress situations has highlighted the need for a clinical rationale and a technology for treating families in crisis.

Several interrelated professional and mental health policy developments have accompanied the ever-growing interest in brief family crisis intervention, including research into such subjects as coping behavior, precipitating stress factors, the use of time-limited and task-oriented problem solving, and waiting-list problems. Other developments include the depopulation of state mental hospitals, which has increased the need for emergency mental health services; recurrent personnel and financial constraints, as in the reluctance of insurance companies to reimburse vendors for long-term treatment; increased emphasis on evaluation, accountability, and related cost-benefit issues; concern about client dropouts; growing awareness of the relevance of crisis intervention services to certain ethnic groups; the contributions of the newer behavioral, humanistic, and other eclectic perspectives to problem-solving and action-oriented coping repertoires; and of course, the enormously accelerated increase in family-oriented therapies (Pardes and Pincus, 1981).

The development of family therapy has been reviewed by Sherman (1979). Mental health professionals are increasingly turning to family therapy as a means of helping to solve problems in psychosocial functioning. The frequency with which papers on family therapy are presented at meetings of mental health professionals, the growing number of centers offering training in family dynamics, and the evident congeniality of both the technique and the approach with the principles associated with the community mental health movement all indicate that family therapy is firmly established in the practice technologies of mental health professionals. Also important is the burgeoning interest in nonkinship support networks and other group social systems. Crisis intervention personnel are now more aware of these systems and have begun to enlarge their thinking about the crisis experience and the use of the family system as a therapeutic context (Speck and Attneave, 1973; Rueveni, 1975).

Time Limits

Since this chapter presents a brief, time-limited approach to family crisis intervention, I want to consider brief therapy in general and time limits in particular. Crisis intervention services are usually brief, but as indicated below, not all brief therapy is to be equated with crisis intervention. Crisis intervention may involve a specific or approximate number of interviews or weeks of treatment as part of the treatment arrangement. Several rationales have been offered for the desirability of time limits in therapy. One commonly advanced argument is that time limits may increase the client's and the worker's motivation. The question of how brief is brief treatment, while seemingly simple, is actually very complex. Some consider brief treatment to consist of a single session, others think it should involve about six sessions, while still others define brief therapy as extending up to twenty or even forty interviews. A nationwide study of crisis-oriented treatment in family services and children's psychiatric services demonstrated that from 80 to 90 percent of all planned short-term cases were seen for up to twelve interviews over a period of up to three months (Parad and Parad, 1968). A planned short-term treatment (PSTT) approach involves the preplanning of a specific number of interviews or weeks of treatment within the first or second session with the client or family.

Bloom (1980) recently reviewed a number of studies concerning PSTT. Citing the benefits of brief crisis-oriented therapy, he argues that "an hour spent with the client at the time of crisis has the same potential benefit as perhaps ten hours spent with that same client after that enhanced state of readiness to change has passed" (p. 114). Bloom suggests that the renewal of interest in PSTT has been influenced by at least three developments: issues relating to efficiency, changing concepts and approaches to psychotherapy, and the conclusion drawn by many researchers that PSTT is generally as effective as long-term and open-ended treatment is and often even more effective.

A census of family service agencies concluded that planned short-term treatment is generally cost effective, thus suggesting that PSTT not only can reduce the number of dropouts from treatment but can improve treatment outcomes in less time than that involved in traditional open-ended services (Beck and Jones, 1973). In a perceptive article on the historical background and future of brief psychotherapy, Marmor (1979) concludes that "the trend of the future can be expected to be toward short-term therapies" (p. 149). This position is supported by an in-depth review of research on brief and crisis-oriented therapies that concludes that "comparative studies of brief and unlimited therapies show essentially no difference in results" (Butcher and Koss, 1978, p. 758).

The issue of time and timing is now a moot question in crisis counseling. There seems to be general agreement, based on practice-derived wisdom, that there should be early access to help and that help is best timed at the onset of a crisis experience. But such issues as how many contacts there should be, how they should be spaced, and for what duration for each individual, family, or other small group are less settled. Mental health practice tends to be flexible and is often based on matters of expediency as well as on the style and temperament of practitioners. There seems to be no magic in the six-week pattern of crisis first suggested by Caplan, although in a nationwide study six was the modal number of interviews used in PSTT crisis-oriented programs (Parad and Parad, 1968). There are, of course, many variations in practice, from marathon groups to once-a-week sessions over six to twelve weeks. Any additional light on the optimal number, frequency, and spacing of treatment contacts would be useful to those interested in both crisis intervention and brief therapy.

The paradigm presented in Table 1 attempts to clarify the use of the crisis approach and the structured use of time in mental health practice. As indicated in this paradigm, the following are four logical service categories with respect to the dimensions of crisis and time:

1. PSTT crisis-oriented services (much crisis intervention work would fall within this cell).
2. Non-PSTT crisis-oriented services (the crisis may afford an entry into open-ended and long-term therapy).
3. PSTT noncrisis-oriented services (many forms of brief ther-

Table 1. Use of the Crisis Approach and the Time Dimension in Mental Health Practice.

	PSTT	*Non-PSTT*
Crisis Oriented	1. Early accessibility at time of request for help (within twenty-four to seventy-two hours of the "cry for help") 2. Use of PSTT limits (specific number or approximate range of interviews or weeks—determined at intake—to be utilized during crisis response and resolution phases) 3. Use of task-centered techniques 4. Focused attention to crisis configuration (precipitating event, perception of threat, response, and resolution) (++)	1. Early accessibility at time of request for help (within twenty-four to seventy-two hours of the "cry for help") 2. Open-ended orientation toward time dimension; duration of contact may be informally brief (no time contract made during intake phase, that is, first or second interviews; or contact may be "long-term": crisis intervention may be regarded primarily as point of entry into an extended treatment service 3. Some attention to elements of crisis configuration (+–)
Noncrisis Oriented	1. May be short or long waiting period 2. Use of PSTT limits: contract for specific predetermined number of interviews, determined at intake 3. Use of task-centered or goal-oriented techniques 4. No special attention to crisis configuration (–+)	1. May be short or long waiting period 2. Open-ended orientation toward time dimension; no use of PSTT limits 3. No special attention to crisis configuration 4. May be oriented to specific or diffuse goals (––)

apy are offered in human service programs; see Budman, 1981).

4. Services that are neither PSTT nor crisis-oriented.

This paradigm clarifies a point all too frequently confused by many practitioners, namely, that not all brief service programs are oriented to a crisis framework and not all crisis-oriented pro-

programs are geared exclusively to brief service, let alone to planned short-term approaches.

Family Crisis Therapy

Crisis workers are now attracted to a variety of family therapy modalities. Family crisis intervention is useful in solving problems of psychosocial functioning during an acutely stressful period experienced by a relatively intact family, as well as during an acute eruption of stress within a chronically disordered family. Of course, in the latter instance, only one member of the disordered family may be presented as the emotionally disturbed or mentally ill "identified patient." Family-oriented crisis intervention is practiced in a broad spectrum of outpatient psychiatric clinics, as well as in institutional settings, including crisis hostels, halfway houses, and detention facilities. It may also be the treatment of choice for mentally disordered persons decompensating after discharge from a state hospital.

A number of researchers have inquired into experimental crisis-oriented and time-limited programs in hospitals, psychiatric clinics, family service agencies, police departments, protective services, and other human service settings. From the perspectives of psychiatry and social work, Langsley and Kaplan (1968) combined the elements of time limits, family therapy, and crisis intervention into an action-research project that produced an effective alternative to hospitalization (Langsley, Machotka, and Flomenhaft, 1971; Langsley, 1980). Liberal use of referrals to other social services helped to link the family with an ongoing social support system, thus affording continuity of care. In addition, psychotropic medication was used with appropriate medical and nursing supervision. The identified patient was often considered the family's spokesperson, and his or her behavior was defined as the family's way of crying out for help at a time of crisis (Langsley and Kaplan, 1968).

Also noteworthy is the research reported by Rubinstein (1972), who found that by mobilizing family support, a mental health team was generally able to help resolve the patient's crisis without resorting to hospitalization. Rubinstein's approach also stresses the concept that the family should and can share responsibility for the patient's treatment. Other investigators have similarly emphasized that crisis intervention works best when "the family is the patient," even though we are a long way from determining when it is most efficacious to see the family together and when one should work primarily with the identified patient (Langsley, 1972).

Moreover, I must emphasize that the full benefits of family-oriented crisis intervention programs can be realized on a long-range basis only when outpatient clinical services are supplemented and reinforced by adequate community support systems that include properly supervised psychotropic medication; employment and job-training opportunities; income maintenance provisions; a spectrum of housing resources (independent living arrangements, halfway houses, crisis hostels, foster care, and other residential facilities geared to the individual's rehabilitation potential); and involvement of families and significant others in the person's social network. Current experience offers overwhelming evidence for the need to plan for easy-access community crisis programs and for the above-mentioned community care and support services prior to, rather than after, the discharge of large numbers of patients from state mental hospitals (Yarvis, 1975). As for criteria for case selection, families with chronic disturbances, as well as those with acute problems, have apparently been helped by crisis-oriented approaches. In my pragmatic view, the question of criteria has more to do with clients' needs, therapeutic goals, and the mental health worker's stance than with clinical diagnostic labels.

Conceptual Framework

Having reviewed the elements of time and crisis and the relevance of family crisis intervention for community mental health programming and practice, I will now present a framework for viewing the family in crisis. This framework derives from a preliminary paradigm developed with colleagues at the Family Guidance Center at the Harvard School of Public Health in order to further the center's goal of studying how families cope with selected stress situations (prematurity, congenital abnormality, the birth of twins, and so on) commonly encountered and routinely reported in public health programs (Parad and Caplan, 1965). The framework has been found useful in studies of family functioning in its relationship to mental health. In this conceptual framework, data about family functioning are analyzed under the following basic classifications:

First, in relation to the structural and functional parts of family life, we attend to three interdependent subsystems: value orientations, communication styles, and role networks. Collectively, these comprise the family's *life-style.* Values, like family rules, are usually implicit, not explicit. They refer to shared premises, commonly held beliefs, and attitudes about what is to be cherished, how much, and in what order, and they thus influence the family's allocation of time, money, status, and affectional rewards. What the family thinks and believes influences another interdependent part of the family system, namely, the family's communication style.

Assessment of family communication style reveals what messages are important enough to be transmitted and received, as well as how they are transmitted. The degree of importance attached to each message unit is determined by the family members' value orientations. Some families are relatively comfortable in expressing angry and judgmental feelings but much less comfortable in expressing the tender feelings that these angry feelings often mask. In many families, analysis of recurrent uproars often reveals that overdetermined hostile expressions mask areas of tenderness and extreme vulnerability.

The last interrelated subsystem pertains to the role network. Who expects what of whom? Who does what? This subsystem of reciprocal expectations and loyalties mediates the value subsystem, that is, what people feel and believe, along with the communication network subsystem, that is, what messages and signals are considered worth sending and how they are sent. Overtly? Covertly? And with what combination of words, symbols, and nonverbal gestures?

Second, *intermediate problem-solving mechanisms* are coping devices triggered by the actual impact of crisis. They are called intermediate to emphasize the temporary dynamic nature of processes in flux, as compared with the relative stability of family life-style. Intermediate mechanisms are various transactional, interactional, and intrapersonal methods for coping with the emotional difficulties associated with stress. These may be negative—scapegoating, emotional neglect, and so on—or positive, such as use of family and neighborhood social network resources, and adequate worry and grief work. Above all, these mechanisms are a series of attempts at problem solving through trial and error. In dealing with dysfunctional and disordered families, the clinician's role is to point out that faulty mechanisms involving "error" are often repeatedly used despite the great pain and discomfort that they produce in family members and the identified patient.

Third, *the need-response pattern* affords a dynamic assessment of the mental health of an individual family member within the context of family interaction processes, thereby furnishing a conceptual linkage between family functioning and the individual's mental health. Several basic human needs are considered relevant to mental health, including love for one's own sake, a balance between support and independence with respect to tasks, a balance between freedom and control with respect to instinctual expression, and the availability of suitable role models. In studying the response to these categories of need, one can observe three separate but interlocking phases: (1) the *perception* of the individual's needs by other family members and by the culture of the family; (2) the *respect* accorded to these needs as being worthy of attention; and (3) the *satisfaction* of such needs to the extent possible in the light of available family resources. The need-response pattern, which may be altered during a period of crisis, becomes an instrument for assessing the family solution of problems posed by the crisis. In research terms, family life-style elements may be considered as antecedent variables, intermediate problem-solving mechanisms as intervening variables, and the need-response pattern with its triad of perception, respect, and satisfaction of needs as a consequent or outcome variable.

My main thesis is that important changes occur in the

family during a crisis period with respect to the future mental and social functioning of individual family members and the family as a group. Thus, as outlined in Table 2, the need-response pattern may be approximately the same (T4) as that which prevailed prior to the crisis (T4b); it may be at a lower level when the crisis adversely affects the family (T4c); or it may reflect a higher level of functioning (T4a) when the response to crisis is in terms of challenge and opportunity rather than just danger.

The crisis intervention worker's basic task is to help family members change those affective (feeling), cognitive (thinking), and behavioral (doing) patterns that hinder effective value clarification and rule making, as well as to encourage constructive communication and appropriate role behavior. I thus find it essential to develop a judiciously eclectic approach that attends to these domains of human functioning (feeling, thinking, and doing) in order to help family members mobilize the resources that will unblock and enhance performance in these vital areas. Recent publications indicate that eclecticism, while perhaps regarded pejoratively in some quarters, is a fact of the mental health professional's life (Jayaratne, 1978; Lazarus, 1976). Sherman (1977) refers to the impact of scientific eclecticism by saying that "a cloudburst of valuable concepts has pelted innovators in family treatment" (p. 437).

In practice, most crisis intervention workers are probably eclectic. Although they may not formally label their theoretical orientations as eclectic, they pragmatically recognize that (1) no single theory exists to explain all clinical phenomena, nor is such a theory ever likely to exist; (2) different clinical approaches—or different "eclectic" blends—work well with different clients; and (3) different approaches may be used with the same client at different times. In my opinion, then, a disciplined eclecticism utilizing psychodynamic, humanistic, and behavioral theories and techniques can facilitate a new synthesis of interlocking modes of clinical intervention. However, unraveling the puzzle of what makes people change and what makes some people responsive to some approaches and not others is beyond the scope of the present chapter.

Utilizing an eclectic approach to family therapy, Steidl

Table 2. Theoretical Framework for Viewing Families in Crisis

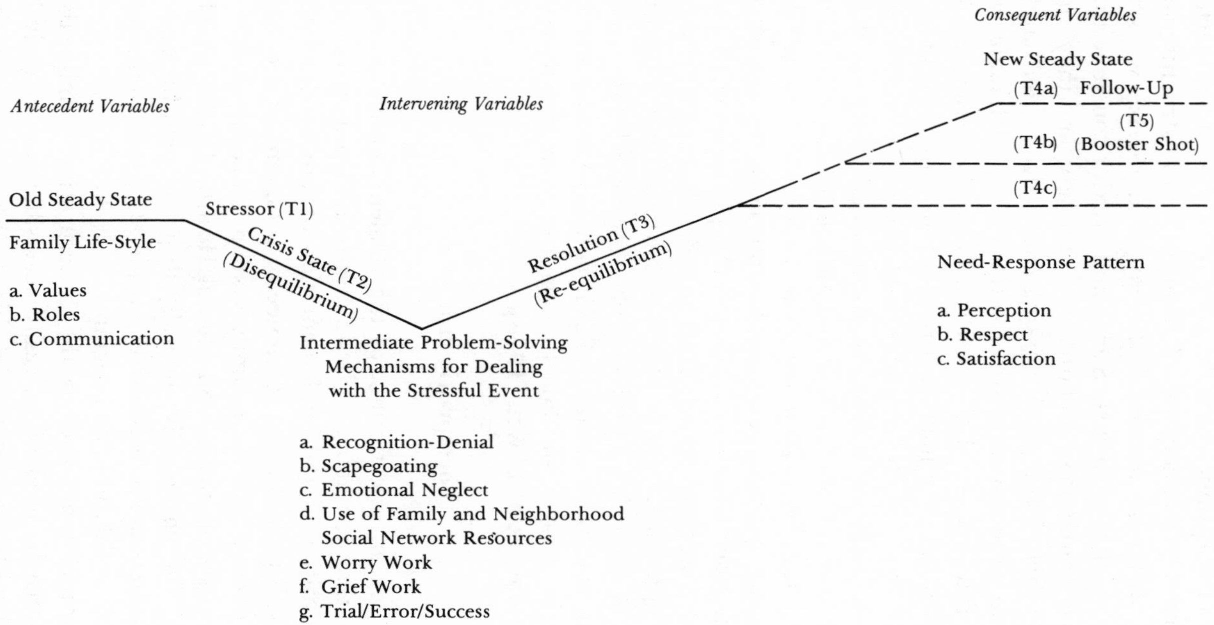

Note:

T1 = Impact of Stressor (Stress Perception)
T2 = Crisis (Upset) State (Stress Response)
T3 = Resolution/Recovery Phase
T4 = New Steady State (or New Equilibrium, T4a, T4b, or T4c)
T5 = Follow-Up (Booster Shot)

and Wexler (1977) underscore the need for different approaches because there are so many varied forms of family structure and pathology, different forms of therapy, and diverse ways in which human change occurs. Steidl and Wexler conclude that there is no overarching or metatheory of therapy, and they urge clinicians to "develop a good working knowledge of the variety of models in order to do justice to the variety of families we see" in clinical practice (1977, p. 195). In their overview, Steidl and Wexler outline the main features of four important models of family therapy: (1) the communication approach, emphasizing cognitive and affective themes, as exemplified in the work of Watzlawick and his associates at the Mental Research Institute in Palo Alto, California (Watzlawick and others, 1967); (2) the psychodynamic approach, also emphasizing cognitive and affective themes, especially those related to loss phenomena, as illustrated by the work of Paul (1976) and Framo (1965); (3) the structural approach, emphasizing behavioral and affective themes, as in Minuchin's problem-solving approach (Minuchin, 1974; Minuchin and Fishman, 1981); and (4) the systems approach, relying heavily on didactic cognitive themes and exemplified by the work of Bowen (1978).

Therapeutic Principles

Utilizing an eclectic mix of the elements noted above, I will now outline a number of basic interrelated principles concerning the initiation and implementation of family crisis intervention. I will make special reference to problems of mentally disordered persons and their family systems since, according to the President's Commission on Mental Health (1978a, 1978b) problems of the chronically mentally ill person and his or her significant others are now priority considerations in community mental health legislation and programs.

Of prime importance is the concept that family crisis treatment must be immediate, easily accessible, and effectively coordinated with early and quick biopsychosocial assessment. In other words, the traditional approach of prolonged history taking and extended diagnostic study is quite contrary to the crisis approach. In traditional long-term modalities the clinician may typically elicit information from "healthy" family members about the "ill" patient. There is often an implicit expectation aroused in family members that the expert ("doctor-magician") will provide a solution to the family's problem and rid it of either the deviant behavior or the person causing it.

By definition, the crisis worker makes a strong commitment to treating the family as a group—as a small-scale social system—often in the natural social habitat of the home setting. With rare exceptions involving the very high-risk suicidal or homicidal person, outpatient family crisis therapy is regarded as a far more desirable treatment alternative than hospitalization. Ideally, the family, not the identified patient, is the client.

The disordered behavior of the identified patient is conceptualized as a cry for help, representing the result of blocked communication, of absence of warm contact, or of lack of subgroup alliances among family members; the patient's presenting problem is regarded as a reflection of treatable problems in family interaction.

The worker confronts the family with the main cognitive, affective, and behavioral tasks that must be addressed and offers advice on how to carry them out. The worker makes liberal use of contracts, encouraging working agreements among family members to deal with problems through a here-and-now interactional approach. He uses a variety of eclectic techniques, including sculpting, psychodrama, modeling, and whatever else might work.

Well before the end of the first interview, the worker is likely to plan a second session, either in his office or the patient's home. In order to gain the family's collaboration, he seeks sanction from the family power figure, perhaps one of the parents, a grandparent, or an older sibling. He reviews goals and specific means for reaching them; encourages feedback concerning what has been accomplished thus far; negotiates regarding family members' expectations; makes sure that homework assignments are clear, relevant, and achievable; and, mindful of the power of the self-fulfilling prophecy, arouses hopeful expectancies to help the family improve its functioning.

To recapitulate, this framework involves antecedent (family life-style) variables, intervening (intermediate problem-solving) variables, and consequent (need-response) variables as an approach to the observation, study, and treatment of the family in crisis. Follow-up interviews (T5 in the theoretical framework presented in Table 2) can have a reenforcing effect and thus enhance the new postcrisis need-response pattern, provide feedback to increase consumer input into crisis-oriented mental health delivery systems, afford a safeguard in case the time limits used were not adequate for the family's needs, and aid systematic research on cost effectiveness and other issues.

When family crisis intervention is implemented, the following specific steps should be taken, along with appropriate efforts at involving family members in each stage: (1) search for the precipitating event and its perceptual meaning to the family members; (2) look for the coping means used by the family and appraise the extent to which these have or have not been successful; (3) search for alternative ways of coping and the resources that might improve the situation, while actively soliciting suggestions from family members; (4) review and support the family members' efforts to cope in new ways, with evaluation of results in terms of day-to-day living experiences; (5) assist toward the early termination that has been planned in the initial contract with the family; and (6) plan and conduct a follow-up or booster-shot session. Throughout this process, the family worker actively defines the goals of the family crisis session and the means that can be used for goal achievement. The worker must energetically focus on the relevant issues and attend to the stages outlined above.

Influenced by the communications and psychodynamic orientations as well as by Bowen's (1978) systemic concepts relating to family fusion and individual autonomy, I am, on the basis of my assessment of the family, active, planfully directive, goal-oriented, selectively risk-taking, and often assume a problem-solving stance similar to Minuchin's (1974) approach to structural family therapy.

Case Examples

An excerpt from the case history of the A family illustrates my theoretical perspectives on family values, roles, and communication as systemic focuses in short-term crisis intervention.

> The A family consisted of Sam, nineteen, a younger sister, three older brothers, his mother, and his father. Mrs. A earned more money than her husband, a source of some concern. The three older brothers, who as adolescents had serious problems with drugs, wore long hair and had trouble with the law; all had finally moved almost next door to the parental home to settle down with their wives and raise families. This is an enmeshed family illustrating Bowen's (1978) theory of the undifferentiated ego mass, with all four sons working with the mother in a small family business.
>
> Sam had been rushed to a local hospital after taking all the pills he could find in his mother's medicine chest. This was Sam's *seventh* suicidal attempt through overdosing. Mother had just given Sam a job in the family business, and when Sam did not behave responsibly, mother angrily threatened that Sam would be fired. This precipitated Sam's suicidal gesture. Immediately after ingesting the pills, Sam called a hot line. Unfortunately, the line was busy. Fortunately, he had enough presence of mind to call a local clergyman, a friend of the family, who immediately came to the house and rushed Sam to the hospital where his stomach was pumped. Sam's parents were interviewed by hospital staff only as sources of information for history-taking purposes.
>
> A few days after Sam's brief stay in the hospital, I initiated family crisis therapy with Sam, his parents, and his younger sister. After an initial period of anxious mumbling, Sam began to open up in

response to a sculpting exercise in which he was asked to portray his father and mother in relation to himself (Papp, 1976). His first sculpting exercise placed father in a mildly threatening position, with father's fist near Sam's head. Impressed by Sam's beginning efforts at communication, father responded surprisingly by saying, "I'll show you the way it really is; in your eye, I think you view me this way," and proceeded to resculpt the family interaction by making his hand into claws menacing his son's throat. When asked how this felt, Sam was at first quiet, but in response to my insistence, brought out his anger against father and his feeling that mother passes the ammunition to father, who then shoots it at him. In the ensuing flooding of emotion, father began crying, saying that he and Sam had a long history of fighting and he wanted to end the battle. Sam said, "You always notice what I do that is bad, not when I do something that is good." In an attempt at *value clarification,* I asked for a discussion of the good/bad issue. Mother said, "My idea of your being good is when you are concerned with us; you're bad when you are concerned with you." I concentrated on this kind of value confrontation for several minutes. It was clear Sam's need for autonomy paralleled father's need for freedom to be himself and plot his own direction in life.

In relation to the *communication subsystem,* I encouraged open expression of feelings, and father was able gradually to become much less judgmental in his approach toward his son, validating son's desire for self-direction. In this interview, mother was not able to validate her son's feelings beyond a few cliché responses.

In relation to *role patterning,* it was obvious that expectations were not clear as to who does what. Sam's abortive efforts at going to a local college were frowned upon because the college he had attended was not his parents' choice. When asked directly what he wanted to do, he told his parents, "to carry out my wishes, not yours!" In subsequent discussions, it became obvious that Sam was in part acting out his father's anger against his mother. His suicidal attempt was formulated as a *cry for help* regarding his wish that he simply not be. We discussed how Sam had turned his anger against himself instead of expressing it directly. Did Sam think he was so bad he had to destroy himself?

Attempts at crisis resolution culminated in a series of integrative problem-solving discussions relating to Sam's proclaimed need to carry out his own wishes to leave home and enroll in a college to pursue his studies and grow up. I supported Sam in his struggle for individuation, and I modeled for the parents how they, too, could encourage Sam in his new efforts at independence.

Especially noteworthy is the fact that Sam's family was not included in Sam's hospital treatment plan, even though the family would have been responsive to an outreach effort. I attempted to move family functioning away from pseudointegration, which had involved the parents in an unhealthy, wavering alliance against the children, toward a more facilitating and validating type of integration that would lead to greater recognition of Sam's growing autonomy. In a later discussion, while encouraging the parents to deal directly with their own mid-life transitional crises, I emphasized the similarity between the developmental tasks with which the adolescent was struggling and those with which the parents were struggling; I was thus working actively toward intergenerational problem solving. However, as is typical in brief family crisis intervention (perhaps also in long-term family treatment?), I was willing to settle for limited, but positive goals.

The second case briefly illustrates crisis intervention with a family where the identified patient, Anna K., had been hospitalized with a diagnosis of paranoid schizophrenia.

The K family consisted of the identified patient, Mrs. Anna K, age thirty-four, born in Hungary, from a strongly religious background; her son

Tom, nine, from her previous marriage; and her common-law husband, Herb, thirty-five, also divorced, self-described as a "backsliding" Irish-Catholic whose parents were both alcoholics.

Videotaped demonstration interviews were held in front of selected staff members at a state hospital (just prior to Mrs. K's anticipated release to home) in order to demonstrate the relevance of a family crisis approach to the community mental health aftercare program to which Mrs. K was being discharged. Mr. K and their son, Tom, had *not* been previously seen by hospital staff, although they had been visiting Mrs. K daily during the ten-day period of her hospitalization! Mrs. K had responded well enough to psychotropic medication and the protective milieu of the hospital to be ready for a trial visit. Mrs. K began the interview by explaining that about two weeks ago, she had begun to feel anxious and overwhelmed and was afraid that the "force" (from the movie "Star Wars") would harm her. She had experienced a psychotic episode about two years ago at the time of her divorce. To cope with her fears, she sobbingly revealed, she had called a friend who told her not to let her imagination take over. She then tried to cope by drinking coffee and smoking cigarettes to calm her nerves, but these attempts were to no avail. Despairing, she then tore off all her clothes, screamed at her terrified son Tom, ran out of the house, and with a bright red lipstick scribbled "HELP!" on her car's windshield, literally crying for help; clearly she was experiencing an intense emotional crisis of abandonment.

Detailed discussion with Herb and Anna revealed that just prior to this episode, there had been terrible fights between them because Herb had been dating another woman. Anna, according to Herb, had been sexually unresponsive and generally distant, though Herb really loved her. He said he couldn't communicate with her, and Anna said, "You never try!" The following is a brief interview excerpt:

Herb [to Anna]: I try, but you don't listen.

Anna: I put my faith in the Lord.

Herb: [angrily] That's a lot of crap, and you know it!

Therapist: Herb, you said when you were a kid, your parents would drink and fight?

Herb: Yes, you better believe it, and they would throw me and my brother and sister out of the room. Nothing ever got settled.

Therapist: Are you repeating the same patterns?

Herb: I don't understand—how do you mean?

Therapist: I mean the pattern of being excluded.

Anna: [touching Tom tenderly] Herb drinks and smokes pot when he's angry and stays away from me.

Therapist: [observing Anna who is hugging and looking at Tom while talking to Herb] Anna, are you aware of what you're doing?

Anna became aware she is attending to Tom as Herb is talking to her. And Herb immediately noticed that Anna did not make eye contact while talking to him. Anna smiled inappropriately.

Herb: [surprised] Anna, you don't even look at me!

Subsequent discussions focused on the couple's *communication* pattern and the *triangulation* that was occurring and how Herb felt shut out. He then related how depressed that made him and how he would handle his feelings by drinking, pot smoking, and going out with other women. But, he repeated, he loves Anna and Tom, and doesn't want to break up the family.

In response to the worker's interpretation of how Anna and Herb hurt each other ("we often hurt the very ones we love the most"), Anna and Herb engaged in a tender dialogue, embraced, cried, and poignantly discussed plans for the future.

In another discussion, we talked about how Tom, confused by the events that had preceded Anna's hospitalization, had blamed himself for mother's illness, asking if he had been "bad." Herb, talking directly to Tom, explained that Tom had nothing to do with mother's illness, and Tom visibly relaxed.

Hospital staff agreed on carrying out a bio-psychosocial plan with the K family, including continued medication for Mrs. K with supervision by the public health nurse; conjoint interviews with Anna and Herb by the community care social worker to maintain good communication between them—specifically to avoid the feeling of being shut out (to which both Herb and Anna were vulnerable); and family interviews (including Tom) to encourage shared recreational and social activities for the family as a group.

In the treatment encounter, there should be a balance of support and confrontation to help achieve the goal of action-oriented problem solving at a time of family crisis. The focus is often—but not always—on planned short-term contracting, on setting specific and achievable goals, on clarifying who will do what, on the use of homework assignments between interviews, and on an exploration of reasons for success and failure in carrying out homework tasks. Flexibly spaced interviews are arranged to support completion of the treatment contracts. Follow-up interviews frequently have a booster-shot effect during the postcrisis period. Keeping in mind the life cycle through which the family evolves, the therapist focuses on marital, parent-child, and sibling subsystems, in addition to viewing the family system as a whole.

Community Care

In response to the continuing depopulation of state mental hospitals, there have been a number of innovative attempts to apply a family-oriented crisis approach to the community care of mentally disordered persons. The Southwest Denver Mental Health Service affords a promising example of this trend by using rapid tranquilization, offering nonhospital care through family sponsors (who are on the payroll of the Southwest Denver Center), making frequent home visits, drawing upon a large cadre of volunteers, arranging special homes for constant observation in the case of acutely psychotic or suicidal or potentially dangerous clients, and operating within a social system framework rather than following a purely psychodynamic ideology (Polak, 1978). In this attempt at creatively designing family-oriented care of the mentally disordered, hospitalization gives way to a community system of carefully selected family settings. Mechanic (1980) has emphasized the need for comprehensive systems of service to aid the family in meeting crises relating to mental disorder. We urgently need further models that incorporate the social system perspectives of Jones and Polak (1968) and utilize the techniques developed by family crisis workers who are comfortable working with the emotionally disturbed and mentally disordered in their own homes or in substitute community settings.

There is also great need for further training and administrative changes if the family-oriented community programs suggested here are to achieve fruition. There are formidable obstacles. First, I have often encountered resistance from senior staff members toward work with families. Often cast in the role of rebels, new staff members may have to fight to be allowed to do family crisis intervention. Second, involving families at the time they request hospitalization or rehospitalization of the identified patient is particularly difficult in the face of bureaucratic opposition—overt or covert (Framo, 1976). Yet, at times, the initial process of family involvement can be extremely simple.

I recently learned about the typical practices followed by different staff members in a university-sponsored outpatient emergency clinic that serves large numbers of emotionally disturbed and mentally disordered persons who are variously self-referred, brought in handcuffed by the police, or shepherded into the crowded emergency waiting room by anxious family members. In one situation, for example, a senior staff member would emerge from his office, ask the nurse, "Who is the next patient?" and proceed to interview that person alone in his office, even though the patient had been accompanied to the emergency room by his significant others. (Or, as in the case of Sam, staff may view other family members primarily as sources of background information rather than as collaborative agents of change.) In dramatic contrast, however, a young staff member, trained in the techniques of family crisis intervention, would request that all members of the family who were with the identified patient accompany him to the office to discuss and deal with the *family* problem. Quite a contrast! Differences in therapeutic ideology are immediately reflected in therapists' initial approaches to the family.

Ongoing family crisis intervention with emotionally upset and mentally disordered individuals, and particularly with the psychotic-level family, is not easy work. Constantly expected to give sustenance as they implement the concept of the social support system, family crisis interveners themselves need support. For, as we well know, there are mental health hazards in this work. To cope with them, staff members need opportunities for respite, for additional training and supervision, for staff development seminars, and for a favorable work milieu in which they can share their clinical experiences, both their failures and their successes.

Drawing on my early work in family-oriented crisis intervention with Gerald Caplan and other Harvard colleagues, I have attempted to update the conceptual framework and family crisis intervention principles that characterize my present approach to families in crisis. I have outlined an approach that relies on the structured use of time limits; the understanding of family dynamics within a systems perspective; the use of the family life-style concept, with attention to its three components (values, roles, and communication); the appreciation of the intervening problem-solving mechanisms used by families to cope with crisis events; and the relevance of the need-response pattern as a way of measuring the success of these coping efforts. Finally, I have outlined the use of various action therapy techniques within an eclectic framework aimed at dealing with the cognitive, affective, and behavioral components that comprise the phenomenology of crisis intervention.

I conclude with the hope that mental health professionals will undertake the research so urgently needed in the field of family crisis intervention. While such intervention is increasingly employed in dealing with mental health emergencies in outpatient, inpatient, and community care services, it is unfortunate that the Langsley-Kaplan (1968) project and a few other studies, such as the inquiry into short-term family therapy outcomes (Parsons and Alexander, 1973), remain exceptional. Most of the literature offers descriptions of programs and techniques rather than well-designed research aimed at systematic, scientific study of such persistent problems as the criteria for seeing the family as a group, the relevance of ethnic and other sociocultural factors, differences between those families who accept and those who decline family crisis therapy, the types of skills and worker temperaments associated with the effective recruitment of families into ongoing family crisis intervention, and—perhaps above all—specification of treatment methods that will lead to adaptive crisis coping and improved need-response patterns. This field badly needs objective, differential measurement of the efficacy of outpatient family crisis approaches as compared with other therapeutic modalities, both inpatient and outpatient, including individual-centered and long-term therapy for persons in crisis. More specifically, we need to focus on the relationship of such variables as immediacy of treatment, frequency of interviews, degree of family involvement, and type of treatment approach to outcome (Umana and others, 1980). And ideally, longitudinal studies could profitably investigate how treated families, as compared with untreated ones, cope with future crises.

References

Beck, D. F., and Jones, M. A. *Progress on Family Problems.* New York: Family Service Association of America, 1973.

Bloom, B. L. "Social and Community Interventions." *Annual Review of Psychology,* 1980, *31,* 111-142.

Bowen, M. *Family Therapy in Clinical Practice.* New York: Jason Aronson, 1978.

Brown, V. "The Community in Crisis." In G. Jacobson (Ed.), *New Directions for Mental Health Services: Crisis Intervention in the 1980s,* no. 6. San Francisco: Jossey-Bass, 1980.

Budman, S. D. (Ed.). *Forms of Brief Therapy.* New York: Guilford Press, 1981.

Butcher, J. N., and Koss, M. P. "Research on Brief and Unlimited Therapies." In S. L. Garfield and A. E. Bergin (Eds.), *Handbook of Psychotherapy and Behavior Change.* New York: Wiley, 1978.

Framo, J. "Rationale and Techniques of Intensive Family Therapy." In I. Boszormenyi-Nagy (Ed.), *Intensive Family Therapy.* New York: Harper & Row, 1965.

Framo, J. "Chronicle of a Struggle to Establish a Family Unit Within a Community Mental Health Center." In P. Guerin (Ed.), *Family Therapy.* New York: Gardner Press, 1976.

Jayaratne, S. "A Study of Clinical Eclecticism." *Social Service Review,* 1978, *52* (4), 584-595.

Jones, M., and Polak, P. "Crisis and Confrontation." *British Journal of Psychiatry,* 1968, *114,* 169-174.

Langsley, D. G. "Crisis Intervention." *American Journal of Psychiatry,* 1972, *129* (6), 734-736.

Langsley, D. G. "Crisis Intervention and the Avoidance of Hospitalization." In G. Jacobson (Ed.), *New Directions for Mental Health Services: Crisis Intervention in the 1980s,* no. 6. San Francisco: Jossey-Bass, 1980.

Langsley, D. G., and Kaplan, D. M. *Treatment of Families in Crisis.* New York: Grune & Stratton, 1968.

Langsley, D. G., Machotka, P., and Flomenhaft, K. "Avoiding Mental Hospitalization: A Follow-Up Study." *American Journal of Psychiatry,* 1971, *127,* 1391-1394.

Lazarus, A. A. (Ed.). *Multimodal Behavior Therapy.* New York: Springer, 1976.

Marmor, J. "Short-Term Dynamic Psychotherapy." *American Journal of Psychiatry,* 1979, *136,* 149-155.

Mechanic, D. *Mental Health and Social Policy.* Englewood Cliffs, N.J.: Prentice-Hall, 1980.

Minuchin, S. *Families and Family Therapy.* Cambridge, Mass.: Harvard University Press, 1974.

Minuchin, S., and Fishman, H. C. *Family Therapy Techniques.* Cambridge, Mass.: Harvard University Press, 1981.

Papp, P. "Family Choreography." In P. Guerin (Ed.), *Family Therapy: Theory and Practice.* New York: Gardner Press, 1976.

Parad, H. J., and Caplan, G. "A Framework for Studying Families in Crisis." In H. J. Parad (Ed.), *Crisis Intervention: Selected Readings.* New York: Family Service Association of America, 1965.

Parad, H. J., and Parad, L. G. "A Study of Crisis-Oriented Planned Short-Term Treatment, Parts I and II." *Social Casework,* 1968, *49* (6) and (7), 346-355 and 418-426.

Parad, H. J., Resnik, H. L. P., and Parad, L. G. (Eds.). *Emergency and Disaster Management: A Mental Health Sourcebook.* Bowie, Md.: Robert J. Brady, 1976.

Pardes, H., and Pincus, H. A. "Brief Therapy in the Context of National Mental Health Issues." In S. H. Budman (Ed.), *Forms of Brief Therapy.* New York: Guilford Press, 1981.

Parsons, B. V., and Alexander, J. F. "Short-Term Family Intervention: A Therapy Outcome Study." *Journal of Consulting and Clinical Psychology,* 1973, *41,* 195-201.

Paul, N. "Cross-Confrontation." In P. Guerin (Ed.), *Family Therapy.* New York: Gardner Press, 1976.

Polak, P. "A Comprehensive System of Alternatives to Psychiatric Hospitalization." In L. Stein and M. A. Test (Eds.), *Alternatives to Mental Hospital Treatment.* New York: Plenum, 1978.

Polak, P., and Jones, M. "The Psychiatric Non-Hospital: A Model for Change." *Community Mental Health Journal,* 1973, *9,* 123-132.

President's Commission on Mental Health. *Report to the President.* Vol. 1. Washington, D.C.: U.S. Government Printing Office, 1978a.

President's Commission on Mental Health. *Report to the President.* Vol. 2. Washington, D.C.: U.S. Government Printing Office, 1978b.

Redl, F. "Strategy and Techniques of the Life Space Interview." *American Journal of Orthopsychiatry,* 1959, *31* (1), 1-18.

Rubinstein, D. "Rehospitalization Versus Family Crisis Intervention." *American Journal of Psychiatry,* 1972, *129* (6), 91-96.

Rueveni, U. "Network Intervention with a Family in Crisis." *Family Process,* 1975, *14* (2), 193-203.

Sherman, S. "Family Treatment." In J. B. Turner (Ed.), *Encyclopedia of Social Work.* Washington, D.C.: National Association of Social Workers, 1977.

Sherman, S. "Family Therapy." In F. Turner (Ed.), *Social Work Treatment: Interlocking Theoretical Approaches.* New York: Free Press, 1979.

Speck, R. V., and Attneave, C. L. *Family Networks.* New York: Pantheon, 1973.

Steidl, J. H., and Wexler, J. P. "What's a Clinician to Do with so Many Approaches to Family Therapy?" In E. G. Pendagast (Ed.), *The Family,* 1977, *4* (2), 190-197. New Rochelle, N.Y.: Center for Family Learning.

Umana, R. F., and others. *Crisis in the Family.* New York: Gardner Press, 1980.

Watzlawick, P., and others. *Pragmatics of Human Communication.* New York: Norton, 1967.

Yarvis, R. "Crisis Intervention as a First Line of Defense." In *Psychiatric Annals Reprint.* New York: Insight Communications, 1975.

Chapter 18

Primary Prevention of Emotional Disorders in School Settings

Helen Z. Reinherz

Primary prevention in mental health has recently been described as "an idea whose time has come" (Goldston, 1977). Ideas, however, do not spring up fully grown. There must be a history of initiation, growth, and development. The background for interest in primary prevention in the mental health field, as well as the direction for emerging programs, is lineally descended from the pioneer work of Caplan (1961, 1964, 1969), with the major definitions of primary prevention and the thrust toward programming for children arising directly from his writings. Furthermore, these seminal works identified the school as a major arena for preventive efforts. They also introduced interdisciplinary programs that foreshadowed the current dual trend toward strengthening the coping capacities of children and advocating the modification of the environments in which children develop.

Note: The author wishes to thank Cheryl Gracey for her editorial assistance, Joseph Regan for his suggestions, Christine Johnson and Lori Gamzon Winer for their help with the bibliographical research, and Faye Lavrakas and Mary Sullivan for their work on the manuscript. The completion of this work was made possible in part by National Institute of Mental Health grant 5-R01 MH-27458.

Although there have been many recent efforts to define primary prevention (Cowen, 1977b; Bloom, 1977; Reinherz, 1979a), one definition is most frequently cited: "Primary prevention aims at reducing the incidence of new cases of mental disorder in the population by combatting harmful forces which operate in the community and by strengthening the capacity of people to withstand stress" (Caplan, 1974, p. 189). This definition allows for programs of health promotion that include enhancement of affective and cognitive functioning. In this approach, mental health is viewed as ranging on a continuum from positive well-being to emotional disorder.

As one moves from the area of definition to a review of programs reported in the recent literature, two major program thrusts are clearly visible: (1) programs to enhance capacity to withstand stress and build competency and (2) programs to alter environments, whether community, institutional, or familial. Schools as institutions afford the opportunity for both approaches and therefore offer an important avenue for addressing the needs of children, a population singled out by the President's Commission on Mental Health (1978) as among the most vulnerable and underserved.

Schools as Settings for Programs of Primary Prevention

Schools have been characterized as "high-impact" environments (Cowen, 1977a). They have also been identified as among the primary agents of socialization (Bronfenbrenner, 1974) and as one of the "key integrative social systems" (Bower, 1977). Within the natural settings of schools, programs of primary prevention can be introduced to children more easily than they can within the child's other major environments, that is, the family and the neighborhood. Schools afford the institutional structure to reach children with programs aimed at primarily healthy populations. They also provide a chance to develop a range of programs for the potentially "at risk" child without the stigmatization that adds a heavy burden to already vulnerable children.

An important policy trend that has emerged in the mid

and late 1970s is the increased role of school systems as gatekeepers for mental health referrals and even as providers of services formerly delivered by mental health agencies. With the passage of right to education laws (for example, P.L. 94-142), an increasing number of school programs began to be provided for handicapped children with special needs. Through screening programs, children handicapped by health or other developmental problems can now be identified and evaluated, and remedial programs can be offered (Reinherz and Griffin, 1977). Services provided to physically handicapped children may be considered part of preventive mental health efforts, since untreated physical problems can have emotional consequences (Caplan, 1961; Reinherz, 1980). Above all, schools must be considered as institutions that have the latent capacity for promoting competence in children in both social growth and achievement. A major goal that has yet to be achieved is the provision for *all* children of an educational experience that is truly positive and ego enhancing (Bower, 1969).

Although the ultimate targets of programs of primary prevention in school are children, they live in a world in which they encounter parents, teachers, siblings, peers, and the environments of home and school. The school and family are important ecological systems that interact with the child (Bronfenbrenner, 1974) and may themselves be targets of prevention programs. Thus, four major target areas are identified in this paper: children, school personnel, parents, and the school environment.

The programs to be discussed represent three major models illustrating current approaches to primary prevention: (1) programs to promote positive mental health through building and enhancing competency, (2) programs of prevention through environmental and system change, and (3) programs providing protection for specific groups. (The programs to be discussed do not include populations of previously identified emotionally disturbed children. Once the diagnosis of emotional disturbance is made, the program is clearly one of secondary prevention.) Each is conceptualized as having major impact on the ultimate prevention of emotional breakdown in children. All are addressed to specific populations and systems. As will be apparent, each has a rationale for its design and implementation. The criteria for selecting specific programs in the subsequent sections of the paper include their adherence to a conceptual framework that specifies the intervention and the intended outcomes. This chapter identifies major exemplars of current program types, without attempting to provide exhaustive coverage of all existing programs.

Children as Targets of Primary Prevention

The designing of programs to build and enhance coping capacity in children is an ever-growing theme in recent primary prevention literature (Bloom, 1977; Cowen, 1977b). As already indicated, this view of primary prevention as promotion of positive mental health as well as deterrence of mental illness was clearly present in the work of Caplan (1961). It has been carried forward most strongly in the relatively youthful field of community psychology (Cowen, 1973), but all the mental health professions, including social work, have strong adherents to this approach (Reinherz, 1979b; Bloom, 1979).

Interest in competence and competence training is highly indebted to Ojemann's early work (1961). In the 1940s Ojemann began to develop "causal" teaching curricula based on observations linking noncausal thinking and emotional problems in children. Children exposed to this approach seemed better able to generalize knowledge, weigh alternative solutions, and understand human behavior. A study by Griggs and Bonney (1970) revealed that children who participated in a program using Ojemann's curriculum had significantly higher scores on measures of peer acceptance, self-ideal congruence, and general adjustment than did matched controls. Although Lemle (1976) has criticized the research design and the primarily cognitive measures used to evaluate Ojemann's programs, this work offers a conceptual cornerstone for one of the most important models of primary prevention in the schools.

The work of Spivack and Shure (1977) is within the general competence model initiated by Ojemann. The broadened objectives of this program, targeted at Head Start children, included solving interpersonal problems, increasing sensitivity to others, and understanding the effect of one's behavior on others. It has been reported that the positive results of this program, which included increased capacity to see alternative solutions to interpersonal situations, extended to children's behavior at home (Shure, 1979).

In the affective domain, a number of preventive programs have been initiated (Cooper, 1980). A key concept applicable to such programs is Hollister's neologism *strens* (1977), coined to serve as an antonym to *trauma* and to represent experiences that enhance growth and facilitate coping. Several programs of affective education have emerged. Among the programs most often cited is the Human Development Program (Bessell, 1972). This program has three units designed to enhance awareness of self, understanding of one's abilities, and competence in social interaction. The program, often called "the magic circle," is based on the encounter group model in which small groups of children interact with their teacher and with each other. Curricula have been developed for specific age groups from preschool through high school. Although the number of individuals trained in Bessell's method is said to exceed 30,000, there have been few reports of evaluations of the program (Lemle, 1976).

A positive and realistic self-concept is an important component of mental health, and several programs have directed their efforts toward enhancing self-concept. Schulman, Ford, and Busk (1973), for example, developed teaching units and administered them to students in the sixth, seventh, and eighth grades. Children in the experimental group were found to have made more positive change in their self-evaluation of academic and social skills than did the controls. An important development in recent years is the growing emphasis on integration of the cognitive and affective domains. Competency is seen as at least a necessary (if not sufficient) condition of positive mental health. A group of programs and curricula, variously described as "confluent, humanistic, or psychological education" (Kuriloff and Rinder, 1975), have been developed to illustrate this interdependence. As an example of this method, Rustad and

Rogers (1975) developed a seminar open to junior and senior high school students that met for twelve weeks. The program, entitled "Psychology of Counseling," was planned to operationalize cognitive developmental concepts. It concentrated on teaching adolescents to listen actively and empathically to others. Role taking was used to enhance students' ability to understand the concerns and feelings of others and to act in consonance with this understanding.

A final example of a program promoting positive strengths is one reported by Yee and Lee (1977) in which students of Asiatic descent were helped to view the positive qualities of their cultural and ethnic heritages. Participants gained emotional support through group discussions with other youths of similar backgrounds. The important principle of peer support for youngsters of all ages is illustrated by this program.

But what about programs for especially vulnerable groups? In a paper addressed to school psychologists, Caplan (1969) discussed the conceptual link between primary prevention and the theory of crisis. According to this paper, crises offer children the opportunity to reach a new, healthier equilibrium; however, if crises are not resolved favorably, they may result in mental disorder or an increased future likelihood of mental disorder. "Crises" may be expectable biological or psychosocial transitions, such as entering school or becoming an adolescent, or they may take the form of accidental happenings or traumas occurring in a child's life—for example, illness, death in the family, or natural disaster.

A number of schools and mental health services have collaborated in providing programs to ease the transition into school (Caplan, 1969; Signell, 1972). More recently have come reports of programs that helped children to cope with the accidental deaths of two classmates (Meyers and Pitt, 1976) and with the consideration of death in general (Nelson, Peterson, and Satore, 1975). Although some of the programs listed above deal with children already subjected to trauma, they can still be considered as primary prevention since they are directed to nonpatient populations with the aim of diminishing the incidence of emotional problems that could result from exposure to death and the experience of bereavement.

School Personnel as Targets and Agents of Primary Prevention

Teachers and administrators may be seen as target groups to be influenced or changed in order to promote mental health and prevent mental illness in the children in their care. They may also be seen as implementers and agents of primary prevention. This dual view emerges clearly in current programs, which show an increasing trend toward encouraging school personnel to more actively generate and implement mental health programs.

Teachers and Primary Prevention. Teachers are the professionals with the most direct contact with children and, second only to parents, have the potential of exerting the greatest influence on them. Programs of primary prevention utilize several methods to reach teachers, with in-service training (consisting of lectures and workshops) and consultation by mental health professionals being the most frequently reported. The goals of these approaches are to promote positive mental health attitudes, including self-awareness in teachers, and to improve understanding and management of behavior in the classroom. Objectives also include the training of teachers to implement specifically designed affective and cognitive curricula to enhance and promote children's competence. Finally, these programs may have the goal of training teachers to identify at-risk children and situations so that they can more effectively understand and work with children who are in the midst of psychosocial or situational crises.

An emerging trend in the training of teachers as effective interveners in primary prevention involves teaching content, skills, and techniques for use in the classroom with a focus on teachers' self-awareness and interpersonal skills. Kennedy and Seidman (1972) reported their experience in conducting workshops on classroom management and human relations. Teachers participating in the program reported increased self-awareness of the negative techniques they had formerly used to control children. Although contingency techniques were more easily accepted, the workshop participants were "willing to engage in self-appraisal and to assess honestly relations with students, parents, and among themselves" (p. 74).

Multari (1975) used an experimental approach with elementary school teachers, contrasting a didactic lecture series on child behavior with a model combining the same didactic material with "group psychotherapy" sessions for teachers. Teachers participating in the combined didactic and psychotherapeutic sessions were said to be more sure of themselves and their approach to pupils than those attending only lectures. Most important, pre- and postmeasures indicated a clearer understanding of the etiology of children's behavior by teachers in the combined program. Adolescents can provoke particularly strong reactions from school personnel. Coleman (1972) reported a series of seminars on adolescent behavior conducted for teachers by a mental health agency. Objectives included increased understanding of individual adolescent behavior in a broad social and community context, as well as of the teachers' own reactions and feelings toward adolescent problems. Although not extensively evaluated, the approach was considered helpful by the participants.

Mental health consultation is a technique brought to its major development by Caplan (1970). It is one of the methods most frequently used by mental health professionals to help teachers deal with the mental health problems of their pupils. In spite of stylistic and theoretical modifications (Carter and Cazares, 1976), the Caplan model continues to be the most commonly used (Kadushin, 1977). Several criticisms, however, have been leveled at mental health consultation in school settings. It has been suggested, for example, that teachers feel intimidated by the "expert" aura of the mental health consultant. (Ironically, some mental health consultants fault teachers for demanding immediate advice on a particular child's problem rather than being willing to involve themselves in broader discussions that might lead to more positive functioning of the consultee (teacher) in his or her professional role.) In the original formulation by Caplan (1970), the consultee is always to be treated by the consultant as a professional person with a professional problem in a manner that is inherently ego supportive. The importance of interacting with the consultee as a fellow professional is underscored by experience in the field.

Studies reported by Schulman and others (1973-1974) indicate that a "problem-solving" approach to consultation leads teachers to take positive attitudes toward themselves and their professional roles in dealing with mental health issues, including prevention. One evaluation also reported that teachers valued the personal self-awareness aspect of the problem-solving process over a predominantly case (individual child) approach (Silverman, 1974), a finding that offers promise of a broader orientation in teachers' views of the consultation process. It is clear that teachers have an important role to play in all preventive activities; their continued training and involvement in carrying out positively evaluated programs should remain a high priority in primary prevention.

School Administrators and Primary Prevention. Since administrative agreement is usually essential in mounting new programs, administrators are often involved in sanctioning efforts of primary prevention in the schools. While the literature presenting detailed descriptions of administrative involvement in primary prevention is sparse, there are a few examples of such involvement. For instance, a mental health consultation program was established within one school system to prepare administrators and staff to deal with racial integration (Prunty, Singer, and Thomas, 1977). The goals of the program included the reduction of racist attitudes and increased awareness of ethnic, racial, and cultural differences. Although evaluations were available only from the program participants, the result indicated an increased amount of communication and peer acceptance among staff members.

Parents and Their Role in Programs of Primary Prevention

The institutions of family and school form the major worlds of the child. Thus, school programs of primary prevention in which the family (specifically parents) can be involved along with their children should provide the greatest impact on mental health, and a number of such programs have in fact been designed. In some, parents and parental attitudes are seen as the targets for change. Change in parental attitude and understanding of children is the intermediate goal, the ultimate goal being a positive effect on the children themselves through change in their immediate family environment. Parents can also be considered as active agents of health promotion and primary prevention or even as partners with the schools in leading classes and groups.

DeRosis (1969) has described a series of parents' groups organized through public schools in New York City. The goal of the program was to prevent learning and behavior problems. The group was initiated by a psychiatrist (DeRosis) who acted as group coordinator. Major emphasis was placed on positive coping and appropriate actions in handling everyday problems of childrearing. An outgrowth of the initial program was the establishment of training groups for school personnel to carry out similar programs for parents.

Several programs involving mothers were established by a public health department in collaboration with schools in St. Louis County. One of these was an ambitious effort in which parents were offered peer-led education groups or a dual program combining the education program and the school mental health service. According to reports issued two and one-half years later, programs resulted in fewer problems among children whose parents participated as compared to control groups that received no services (Glidewell, Gildea, and Kaufman, 1973). Stringer (1969) reported the serendipitous finding from interviewing mothers for other research purposes that parents benefited from a program of supportive contacts with caseworkers who reinforced behaviors productive of mental health in children. It was recommended that the practice be institutionalized and that such services be offered to all mothers of children entering school.

Parents have also been active participants in several programs to foster the development of children's interpersonal competency. Spivack and Shure (1977) have used parents, as well as teachers, as trainees in their programs to develop problem-solving thinking in young children. Parents were also actively involved by Kellam and others (1975) in their systemwide intervention in a Chicago neighborhood. In addition, there has been at least one explicit example of primary prevention in which parents were formally utilized as "helpers" within the public school classroom. Dinkmeyer and Ogburn (1974) describe a program designed for kindergarten and early primary grades in which one goal was to educate parents in effective understanding of and interaction with their own children as they participated in classroom teaching. In this program, teachers could provide clear role models for parents.

Finally, a series of programs has been designed to provide group educational approaches to parents for transitional "crisis" periods such as a child's entrance into kindergarten. Signell (1972) reported on a series of small-group discussions with parents. These were initially led by mental health workers providing anticipatory guidance about problems to be expected at school entry. The author observed that participating mothers reported enhanced ability to help their children cope with similar loss and separation situations. Ultimately this preventive approach had a multiplier effect, as mothers who had participated assisted other mothers in helping their children to make transitions. Additionally, a number of parents became group leaders in subsequent years.

There are a number of clear benefits that result from parental participation. Programs of cognitive development and enrichment for children have shown little staying power without active parental involvement (Bronfenbrenner, 1974). Such participation should be even more important in programs involving children's self-understanding and social interaction. Additionally, Berlin (1975) has noted that parental involvement is of immeasurable benefit to parents themselves, who gain self-esteem and a sense of potency from participation.

The School Environment: Implications for Primary Prevention

There is increasing recognition of the impact that the school as a social environment can have on the healthy development of children. However, difficulties in specification and measurement of key variables, as well as a lack of accumulated examples of successfully implemented programs, have constituted major obstacles to full program development. In order to develop appropriate primary prevention programs to build healthy environments in schools, there must be agreement on major environmental variables, as well as on appropriate instruments to measure them. Cowen (1977a) optimistically suggests that such a beginning has been made, referring to the pioneer work of Barker and Gump (1964), who identified school size as a major variable, and Kelly (1977), whose studies established a series of social climate clusters applicable in diverse social settings. Such studies constitute only the beginning of efforts to understand the impact of environments on the development of children.

The successful launching and full implementation of programs of environmental change are particularly difficult in that such programs challenge established patterns and cherished procedures. It is easier to introduce a discussion group for parents or even to add an affective education course for kindergarten children than to achieve structural institutional change of any substance. Also, the areas to be addressed—those comprising the child's environment—reach deeply into many potentially sensitive aspects of school and community. It is understandable, therefore, that this program model offers the smallest number of examples of successfully implemented programs.

Environmental variables to be addressed in programs of primary prevention include such physical aspects as the design, general ambience, and age of schools. Other physical variables include equipment and material resources. The environment also encompasses human aspects, such as the style of administration, the teacher-pupil ratio, the number of students in the school, their age range, and the degree to which the school is child or adult centered. Another variable of particular interest in the past decade has been whether schools are traditional (closed) or modern (open). This concept of "openness" includes physical openness—in some cases the absence of walls between classrooms—as well as informality in teaching style. It also includes whether there are provision for multiage and interest groupings of students and consideration of children's individual learning styles.

There are even more subtle aspects of school environments that are still in the process of conceptualization and measurement. Trickett and Moos (1974) have measured individual high school class environments, finding more satisfaction where a close student-teacher relationship existed. But the complexity of these issues is illustrated by the finding that students in environments high in competition—a "negative" characteristic—learned more than those in less competitive situations.

An important issue emerging from examination of the environmental characteristics of schools is that of individual and environmental fit. Although a particular structure may enhance learning and competence for some children, others may fare poorly in the same situation. In several studies of open versus closed environments, Allinsmith and Grimes (1961) and Reiss and Dydhalo (1975) concluded that specific personality types such as distractible and anxious-compulsive children fared less well with loosely structured curricula and open-space classrooms compared to their peers without such problems. This ecological perspective, encompassing person *and* environment, offers important guidelines for programming and planning (Bloom, 1979).

A final consideration in viewing social environments is to include the broader environmental contexts of neighborhood and city as they affect the healthy development of children. Bronfenbrenner (1974) has noted in reviewing early childhood programs that no program to promote competence can combat the deleterious effects of true poverty. Children from the lowest social classes exposed to deprivation of all kinds cannot be expected to flourish without broader social change.

Implementation of Change in the School Environment. There are as yet only a few examples of primary prevention programs involving environmental change in school systems. This is true in spite of promising beginnings in a number of areas of research. The few programs clearly identified appear to be directed at specific aspects of the environment, with the possible exception of Kellam's project in Chicago, which involved work at various administrative levels and with various target groups, including children, teachers, and parents (Kellam and others, 1975). Although dreams of social engineering for optimal positive development of children may continue, from a realistic perspective mental health workers will have to assume both a more activist stance and a more politically sophisticated approach than they have in the past (Iscoe, 1974). To effect systems change, they must learn to collaborate with the administrators of systems, political policy makers, other professionals —educators, architects, lawyers—and other people with influence in the community.

The work of Prunty, Singer, and Thomas (1977) cited earlier had the goal of developing healthy attitudes toward racial integration on the part of the administrators, teachers, and staff of a large school. It illustrates one approach to establishing a viable role for mental health professionals in a situation of political and community controversy. This program was initiated after the decision to integrate the school had been made; school and mental health personnel did not have an active role either in decision making or in implementation of the policy. In contrast collaboration of mental health consultants and educators in planning for implementation of school desegregation is described by Bradshaw and others (1972). In this model the authors describe a *charrette,* that is, a temporary organization established to involve school personnel, students, and their parents in the planning and actual logistics of desegregation of county high schools. Here the primary prevention mission was focused on facilitating actions that would lead to an orderly opening of the schools.

The need for research is nowhere more evident than in the area of programs of primary prevention aimed at changes in the child's school environment. Administrators can in fact be influenced by documented findings that buttress proposed ideas. For example, after several years of research in a school system (Griffin and Reinherz, 1969), my colleagues and I presented findings of harmful effects to children of nonpromotion policies (that is, retaining children in the same grade level). This resulted in a policy change in the school system that called for early decision making concerning children's capacity to cope with formal learning. It also resulted in implementation of flexible class assignments for groups and individual children. Although this was a relatively modest study, the resulting changes could make a difference to a number of children, affecting their subsequent experiences within the school system, so crucial to the development of competency, self-esteem, and good mental health.

An ambitious proposal for establishing mental health programming at all levels, including primary prevention, was developed by Braverman (1976). This author envisioned a "department of human development" in school systems that would be responsible for designing and implementing courses and programs to promote self-knowledge and foster emotional growth in children. Although an interesting idea, particularly if carried out with interdisciplinary collaboration, this innovation remains a future goal.

Status and Future of Primary Prevention in the Schools

For over two decades, concepts and programs of primary prevention of emotional problems in schools have been discussed, endorsed, and occasionally applied. Discussion in professional meetings, articles, and workshops has often been enthusiastic, even evangelical. Proponents of primary prevention have often appeared to have the fervor of a band of true believers (Reinherz, 1979a). In the past few years, more nonbelievers have been recruited to the prevention cause as primary prevention has received more general attention and, most important, some federal funding.

Although programs of secondary and even tertiary prevention outnumber those of primary prevention in school settings, a number of programs are currently in place. The ones reported in the recent literature are mostly those that teach children skills believed to aid in self-understanding, self-acceptance, and interpersonal competence. Both teachers and parents are often used as leaders for such projects. In turn, several of the programs attempt to enhance the competence of these adults in the same spheres as the children. Moreover, mental health consultation is still practiced in schools. There are criticisms of the traditional methods of consultation, yet the original models are still ascendent. Reports of relatively high consumer satisfaction continue to be presented. It is in the area of influencing and changing the social environment of the school to foster optimal development that there are the fewest examples of program implementation. Here the proselytizing becomes more fervent, but the experienced reader realizes that the task has become more arduous.

Future of Programs from Ideas to Service Delivery. The problems of bringing promising ideas from initial germination to fruition include those that are inherent in the introduction of all new approaches and programs, in addition to those that pertain to the philosophically and fiscally conservative period of the late 1970s and early 1980s. An important aid to success in altering school environments is the reaching and mobilization of appropriate constituencies in schools and the broader social and political communities to provide leverage to implement programs. These are tasks of high order and require finely honed community development skills. Clearly, there is a pressing need to develop sophisticated community workers with a high level of political competence.

For programs to work they must have widespread institutional acceptance. There also must be sufficient institutional capacity to carry out the programs. The most successful programs cited in this chapter combine the efforts of school personnel, teachers, parents, and mental health "experts." Teachers and parents no longer easily accept being passive recipients of advice and information. They expect to take an active role in the lives of children. The current move in the direction of philosophical and fiscal conservatism presents another obstacle. It has become increasingly difficult to promote programs promising the intangible "prevention" when the watchwords of communities have become "fiscal responsibility" and "back to basics."

Allied to the specific problems enumerated above is that faced by all proponents of prevention. The cold fact is that there is only the beginning of longitudinal research to identify populations, subgroups, and situations predictable enough of future problems (except in the most obvious sense, for example, children of psychotics) to form a firmly documented, truly at-risk group (Reinherz and others, forthcoming). Compounding the embarrassment of preventers is the scarcity of carefully designed longitudinal evaluations of the effects of interventions (Reinherz, 1979b).

Future Objectives for Primary Prevention in Schools. First, more effort and time must be spent in reaching and mobilizing constituencies in schools and communities to foster programs of primary prevention. A cadre of talented mental health workers from a variety of disciplines (most often social work, psychology, and nursing) have been trained in community prevention skills in the past few years, and the beginnings of their work are being reported in national professional meetings. Such work is sorely needed and should be continued and expanded in the future. Second, the concepts of primary prevention, along with knowledge and practice in intervention skills, need to be incorporated into teacher-training programs. It is possible that, with such training, a new group of teacher-preventers could be developed to think and work in a health promotion and prevention modality and to disseminate their understanding and skills. Teachers have the greatest opportunity to reach all children. Third, research into guideposts to "at riskness" in children and research evaluation of programs should be both encouraged and actually utilized. Scholars of prevention research methods should be developed in all the major mental health training programs.

It is only after we have taken such steps that the dream of providing an optimal environment to foster healthy development of all children and to discourage development of dysfunctional behavior will become a reality.

References

Allinsmith, W., and Grimes, J. W. "Compulsivity, Anxiety, and School Environment." *Merrill-Palmer Quarterly,* 1961, 7, 247-261.

Barker, R. G., and Gump, P. *Big School, Small School.* Stanford, Calif.: Stanford University Press, 1974.

Berlin, T. N. "Some Models for Reversing the Myth of Child Treatment in Community Mental Health Centers." *Journal of American Academy of Child Psychiatry,* 1975, *14* (1), 76-94.

Bessell, H. "Human Development in the Elementary School Classroom." In S. Solomon and B. Berzon (Eds.), *New Perspectives on Encounter Groups.* San Francisco: Jossey-Bass, 1972.

Bloom, B. L. *Community Mental Health: A General Introduction.* Monterey, Calif.: Brooks/Cole, 1977.

Bloom, M. "Social Prevention: An Ecological Approach." In C. B. Germain (Ed.), *Social Work Practice: People and Environments.* New York: Columbia University Press, 1979.

Bower, E. M. "Slicing the Mystique of Prevention with Occam's Razor." *American Journal of Public Health,* 1969, *59* (3), 478-484.

Bower, E. M. "Mythologies, Realities, and Possibilities." In G. W. Albee and J. M. Joffee (Eds.), *Primary Prevention of Psychopathology.* Vol. I. Hanover, N.H.: University Press of New England, 1977.

Bradshaw, W. H., and others. "Mental Health Consultants in an Educational Charrette." *Psychiatry,* 1972, *35* (4), 317-335.

Braverman, J. "The School System as the Vehicle of Preventive Psychiatry." *Canadian Journal of Public Health,* 1976, *67* (1), 61-63.

Bronfenbrenner, U. "Is Early Intervention Effective?" *Teachers College Record,* 1974, *77* (2), 279-304.

Caplan, G. (Ed.). *Prevention of Mental Disorders in Children.* New York: Basic Books, 1961.

Caplan, G. *Principles of Preventive Psychiatry.* New York: Basic Books, 1964.

Caplan, G. "Opportunities for School Psychologists in the Primary Prevention of Mental Disorders in Children." In J. A. Bradman and A. D. Spiegel (Eds.), *Perspectives in Community Mental Health.* Hawthorne, N.Y.: Aldine, 1969.

Caplan, G. *The Theory and Practice of Mental Health Consultation.* New York: Basic Books, 1970.

Caplan, G. *Support Systems and Community Mental Health.* New York: Behavioral Publications, 1974.

Carter, B. D., and Cazares, P. R. "Consultation in Mental Health: A Review of the Literature, 1972-1976." *Community Mental Health Review,* 1976, *1* (5), 1-13.

Coleman, R. F. "Seminars for Teachers of Adolescents." *Journal of School Health,* 1972, *42* (6), 345-347.

Cooper, S. "Affective Education and Prevention in Mental Health." *Journal of Prevention,* 1980, *1* (1), 24-34.

Cowen, E. L. "Social and Community Interventions." *Annual Review of Psychology,* 1973, *24,* 423-472.

Cowen, E. L. "Baby-Steps Toward Primary Prevention." *American Journal of Community Psychology,* 1977a, *5* (1), 1-22.

Cowen, E. L. "Primary Prevention Misunderstood." *Social Policy,* 1977b, *7* (5), 20-27.

DeRosis, H. A. "A Primary Preventive Approach Program with Parent Groups in Public Schools." *Journal of School Health,* 1969, *39* (2), 102-109.

Dinkmeyer, D., and Ogburn, K. D. "Psychologists' Priorities: Premium on Developing Understanding of Self and Others." *Psychology in the Schools,* 1974, *11* (1), 24-27.

Glidewell, J. C., Gildea, M. C. L., and Kaufman, M. K. "The Preventive and Therapeutic Effects of Two School Mental Health Programs." *American Journal of Community Psychology,* 1973, *1* (4), 295-329.

Goldston, S. E. "An Overview of Primary Prevention Programming." In D. C. Klein and S. E. Goldston (Eds.), *Primary Prevention: An Idea Whose Time Has Come.* Department of Health, Education, and Welfare Publication No. (ADM) 77-447. Rockville, Md.: National Institute of Mental Health, 1977.

Griffin, C. L., and Reinherz, H. "Prevention of the 'Failure Syndrome' in the Primary Grades: Implications for Intervention." *American Journal of Public Health,* 1969, *59* (11), 2029-2034.

Griggs, J. W., and Bonney, M. E. "Relationship Between 'Causal' Orientation and Acceptance of Others, 'Self-Ideal Self' Congruency, and Mental Health Changes for Fourth- and Fifth-

Grade Children." *Journal of Educational Research,* 1970, *63* (10), 471-477.

Hollister, W. G. "Basic Strategies in Designing Primary Prevention Programs." In D. C. Klein and S. E. Goldston (Eds.), *Primary Prevention: An Idea Whose Time Has Come.* Department of Health, Education, and Welfare Publication No. (ADM) 77-447. Rockville, Md.: National Institute of Mental Health, 1977.

Iscoe, I. "Community Psychology and the Competent Community." *American Psychologist,* 1974, *29,* 607-613.

Kadushin, A. *Consultation in Social Work.* New York: Columbia University Press, 1977.

Kellam, S. G., and others. *Mental Health and Going to School: The Woodlawn Program of Assessment, Early Intervention, and Evaluation.* Chicago: University of Chicago Press, 1975.

Kelly, J. G. *The High School: Students and Social Contexts in Two Midwestern Communities.* Community Psychology Series, No. 4. New York: Behavioral Publications, 1977.

Kennedy, D. A., and Seidman, S. B. "Contingency Management and Human Relations Workshops: A School Intervention Program." *Journal of School Psychology,* 1972, *10* (1), 69-75.

Kuriloff, P., and Rinder, M. "How Psychological Education Can Promote Mental Health with Competence." *Counselor Education and Supervision,* 1975, *14* (4), 257-267.

Lemle, R. "Primary Prevention of Psychological Disorders in Elementary and Intermediate Schools." *Journal of Clinical Child Psychology,* 1976, *5* (2), 273-278.

Meyers, J., and Pitt, N. W. "A Consultation Approach to Help a School Cope with the Bereavement Process." *Professional Psychology,* 1976, *7* (4), 559-564.

Multari, G. "A Psychotherapeutic Approach with Elementary School Teachers." *Community Mental Health Journal,* 1975, *11* (2), 122-128.

Nelson, R. C., Peterson, W. D., and Satore, R. L. "Issues and Dialogues: Helping Children to Cope with Death." *Elementary School Guidance and Counseling,* 1975, *9* (3), 226-232.

Ojemann, R. H. "Investigations on the Effects of Teaching an Understanding and Appreciation of Behavior Dynamics." In

G. Caplan (Ed.), *Prevention of Mental Disorders in Children.* New York: Basic Books, 1961.

President's Commission on Mental Health. *Report to the President.* Vol. 1. Washington, D.C.: U.S. Government Printing Office, 1978.

Prunty, H. E., Singer, T. L., and Thomas, L. A. "Confronting Racism in Inner-City Schools." *Social Work,* 1977, *22* (3), 190-194.

Reinherz, H. Z. "Primary Prevention in Community Mental Health: Holy Grail or Empty Vessel?" In A. Katz (Ed.), *Community Mental Health: Issues for Social Work Practice and Education.* New York: Council on Social Work Education, 1979a.

Reinherz, H. Z. "The Evaluation of Programs of Primary Prevention: How Can We Know if They Make a Difference?" Louisville, Ky.: Council on Social Work Education Project on Prevention in Social Work Education, 1979b.

Reinherz, H. Z. "Primary Prevention of Emotional Disorders of Children: Mirage or Reality?" *Journal of Prevention,* 1980, *1* (1).

Reinherz, H. Z., and Griffin, C. L. "Identifying Children at Risk: A First Step to Prevention." *Health Education,* 1977, *8* (4), 14-16.

Reinherz, H. Z., and others. "An Epidemiological Study of the Behavior Problems of Young Children." In S. A. Mednick and M. Harway (Eds.), *Longitudinal Research in the U.S.,* forthcoming.

Reiss, S., and Dydhalo, N. "Persistence, Achievement, and Open Space Environments." *Journal of Educational Psychology,* 1975, *67,* 506-513.

Rustad, K., and Rogers, C. "Promoting Psychological Growth in a High School Class." *Counselor Education and Supervision,* 1975, *14* (4), 277-285.

Schulman, J. L., Ford, R. C., and Busk, P. "A Classroom Program to Improve Self-Concept." *Psychology in the Schools,* 1973, *10* (4), 48-56.

Schulman, J. L., and others. "Mental Health in the Schools." *Elementary School Journal,* 1973-1974, *74,* 48-56.

Shure, M. B. "Training Children to Solve Interpersonal Problems: A Preventative Mental Health Program." In R. F. Muñoz, L. R. Snowden, and J. G. Kelly (Eds.), *Social and Psychological Research in Community Settings: Designing and Conducting Programs for Social and Personal Well-Being.* San Francisco: Jossey-Bass, 1979.

Signell, K. A. "Kindergarten Entry: A Preventive Approach to Community Mental Health." *Community Mental Health Journal,* 1972, *8* (1), 60-70.

Silverman, W. H. "Some Factors Related to Consultee Satisfaction with Consultation." *American Journal of Community Psychology,* 1974, *2* (3), 303-310.

Spivack, G., and Shure, M. B. "Preventively Oriented Cognitive Education of Preschoolers." In D. C. Klein and S. E. Goldston (Eds.), *Primary Prevention. An Idea Whose Time Has Come.* Department of Health, Education, and Welfare Publication No. (ADM) 77-447. Rockville, Md.: National Institute of Mental Health, 1977.

Stringer, L. A. "Research Interviews with Mothers as Entry into Primary Prevention." *American Journal of Public Health,* 1969, *59* (3), 485-489.

Trickett, E. J., and Moos, R. H. "Personal Correlates of Contrasting Environments: Student Satisfaction in High School Classrooms." *American Journal of Community Psychology,* 1974, *2,* 1-12.

Yee, T. T., and Lee, R. H. "Based on Cultural Strengths, a School Primary Prevention Program for Asian-American Youth." *Community Mental Health Journal,* 1977, *13* (3), 239-248.

Chapter 19

Serving the Underserved Through Rural Mental Health Programs

Morton O. Wagenfeld
Lucy D. Ozarin

The superiority of rural life is one of the most durable and cherished myths of Western civilization. Cities have been characterized as sinkholes of sin, degradation, and assorted social evils and held up to invidious comparison with the virtues of pastoral existence (Srole, 1977; Flax and others, 1979; Wagenfeld, 1982). Only recently have serious challenges to this view come forth. What Harrington (1962) has termed the "invisible poverty" of rural America has become much more visible. Recognition is growing that the problems of rural America at least rival, and in some cases surpass, those of the cities. The President's Commission on Mental Health (1978b) appointed a work group to study and report on the mental health needs of rural America. This special concern with rural areas is reflected also in the Mental Health Systems Act passed by Congress in 1980. The mental health needs of rural America can best be understood in the context of its sociology, demography, and social problems.

Sociology of Rural America

Within its 200-year span of history, the United States has changed from an agricultural country to an urban, industrialized nation. Although the majority of the population and much of its ethos are now urban, nearly one quarter of the population lives in rural or semirural areas, and a strong nostalgia for rural life still exists.

The tapestry of rural America is exceedingly difficult to discern. While at some point the referent *rural* may have had a uniform connotation, this is certainly not the case today. Rural America—to the extent that one can describe it—is very heterogeneous and is differentiated by geographical, religious, and economic divisions (Hassinger, 1976). The rural America of Maine fishing villages differs in values and social organization from that of farmers and ranchers in the Midwest or intermountain West. The economic bases also vary: fishing and tourism in New England, lumbering in the Northwest, and agriculture in the Midwest. Finally, any attempt to uniformly characterize an area such as the rural South is likely to miss important distinctions. The Tidewater, the Piedmont, and the Delta are regions with differing values and heritages. Given these distinctions and qualifications, it is tempting to conclude that no generalizations are possible. To do so, however, would be to gloss over significant cultural, geographical, and demographic characteristics that appear to distinguish rural from urban populations.

One important distinction pertains to population dynamics. While the absolute population of the United States has increased in this century, most rural areas have experienced large-scale declines. These reductions generally have resulted from increased mechanization of agriculture and mining, with a consequent lowered need for large labor pools. The out-migration to urban areas, however, has been selective and has involved mainly the young, the productive, and the better educated. The net result is that rural areas have disproportionately large numbers of dependent persons: the very young and the elderly. This underscores the basic dilemma of rural America. On the one hand, the decline of agriculture has resulted in a shrinking economic base and chronic poverty. Data indicate that poverty in rural areas is more serious and extensive than in comparable urban settings (Tweeten, 1970; U.S. Department of Commerce, 1973). The overrepresentation of dependent persons creates a heavy demand for ameliorative human services. The chronic poverty of rural areas, on the other hand, has made it difficult to fund and maintain these programs. In addition to their greater number of age-dependent persons, rural areas are inhabited by large numbers of the disabled, the less well educated, racial and cultural minorities, and migrant workers (Baumheir and others, 1973; Reul, 1974; U.S. Department of Labor, 1970). It is interesting to note that many of these groups were also singled out by the President's Commission on Mental Health (1978b) as being in particular need of mental health services.

Recent demographic evidence suggests that the traditional emphasis on rural population decline and its consequences may be simplistic. Although certain rural regions (the Corn Belt, the Great Plains, the Mississippi Delta) continue to experience population declines, others (for example, the Rocky Mountains, the Upper Great Lakes, southern Appalachia, and Florida) have shown strong growth. This population turnaround is due to the increased economic vitality of some rural areas, the modernization of roads and communication systems, and a preference for rural living. It was emphasized previously that population decline produces problems related to high dependency ratios and a diminished fiscal ability to provide necessary social services. Growth, too, can create difficulties by straining already thin community resources and by introducing new and, often, conflicting values into a traditional social structure. A number of rural communities in the intermountain west have experienced rapid growth as a result of energy development, and there have been studies of the impact of this change on both residents and migrants (Davenport and Davenport, 1979, 1980; Uhlmann, 1981).

A fundamental consideration in understanding rural America and its mental health problems lies in the appreciation of its culture and values (Flax and others, 1979; Wagenfeld and

Wagenfeld, 1981). Values are an integral part of culture. Basically defined, they refer to culturally held definitions of reality, what is considered to be right and proper, the nature of man and human relationships, and concepts of time, fate, and the relationship of man to nature. Values become internalized within the personality system in two ways: through contact with primary groups (for example, the family) in earliest life and through secondary group contacts with peers, school, church, and so on in later life. These values provide guides for conduct and ways of seeking solutions for problems posed by the environment and the requirements of the social system. A crucial point about values and value systems is that they are so "taken for granted" that they are seldom made explicit or questioned unless they clash with competing systems. In most societies, a common core of values exists to which all, or nearly all, the members subscribe. Large, industrialized societies, however, are characterized by a diversity of subcultural groups based on regional, racial, ethnic, age, occupational, or social-class differences. The values of these subcultures can, and often do, conflict with those of the dominant society. These points assume salience when we consider that most practitioners in the health and human services are products of the dominant value perspective in our society: the white middle class. To the extent that the caregivers' value perspectives differ from those of their clients, a situation of conflict exists. This is a crucial—and often overlooked—problem.

If rural America is an exceedingly heterogeneous entity, to what extent can one reasonably assert that there is a core of values common to that segment of our country? At the abstract level, rural values tend to emphasize several themes: man's subjugation to nature, fatalism, an orientation to concrete places and things, a view of human nature as basically evil, human activity as a matter of being rather than of doing, and human relationships based on personal and kinship ties. Sociologically, the last would represent an emphasis on primary, as opposed to secondary, relationships. At another level, the culture of rural America, particularly among the poor, can also be described as a "folk culture." In contrast to general cultures, folk cultures are acquired through personal contact, by word of mouth, and through the emulation of role models. For those participating in a rural folk culture, the soil and its products are more than just a livelihood. Style of life, expectations, and even personality are related to the land.

Whether one is talking about Appalachian whites, residents of Martha's Vineyard in Massachusetts, Native Americans, the Spanish speaking and Spanish surnamed, or blacks, the common experience of rural residence would appear to result in a common core of values. Rural people (relative to urban people) are more conservative, religious, puritanical, work oriented, ascetic, ethnocentric, isolationist, intolerant of heterodox ideas and values, prejudicial, uninformed, authoritarian, and family centered (Hassinger, 1976).

An important correlate of rural values is the nature of rural communities and social organization. Rural communities tend to be trade centers that traditionally have functioned as places of professional and commercial services for well-defined hinterland populations. Rural communities tended to be small in geographical area and population because of the limited transportation technology and the general scale of organization when they were established. These communities were for the most part unspecialized and relatively homogeneous, focusing around the general store, a general medical practitioner, citizen's government, and farmer-preachers. The normative consequences of this type of social organization were noted by Hassinger (1976, p. 169): "On the basis of this mode of organization, interaction among people in town-country communities tended to be face-to-face and informal. Incumbents of public offices and boards were generally selected on the basis of personal characteristics and family background rather than on the basis of issues or political ideologies. Occupants of leadership positions represented the 'backbone' consensus of community norms of behavior. Professionals, including county agents, school teachers, and doctors, were expected to conform to the norms of the community."

It has been noted that a person is typically not aware of his or her values unless they are challenged. However, rural values often conflict openly with the white, middle-class core values of the larger society. According to Mazer, a psychiatrist practicing in a rural area of Massachusetts, one of the major sources of stress for the area's people is the very fact that their values often differ from those of the larger society. Mazer (1976, p. 41) notes: "The assumptions which guide their lives are challenged daily by what they see on television or read in the newspapers that reach the island. Perhaps more important, their assumptions about life are challenged massively each summer when their values come into conflict with those of their summer visitors, who are many times their number."

Mazer's analysis of life on Martha's Vineyard is generally applicable to all rural areas confronted with conflicting beliefs and assumptions. While residents of other areas, more geographically isolated and less popular than Martha's Vineyard, may not experience the same direct confrontation of value systems, mass communication media have penetrated all parts of the country and reduced the isolation of rural America. Furthermore, improved road networks have considerably shortened travel time to urban centers. The friction between value systems creates stresses that may pertain to the etiology of mental disorders and certainly to the delivery of mental health services. The boomtowns of the intermountain West—small, rural communities undergoing explosive growth as a result of coal development—are almost a laboratory situation of this type of value conflict (Davenport and Davenport, 1980).

The traditional assumption that there is a low prevalence of mental disorder in rural areas is being questioned. An extensive review of the literature on psychopathology in rural areas can be found in Wagenfeld (1982), who concluded that, despite the mythology of the superiority of rural life, evidence from the United States and other countries suggests that rates of mental disorder are *higher in rural areas.* Although definitive conclusions are not yet possible, the greater stress associated with poverty, unemployment, poorer physical health, and the inability of traditional institutional structures and value systems to satisfy needs and aspirations may be etiologically associated with psychiatric disorder.

The bulk of evidence suggests that rural areas suffer from the dual disability of a high prevalence of health and social problems, and limited fiscal and other resources to launch ameliorative programs. A third element must also be considered. Even if adequate fiscal and programmatic resources were available, are there certain aspects of rural life and value systems that would militate against the delivery of needed services? Wagenfeld (1977) and Flax and others (1979) have suggested that a series of provider and client barriers do exist. With regard to providers, a major impediment is the urban model of service delivery. Most practitioners have been trained in urban universities and are oriented toward providing specialized care for a largely urban, white, and affluent clientele. Caregivers are also accustomed to the "therapeutic incognito" of urban practice. The realities of rural life, as Mazer (1976) has so aptly pointed out, are quite different. With regard to clients, he notes that "rural clients are more interested in help with specific problems and relief of symptoms than they are with more abstract and distal notions of self-fulfillment characteristic of long-term reconstructive therapies" (p. 63).

In summary, a picture has been presented of a large segment of our rural population with high rates of health, mental health, and human service problems. Ironically, because of rural America's pervasive poverty, it is less able to launch or support ameliorative programs than are urban areas. In addition, where such programs are available, they are often less than optimally successful because of provider and client barriers to service delivery.

Mental Health Services in Rural Areas

It is a fundamental principle that successful service delivery systems allow persons seeking help to reach and to be provided with appropriate and acceptable assistance. This entire process is enmeshed in a complex sociocultural matrix. One can hardly overemphasize the idea that effective service delivery must be *culturally syntonic*—consonant with the needs, perceptions, and values of those being served.

For a number of years, the delivery of mental health services to rural areas has been the focus of a work group at the National Institute of Mental Health (NIMH). This group concluded that data were lacking on the nature of mental health delivery problems in rural America. Two major tasks were planned. The first was a comprehensive review of the literature on health, mental health, and human services problems in rural areas (Flax and others, 1979). Second, together with the Mitre Corporation, which had received an NIMH grant to study the management and development of research, a survey of rural mental health practitioners was conducted to identify the major constraints to service delivery. Five key problems were identified: transportation, recruitment and retention of personnel, interagency collaboration, government rules and regulations, and community advocacy (Cedar and Salasin, 1979). Solutions to these problems have been found, to varying degrees, in some places. They are described in the remainder of this chapter.

Transportation. Distance and sparsely distributed population create problems in service delivery. Mental health centers (or clinics or hospitals) serving a rural population have therefore established satellites to bring service closer to people and lessen staff travel time. The satellite may be a fixed physical site with service five days per week or a transient site with one or more service days per week or month. While satellites bring provider and client closer together, only certain services, such as outpatient and emergency services, may be feasible. Inpatient or partial hospitalization services may not be possible because of lack of facilities and staff resources. Satellites also increase operation costs due to additional expenses for rent, telephones, and staff travel to the main office. Another consideration when a single professional or a small group are on call constantly is staff burnout. The Eastern Montana Community Mental Health Center (CMHC), established in 1967 and serving seventeen counties with 100,000 people scattered over 49,000 square miles, has developed some unique solutions to these constraints. Since the distance from the central office to the most distant satellite is over 200 miles, outpatient, emergency, and consultation-education services have been made available at nine fixed and itinerant sites, including three main offices. Partial hospitalization is provided at three sites. Inpatient and transitional care is available in Miles City, which is the administrative hub, but sixteen small general hospitals located throughout the vast area will also admit psychiatric patients.

While home visits may be important in some situations, bringing clients to the center is the more usual pattern. Many demonstrations of rural transportation systems have been accomplished, and each has advantages and disadvantages. Since a number of agencies concerned with the aged, the mentally retarded, and welfare and health in a given locality may need transportation for clients, coordination is essential to avoid duplication and to maximize funds and resources. A central dispatch office to administer the system under private nonprofit or public auspices has been shown to be feasible. For example, the Trend Community Mental Health Center in Brevard, North Carolina joined with three other human service programs (child daycare, a retardation program, and social services) to purchase three vans and operate them in one county of its catchment area. Under this arrangement, the CMHC notified a designated van driver that transportation would be needed for an individual on the following day. After several years, the CMHC has purchased its own van but still uses the joint transportation arrangement as needed. It is likely that ongoing public support will be necessary to sustain the collaborative system (Allard, 1979; U.S. Department of Agriculture, 1978).

Recruitment and Retention of Personnel. Professional people are usually trained in urban areas and they tend to remain there. Studies have shown, however, that professionals who grew up in rural areas are more likely to practice in them than professionals from urban areas (Dunbar, McKelvey, and Armstrong, 1980). Rural mental health facilities often have difficulty in attracting and retaining professional staff, especially psychiatrists, and it is not surprising that these centers have fewer professional staff than urban ones (Longest, Konan, and Tweed, 1979). Survey data have also found that rural staff members have a different ideological perspective in that they emphasize concerns with community development and the community basis of mental disorders more than their urban counterparts (Jones and others, 1976). These factors strongly influence service programming.

A rural center, since it may be an area's only resource for professional personnel, may be required to function as a family service agency, to provide consultation to local medical practitioners, to serve as the secretariat for local councils on aging, or to establish needed services not otherwise available (for example, senior nutrition and speech and hearing services). As an example of such multifocal activity, the High Plains Comprehensive CMHC in Hays, Kansas, serving twenty counties with 132,000 people scattered over 20,000 square miles in northwestern Kansas, established the Area Agency on Aging for eighteen of its counties. The United Counseling Service of Bennington County (Vermont) initiated and maintained a nutrition program for senior citizens in its county for two years until the local area office on aging could assume this responsibility. The Counseling Center in Bangor, Maine operates a home health service in four rural counties with a staff of more than ninety professional and support personnel.

The limited number of mental health professionals, especially psychiatrists, in rural areas requires that administrative and clinical practices be arranged to maximize the use of professional time, that the levels of skill needed for specific tasks be carefully delineated, and that special attention be given to quality of care procedures. It may be possible to supplement CMHC staff with local general practitioners and with consultants, for example, a child psychiatrist. However, this pattern is expensive and recruitment may be difficult. The West Alabama Mental Health Center in Demopolis, Alabama, serving five predominantly black rural counties, utilizes contract services of general physicians as one way of overcoming professional staff shortages. No psychiatrist practices in this catchment area, but a consultant psychiatrist provides regular visits to each county.

Persistent and widespread efforts to recruit professional staff usually are successful. The involvement of training institutions is particularly helpful. Some, in fact, notably in social work, are concentrating on training professionals for rural practice (Eastern Washington University, West Virginia University, Washington University in St. Louis, and Western Michigan University). Once recruitment has been successful, retention is vital. It may be useful to regard the tenure of a professional as time limited, though one would hope for a minimum of three to five years. It may take six to twelve months for nonindigenous professionals to adapt to the local culture. If this process is not successful, both the professional and the agency will perceive the need for separation. Hence, a carefully planned orientation period is necessary. The agency administration must also find ways to support professional staff. A professional stationed alone at a satellite requires contact with other professionals and should be brought to the central office at regular intervals for staff meetings and in-service training.

Continuing education is now required for professional groups. The rural agency must provide such opportunities either by organizing programs that will meet professional requirements or by allowing educational leaves. Both are probably necessary and they require adequate funds. Agency boards and management must see continuing staff education as a necessary expenditure to maintain staff morale and to improve clinical services. Flax and others (1979) provide a useful review of the literature on options in this area.

The role of natural support systems in maintaining mental health has been given much emphasis (Caplan and Killilea, 1976; President's Commission on Mental Health, 1978a). It has been suggested that the natural support system of friends and neighbors is stronger in rural than in urban areas and could be part of the coordinated community effort to assist those in need. Several research projects are investigating the potential utility of rural support systems. Vallance (1977) has explored rural indigenous caregiving networks for primary prevention. His assumptions were that people who have mental health problems turn first to friends, relatives, clergymen and others whom they trust and that these "natural caregivers" can be identified and made more effective through training in helping skills. Morical (1975), at the University of Wisconsin at Menominee, explored training for rural housewife peer counselors, who would work in a variety of community agencies to help meet the needs of other rural housewives with such concerns as loneliness, breakdown in family communications, changing life-styles, grief, widowhood, and divorce.

Interagency Collaboration. Human service resources in rural areas are notably scarce, and the collaboration of existing agencies is essential for their clients. It is common in small communities for agency staff to know each other on a social as well as a professional basis so that mutual trust and respect may be easier to create than in urban settings. Informal collaboration is also probably more usual—telephone calls and hallway consultations will be more common than formal conferences. Since different agencies may be working with the same families and individuals, many areas also utilize regular meetings of the human service agency staffs, including the police or sheriff and court personnel.

The Aroostook CMHC in Presque Isle, Maine, which serves a single county of 6,400 square miles with 100,000 people (the largest town has only 11,000 people), has a contract with the state Human Services Department to provide aftercare for patients discharged from the state hospital over 150 miles away. This center also utilizes fourteen full-time staff to provide consultation services for schools through contracts with school districts. The Cooperative Extension Service of the U.S. Department of Agriculture, which has the improvement of rural living as a major objective, has representatives in every county of the United States. This organization, delivering services at the grass-roots level and in contact with large numbers of citizens of all ages, devotes considerable effort to education about concerns related to mental health, such as stress management, parenting, and substance abuse. Yet formal working relationships with mental health agencies are reportedly few in number. The Community Support System Core Service agency (a division of Catholic charities) in Utica, New York arranges case management services for chronic mental patients. In conjunction with the local YWCA, the county Cooperative Extension Service, operating under contract, provides social skill classes to small groups on personal grooming, food preparation and nutrition, budgeting, and the use of community resources.

Many mental health centers, in keeping with federal legislative mandates (P.L. 88-164 and P.L. 94-63), collaborate with related agencies by affiliation agreements and contracts that may or may not include the exchange of funds. Among the affiliating agencies are mental health associations, childcare agencies, school systems, courts, private nonprofit social agencies, and health departments. A program of "linkages" between federally funded primary care health programs (PCHPs) (two thirds of which are in rural areas) and mental health facilities is currently being expanded. This federally subsidized effort at coordination supports a mental health professional who is stationed at the PCHP to provide consultation and training for the health staff, as well as assess patients to determine their need for mental health services and possibly to refer them to the mental health center. This professional has a foot in each agency and serves as a link between them. The 1980 Mental Health Systems Act authorizes the expansion of this linkage program. An example of PCHP-CMHC coordination is in Morgantown, West Virginia, where the Valley CMHC established linkages with two federally assisted rural ambulatory care centers, one twenty-five miles away in Blacksville and the other in Fairmont, twenty miles away. A CMHC satellite is also located in Fairmont. Each health center has employed a linkage staff member, who serves as a liaison to the CMHC. Referrals flow freely in both directions, and the linkage workers visit the CMHC regularly.

Notwithstanding the successes noted above, interagency coordination has been extensively researched (Morrill, 1976), and the difficulties have been made evident. A recent review of the literature (Broskowski, 1980) indicates that forces promoting linkage are the need for survival, growth, or stability; increased efficiency and effectiveness; and the preference for cooperation over competition for scarce resources. Forces inhibiting linkage are concern for lost autonomy, costs of maintaining a linkage, incompatible goals or philosophies, and incentives to compete for scarce funds.

Government Rules and Regulations. Rural providers frequently complain that governmental regulations and guidelines are written for urban rather than rural areas. It is not clear whether the regulations are discriminatory in themselves or whether it is their manner of interpretation by the bureaucracy. An example is the requirement that federally supported CMHCs (P.L. 94-63) convene monthly board meetings. However, when the main office of a center is located 200 miles from its furthest county, this may not be possible, especially during northern winters. Nevertheless, an executive committee of the board could meet monthly, or meetings could be rotated among areas where a quorum is likely to be obtained. A more serious problem occurs with third-party reimbursement for services whose fees are set "in keeping with local practice." This places the rural center at a marked disadvantage since urban charges are usually higher, even though the unit cost per service tends to be higher in a rural area because of the need to maintain multiple sites, staff travel time, and so on. Clearly, more study is needed to document whether regulations and/or their interpretation indeed discriminate against rural providers.

Community Advocacy. In a democratic society, government is fashioned to respond to the will of the people. This occurs through elected representatives at local, state, and federal levels. Legislators receive many and varied requests to meet individual or collective needs; a request backed by the support of a large constituency obviously will receive priority over that of an individual. It appears easier to organize a major constituency in urban areas, where people live closer together and are more available to lobby about certain issues. For instance, a city of 100,000 has more mentally retarded persons than a county of only 10,000 and can muster more parents to petition a board of education or supervisors to provide needed services that will be supported by a greater array of potential resources. Nevertheless, community organization is possible in rural areas. As evidence, there presently exist more than 300 rural or part-rural CMHCs with community boards and 650 federally supported rural primary care health programs with similar citizen participation.

Public information and education are essential to community advocacy. Since rural areas may not have their own radio or television stations or even a daily newspaper, other means to communicate must be found. Possibilities include the publications of organized groups such as churches, PTAs, farm groups, and professional or fraternal organizations. Interested, committed leadership and the involvement of influential people at the local level are essential.

Once a mental health service is established, continuing advocacy will be necessary to keep it alive and functioning. This advocacy will be needed to ensure regular input of funds and resources and to deal with the constraints described above. A strong board will be the mental health center's major advocate. In order to fulfill its policy function, it will need a constant flow of information from both the staff and the community. Staff will provide the clinical expertise, while the board must be open to the needs and concerns of the community. The board-staff relationship, as well as the relationship between mental health center staff and the staff of other agencies, will be strong factors in developing advocacy and securing support for effective mental health service programs. The awareness and responsiveness of staff to community needs and demands will largely determine the center's effectiveness as a mental health agency and perhaps even whether it survives or not.

The Bi-State Mental Health Foundation, a nonprofit corporation based in Ponca City, Oklahoma, is an example of effective community advocacy.* The center operated by the foundation provides comprehensive mental health services to six counties in north central Oklahoma and one county in south central Kansas. It is an outgrowth of a guidance clinic organized in Kay County, Oklahoma in 1954 by a group of interested citizens; since its inception, the center and the community have enjoyed close working relationships based on an understanding of each other's needs. Center staff, through frequent formal and informal contacts, helped gain community acceptance of services and programs. Community groups, in turn, helped initiate new inpatient mental health services, as well as innovative programs in speech, hearing, and educational therapy. Until federal funding

*We are indebted to Edwin Fair, psychiatric director of the foundation for a description of this unique program. For a more extensive description, see Fair (1981).

was terminated, the foundation operated a separate department of pastoral services that provided direct treatment, continuing education, and consultation programs for clergy.

Rural America—as an underserved and often overlooked segment of our society—has a unique set of problems and needs in the area of health and human services and, particularly, in mental health service delivery. This was specifically recognized in the report of the President's Commission on Mental Health (1978a), which singled out several populations in special need: children, the elderly, the poor, and minorities. Many of these populations are found in disproportionately large numbers in rural areas. The 1980 Mental Health Systems Act names as priority populations the same groups mentioned in the commission report but explicitly adds *rural people* for the first time in any federal mental health legislation.

In spite of formidable problems, mental health services are being made available to rural people. Much remains to be done, but a good start has been made. Issues of transportation, personnel recruitment, interagency collaboration, government rules and regulations, and community advocacy must be resolved. By jointly focusing on these concerns, practitioners and researchers can help develop more effective service delivery systems for persons residing in rural areas.

References

Allard, M. A. "Rural Transportation for Human Services—A Guide for Local Agencies." Rockville, Md.: Division of Mental Health Service Programs, National Institute of Mental Health, 1979.

Baumheir, E. C., Derr, J. M., and Gage, R. W. *Human Services in Rural America: An Assessment of Problems, Policies, and Research.* Denver, Colo.: Center for Social Research and Development, University of Denver, 1973.

Broskowski, A. "Evaluation of Primary Health Care Project—CMHC Linkage Initiative." National Institute of Mental Health Contract No. 278-79-0030 (OP), 1980.

Caplan, G., and Killilea, M. *Support Systems and Mutual Help:*

Multi-Disciplinary Explorations. New York: Grune & Stratton, 1976.

Cedar, T. B., and Salasin, J. *Research Directions for Rural Mental Health.* McLean, Va.: Mitre Corporation, 1979.

Davenport, J., and Davenport, J., III (Eds.). *Boom Towns and Human Services.* Laramie: University of Wyoming Press, 1979.

Davenport, J., III, and Davenport, J. *The Boom Town: Problems and Promises in the Energy Vortex.* Laramie: University of Wyoming Press, 1980.

Dunbar, E., McKelvey, J., and Armstrong, L. "Characteristics of Workplace and Workers in Rural Mental Health Settings." Region X Human Resource Development Task Force, Department of Health, Education, and Welfare, 1980.

Fair, E. "Community Support and Involvement in a Rural Mental Health Center." In M. O. Wagenfeld (Ed.), *New Directions for Mental Health Services: Perspectives on Rural Mental Health,* no. 9, 1981.

Flax, J. W., and others. *Mental Health and Rural America.* Department of Health, Education, and Welfare Publication No. (ADM) 78-753. Washington, D.C.: U.S. Government Printing Office, 1979.

Harrington, M. *The Other America.* New York: Penguin Books, 1962.

Hassinger, E. W. "Pathways of Rural People to Health Services." In E. W. Hassinger and L. R. Whiting (Eds.), *Rural Health Services: Organization, Delivery, and Use.* Ames: Iowa State University Press, 1976.

Jones, J. D., Robins, S. S., and Wagenfeld, M. O. "Rural Mental Health Centers—Are They Different?" *International Journal of Mental Health,* 1974, *3,* 77-92.

Jones, J. D., Wagenfeld, M. D., and Robins, S. S. "A Profile of the Rural Community Mental Health Center." *Community Mental Health Journal,* 1976, *12,* 176-181.

Longest, J., Konan, M., and Tweed, D. *A Study of Deficiencies and Differentials in the Distribution of Mental Health Resources in Facilities.* Department of Health, Education, and Welfare Publication No. (ADM) 79-517. Washington, D.C.:

U.S. Government Printing Office, 1979.

Mazer, M. *People and Predicaments.* Cambridge, Mass.: Harvard University Press, 1976.

Morical, L. *Training Trainers of Rural Housewife Peer Counselors.* Report on National Institute of Mental Health Grant No. MH14070, 1975.

Morrill, W. A. "Services Integration and the DHEW." *Evaluation,* 1976, *3,* 1-2.

President's Commission on Mental Health. *Report to the President.* Vol. 1. Washington, D.C.: U.S. Government Printing Office, 1978a.

President's Commission on Mental Health. *Report to the President.* Vol. 3. Washington, D.C.: U.S. Government Printing Office, 1978b.

Reul, M. R. *Territorial Boundaries of Rural Poverty: Profiles of Exploitation.* Lansing: Center for Rural Manpower and Public Affairs, Michigan State University, Cooperative Extension Service, 1974.

Srole, L. "Long-Term Trends in Urban Mental Health: Old Theories and New Evidence from the Midtown Manhattan Restudy." Paper presented at annual meeting of American Psychiatric Association, Toronto, May 1977.

Tweeten, L. *Foundations of Farm Policy.* Lincoln: University of Nebraska Press, 1970.

Uhlmann, J. "Boom Towns: Implications for Human Services." In M. O. Wagenfeld (Ed), *New Directions for Mental Health Services: Perspectives on Rural Mental Health,* no. 9, 1981.

U.S. Department of Agriculture. *Rural Rides: A Practical Handbook For Starting and Operating a Rural Public Transportation System.* Program Aid 1215. Washington, D.C.: Department of Agriculture, 1978.

U.S. Department of Commerce, Bureau of the Census. "Population of the U.S. by Metropolitan–Nonmetropolitan Residence: 1970." In *Current Population Reports, Population Characteristics.* Series P-20, No. 197. Washington, D.C.: U.S. Government Printing Office, 1973.

U.S. Department of Labor. "Highlights of the 1970 Manpower Report to the President." *Manpower,* June 1970.

Vallance, T. *Indigenous Caregiving Networks in Primary Prevention.* Report on National Institute of Mental Health Grant No. MH14883, 1977.

Wagenfeld, M. O. "Cultural Barriers to the Delivery of Mental Health Services in Rural Areas: A Conceptual Overview." Paper presented at the Conference on Rural Community Mental Health, National Institute of Mental Health, Rockville, Md., May 1977.

Wagenfeld, M. O. "Psychopathology in Rural Areas: Issues and Evidence." In P. Keller and J. D. Murray (Eds.), *Handbook of Rural Community Mental Health.* New York: Human Sciences Press, 1982.

Wagenfeld, M. O., and Wagenfeld, J. "Values, Culture, and the Delivery of Mental Health Services." In M. O. Wagenfeld (Ed.), *New Directions for Mental Health Services: Perspectives on Rural Mental Health,* no. 9, 1981.

Chapter 20

Linking Mental Health and Health Care Systems

Anthony Broskowski

The primary focus of this chapter is on the organizational and clinical service issues related to improved coordination between the general health sector and the mental health sector. These specific issues stem from an older and much broader set of concerns pertaining to the relationship between physical health and mental health and from more extensive efforts to improve coordination among all types of human services.

Emanating from concerns with fragmentation, inaccessibility, discontinuity, duplication, and inefficiency of services, major efforts were made in the 1960s and 1970s at all levels of federal, state, and local government to better coordinate and integrate the wide range of human services being provided at the state and local levels. The major efforts in this area were funded by the Department of Health, Education, and Welfare through Services Integration Projects aimed at creating integrated struc-

Note: Parts of this chapter reflect work conducted under National Institute of Mental Health Contract No. 278-79-0030 (OP), Division of Biometry and Epidemiology, Primary Care Research Section; Dr. Jack Burke, government project officer.

tures for policy making, planning, funding, and service delivery. These general concerns for improved coordination of services achieved came to focus on special high-risk target groups and those persons who were likely to have greater than usual problems in gaining access to services and in receiving continuity of care across specialized settings.

Many of these specific concerns were finally brought together by the President's Commission on Mental Health (1978), whose final report and associated appendixes documented the continuing needs of unserved or underserved high-risk groups. The reasons for lack of service included the barriers to care presented by a categorically specialized service delivery system, the poor match between needs and distribution resources (facilities, programs, and service staff), and the continuing stigma associated with mental illness and the utilization of mental health services. Coordinated service delivery strategies were especially recommended for such high-risk groups as chronic psychiatric patients, children, migrants, and the elderly, as well as for rural or poverty-level urban areas, where distance or a lack of resources created special problems of discontinuity and fragmentation.

Research conducted in the earliest days of the neighborhood health centers (NHCs) program demonstrated that the most consistent barrier to the goal of achieving comprehensive health services was, very simply, the lack of mental health services (Langston, 1979). Findings stressed that the lack of available mental health personnel and the general stigma attached to mental illness contributed to the gaps observed between estimated needs, actual demands, and final utilization of mental health services.

As initially passed by Congress, the Mental Health Systems Act (P.L. 96-398) made provision for special grants to "any public or nonprofit private entity which provides mental health services . . . and has in effect an agreement of affiliation . . . with an entity which is a health care center." This "agreement of affiliation" was to describe the common geographical areas to be served, provide for the employment of "at least one mental health professional to serve as a liaison," and give assurances that the mental health entity would make services available to patients referred by the health center. A "health care center" was defined in this law to include "an outpatient facility operated in connection with a hospital, a primary care center, a community health center, a migrant health center, a clinic of the Indian Health Service, or skilled nursing home, an intermediate care facility, and an outpatient health care facility of a medical group practice, a public health department, or a health maintenance organization." Although later repealed by Congress as part of the Reagan administration's Budget Reconciliation Act, these provisions were another expression of a renewed desire at the federal level to promote greater coordination in health and mental health services, training, and research (Burns, Burke, and Kessler, 1981). Now the new block grants for alcohol and drug abuse and for mental health services also allow states to use these funds to support linkages between mental health and primary health care.

Current Efforts Toward Coordination

Coordination of services is obviously needed, given the realities that have been uncovered by epidemiological and service utilization studies. These studies indicate that the greatest amount of mental health care is already being provided by the primary care service sector. Regier, Goldberg, and Taube (1978) estimate that approximately 54 percent of all persons with mental health disorders who receive treatment are treated exclusively in the primary care sector. Only 15 percent of all those persons with diagnosed mental health disorders (3 percent of the total population) receive services in such specialty mental health settings as community mental health centers (CMHCs), psychiatric hospitals, and private offices of mental health professionals. Furthermore, research indicates other critical patterns: A significant percentage of the primary care physician's case load consists of patients with significant mental health problems as their chief or secondary complaint; there is a positive correlation between the utilization of medical services and the presence of psychiatric problems; a significant percentage of clients in mental health settings have undetected medical problems, some of which could readily account for their emotional or cognitive disorders; and psychological factors may affect levels of susceptibility to physical disease, influence the severity of somatic symptoms, or mitigate against the efficiency and effectiveness of medical interventions.

An excellent review of the literature on the relationship of health and mental health disorders has recently been written by Hankin and Oktay (1979). In addition to documenting the high prevalence of mental disorders seen in primary care settings, their review examines the different hypotheses to account for the relatively high rate of medical service utilization by persons with psychiatric problems. Emotionally disturbed persons may have a lower tolerance for symptoms of physical illness or greater "propensities to seek medical care" (Hankin and Oktay, 1979). Also, they may be more likely to "somaticize" their psychological problems, or they may actually contract more diseases than less psychologically disturbed persons. For reasons not well understood, psychological and environmental stresses may increase susceptibility to germs or make one more accident prone (Broskowski and Baker, 1974). Another reason for the correlation of emotional problems and medical care utilization is that patients with emotional problems probably experience fewer feelings of shame when they seek care in a primary health care setting rather than in a mental health setting (Hankin and Oktay, 1979). Finally, although not explicitly hypothesized by Hankin and Oktay, the findings that persons with emotional problems tend to use medical services at a higher than average rate can be partly explained by economic incentives. A visit to an internist for back pain and "tension" is more likely to be reimbursed, depending on the diagnosis and treatment reported to the insurance company, than a visit to a community mental health center.

Literature on the physician's management of emotionally disturbed patients in primary care settings has also been reviewed by Hankin (1980). She found that there is a heavy reliance on the use of psychotropic medication, and, in many cases, on brief counseling. However, Hankin reports that there is very little well-conducted research on the intensity, appropriateness, and effectiveness of these techniques of patient management. Clearly the pace and volume of services in primary care settings preclude the use of specialized diagnostic and treatment methods typically found in specialty mental health settings. The National Ambulatory Medical Care Survey shows that the nonpsychiatric physician spends an average of thirteen minutes for each patient's visit (Hankin and Oktay, 1979).

Related to the epidemiological literature reviewed by Hankin and Oktay is the growing literature on behavioral medicine and those environmental and behavioral factors related to the population's general level of health or specific diseases. Stress, diet, exercise, smoking, and a host of psychological factors are being implicated in an increasingly greater range of medical disorders previously thought to be related exclusively to genetic, biological, or chemical factors (Houpt and others, 1979; Stone, Cohen, and Adler, 1979; Goplerud, 1981). Greater awareness of the role of psychological and behavioral factors in general health and medical care will continue to suggest the need for greater cooperation between specialty mental health professionals and both general and specialty medical professionals.

In addition to the current realities of epidemiology, service utilization, and patient management practices, there is continuing pressure to reexamine and change existing methods of service organization and financing. Health maintenance organizations (HMOs), health care foundations, group practice, and new cost containment and financial incentive systems are receiving great attention. The heavy utilization of medical services by persons with psychiatric problems suggests that significant cost savings may be realized when less expensive and more appropriate mental health services are made available as an alternative to expensive and unnecessary medical services. The extensive literature and research related to these issues have been discussed under the rubric of "cost offset" and are reviewed by Jones and Vischi (1979) and by Mumford, Schlesinger, and Glass (1981). Also related to the accessibility and cost of services is the continuing trend to shift services from expensive institutional settings to ambulatory, community-based settings or to provide home-based care. More leaders in society also seem willing to balance the need for highly specialized medical care of acute conditions against the need for secondary and tertiary levels of care for chronic medical and psychiatric conditions.

In addition to service delivery and service-financing concerns, there are efforts to integrate the health and mental health sectors in areas of planning (Hagedorn, 1981), training (Hollen, Ehrlich, and White, 1981; Adams, Chapter Twenty-Four in this volume), and research (Guerra and Aldrete, 1980).

Before examining specific strategies to achieve broad-scale delivery coordination, however, it would be useful to synthesize these trends by portraying them as potential benefits to consumers, staff, and funding sources. Table 1, based on earlier work by Borus and others (1980) and Burke, Burns, O'Flaherty, and Broskowski (1980) – and adapted by Broskowski (1980a, 1980b)–summarizes the major benefits for patients of better health and mental health linkages: improved case finding and diagnosis, increased comprehensiveness and efficiency in service utilization, and improved continuity, compliance, and satisfaction. A more detailed review of the literature documenting these benefits has been done by Broskowski (1980b) and Marks and Broskowski (1981). In addition to these clinical benefits, there is a possibility of financial savings when mental health services are provided to heavy but inappropriate users of health care services (Cummings and Follette, 1968; Jones and Vischi, 1979; Mumford, Schlesinger, and Glass, 1981). Problems will remain, however, in measuring the actual size of this cost offset and in understanding the cause-effect relationships that account for it. These issues will be reexamined in the final section of this chapter when the needs for future research in the area of coordinated health and mental health care will be discussed.

Models for Coordination

Efforts at coordination are taking place at multiple levels, including federal, state, and local training, research, and service institutions. To guide our understanding of this complex array of efforts, let us consider several general and specific models for

Table 1. Benefits of Health and Mental Health Linkages.

1. *Improved Case Finding*
   a. Improved detection of mental health problems by primary care providers
   b. Improved ability to detect needs of special populations and high-risk groups (for example, the elderly, the poor, and the bereaved)
   c. Increased diagnostic precision through education and consultation by mental health staff
   d. More appropriate utilization of both types of services, particularly by special populations and high-risk groups
2. *Increased Successful Referrals*
   a. Less stigma to service
   b. Decreased waiting
   c. Improved physical or geographical accessibility
   d. Reduced mystery to the process of mental health services
3. *Improved Coordination Between Health Staff and Mental Health Staff*
   a. Improved coordination among staff and their special skills and services
   b. Improved medical care for psychiatric patients
   c. Increase in family-oriented health and mental health care
   d. Increase in appropriate balance of medication and counseling for primary care patients
4. *Improved Follow-Up*
   a. Improved continuity over time, within families, and across providers
   b. Improved patient compliance with treatment regimen, less "shopping."
   c. Increased patient satisfaction

coordination. Like all models, the ones we review are intended to simplify reality by stressing a few major dimensions while ignoring others. Thus, a model's simplicity can make it seductive at the same time as it guides learning and further research.

Generic Models. The early Services Integration Projects stimulated the building of several generic models to conceptualize coordinated services. For example, Gans and Horton (1975) developed a taxonomy of administrative and direct service linkage mechanisms or exchanges that could occur among multiple agencies. They classified each mechanism according to the resources and time needed for its development and its potential impact on access, continuity, and efficiency of services. For the most part, administrative linkages, such as joint budgeting, planning, funding, and consolidated personnel administration, require long periods of time to implement, and their high cost may negate the benefits achieved (John, 1977). However, several types of administrative linkage are more readily instituted than others and are hypothesized to have a considerable impact on services and in particular to facilitate joint purchase of services, colocation of autonomous staff, and joint staff training.

Direct service linkages require shorter implementation periods (Gans and Horton, 1975) than do administrative ones. "Core service" linkages involve cooperative outreach, intake, diagnosis, referral, and follow-up services. Ongoing "case consultation" linkages use case conferences, multidisciplinary treatment teams, and case managers to coordinate the provision of services by multiple but autonomous service providers. Both types of service linkages can increase access and comprehensiveness of services, but little is known about their ultimate impact on the outcome or effectiveness of service delivery (John, 1977).

In contrast to this detailed interorganization typology, other generic models use a "single-solution" approach. They create a single, one-stop, multiservice agency; establish a community-wide, computerized information and referral system; or start a case management and service-brokering agency supported by members' dues, analogous to the American Automobile Association (Long, 1974). Another model developed by Spencer (1974) attempts to define the "horizontal" linkages needed to fill the gaps commonly found in the direct service system, as well as the "horizontal" linkages needed to reduce the common and unnecessary duplication of administrative and support services. Spencer's model also addresses the "vertical" linkages needed by the various branches and levels of federal, state, and local funding and regulatory agencies.

Another approach is to distinguish the varying levels and settings of care needed for different types of clinical problems and population sizes. Macht (1975) and Borus and others (1975) conceptualized four levels of integrated care. Level I (primary care) would consist of direct clinical outpatient services, consultation and education, preventive efforts, crisis intervention, and aftercare programs. These would be delivered within organized health or multiservice centers serving 10,000 to

50,000 persons at the neighborhood level. Level II (acute secondary care) would include short-term hospitalization, along with direct and consultation services in community hospitals or CMHCs; it would cover a "service area" population of up to 200,000 persons. Level III (extended secondary care) would occur in the same settings as Level II services but would include specialized inpatient care of less than twelve months and more specialized outpatient services. Finally, Level IV care (chronic, tertiary, and custodial services) would be provided at regional facilities that encompassed a minimum of two service areas. The success of this staged system of care would rely heavily on linkages between service providers both within and across levels of care.

At this point, we might turn to specific models or mechanisms that operate at the level of primary mental health or health services (Level I). The pertinent models include those that generalize across settings and those that are specific to particular types of settings or interorganizational agreements.

Setting-Specific Models. One of the earliest models for analyzing the patterns of existing relationships between neighborhood health centers (NHCs) and community mental health centers (CMHCs) was developed by Borus and his colleagues (Borus and others, 1975; Borus, 1976). Using a study of nineteen NHCs with mental health programs in the Greater Boston area, these authors developed four models to classify each NHC, based primarily on its relationship to a local CMHC or mental health clinic.

The most prevalent model is called Joint Endeavor. In it, the NHC houses the neighborhood mental health program and directly employs some mental health staff, usually indigenous paraprofessionals. Additional professional staff are employed by the local CMHC and delegated to work at the NHC. These Joint Endeavor NHC programs have varying degrees of independence from the CMHC and provide varying degrees of specialized backup services to one another. The Autonomous NHC model is a mental health program funded and run exclusively by the NHC. Staff and services may be either part time or full time, depending on the NHC funds available for services. These NHCs may have a nonmonetary liaison to the local CMHC, presumably for purposes of referring patients to more specialized care. When all the mental health staff are CMHC employees but they are located within the NHC, the model is called a Community Mental Health Outpost. Finally, the Consultative Model, instead of having a mental health program within the NHC, has a "working alliance" with a nearby CMHC satellite that serves the same area solely for purposes of case consultation and referral to the CMHC.

While the models presented by Borus and others (1975) and Borus (1976) are specific to NHC and CMHC linkages, they do not specify the interaction mechanisms between the centers involved. Integrated care teams, case managers, and a joint record of health and mental health may be maintained, but these mechanisms are not related to any particular model. The main determinant of each model appears to be who hires the mental health staff or contributes it to the program. Contributions of space, funds, and other resources receive little consideration.

Morrill (1972) has suggested the "family health care team" as the most appropriate model for mental health care in an NHC. Similarly, Coleman and Patrick (1976) have recommended a "team collaboration model" for use in HMOs. These two team models differ, however, in that Morrill proposes an egalitarian role for the mental health specialist, while Coleman and Patrick (1976) place the primary care physician in the central role of providing most of the necessary mental health services; the mental health professional would be used only for special referrals. Other mechanisms briefly discussed by Coleman and Patrick (1976) are using psychiatric consultants, educating primary care clinicians, and instituting a full-time program similar to the Autonomous Model of Borus and others (1975). But all these approaches are dismissed by Coleman and Patrick as ineffective in the long run, since each would perpetuate a fragmented and specialized system.

In a recent review of HMO-provided mental health services, Budman (1981) describes three models: (1) the integrated health and mental health primary care team; (2) the separate mental health department within the HMO; and (3) a fee-for-service or per-capita contract between the HMO and one or more private mental health professionals or an organized CMHC. Based on various concerns for staff acceptance, cost control and quality assurance, Budman prefers the second model, acknowledging that the choice is often determined by such other factors as the availability of generalists and specialists and start-up costs.

With regard to the details of linkage mechanisms, Burns (1980) itemized eleven specific mechanisms for coordination in a successful Joint Endeavor model (see Table 2). A highly generalizable approach to coordination, applicable across a wide

Table 2. Mechanisms of Health and Mental Health Interaction at the Provider Level.

Mechanism	*Examples of Applications*
1. Single medical record	Formal communication among providers
2. Multidiscipline health care team	Multiproblem families with health and mental health problems are frequently presented
3. Ease of referral to mental health services	Open intake system by mental health service
4. Case-centered consultation	Health provider requests for advice on management of patients
5. Center committees	Medical records, various task forces
6. In-service education	Series on alcoholism, child development, infant-parent relationships
7. Joint patient interviews	Modeling assessment approaches for health providers
8. Collaborative program	Preschool screening, obesity group, medication clinic
9. Client-centered consultation	Pediatric nurses counseling adolescent mothers meet with psychiatrist regularly
10. Liaison to units	A pediatrician attends the child mental health intake meeting
11. Collaborative research	A study of internists' patterns for prescribing tranquilizers

Source: Burns (1980).

range of local settings, was developed by Pincus (1980). According to this model, linkages between health and mental health services vary along three broad dimensions: the contractual agreement, the functional integration of services, and the educational services. Pincus describes six models for types of linkages in terms of their relative emphasis on one or more of these dimensions.

Model 1, "agreement," emphasizes the purely contractual relationship between a health facility and a mental health facility, usually limited to the clinical services to be provided by each party to the contract. Clinical services are provided on a referral basis, and the patient has the major responsibility for connecting the two systems. Formal and informal referral patterns in private practice are both typical of Model 1 linkages. Contracts between HMOs and CMHCs for purchase of mental health services also illustrate Model 1 linkages.

Model 2, "triage," also emphasizes contractual agreements, but there is in addition a significant functional component, namely, designated staff members who provide assessment, triage, and referral as well as ease follow-up and information flow. Triage linkages also provide for informal consultations and case conferences. The primary care center–CMHC linkage initiative sponsored by the Alcohol, Drug Abuse and Mental Health Administration and the Health Services Administration is an example of Model 2 linkages (Broskowski, 1980a, 1980b; Marks and Broskowski, 1981).

Model 3, "service delivery team," establishes a mental health unit within the primary health care facility. This type of linkage places maximum emphasis on the functional integration of services. The mental health unit provides assessment and limited treatment, which is supplemented by services from other agencies or teams. As in the triage model, the educational elements are only coincidental and secondary to the emphasis on the functional services. As examples of the service delivery team, Pincus (1980) lists a variety of group health plans and HMO programs (see Budman, 1981).

Model 4, "consultation and service," emphasizes mental health educational and consultative services to improve the expertise of the primary care provider in the diagnosis and treatment of mental illness. Specialty care is provided by the specialist only when necessary. In Model 4, functional and educational aspects are combined, with more emphasis placed on the functional consultation. Contractual agreements are usually informal. Illustrations are found in teaching hospitals with consultation-liaison services.

Model 5, "supervision and education," places primary emphasis on educational aspects, with little or no direct service provided by referral to specialty staff. Contractual issues are minimal. Continuing medical education programs in psychiatry for nonpsychiatric physicians and some programs in undergraduate and graduate medical education are examples of this type of linkage.

Model 6, "integrated health care team," combines all three dimensions of linkage. Mental health specialists are integrated into the day-to-day practice of the primary care facility, and they provide direct services, referral, consultation, and continuing education for primary care staff. Pincus (1980) cites a particular HMO, a neighborhood health center, and a family practice group as examples.

Based on a comprehensive review of the literature and a questionnaire survey of forty-seven sites funded by Bureau of Community Health Services (BCHS) to link CMHCs and Primary Health Care Projects (PHCPs), Broskowski (1980a, 1980b) developed a classification scheme to account for variations in the operation of the agreements between the two kinds of agencies. Deliberately simplified to guide further research and technical assistance, this scheme proposes two essential dimensions: *symmetry,* that is, the degree to which the linked partners are balanced with respect to their relative contribution and control of coordinated resources; and *interaction,* or the intensity, frequency, and levels of exchange taking place through the agreement. These two dimensions are critical in developing a new linkage as well as in its maintenance over time. While partially validated by the survey research, literature review, and seven site visits, this model, as well as others described earlier, warrants further research.

Developing and Maintaining Coordinated Care

The selection of a particular model or mechanisms for linking health and mental health programs will depend upon numerous considerations. Pincus (1980) emphasizes the characteristics and needs of the people served, geographical and cultural constraints, the location and auspices of services, available financing mechanisms, staff attitudes and philosophy of care, and level of care desired. Thus, models emphasizing educational elements will not work in fee-for-service settings since consultation, supervision, and education are not reimbursable activities.

Broskowski (1980b), in a review of 200 theoretical articles, case studies, and research reports, emphasizes the importance of both clinical and administrative factors in planning, implementing, and maintaining an effective linkage between two or more organizations or units within a single organization. These factors were further differentiated according to whether they reflected environmental conditions, interorganizational comparisons, or intraorganizational capacities on the part of each setting. Finally, a developmental perspective is required as the field of forces changes from the earliest period of no linkage, through successive stages of linkage development, and on to maturity.

A number of forces are found to support or promote the development of linkage:

- Interdependency based on complementary needs and resources.
- Need for survival and/or growth.
- Efficiency through sharing costs and underutilized resources.
- Effectiveness, particularly for the client with numerous problems.
- Comprehensiveness, particularly gaining access to scarce specialized resources.
- Stability through ties to other sources of stability.
- Preferred ideology of human services is cooperation, not competition.

Forces that can inhibit linkage development are as follows:

- Fear of lost control and lost autonomy of action.
- Explicit and hidden costs of maintaining linkages in terms of time, staff, and other resources.
- Perception of incompatible values, goals, or objectives.
- Incentives to compete for money and reputation.
- Lack of awareness of the benefits of a linkage.
- Lack of administrative and/or clinical skill or knowledge needed to develop, implement, and maintain linkages.

Given these facilitating and inhibiting forces, several critical dimensions must be understood for purposes of planning, implementing, and maintaining linkages:

- The level(s) at which a linkage is developed, including clients, staff, middle management, executives, board members, and/or high levels of governmental funding and regulatory agencies.
- The type of exchanges that take place across a linkage, including the exchange of services, money, personnel, or other resources and support services.
- The degree of standardization of the units of information being exchanged.
- The frequency or extensiveness of the exchange(s).
- The formality of the linkage agreement.
- The degree of continuous maintenance and explicit management required by the linkage.
- The degree of reciprocity in costs and benefits among the parties to the agreement.
- The degree to which the linkage is voluntary or mandated.
- The degree of complexity inherent in the linkage by virtue of the combination of factors on the dimensions listed above.

The complexity of linkage development suggests why it is so seldom attempted and effectively maintained, despite the benefits it has to offer. Tables 3 and 4 summarize the variables deemed important in the theoretical and research literature (Broskowski, 1980b). Because of the overwhelming complexity of considering so many variables and combinations, it is critical

Table 3. Environmental and Intraorganizational Conditions That Inhibit or Facilitate Interorganizational Relationships.

		Effect on Interorganizational Relationships		
I	*Environmental Conditions*	*Inhibitory*		*Facilitative*
	a. Resource amount	Abundance		Scarcity
	b. Resource location	Randomized		Organized
	c. Rate of change	Placid	Turbulent	Intermediate
	d. Complexity	Low	High	Intermediate
	e. Predictability	High	Low	Intermediate
II	*Intraorganizational Conditions*			
	a. Amount of resources	Abundant	Scarce	Intermediate
	b. Control over resources	High		Low
	c. Leadership style	Insular/Orthodox		Exploratory/ Innovative
	d. Core technology	Intensive	Mediated	Linked
	e. Internal coordination	Weak		Strong
	f. Information capability	Primitive		Advanced

that linkage strategies be based on a process of slow implementation that is focused on well-defined goals. Assuming that the influence of the thirty-two variables noted in Tables 3 and 4 is valid, then human service agencies already start at a disadvantage in developing linkages with one another. Specifically, health and mental health agencies are characterized by complex, intensive technologies, they use high levels of specialization, and they require a great deal of internal control over their own resources. An agency's informational requirements are not simple, and information-processing capabilities are generally not well developed (Broskowski and Attkisson, forthcoming). Finally, the general environment of human services is characterized by multiple and conflicting levels of control and management. Turbulent change and low predictability are endemic. Paradoxically, the more that external forces attempt to control and regulate a health agency, requiring it to be responsible and accountable for more and more details, the less inclined its leadership will be to sacrifice control through a potentially risky linkage.

Table 4. Interorganizational Conditions that Inhibit or Facilitate Interorganizational Relationships.

Interorganizational Conditions	*Effect on Interorganizational Relationships*		
	Inhibitory		*Facilitative*
I. Comparative			
A. Entities involved	Many		Few
B. Dependency	None	Asymmetrical/unilateral	Reciprocal
C. Prior experience	Negative	None	Positive
D. Goals/domains	Competitive	Identical	Complementary
E. Auspices	Antagonistic	Neutral	Supportive
F. Sanctions	None	Required	Voluntary
G. Philosophy/values	Conflictual	Similar	Identical
H. Complexity	Dissimilar		Similar
1. Size	Dissimilar		Similar
2. Structure	Dissimilar		Similar
3. Technologies	Dissimilar		Similar
II. Relational			
A. Planning/negotiations	Unilateral		Reciprocal
B. Implementation	Sudden/sporadic		Gradual
C. Dimensions of exchange			
1. Benefits	Unequal		Equal
2. Units	Heterogeneous		Standardized
3. Levels	Few	Many	Intermediate
4. Information	Little		Mutual feedback
5. Rate	Seldom		Frequent
6. Distance	Great		Small
D. Commitment/formality	Unmanaged		Managed

Interorganizational relationships between health and mental health must be built slowly and must be based on the complementary and reciprocal needs of both organizations and their clients. Simple and well-defined goals should be mutually arrived at and agreed upon in writing. Both organizations need to be explicit with regard to their motivations and ultimate goals. Clear delineation of each organization's administrative and clinical responsibilities and authority should be specified in the early stages. Details regarding the exchange of information, money, or personnel need to be considered. Successive discussions should be reduced to writing for review and further revisions.

After its initial planning, a linkage is best implemented on a gradual but firm schedule. Linkages need clear and unambiguous support by the top management as well as the line staff. If "linkage" personnel are to be hired, particular attention should be paid to the compatibility of such personnel with the staffs of both agencies. Staff who engage in boundary-spanning roles are commonly subject to the pressures and strains that can exist at any level between two organizations. Boundary-spanning jobs require experience, maturity, and the ability to earn the respect of staff in both organizations. Ongoing clinical and administrative supervision and support are critical. Information to monitor the relationship should be identified, collected, and routinely shared by both parties.

Even under these idealized circumstances, line staff and directors will need to be flexible and patient. Environmental barriers, in the form of nonsupportive funding or regulatory prohibitions, must be overcome. Flexibility, consistency, and predictability on the part of government funding sources would help enormously. Higher-level governmental executives will have to develop and maintain linkages across their own boundaries so that the burdens of experimentation, risk, and lost autonomy are not limited to the front-line staff.

Published case studies and information gathered at the seven program sites visited by Broskowski and his colleagues reinforce the theoretical literature and raise additional concerns. For example, case studies by Earls (1979), Schniewind (1976), and Lowenkopf and Zwerling (1979) identify additional but related environmental, administrative, and clinical concerns. Furthermore, Schniewind (1976), Gilchrist and others (1978), and Burns (1980) highlight the developmental nature of a linkage agreement and the linkage worker's job duties. The issues from these and other case studies are summarized in Table 5. These

Table 5. Factors Affecting Health and Mental Health Coordination.

A. *Environmental Conditions*
   1. Community stability or turbulence
   2. Levels of government and intergovernmental issues
      a. Barriers in statutes, rules, and regulations
      b. Technical assistance and support
   3. Other community resources or barriers

B. *Administrative Concerns*
   1. The administrative planning process: specific and incremental
   2. Administrative leadership, support, and control
   3. Fiscal considerations; who receives funds, who pays what costs
   4. Facilities, personnel policies, and other logistical supports (phone, travel, and so on)
   5. Mechanisms for administrative integration and feedback (committees, reports, and so on)

C. *Clinical Concerns*
   1. Recruiting appropriate staff, gaining entry, developing relationships, clarifying expectations and stereotypes
   2. Range of services and activities to be provided by each staff
   3. Clinical authority and responsibility, and who supervises whom
   4. Professional identification and specialized career development; interprofessional rivalry
   5. Technologies, language systems, and ideologies (for example, social, medical, or biopsychosocial models)
   6. Mechanism for frequent, case-oriented clinical integration and feedback (consultations, record systems, and so on)

fourteen areas of concern were reported to be critical to the ultimate success or failure of many efforts at health and mental health coordination (Broskowski, 1980b). Again, they all occur simultaneously, with no clear priorities or well-defined solutions that apply in all circumstances.

Recommendations for the Future

The potential benefits of coordinated care, coupled with the complexities of achieving it, suggest the need for a full range of future actions. For convenience, we have arbitrarily organized these actions into three domains: epidemiology and treatment research, organizational and financial initiatives, and professional training and development.

Epidemiology and Treatment Research. Further research is needed to estimate the incidence, prevalence, and distribution of conjoint health and mental health problems. Hankin and Oktay (1979), Regier (1980), and others indicate that estimates vary according to the criteria and methods of research that are used. For example, reliable and valid screening and assessment instruments are needed to estimate the prevalence of psychiatric disorders appearing in primary care settings and of medical disorders in mental health settings. Further, environmental and behavioral correlates of conjoint health and mental health problems must be identified. Developmental patterns may also exist that would suggest prevention strategies.

Treatment research is needed to compare the relative effectiveness of alternative intervention strategies, such as brief counseling by primary care physicians, changes in patients' behavioral life-styles, or modifications in their personal support systems or environments. Currently, research is being conducted on the impact of a wide range of attitudes, emotions, and behaviors on various physical disease processes, such as hypertension and cancer.

As a part of treatment research, studies of service utilization and patient management will elucidate current practices. For example, are there particular patterns of medical services that are overused or misused by emotionally disturbed patients? Studies that bridge the areas of treatment impact and financing need to examine the size and causes of the "cost-offset" effect, that is, the reduction of health care service utilization following even brief mental health interventions. Mumford, Schlesinger, and Glass (1981) have pointed out many difficulties in the valid interpretation of such effects. But certainly, to the extent that inappropriate health services utilization can be reduced at no loss of health to the consumer, mental health providers could expect to be allocated some of the savings in the reallocation of financial savings. Numerous logical and methodological problems remain to be solved (Jones and Vischi, 1979). Well-controlled research may show a cost savings for particular subgroups of patients or problems (Goldberg and others, in press). Another area of needed treatment research is the development of patient management protocols for prevalent psychological-medical disorders. Walker (1981), for example, has emphasized the need to understand behavioral emergencies so that better patient assessment and treatment intervention can be instituted in general hospital emergency rooms.

Organizational and Financial Research. Continued organizational research and technical assistance are needed to improve the accessibility, continuity, and effectiveness of health and mental health care. For example, the effectiveness of health education and promotion and prevention campaigns is still poorly understood.

Organization research must be coupled with treatment research to evaluate the effectiveness and efficiency of strategies that rely on linkages between existing specialty organizations, such as CMHCs and neighborhood health centers. Broskowski (1980b) suggested that longitudinal cohort studies be conducted to achieve a better understanding than is possible through single-time questionnaire surveys. Cohorts served in different types of settings could yield information about the influence of service setting characteristics. Five types of cohorts could be studied:

1. Patients treated by liaison staff in health settings formally linked to specialty mental health settings (called linkage sites).
2. Patients in linkage sites not seen or treated by liaison staff.
   a. Patients with clear psychiatric diagnoses.
   b. Patients without clear psychiatric diagnoses.
3. Patients in health settings that do not have active linkages (formal or informal) with mental health settings and do not have mental health staffs of their own.
4. Patients seen in CMHCs with no formal or informal linkages with primary health care settings. (Does a linkage increase access above what CMHCs can do alone?)
5. Patients seen in health settings where there is some minimal

mental health staff but no sources of referral to mental health settings for backup services.

Studies using cohorts from these five settings could examine their sociodemographic and clinical characteristics, the pattern of services provided (time and amount), the providers of each service type, referral sources, and disposition data.

Once utilization studies have been conducted, it is feasible to analyze the relationship of services utilized, or not utilized, to patient outcomes. The difficulties of conducting patient outcome studies have been well described in other publications (Attkisson and others, 1978). The point to be emphasized here is that greater efficiency and specificity in examining pertinent outcomes in both the health and mental health domains will be possible only after the interaction of patient characteristics and service utilization patterns is well understood. Utilization studies can also be extended to determine if the cost-offset effect in health and mental health linkage sites is as extensive as that reported in HMOs and other highly integrated health and mental health care settings. Even if the agencies do not directly benefit from the savings, utilization offset may also be attractive to directors and staff because they can improve staff working conditions and/or reduce morale problems and service pressures on overworked primary health care providers.

Many of the organizational linkage models reviewed earlier need to be evaluated and compared on such criteria as accessibility, effectiveness, continuity, and costs. Technical solutions to some of the commonly reported problems with interorganizational linkages, such as agreeing on the scope of duties, responsibilities, and authority of the clinical liaison staff, need to be field tested and disseminated (Broskowski, 1980b).

Professional Training and Development. The administrative and clinical skills to implement and maintain interorganization linkages are generally underdeveloped. Current and prospective professional liaison staff need training in entry and relationship-building skills, in procedures for clarifying supervision and clinical authority relationships, and in specific skills in detection, differential diagnosis, and case consultation.

Training for administrators also needs to be studied. For example, how does an agency best recruit and supervise qualified liaison staff? What are the organizational correlates of treatment continuity and of efficient team management? What types of personnel policies, fiscal incentives, patient records, and statistical information systems are needed to maintain an effective interagency linkage? What types of patient referral and treatment scheduling systems will maintain continuity across separate agencies or specialty units within a multiservice organization?

Even before working together as employees or private practitioners, personnel must develop attitudes and skills that promote better coordination. The chapter by Adams in this volume provides one example of a pertinent multidisciplinary training program. Similar programs are developing in other educational and field-based training sites (Authier, 1981; Hollen, Ehrlich, and White, 1981). Nevertheless, interdisciplinary rivalries will continue to be barriers to well-coordinated patient care. For example, family medicine specialists may be seen as threats by general psychiatrists, who, in turn, may strive to maintain professional ascendancy over behavioral scientists as the latter groups press for a more equitable share of professional privileges and patient revenues. In fact, competition for decreasing training funds and treatment revenues may be the biggest barrier to improved linkages between health care and mental health care. In the meantime, we must continue training efforts to reduce such rivalries, clarify mutual expectations, improve referral practices, and share limited resources.

A major development in the next decade will be the building of linkages between the two domains of health and mental health. On the one hand, epidemiological service utilization studies and economic scarcity suggest that continued specialization or competition will have serious negative consequences for patients and professionals alike. On the other hand, an enthusiastic effort to bridge over long-standing separations is likely to stimulate new clinical knowledge and a renewed faith in our professions by the public. Presidential and congressional interest in block grant funding mechanisms can either stimulate more intense competition between the health sector and the mental health sector for the scarce service dollar or promote local-level coalitions that will make more efficient use of dollars. We cannot believe that competition will be helpful for either sector.

References

Attkisson, C., and others (Eds.). *Evaluation of Human Service Programs.* New York: Academic Press, 1978.

Authier, J. "Integrated Medical Training: A Family Focus." In A. Broskowski, E. Marks, and S. Budman (Eds.), *Linking Health and Mental Health: Coordinating Care in the Community.* Beverly Hills, Calif.: Sage, 1981.

Borus, J. "Neighborhood Health Centers as Providers of Primary Mental Health Care." *New England Journal of Medicine,* 1976, *295,* 140-145.

Borus, J., and others. "The Coordination of Mental Health Services at the Neighborhood Level." *American Journal of Psychiatry,* 1975, *132,* 1177-1181.

Borus, J., and others. *Coordinated Mental Health Care in Neighborhood Health Centers.* Department of Health and Human Services Publication No. (ADM) 80-996. Washington, D.C.: U.S. Government Printing Office, 1980.

Broskowski, A. "Literature Review on Interorganizational Relationships and Their Relevance to Health and Mental Health Coordination." Contract No. 278-79-0030 (OP). Rockville, Md.: National Institute of Mental Health, 1980a.

Broskowski, A. "Evaluation of the Primary Health Care Project –Community Mental Health Center Linkage Initiative; Final Report." Contract No. 278-79-0030 (OP). Rockville Md.: National Institute of Mental Health, 1980b.

Broskowski, A., and Attkisson, C. *Information Systems for Health and Human Services.* New York: Academic Press, forthcoming.

Broskowski, A., and Baker, F. "Professional, Organizational, and Social Barriers to Primary Prevention." *American Journal of Orthopsychiatry,* 1974, *44,* 707-719.

Budman, S. "Mental Health Services in the Health Maintenance

Organization." In A. Broskowski, E. Marks, and S. Budman (Eds.), *Linking Health and Mental Health: Coordinating Care in the Community.* Beverly Hills, Calif.: Sage, 1981.

Burke, J. D., Burns, B. J., O'Flaherty, H., and Broskowski, A. "Linkage Relationships in the Federal Health-Mental Health Linkage Initiative: Clinical and Organizational Aspects." Paper presented at annual meeting of the American Psychiatric Association, San Francisco, Calif., 1980.

Burns, B. "Neighborhood Health Center Model." In National Institute of Mental Health Series DN No. 2, *Mental Health Services in Primary Care Settings.* Department of Health and Human Services Publication No. (ADM) 80-995. Washington, D.C.: U.S. Government Printing Office, 1980.

Burns, B., Burke, J., and Kessler, L. "Federal Efforts to Promote General Health-Mental Health Coordination." In A. Broskowski, E. Marks, and S. Budman (Eds.), *Linking Health and Mental Health: Coordinating Care in the Community.* Beverly Hills, Calif.: Sage, 1981.

Coleman, J., and Patrick, D. "Integrating Mental Health Services into Primary Medical Care." *Medical Care,* 1976, *14,* 654-661.

Cummings, N., and Follette, W. "Psychiatric Services and Medical Utilization in a Prepaid Health Plan Setting (Part II)." *Medical Care,* 1968, *6,* 31-41.

Earls, F. "Experience in Primary Mental Health Care." *Journal of the National Medical Association,* 1979, *71,* 779-782.

Gans, S., and Horton, C. *Integration of Human Services.* New York: Praeger, 1975.

Gilchrist, I., and others. "Social Work in General Practice." *Journal of the Royal College of General Practitioners,* 1978, *28,* 675-686.

Goldberg, I., and others. "Utilization of Medical Services After Short-Term Psychiatric Therapy in a Prepaid Health Plan Setting." *Medical Care,* in press.

Goplerud, E. "The Tangled Web of Clinical and Epidemiological Evidence." In A. Broskowski, E. Marks, and S. Budman (Eds.), *Linking Health and Mental Health: Coordinating Care in the Community.* Beverly Hills, Calif.: Sage, 1981.

Guerra, F., and Aldrete, J. *Emotional and Psychological Re-*

sponses to Anesthesia and Surgery. New York: Grune & Stratton, 1980.

Hagedorn, H. "Coordinating Health and Mental Health Planning." In A. Broskowski, E. Marks, and S. Budman (Eds.), *Linking Health and Mental Health: Coordinating Care in the Community.* Beverly Hills, Calif.: Sage, 1981.

Hankin, J. "Literature Review on Management of Emotionally Disturbed Patients in Primary Care Settings." In National Institute of Mental Health Series DN No. 2, *Mental Health Services in Primary Care Settings.* Department of Health and Human Services Publication No. (ADM) 80-995. Washington, D.C.: U.S. Government Printing Office, 1980.

Hankin, J., and Oktay, J. *Mental Disorder and Primary Medical Care: An Analytic Review of the Literature.* Department of Health, Education, and Welfare Publication No. (ADM) 78-661. Washington, D.C.: U.S. Government Printing Office, 1979.

Hollen, L., Ehrlich, R., and White, S. "Integrating Health-Mental Health Training." In A. Broskowski, E. Marks, and S. Budman (Eds.), *Linking Health and Mental Health: Coordinating Care in the Community.* Beverly Hills, Calif.: Sage, 1981.

Houpt, J., and others. *The Importance of Mental Health Services to General Health Care.* Cambridge, Mass.: Ballinger, 1979.

John, D. *Managing the Human Services System: What Have We Learned From Services Integration?* Rockville, Md.: Project SHARE Monograph Series, No. 4, 1977.

Jones, K., and Vischi, T. "Impact of Alcohol, Drug Abuse and Mental Health Treatment on Medical Care Utilization: A Review of the Research Literature." *Medical Care* (Supplement), 1979, *17,* (12), 1-82.

Langston, J. "The Neighborhood Health Center Program." In J. G. Abert (Ed.), *Program Evaluation at HEW, Part I.* New York: Marcel Dekker, 1979.

Long, N. "A Model for Coordinating Human Services." *Administration in Mental Health,* 1974, *1,* 21-27.

Lowenkopf, E., and Zwerling, I. "Psychiatric Services in a Neighborhood Health Center." *American Journal of Psychiatry,* 1979, *127,* 916-920.

Macht, L. "Beyond the Mental Health Center: Planning for a Community of Neighborhoods." *Psychiatric Annals,* 1975, *5,* 56-69.

Marks, E., and Broskowski, A. "Community Mental Health and Organized Health Care Linkages." In A. Broskowski, E. Marks, and S. Budman (Eds.), *Linking Health and Mental Health: Coordinating Care in the Community.* Beverly Hills, Calif.: Sage, 1981.

Morrill, R. "A New Mental Health Services Model for the Comprehensive Neighborhood Health Center." *American Journal of Public Health,* 1972, *62,* 1108-1111.

Mumford, E., Schlesinger, H., and Glass, G. "Reducing Medical Costs Through Mental Health: Research Problems and Recommendations." In A. Broskowski, E. Marks, and S. Budman (Eds.), *Linking Health and Mental Health: Coordinating Care in the Community.* Beverly Hills, Calif.: Sage, 1981.

Pincus, A. "Linking General Health and Mental Health Systems of Care: Conceptual Models of Implementation." *American Journal of Psychiatry,* 1980, *137,* 315-320.

President's Commission on Mental Health. *Report to the President.* Vol. 1. Washington, D.C.: U.S. Government Printing Office, 1978.

Regier, D. "The Nature and Scope of Mental Health Problems in Primary Care." In National Institute of Mental Health Series DN No. 2, *Mental Health Services in Primary Care Settings.* Department of Health and Human Services Publication No. (ADM) 80-995. Washington, D.C.: U.S. Government Printing Office, 1980.

Regier, D., Goldberg, I., and Taube, C. "The De Facto U.S. Mental Health Services System." *Archives of General Psychiatry,* 1978, *35,* 685-693.

Schniewind, H. "A Psychiatrist's Experience in a Primary Health Care Setting." *International Journal of Psychiatry in Medicine,* 1976, *7,* 229-240.

Spencer, L. "The Federal Approach to Services Integration." *Urban and Social Change Review,* 1974, *7,* 7-13.

Stone, G. C., Cohen, F., and Adler, N. E. (Eds.). *Health Psychology—A Handbook: Theories, Applications, and Challenges of a Psychological Approach to the Health Care System.* San Francisco: Jossey-Bass, 1979.

Walker, E. "Behavioral Emergencies in Medical Settings." In A. Broskowski, E. Marks, and S. Budman (Eds.), *Linking Health and Mental Health: Coordinating Care in the Community.* Beverly Hills, Calif.: Sage, 1981.

Chapter 21

Evaluating Community Mental Health Programs

Herbert C. Schulberg

A unique feature of community mental health program development has been its quest for meaningful approaches to accountability. Few other human services have been subjected to as much internal and external pressure to develop evaluation procedures as have these burgeoning service delivery systems. Although the initial 1963 Community Mental Health Centers Act contained no statutory assessment requirement, a considerable amount of evaluation of these centers was undertaken, if only at simple levels (Majchrzak and Windle, 1980). The Community Mental Health Centers Amendments of 1975 did establish compulsory quality assurance procedures, and the Mental Health Systems Act of 1980 mandated specific performance measures to assess productivity, effectiveness, and fiscal viability. Much of the Mental Health Systems Act was, unfortunately, scuttled by the 1981 congressional tax legislation, and it is doubtful whether federally designed performance measures will be instituted during the Reagan administration.

Despite this policy setback, the need for accountability in the field of community mental health remains unchallenged. Some have even suggested that evaluations will assume increased significance under block grant appropriations, but at the state rather than at the federal level. The thesis of this chapter, therefore, is that program evaluation in the community mental health field is intrinsic to planning and management; its utility and significance are not dependent on specific federal legislation. While the focus of evaluation may fluctuate with changing environmental mandates and refinements in the technology of assessment, accountability nevertheless remains a key organizational function, and the following chapter reviews important issues pertaining to the evaluation of community mental health programs. Particular attention will be paid to assessing recently developed services for the chronically mentally ill—services whose efficacy especially needs to be determined in the face of impending budgetary reductions.

Human service organizations evaluate their policies and programs only periodically, if at all. They tend to maintain established practices with only minimal concern about their propriety and/or effectiveness since funding is usually continued regardless of whether client improvement can be demonstrated. However, as already noted, community mental health centers (CMHCs) have come under intense pressure to function as self-evaluating organizations that carefully link planning, service delivery, and assessment (Schulberg, 1977). Although these three functions have often been seen as discrete components in an ongoing cycle of program operation, such arbitrary distinctions are beginning to fade. Administrators and researchers, therefore, are beginning to struggle with questions that address concerns in each of these realms. As this process unfolds, choices must be made regarding which evaluative categories are most relevant to a community mental health program's development and even its very survival. The complexity of the selection process is evident in the fact that the administrator of a publicly funded program must consider his or her accountability to the patient, the clinician working with the patient, the center's administrative staff, county and state administrators, appropriate legislative bodies, and the general public. With the needs of these diverse bodies in mind, evaluation may be undertaken at one or more of the following levels:

1. Assessment of effort: How are staff utilized and how do the patterns of their utilization compare with local or national standards?
2. Assessment of effectiveness: What outcomes have the program's efforts produced?
3. Assessment of adequacy: To what extent has the community's problem been solved by this program?
4. Assessment of efficiency: Can the same outcome be achieved at lower cost?

Each type of question is answered with different kinds of data. Administrators, therefore, must specify their information needs with some precision if the evaluator's contribution is to be relevant. A review of present mental health evaluation activities leads to the encouraging conclusion that data needs are in fact being expressed in increasingly refined and researchable ways. For example, most administrators now recognize, at least superficially, that they cannot pose global inquiries about their program's worth. The repeated admonition in evaluation literature that program objectives must be specified before assessment can be initiated seems to be paying off at last. It is particularly significant that in the present period of fiscal austerity, increased attention is being paid to assessments of efficiency and cost benefit. Although mental health practitioners have long viewed the economic perspective as irrelevant and even dehumanizing, their resistance to that perspective is crumbling under the combined weight of legislative demands for fiscal data and the improved capabilities of management information systems. Thus, in addition to growing demands for the assessment of performance and effectiveness, administrators are simultaneously being required to justify fiscal support in the light of criteria more familiar to the world of business than of human services (Frank, 1981).

Assessment of Effort

The two questions of whether appropriate clientele are being served by community mental health centers and of the extent to which client needs are being met have provoked considerable debate over the years. There have been numerous studies of whether economically disadvantaged and minority groups, for example, are overtly or covertly dissuaded from seeking psychiatric care, and whether their treatment attrition rates differ from those of other clinical groups (Tischler and others, 1975; Rosen, Olarte, and Masnick, 1980). Evaluative procedures are needed, therefore, to clarify which groups are being treated and whether the volume of resources expended by community mental health centers for their care is consistent with public priorities.

This form of program accountability is classified as the evaluation of effort, and such studies are performed on the premise that a patient's participation in care will result in a positive outcome. Client count data, along with measures of how staff spend their time, have long been collected through the annual "Inventory of Comprehensive Community Mental Health Centers" conducted by the National Institute of Mental Health (NIMH). In fact, the series of Mental Health Statistical Notes produced by NIMH's Division of Biometry and Epidemiology has, on the basis of this and similar inventories, provided a meaningful picture of service utilization trends and shifts in the patient population being treated within psychiatric facilities. Nevertheless, it appeared several years ago that evaluation of effort would take second place to outcome studies. Surprisingly, however, evaluation of effort emerged with renewed vigor in the defunct 1980 Mental Health Systems Act under the label of "performance" measurement. This development reflected both the continuing conservatism of program directors and lingering difficulties in the design of outcome studies.

Analyses by Connolly and Deutsch (1980) and Keppler-Seid, Windle, and Woy (1980) of the rationale for and implications of utilizing performance measures emphasize the complexities and limitations of these measures. Nevertheless, four of the thirteen performance indicators selected by NIMH pertained to CMHC "accessibility" or admission patterns. They were the rates of minority members, persons under age eighteen, and persons over age sixty-five per 100,000 community residents admitted as patients, and the number of severely mentally disabled persons as a proportion of the CMHC's total case load. A similar approach to the assessment of effort based upon service delivery patterns is utilized in the state of Colorado. Miller and Wilson (1981) reported that mental health centers receiving state funds in Colorado must fulfill performance contracts that incorporate such criteria as number of admissions by age group, number of minorities served, and number of severely disabled served.

It is conceivable that experience with these initial performance measures could lead to additional and more detailed indexes of whether appropriate clientele are being effectively served in CMHCs. This approach to accountability must be taken cautiously, however, since increased program effort may or may not signify that enrolled groups are benefiting from CMHC interventions. Given the predilection of administrators and others to reify body counts, prudent interpretation of performance measurements is essential.

Assessments of effort that focus on whether a CMHC is serving appropriate clientele are likely to be increasingly influenced by epidemiological analyses of case prevalence. Community studies of how many and what types of persons need psychiatric care (which is the denominator in need assessment ratios) have been conducted for many years with the hope that improved diagnosis and treatment of mental disorders will ensue from a better understanding of their patterns of occurrence. However, even the most rigorous of these earlier investigations suffer from the ambiguity of whether mentally disordered persons uncovered through household interviews—for example, those classified in the Midtown Manhattan and Sterling County studies as manifesting severe impairment—resemble patients seen in caregiving facilities. In recent years, however, epidemiologists have begun to assess "caseness" in community surveys with the same structured interviews as are used by clinicians to achieve research diagnoses. Thus, Weissman and Myers (1978) employed the Schedule for Affective Disorders and Schizophrenia (Endicott and Spitzer, 1978) in determining the prevalence of depression among New Haven residents, a strategy that permitted them to interpret their findings about psychiatric needs in the community with greater validity than was true previously. Through the present NIMH Epidemiologic Catchment Area grant program, which is utilizing the Diagnostic Interview Schedule (Robins and others, 1981) to establish "caseness," community studies of psychiatric incidence and prevalence will become increasingly common and pertinent for determining true population needs. Their findings have significant potential for influencing the performance standards to be used in assessing the relevance and adequacy of CMHC services for particular at-risk populations.

Assessment of Effectiveness

The 1963 Community Mental Health Centers Act shifted psychiatric care away from inpatient settings in distant, large institutions to ambulatory facilities in local, smaller settings. Because of the major restructuring entailed in this transfer, there was considerable pressure to determine whether patients indeed benefited from this altered pattern of service delivery. If primary prevention programs grow during the coming years, there will be similar pressure to assess their efficacy. Furthermore, as it has become apparent that the major portion of America's care for emotionally disturbed persons occurs within the general health sector rather than within the specialty psychiatric system, the need to ascertain the benefits and liabilities of this reality have also become crucial.

In the early 1980s legislative pressures rather than clinical and administrative concerns have come to dominate the realm of program accountability, and these pressures will inexorably move the mental health system from process to outcome evaluations. This development is perhaps best exemplified by Congress' controversial effort to limit national health insurance coverage to those psychiatric services that are proved efficacious, appropriate, and safe in clinical trials to be conducted over the next few years.

While administrators, clinicians, and researchers generally acknowledge the theoretical usefulness of outcome evaluations, they also express considerable caution about our present ability to conduct such assessments. After reviewing strategies for measuring the quality of medical care, McAuliffe (1979) concluded that outcome measures lack the face validity claimed for them, often exclude many relevant effects of care, and are based on data of poor quality. He also contended that factors unrelated to the medical care system account for more of the outcome variance than do measures of medical inputs. In their reasoned analysis of the 1980 Mental Health Systems Act provision for performance contracting, Keppler-Seid, Windle, and Woy (1980) also emphasized the complexity of utilizing outcome measures. Different criteria are meaningful to different users of the information, and the authors suggest that research is needed to validate performance indicators for a variety of client types and against a variety of treatment outcome dimensions.

Concerns about the validity and utility of outcome evaluation are surely appropriate, but it will receive growing priority as clinicians are pressured to demonstrate program effectiveness. As this occurs, the methodological issues still plaguing outcome studies will very likely be resolved, and the cost-benefit ratio of evaluating the service delivery system's effectiveness should improve markedly; that is, the value of the information yielded by these studies for decision-making purposes should begin to surpass their fiscal costs and scientific compromises (Schulberg, 1981). Given such a prospect, outcome evaluations are reviewed in the following sections from perspectives salient to policy makers, administrators, and clinicians.

Impact Model. Outcome studies must be founded on the theoretical principles that guide the service delivery program. When evaluators poorly comprehend or even disregard the program's underlying rationale, the risk is high of measuring outcomes unrelated to the program's purposes. Alternatively, if administrators and/or clinicians are vague about the program's mode of impacting upon clients, the evaluator's outcome criteria may begin to determine program goals. The significance of this issue can be illustrated with regard to Community Support Programs, which are broad-scale, multilevel interventions aimed at the chronically mentally ill, their families, agency personnel, and the communities in which the chronically ill reside (Turner and Ten Hoor, 1978). Past experience has revealed how difficult it is to specify which variable from an interrelated array is causally related to an observed outcome. The problem of ambiguous causality is compounded in Community Support Programs since interventions may emanate from a variety of agencies, each of whose service volume fluctuates over time. The specific program characteristics accounting for outcome variance may then depend, in part, upon the focal time frame.

To determine whether benefits derive from the unique or interactive contributions of a community support system's many components requires a highly sophisticated multivariate research design (Schulberg and Bromet, 1981). It is unlikely that all demonstration projects can establish and maintain the complex protocols needed for such designs. However, if such considerations confine outcome evaluations to the study of single interventions alone, it is quite likely that the subsequent findings will demonstrate null or trivial effects. The danger exists, therefore, that a complex theoretical model of service delivery will be rejected by faulty research methodology and that necessary large-scale interventions will be prematurely abandoned.

An alternative strategy for evaluating complex impact models is to assign particular multifactorial studies to selected programs with the interest in and capacity for conducting them. Thus, one program could study whether well-designed interorganizational linkages generate more comprehensive care and improved client functioning. A contrasting hypothesis to be studied elsewhere would be that enthusiastic staff commitment is essential for good outcomes. A further hypothesis warranting analysis in a third site would be that client outcome primarily reflects the screening criteria used to select program participants. This strategy would make it feasible to undertake studies of the specific factors affecting outcome and, through their triangulated findings, to move beyond global conclusions.

Target Populations. Evaluations of the benefits generated by CMHCs must consider the several target populations at whom services are directed and the outcome indexes pertinent to each. While clients are the focal concern of most administrators and clinicians, it should be recognized that the families of clients, the communities within which clients reside, and the staff of mental health centers are also populations directly or indirectly affected by mental health service delivery patterns. Outcome studies, therefore, should consider and be designed for all these groups.

The quality and effectiveness of a CMHC's services may vary among its target populations, but too often we assume that all groups benefit from a properly functioning system. Little attention has been directed, however, to the fundamental question of whether a CMHC's services are compatible for all possible beneficiaries. Despite our faith in their congruent—even synergistic—nature, such large-scale undertakings as Community Support Programs for the chronically mentally ill can encounter difficulties because of goal conflicts between clients and communities, clients and families, and families and staff (Schulberg and Bromet, 1981). Similar goal conflicts, and differential outcomes, may also occur as the result of a CMHC's assigning contrasting treatment priorities for young adults, for elderly, acutely, and chronically ill persons, for individuals and families, and so on. Outcome studies, thus, should optimally determine not only whether an individual target group benefits relative to its own needs, but also whether positive or negative interactive patterns develop among the several target groups affected by a program.

Outcome Indexes. The prevailing approach in client outcome studies is to obtain measures of change in the individual's (1) psychiatric status or distress level, (2) social functioning, and (3) satisfaction with treatment. For chronically ill persons, the framework has been extended to include: (4) indexes of vocational functioning and (5) the nature of their physical and social environments. These several dimensions in their totality have been called "quality of life" (Zautra and Goodhart, 1979). Various efforts are now underway to determine whether this can be assessed as a cohesive concept and whether it is best measured through objective or subjective indexes. It is of interest that recent concerns about quality of life and its measures emanate from both professional and political groups. Members of the former group recognize that comprehensive human service interventions require complex outcome approaches, while members of the latter group strive for valid social indicators that will reflect the benefits and problems resulting from social welfare and other legislation. Whether quality of life is similarly construed by professionals and politicians, and by liberals and conservatives, will deserve careful attention as this concept gains wider acceptance.

Psychiatric programs have long viewed the reduction of client symptomatology or distress as their prime treatment goal. CMHCs surely are concerned about this outcome criterion, but they also place emphasis on their clients' social functioning and vocational performance. In fact, one of community mental health's ideological principles is that clinical services should improve clients' interpersonal skills rather than reconstruct their personalities. Community mental health programs pursuing socially oriented client goals would give higher priority to measures of personal adjustment and role skills, and less attention to symptomatology, in assessing service outcomes.

At this point in time, the most progress has been made in refining psychometrically sound measures of client functioning; the least sophistication is evident with regard to indexes of the service delivery system's impact on its staff and on the communities in which clients reside. Measures of family burden are becoming more acceptable, but they still lack the validity and reliability of client-focused instruments. In contrast to the slow but steady progress evident in perfecting outcome indexes appropriate to the study of professional caregiving systems, major difficulties still confront evaluations of diverse self-help groups. Lieberman and Bond (1978) emphasize that the variability in problems presented by self-help participants, as well as differences in the levels of goals pursued by organizations, renders many of the usual indexes inadequate. The continual development of new self-help groups with ever more complex subsystem and suprasystem goals adds further to the problem of criteria standardization. The dilemma of how to assess program outcome is even more critical with regard to primary prevention activities, which often are directed at vague populations and are intended to achieve ambiguous goals.

Data Collection Instruments

The outcomes of services provided to CMHC clients can be investigated on a broad range of instruments. Evaluators may consider pertinent tests and rating scales in the collections prepared by Chun, Cobb, and French (1973), Comrey, Backer, and Glaser (1973), Waskow and Parloff (1975), Hagedorn and others (1976), Hargreaves, Attkisson, and Sorensen (1977), and Buros (1978). It has been suggested previously that community mental health benefits be identified and evaluated in relation to each of the several target populations served. Representative instruments specific to outcome evaluations with clients will be reviewed here.

Psychiatric Status. Because of clinicians' and researchers' long-standing interest in determining the psychiatric status of clients, numerous well-established instruments are available for this purpose. The Brief Psychiatric Rating Scale (Overall and Gorham, 1962) and the Inpatient Multidimensional Psychiatric Scale (Lorr and others, 1962) are commonly used in community treatment outcome studies. Another commonly used instrument is the SCL-90 (Derogatis and Cleary, 1977), which is particularly suited to studies of client functioning in the community. In addition to scales that derive clinical assessments from multidimensional ratings, psychiatric status may also be assessed on unidimensional scales. Examples of this latter approach include the 9-point Levels of Functioning Scale (Carter and Newman, 1976) and the Global Assessment Scale (Endicott and others, 1976), on which client scores may range from 1 to 100. Although lacking the conceptual diversity of multidimensional scales, global ones are easily completed by trained observers. The Levels of Functioning Scale has been particularly useful as a single clinical measure in studies relating client outcome to cost of treatment.

Social Adaptation. American society places considerable emphasis on the nature and quality of interpersonal relationships, and this index has become very significant in assessing a mentally ill person's functioning. The most comprehensive overview of outcome instruments pertinent to this dimension is provided by Weissman (1975), who analyzed the content, manner of administration, and psychometric properties of fifteen scales measuring individual role performance. The Katz Adjustment Scale (Katz and Lyerly, 1963) and the Personal Adjustment and Role Skills Scale (Ellsworth and others, 1968) are the most commonly used of these instruments. Their psychometric properties and the purposes best fulfilled by each are compared by Hogarty (1975). Scales most specifically suited to outcome evaluations with chronically ill persons are the Community Adjustment Form (Test and Stein, 1978) and the Behavioral Repertoire (Datel, Murphy, and Pollack, 1978).

Satisfaction with Treatment. Mental health professionals have traditionally minimized the significance of client satisfaction with care, viewing it as laden with psychodynamic distortions. The clinician's bias has been reinforced by investigations that found differing staff and patient perceptions of which treatment elements produced improvement. But despite continuing qualms about the true meaning of consumer satisfaction and valid procedures for assessing it, the client's perspective is increasingly sanctioned—even required—in outcome studies. Windle and Paschall (1981) emphasize that, from a technical standpoint, validity is increased when the concerns unique to clients are measured and that, politically, the expression of one's views is a right rather than a privilege in a participatory democracy. Perhaps the most sophisticated effort to construct a psychometrically sound, easily administered measure of consumer satisfaction is that of Larsen and others (1979). Through factor analytic techniques, their earlier Client Satisfaction Questionnaire has been reduced from a thirty-one-item multifactorial scale to an eight-item unifactorial one. The retained items are readily comprehensible to, and easily answered by, both acutely and chronically mentally ill persons.

Vocational Performance. Improved vocational performance is a common goal for chronically ill persons, even though only a minority actually obtain gainful employment. Here, program effectiveness can be assessed on such reasonably straightforward measures as whether or not a client is working, the percent of time he is employed, his skill level, his earnings, and so on. More recently, increasingly refined measures are being developed as work comes to be (1) conceptualized as a multidimensional rather than a unidimensional activity and (2) considered in relation to other facets of the person's life-style. Recognition of the complexities underlying the term *work* is particularly needed when assessing a chronically impaired person's progress toward partial or full employment. Thus, Anthony, Cohen, and Vitalo (1978) present a scheme for before-and-after evaluation of the skills of clients in the physical, emotional, and intellectual domains as they pertain to work settings. Criteria are defined for each domain so that reliable assessments may be conducted.

Environmental Conditions. Considerable controversy has been generated as to whether the living conditions of chronically ill persons improve or deteriorate when they leave state hospitals for community settings. Data collection procedures, therefore, are needed to assess the quality of community-based environments. They should distinguish, if possible, the environment's social characteristics from its physical ones, since their quality may well differ. Unfortunately, few instruments exist for such outcome analyses. The best instrument for analyzing the social features of community environments is the Community-Oriented Programs-Environment Scale (Moos and Otto, 1972). Its 102 items are arranged into 10 subscales that measure interpersonal relationships, treatment program, and administrative structure variables. No psychometrically refined instrument yet exists for evaluating physical environments, although efforts to develop such scales are now in progress.

While the previously described indexes and instruments have focused on personality and functional measures of the target populations served, outcome studies during the 1980s will include the economic perspective as well. Mental health practitioners have resisted this approach to evaluation for some time, but fiscal accountability is expected to move from the shadows to the forefront in the next several years. Not only will cost-benefit analyses become more methodologically sophisticated as they increasingly are applied to psychiatric care, but their very rationale will be legitimated rather than attacked. This trend already is evident in the fact that after many years of professional reluctance to accept fiscal criteria as germane to the evaluation of therapeutic interventions, economic studies were assigned a high priority by NIMH's Division of Biometry and Epidemiology in its 1979 "Mental Health Service System Research" grant program. An example of the fiscal analyses that can be expected to appear with growing frequency is Weisbrod, Test, and Stein's (1980) study of the costs and benefits of maintaining psychiatric patients in an experimental community setting. The investigators determined through quantifiable monetary and nonmonetary indexes that the costs of the experimental community program exceeded those of hospital care but that the additional benefits that it produced far surpassed these supplemental costs.

Conducting Evaluations

Having formulated a theoretical impact model suited to the mental health center's service delivery pattern, having selected the target populations for study, and having chosen the indexes on which outcome is to be assessed, the evaluator is then faced with methodological, ethical, and fiscal decisions. They will be considered in the following section.

Research Designs. There is a widespread impression that the ideal, if not only, approach to future mental health program evaluation is through research designs that attempt to validate causal linkages by isolating dependent variables and manipulating independent ones, maximizing the influence of independent variables while minimizing sources of variance, and quantifying the independent and dependent variables. In practice, however, key requirements of this experimental model—or even of quasi-experimental models—cannot be met in evaluating mental health programs. Limitations in the investigator's ability to assign subjects among experimental and control groups, tenuous theoretical linkages between the intervention and the anticipated outcome, uncontrollable sources of variance, and so on have thus renewed interest in alternatives to the experimental approach of the natural sciences.

Given the current political and scientific environment that requires that at least probabilistic conclusions be derived from outcome studies, Cook and Campbell's (1979) analysis of various conceptions of causality assumes particular significance for mental health clinicians and evaluators. Cook and Campbell propose eight principles of causality on the premise that experiments seek to elucidate whether a particular cause, or a restricted set of causes, has an effect. They indicate that experiments do not aim at a comprehensive explanation of all the causal forces determining a particular outcome, nor are they usually aimed at establishing sufficient causes and their necessary counterparts. Rather, in the short term, experiments attempt to examine probabilistic causes.

Cook and Campbell's conception of the experimental study's power is most appropriate to the mental health field, where outcome investigations resembling quasi-experiments rather than scientific experiments are the norm. The resulting data's ability to establish causal attribution may be analyzed within the well-known framework of "threats" to a study's internal and external validity. The two threats of mortality and instrumentation warrant discussion here, since they are receiving increased attention in regard to the quality of outcome data. And it becomes particularly vital to understand the manner in which instruments measure the dependent variables when ethical and/or legal considerations preclude the use of no-treatment control groups.

Mortality is a threat to the validity of causal inference when the observed effect may result from different kinds of subjects dropping out of a particular treatment group during the course of an experiment. Upon posttest, the experimental groups would then be composed of unrepresentative samples, and the results might reflect selective attrition rather than the true effects of treatment. Mental health outcome studies are commonly plagued by this problem. When it occurs, the findings are viewed as biased, on the assumption that nonparticipants at follow-up are primarily poorly adjusting persons. The complexity of this issue is illustrated by Ellsworth's (1979) comparison of the follow-up adjustment of clients from whom information was obtained by mail with the adjustment of nonresponders who subsequently were interviewed by phone. Surprisingly, Ellsworth found that posthospital adjustment was not significantly related to whether or not mail questionnaires were returned. Low response rates were found instead to reflect data collection style and subjects' motivation level. However, Penk and others' (1981) study of this same client sample concluded that when follow-up data are sought from significant others, such data are retrieved less often about poorly adjusted clients than about well-adjusted ones.

Causal attribution also is threatened when altered client functioning might reflect a change in the measuring instrument between pretest and posttest rather than in the treatment's differential impact at each time interval. Outcome studies that gather data at several points in time are vulnerable to unreliable instrumentation since repeated exposure to the same scales may alter the client's conception of the assessed variable. This risk is especially present when treatment focuses on the variable being assessed and seeks to modify the client's understanding of it. The client's standard of measurement may also change over time, and a common metric thus will no longer exist between sets of scores. Edwards and others (1978) examined the effects of repeated testing on change scores in five adjustment scales. They recommend that the SCL-90 be used as the self-assessment instrument because of its very high test-retest reliability (.94) and internal consistency coefficient (.95). With regard to the need to maintain a common metric at all measurement points, Howard (1980) recommends that pretests be administered retrospectively so as to minimize this source of instrument contamination.

In addition to the efforts being directed at improving the validity of quasi-experimental designs, attention is also being focused upon criteria for utilizing qualitative as well as quantitative information. Filstead (1981) defines qualitative evaluation as a paradigm in which assumptions about the social world provide a philosophical and conceptual framework for its study. He considers social processes to be objective, extant, and knowable to all the members of a society through such data-collecting activities as participant observation, unstructured interviewing, diaries, and self-reports. Qualitative evaluation has already found its greatest applications by social system analysts seeking to comprehend the manner in which organizational factors abet or hinder service delivery. Thus, Schulberg and Baker's (1975) study of the changing mental hospital utilized open systems concepts to select intraorganizational and extraorganizational focuses for analysis and triangulated various data sources in deriving conclusions. A similar strategy would be highly relevant for evaluating the key program thrusts of the 1980s. For example, the efforts of policy makers and administrators to more closely link the health and mental health service delivery systems could be readily assessed within this open systems paradigm. Attention would be directed not only to such traditional numerical indexes as continuity of care, accessibility, referral patterns, and resource exchanges but also to such qualitative measures as staff interaction, executive decision making and priority setting, and patterns of intersector cooperation and competition. The joint use of quantitative and qualitative indexes is consistent with Reichardt and Cook's (1979) view that researchers need not adhere blindly to one of the polar-extreme paradigms but can freely choose from both so as to fit the demands of the problem at hand.

Evaluative Perspective. A major decision confronting the evaluator in studies of program effectiveness is the perspective to utilize in judging the client's functioning on entry into treatment and/or at subsequent points in time. The possible vantage points for these judgments include those of the client, a significant other, the therapist, and an independent observer. Some outcome measures can be rated with equal objectivity from any of these perspectives; others are more validly assessed from only one of them (Harty and Horwitz, 1976). Therefore, objectivity, reliability, salience, and cost should all be considered in choosing respondent viewpoints. It should be noted that while theoretically a client's social functioning may best be assessed by a significant other, in practice the client may not provide consent for a relative's or friend's participation in the study. Furthermore, relatives and friends may not be available, or even exist, in the case of chronically ill persons, so that other rater perspectives will need to be substituted.

At a more global level of analysis, the issue of evaluative perspective includes the benefits and limitations of citizen review of program effectiveness. This particular viewpoint was mandated by the 1975 Amendments to the Community Mental Health Centers Act, but in point of fact it has only been minimally incorporated into evaluative practice. Dinkel, Zinober, and Flaherty (1981) reviewed the reasons for low compliance and report that much of it can be attributed to ambiguous federal policies. They offer suggestions for reducing this ambiguity and establishing channels for constructive citizen participation in the evaluation process. However, policy-setting procedures are now being decentralized from the federal to the state levels, and it is unclear how receptive executives and legislators at the latter level will be to citizen involvement that exceeds superficial advisory functions.

Ethical and Fiscal Considerations. While the methodology of outcome evaluations is becoming increasingly refined, their ethical dimensions are generating ever more complex dilemmas. Recent judicial decisions and governmental regulations about the protection of privacy have seriously restricted the manner in which researchers can gain access to subjects and to agency data about them. As a consequence, the evaluator must take greater care to ensure that clients and significant others are providing truly informed consent and that their privacy is maintained. These requirements produce unique concerns in longitudinal follow-ups; for example, the client may provide consent at one point in time but refuse it at later points. If a significant proportion of the follow-up cohort, or even a selected segment of it, exercises this prerogative, the researcher's design may be threatened. Procedures for coping with this circumstance are suggested by Showstack and others (1978).

Another contemporary ethical development complicating outcome studies is the diminished access that evaluators have to agency records without the client's informed consent. Many follow-up assessments, particularly of the quality-monitoring type, are designed and initiated only after clients have terminated treatment. Obtaining informed consent under this condition for chart review and additional data collection creates obvious problems. Such program monitoring becomes even more complicated when the evaluator wishes to complement staff ratings about client functioning with the freshly solicited judgments of relatives and/or friends. Obtaining the client's consent, without implied coercion, for gathering such data is difficult when he or she wishes to "forget" the earlier psychiatric illness. While procedures for coping with these complexities can be readily devised, it must be recognized that the evaluator's resolution of ethics-related dilemmas occurs within the context of profound value choices. A growing literature is considering the role strains and conflicting demands facing the evaluator (Windle and Neigher, 1978; Sheinfeld and Lord, 1981), and the Evaluation Research Society has drafted a code of ethics for those conducting program assessments.

Assuming that evaluators and administrators can properly address a follow-up study's ethical requirements, they must also consider its fiscal requirements. Evaluation funds are always limited, and a cost-efficient research strategy is imperative. Those seeking information upon which to base such a decision should consider the cost estimates derived from Schainblatt's (1980) studies in which inpatient and outpatient care were monitored at several Michigan and Virginia mental health facilities. Using a combination of mail and telephone data collection methods, he incurred a cost of $31 per outpatient for intake and follow-up measures of client distress, social functioning, and satisfaction with treatment. For inpatients, similar follow-up procedures cost $38. An additional expense of $6 per outpatient and $10 per inpatient would be generated if family burden measures were desired as well. Schainblatt's estimates include the cost of collecting and processing outcome, demographic, and service utilization data, and of analyzing basic cross-tabulations.

Policy Implications

Having reviewed several of the key issues affecting the conception and design of accountability systems, we turn now to the question of what role program evaluation will play in the policy-setting process during the decade of the 1980s. The environment of mental health programs consists of incentives and penalties, reinforcements and constraints, mandates and prohibitions. Thus, evaluative data are but one input into a complex policy-setting process in which a host of other factors generally assume equal, if not greater, weight. Sechrest and Mabe (1981) warn against the common myth that evaluation outcomes can produce the binary conclusion that a program is effective or ineffective and that a similarly discrete policy decision is therefore possible. They emphasize that evaluations rarely produce absolute, final answers that allow conclusions to emerge incrementally. Additional obstacles to the direct translation of research findings into policy include the unfamiliarity of policy makers with social science concepts and methodologies, ambiguity about the strength and integrity of treatments utilized in the demonstration program, and unknown cost implications. A particularly troublesome issue is whether the magnitude of achieved effects truly warrants major programmatic change. Sechrest and Yeaton (1981) consider statistical significance alone an inappropriate criterion upon which to gauge the size, no less than the profundity, of an effect, and they propose judgmental and normative alternatives for reaching this decision.

If accountability mechanisms are not the dominant factor in the policy-setting process, under what circumstances will the contributions of evaluation data be maximized and when will they be trivialized? This question can be addressed from many vantage points. My analysis is limited to that of evaluative data's ability to support rather than oppose forthcoming policy.

Few would assert that evaluation is intrinsically objective and devoid of value biases; even fewer would contend that the manner in which its data are utilized is value free. Thus, it is not at all unusual for the same assessment to be cited in support of opposing policies. For example, the same body of psychotherapy research has recently served to advance as well as to disparage the merit of covering this therapeutic modality under national health insurance. The question here is whether differing standards of technical adequacy are needed in evaluations intended to support a proposed policy and in evaluations designed to oppose the policy. This determination should relate to the risk that society wishes to incur by supporting ineffective services, that is, programs wrongly viewed as effective, in contrast to the risk incurred by curtailing truly effective services, that is, programs wrongly judged as ineffective (Schulberg, 1979).

Society's criteria for choosing between the former risks and the latter tend to shift over time. During the initial half of the 1980s, the balance of risk-taking will shift from Congress' earlier willingness to maintain possibly ineffective programs to a much more conservative posture that risks closing effective services. This transition became particularly evident in 1981 when Congress significantly reduced social expenditures and will become evident again if Congress ponders which forms of psychiatric care to include under national health insurance. Given the fiscal implications of this latter decision, legislators will prefer to err on the side of caution rather than to expend hundreds of millions of dollars for treatments that they think to be of limited or unknown utility. The shift toward more rigorous accountability criteria can already be seen in the consensus reached by congressional and Alcohol, Drug Abuse, and Mental Health Administration (ADAMHA) leaders that psychotherapy's effectiveness should be assessed in terms of its scientific "safety and efficacy" rather than within the traditional framework of whether it conforms to "usual and customary practice."

Community mental health program evaluation was largely stimulated by forces external to the field, but it is now sufficiently intrinsic to administrative and clinical tasks that legislative mandates are no longer critical. Program accountability is being pursued at various levels, and this momentum will be sustained during the coming years. The major evaluative focus continues to be at the level of assessing effort, and procedures for measuring such performance are receiving widespread attention. It is possible, however, that effectiveness studies will assume far greater significance in the future. Much of this chapter, therefore, was devoted to the conceptual and methodological issues associated with this more complex evaluative strategy. The need to formulate a theoretical model of how programs impact upon clients was emphasized because the model is so fundamental to the choice of research design, target population, and outcome indexes.

References

Anthony, W., Cohen, M., and Vitalo, R. "The Measurement of Rehabilitation Outcome." *Schizophrenia Bulletin,* 1978, *4,* 365-383.

Buros, O. (Ed.). *The Eighth Mental Measurements Yearbook.* Highland Park, N.J.: Gryphon Press, 1978.

Carter, D., and Newman, F. *A Client-Oriented System of Mental Health Service Delivery and Program Management: A Workbook and Guide.* Rockville, Md.: National Institute of Mental Health, 1976.

Chun, K., Cobb, S., and French, J. *Measures for Psychological Assessment.* Ann Arbor: Institute for Social Research, University of Michigan, 1973.

Comrey, A., Backer, T., and Glaser, E. *A Sourcebook for Mental Health Measures.* Los Angeles: Human Interaction Research Unit, 1973.

Connolly, T., and Deutsch, J. "Performance Measurement: Some Conceptual Issues." *Evaluation and Program Planning,* 1980, *3,* 35-43.

Cook, T., and Campbell, D. *Quasi-Experimentation: Design and Analysis Issues for Field Settings.* Chicago: Rand McNally, 1979.

Datel, W., Murphy, J., and Pollack, P. "Outcome in a Deinstitutionalization Program Employing Service Integration Methodology." *Journal of Operational Psychiatry,* 1978, *9,* 6-24.

Derogatis, L., and Cleary, P. "Confirmation of the Dimension Structure of the SCL-90: A Study in Construct Validation." *Journal of Clinical Psychology,* 1977, *33,* 981-989.

Dinkel, N., Zinober, J., and Flaherty, E. "Citizen Participation in CMHC Program Evaluation: A Neglected Potential." *Community Mental Health Journal,* 1981, *17,* 54-65.

Edwards, D., and others. "Test-taking and the Stability of Adjustment Scales." *Evaluation Quarterly,* 1978, *2,* 275-291.

Ellsworth, R. "Does Follow-Up Loss Reflect Poor Outcome?" *Evaluation and Health Professions,* 1979, *2,* 419-437.

Ellsworth, R., and others. "Hospital and Community Adjustment as Perceived by Psychiatric Patients, Their Families, and

Staff." *Journal of Consulting and Clinical Psychology Monograph Supplement,* 1968, *32,* 1-41.

Endicott, J., and Spitzer, R. "A Diagnostic Interview. The Schedule for Affective Disorders and Schizophrenia." *Archives of General Psychiatry,* 1978, *35,* 837-844.

Endicott, J., and others. "The Global Adjustment Scale: A Procedure for Measuring Overall Severity of Psychiatric Disturbance." *Archives of General Psychiatry,* 1976, *33,* 766-771.

Filstead, W. "Qualitative and Quantitative Information in Health Policy Decision Making." *Health Policy Quarterly,* 1981, *1,* 43-56.

Frank, R. "Cost-Benefit Analysis in Mental Health Services: A Review of the Literature." *Administration in Mental Health,* 1981, *8,* 161-176.

Hagedorn, H., and others. *A Working Manual of Simple Program Evaluation Techniques for Community Mental Health Centers.* Department of Health, Education, and Welfare Publication No. (ADM) 76-404. Washington, D.C.: U.S. Government Printing Office, 1976.

Hargreaves, W., Attkisson, C., and Sorensen, J. *Resource Materials for Community Mental Health Program Evaluation.* (2nd ed.) Department of Health, Education, and Welfare Publication No. (ADM) 77-328. Washington, D.C.: U.S. Government Printing Office, 1977.

Harty, M., and Horwitz, L. "Therapeutic Outcome as Rated by Patients, Therapists, and Judges." *Archives of General Psychiatry,* 1976, *33,* 957-961.

Hogarty, G. "Informant Ratings of Community Adjustment." In I. Waskow and M. Parloff (Eds.), *Psychotherapy Change Measures.* Department of Health, Education, and Welfare Publication No. (ADM) 74-140. Washington, D.C.: U.S. Government Printing Office, 1975.

Howard, G. "Response Shift Bias: A Problem in Evaluating Interventions with Pre/Post Self-Reports." *Evaluation Review,* 1980, *4,* 93-106.

Katz, M., and Lyerly, S. "Methods for Measuring Adjustment and Social Behavior in the Community." *Psychological Reports,* 1963, *13,* 503-535.

Keppler-Seid, H., Windle, C., and Woy, J. "Performance Measures for Mental Health Programs: Something Better, Something Worse, or More of the Same?" *Community Mental Health Journal,* 1980, *16,* 217-234.

Larsen, D., and others. "Assessment of Client Satisfaction: Development of a General Scale." *Evaluation and Program Planning,* 1979, *2,* 197-207.

Lieberman, M., and Bond, G. "Self-Help Groups: Problems of Measuring Outcome." *Small Group Behavior,* 1978, *9,* 221-241.

Lorr, M., and others. "Evidence of Ten Psychotic Syndromes." *Journal of Consulting Psychology,* 1962, *26,* 185-189.

McAuliffe, W. "Measuring the Quality of Medical Care: Process Versus Outcome." *Milbank Memorial Fund Quarterly,* 1979, *57,* 118-152.

Majchrzak, A., and Windle, C. "Patterns of Program Evaluation in Community Mental Health Centers." *Evaluation Review,* 1980, *4,* 677-691.

Miller, S., and Wilson, N. "The Case for Performance Contracting." *Administration in Mental Health,* 1981, *8,* 185-193.

Moos, R., and Otto, J. "The Community-Oriented Programs-Environment Scale." *Community Mental Health Journal,* 1972, *8,* 28-37.

Overall, J., and Gorham, D. "The Brief Psychiatric Rating Scale." *Psychological Reports,* 1962, *10,* 799-812.

Penk, W., and others. "Psychological Aspects of Data Loss in Outcome Research." *Evaluation Review,* 1981, *5,* 392-396.

Reichardt, C., and Cook, T. "Beyond Qualitative Versus Quantitative Methods." In T. Cook and C. Reichardt (Eds.), *Qualitative and Quantitative Methods in Evaluation Research.* Beverly Hills, Calif.: Sage, 1979.

Robins, L., and others. "National Institute of Mental Health Diagnostic Interview Schedule." *Archives of General Psychiatry,* 1981, *38,* 381-389.

Rosen, A., Olarte, S., and Masnick, R. "Utilization Patterns of a CMHC in an Urban Ghetto Area." *Hospital and Community Psychiatry,* 1980, *31,* 702-704.

Schainblatt, A. "What Happens to the Clients?" *Community Mental Health Journal,* 1980, *16,* 331-342.

Schulberg, H. "Issues in the Evaluation of Community Mental

Health Programs." *Professional Psychology,* 1977, *8,* 560-572.

Schulberg, H. "Community Support Programs: Program Evaluation and Public Policy." *American Journal of Psychiatry,* 1979, *136,* 1433-1437.

Schulberg, H. "Outcome Evaluation in the Mental Health Field." *Community Mental Health Journal,* 1981, *17,* 132-142.

Schulberg, H., and Baker, F. *The Mental Hospital and Human Services.* New York: Behavioral Publications, 1975.

Schulberg, H., and Bromet, E. "Strategies for Evaluating the Outcome of Community Services for the Chronically Mentally Ill." *American Journal of Psychiatry,* 1981, *138,* 930-935.

Sechrest, L., and Mabe, P. "Translating Evaluation Research Findings into Health Policy." *Health Policy Quarterly,* 1981, *1,* 57-72.

Sechrest, L., and Yeaton, W. "Assessing the Effectiveness of Social Programs: Methodological and Conceptual Issues." In S. Ball (Ed.), *New Directions for Program Evaluation: Assessing and Interpreting Outcomes,* no. 9. San Francisco: Jossey-Bass, 1981.

Sheinfeld, S., and Lord, G. "The Ethics of Evaluation Researchers: An Exploration of Value Choices." *Evaluation Review,* 1981, *5,* 377-391.

Showstack, J., and others. "Psychiatric Follow-Up Studies: Practical Procedures and Ethical Concerns." *Journal of Nervous and Mental Disease,* 1978, *166,* 34-43.

Test, M., and Stein, L. "Training in Community Living: Research Design and Results." In L. Stein and M. Test (Eds.), *Alternatives to Mental Hospital Treatment.* New York: Plenum, 1978.

Tischler, G., and others. "Utilization of Mental Health Services. I. Patienthood and the Prevalence of Symptomatology in the Community." *Archives of General Psychiatry,* 1975, *32,* 411-415.

Turner, J., and Ten Hoor, W. "The NIMH Community Support Program: Pilot Approach to a Needed Social Reform." *Schizophrenia Bulletin,* 1978, *4,* 319-344.

Waskow, I., and Parloff, M. (Eds.). *Psychotherapy Change Measures.* Department of Health, Education, and Welfare Publication No. (ADM) 74-120. Washington, D.C.: U.S. Government Printing Office, 1975.

Weisbrod, B., Test, M., and Stein, L. "Alternative to Mental Hospital Treatment. II. Economic Benefit-Cost Analysis." *Archives of General Psychiatry,* 1980, *37,* 400-405.

Weissman, M. "The Assessment of Social Adjustment." *Archives of General Psychiatry,* 1975, *32,* 357-365.

Weissman, M., and Myers, J. "Affective Disorders in a United States Community: The Use of Research Diagnostic Criteria in an Epidemiological Survey." *Archives of General Psychiatry,* 1978, *35,* 1304-1311.

Windle, C., and Neigher, W. "Ethical Problems in Program Evaluation: Advice for Trapped Evaluators." *Evaluation and Program Planning,* 1978, *1,* 97-108.

Windle, C., and Paschall, N. "Client Participation in CMHC Program Evaluation: Increasing Incidence, Inadequate Involvement." *Community Mental Health Journal,* 1981, *17,* 66-76.

Zautra, A., and Goodhart, D. "Quality of Life Indicators: A Review of the Literature." *Community Mental Health Review,* 1979, *4,* 1-10.

Chapter 22

Human Resources for Mental Health Services

Harold W. Demone, Jr.

The mental health industry is labor intensive: Approximately 80 percent of its expenditures are for staff salaries and fringe benefits. After a physical plant is completed, capital investments are a relatively minor part of a mental health facility's budget, and most such facilities have relatively little expensive technical equipment. Given the fiscal as well as clinical significance that human resources play in the mental health field, it is vital to understand how policy is established for their production and utilization. In particular what trends may be anticipated during the 1980s? This chapter first considers government's influence on the supply and demand for mental health professionals and then considers issues pertaining to their employment in selected service delivery settings.

Federal Policy Objectives

Two themes dominate current manpower policy: (1) the extraordinary and increasing influence of the federal government and (2) cost control. The earlier issues were the quality, availability, accessibility, and continuity of services; removing the financial barriers to health care; alternative approaches to care; and subsidizing health manpower production. The focus in the 1980s is on saving money, reducing the maldistribution of health services, and enlarging the pool of minority and female mental health workers.

Governmental influence is not an exclusively American phenomenon. In 1979 the nine member nations of the European Economic Community undertook to implement national standards regarding training differentials within the five professions of nursing, medicine, veterinary science, dentistry, and the law. When the decision-making processes of the nine nations and the five professions were tested, it was found that national governmental bureaucracies wielded the greatest authority while the national professional associations were the most active nongovernmental bodies. "Educational interests [played] minor roles" (Orzack, 1980, p. 307).

Efforts to impose cost controls have been relatively consistent for more than a decade, no matter what bureaucracy, president, or political party was in power. By the late 1960s, the Nixon administration had initiated challenges to the traditional health manpower role of the federal government and sought both to phase out and reduce support for various health programs. Congress annually restored funds at varying but declining rates and also began to view manpower problems as selective rather than as absolute. The maldistribution of professionals was openly recognized and legislated solutions were targeted to that end. Political ideology, mythology, and a quasi-projection science provided powerful tools for those seeking to reduce training support.

President Reagan's goal is to eliminate all training programs except for those in research. His special targets include the social and behavioral sciences and the human service professions. This negative ideology contrasts strikingly with the thinking of the 1950s and 1960s when the goal was to meet demand by expanding the supply of core mental health professionals, that is, psychiatrists, clinical psychologists, psychiatric social workers (now called clinical social workers), and psychiatric nurses. Various statutes were aimed at developing, enlarging, and strengthening the teaching capacity of professional schools (Comings, 1978), which, together with professional associations and the Department of Health, Education, and Welfare, were full partners in manpower development.

Priorities and expenditures for human resources in the 1980s will continue to be dominated by the values and budget-balancing tactics of President Reagan and his key advisers. The professional schools and associations are playing increasingly subservient roles. Congress is their only significant ally, and even it is wavering. The overriding objective is to reduce expenditures, and in this respect policy has remained unchanged since the Nixon era. The means to achieve this end are disincentives, market constraints, regulations, restructuring of the health care system, program reductions and eliminations, or some combination of the above (Zubkoff, 1977). References to the findings of supply-side economists are cited after the fact to justify budget-cutting decisions. For example, if professionals are considered individual cost centers, the conclusion can be reached that if fewer researchers or clinicians are produced, less demand will be placed on resources, and expenditures will be reduced.

The federal bureaucracy has responded to successive budget-cutting presidents in several ways. One group has joined the fray with enthusiasm, using quasi-magical formulas to legitimate the politically based conclusion that there is a surplus of human resources. A second group, new to the struggle and lacking skill in economics, has become thoroughly socialized to the surplus mentality and mouths the appropriate language. A third group marches to another tune. It asserts that by controlling the number of professionals, we can anticipate reduced competition among them, higher rates for services, and income maximization for professionals. A fourth group, seeking more program flexibility, rejects the surplus theme. It continues to support maldistribution as an alternative rationale for delivering health care and urges more study. A fifth group, which also rejects the surplus ideology, searches for exceptions to the presidential directives. It seeks allies in Congress, the professions, and the universities. Not surprisingly, this group tries to maintain low visibility in what it sees as a hostile environment. Thus, the many-faceted bureaucracy confuses itself as well as its potential interest group supporters in groping for a national policy. The latter become increasingly disenchanted, alienated, and suspicious of their federal brethren.

In recent years, several key federal reports have analysed human resources in the health industry. They include a statement by the Health Resources Administration (1979b), a memorandum (Klerman, 1977) by the administrator of the Alcohol, Drug Abuse, and Mental Health Administration (ADAMHA), the report of the President's Commission on Mental Health (1978), an ADAMHA task force report on manpower (Alcohol, Drug Abuse, and Mental Health Administration, 1978), the Mental Health Systems Act (1980), a 1980 report of the U.S. Department of Labor, and a 1980 report to Congress by ADAMHA (Department of Health and Human Services, 1980) in a response to a congressional request. Their key objectives will be considered here.

The Health Resources Administration (Health Resources Administration, 1979a) identified five objectives for 1981. The first was to remove incentives for unwarranted growth in the aggregate supply of health professionals. The second was to promote an increased supply of primary care professionals relative to other types of specialists. The third was to increase the availability of health professionals in underserved areas. The fourth was to expand the participation of minorities in the health professions, and the fifth was to promote national health care priorities through targeted special projects, that is, through cost consciousness, care of the elderly and terminally ill, and preventive services.

The federal mental health agencies, all constrained by the same cost control policies, have opted for a dual response to these objectives: While continuing to look for third-party funds and legitimacy, they also press for acknowledgment of selected shortages of mental health professionals in contrast to the surpluses projected for most other health providers. This strategy is evident in Klerman's (1977) memorandum "Policy Analysis and Recommendations Concerning Clinical/Services Manpower and Training Activities of ADAMHA," as well as in the 1980

ADAMHA report to Congress (Department of Health and Human Services, 1980). Five systemic and pervasive deficiencies related to manpower in mental health areas were identified in the report: (1) maldistribution of providers; (2) inefficient utilization of professionals, in that some functions could be performed with equal quality by people with less technical competence; (3) poor needs assessment and demand forecasting, especially for discerning differences at state and local levels; (4) an inadequate manpower information system; and (5) geographical and jurisdictional inconsistencies in professional licensing and credentialing procedures. Cost control, filtered and translated as maldistribution, is preeminent, but more agency flexibility was sought than is evident in the position of the Health Resources Administration (1979a).

The defunct Mental Health Systems Act (1980), primarily directed at service delivery concerns, nevertheless contained twenty-two references to training and retraining. The act asserted that because of the rising demand for mental health services and the wide disparity in the distribution of psychiatrists, clinical psychologists, social workers, and psychiatric nurses, there is a shortage in the medical specialty of psychiatry, and there are also shortages around the other health personnel who provide mental health services. Projections of the Bureau of Labor Statistics ("Careers: Beating Inflation," 1980) regarding job prospects through the end of the 1980s also conflict with the generally pessimistic demand picture. The bureau forecasts a 34 percent growth in the number of jobs expected in this decade for physicians and osteopaths, 34 percent for psychologists, 45 percent for registered nurses, and 19 percent for social workers.

In contrast to other recent reports, the one prepared for Congress by ADAMHA (Department of Health and Human Services, 1980) urged continued federal support of training. For psychologists and social workers, it was recommended that the present production rate be maintained to offset annual attrition and permit modest growth. For psychiatric nursing, ADAMHA recommended an increase in productivity. For psychiatry, it was urged that an effort be made to reverse the trend that sees fewer American medical school graduates entering this specialty.

(The primacy of psychiatry dominates National Institute of Mental Health policy.) However, ADAMHA support would be limited to training professionals for work with underserved populations, that is, children and youth, the elderly, minorities, the chronically mentally ill, and criminals and delinquents. Additional targets include: training workers for understaffed public facilities or for geographical shortage areas, increasing the number of minority mental health specialists, providing education in mental health skills to general and primary health caregivers, training mental health specialists to work closely with professionals in the general health field, and training in preventive techniques.

Projection Models

Bureaucrats required to implement budget-cutting political directives find procedures for quantifying data about human resources highly useful. Hall (1974) outlined four methods for determining health resource requirements: (1) the economic method, (2) the health needs method, (3) the health manpower to population ratio method, and (4) the service target method. The criteria and questions utilized by each method reflect both differing values and content.

The economist asks, What will people and government pay for? In the health needs method, the overarching question is determining what people need to maintain health. The manpower-population ratio develops and extrapolates formulas by various means. Finally, the service target method inquires as to how many services of each kind are necessary to meet health requirements, and this information is then translated into manpower patterns. A complication is that various federal agencies use differing distribution criteria. One simply uses the ratio of psychiatrists to the population, but others include such factors as distance from services, health status of the population, income levels, waiting lists, percent of population below the poverty level, and percent of population over age sixty-five. Another variation compares U.S. manpower-population ratios with those of Western European countries or with successful group health plans in the United States. Still another variation uses expert opinion about the health needs of a population and then establishes manpower ratios for that population. A final variation of the ratio method is to use cost benefits or health benefits as a criterion, that is, to measure the marginal contribution as manpower is increased. All projection models assume that data are accurate and available.

Depending upon the projection model chosen, different analytic competencies are needed. The economists claim an expertise in judging the population's ability and willingness to pay for care; the health professionals claim expertise in determining health needs. Determining manpower-population ratios is probably within the province of several groups. Since service targets encompass health needs, health professionals claim priority over them, but other competencies and skills may be involved as well.

Liptzin (1978) analyzed the various methods for estimating human resource needs and concluded that none allow for future policy shifts, for example, deinstitutionalization of patients or basic changes in financing mechanisms. In fact, none would effectively accommodate major technological advances. The economic method fails to consider the quality, appropriateness, or necessity of the provided service, nor does it take into account the need for continuity of care. The health needs method fails to consider the interest, willingness, or capacity of the nation to pay for the "needed" services. The health manpower ratio method fails to allow for substitutability among professions and does not distinguish differing problems and characteristics among patient groups. The service target method is based upon certain premises as yet unrealized; that is, we are still not certain of the causal relationship between vital services and outcomes, nor is there agreement as to what array of services people truly need. Even if all the problems noted above were to be solved, the data base's adequacy would still need marked improvement.

Liptzin (1978) concluded that the state of the art in manpower projection is complex and confusing. Liptzin is overly generous, and I would agree with Stambler (1976), who describes the projection models as "hazardous" and "foolhardy." Curiously and dangerously, federal policy is increasingly based on such "crystal balling." The 1980 Graduate Medical Education Report (GMENAC) is but one of many examples of this disturbing pattern.

Trends in Supply and Production

The critical but seldom stated facts about NIMH support of mental health training programs is that it peaked in 1969, the year of the final Johnson administration budget. (Federal investment in research and development peaked in 1964 at about 12.5 percent of federal gross expenditure. By 1980, it was about 5.5 percent and dropping. See Price, 1981.) It is noteworthy that even when a subsequent Democratic administration was in power, along with a Congress controlled by Democrats, the expenditure level was not increased. If anything, the claim that there is a surplus of manpower has now been legitimated, since both Republicans and Democrats have apparently reached this conclusion.

The 1978 health manpower legislation, congressionally written with White House support, described the major demon as maldistribution of health services personnel. Thus, in the Carter administration, maldistribution was the popular and politically acceptable explanation for most known human resource problems. Some program cutters preferred a more direct explanation—oversupply of personnel—but the time was not yet ripe for them. While maldistribution hints at oversupply, it allows for exceptions. For example, the President's Commission on Mental Health (1978) concluded: "The major mental health personnel problem facing the country is not one of inadequate numbers. It is, more precisely, one of maldistribution of personnel" (p. 36).

Those who see maldistribution as the problem focus on selective resource shortages and imply that we merely need to shift surplus professionals to pockets of shortage that are variously defined as the poor, the aged, minorities, children and youth, alcoholics and drug abusers, and the populations of inner urban areas and isolated rural areas. A simple summation of these groups will give us a total substantially in excess of 100 percent of the U.S. population but, of course, these groups overlap. Eliminating duplication, it is more realistic to estimate that two thirds of our population are victims of resource maldistribution. The 1980 Mental Health Systems Act defined the unserved and underserved as the chronically mentally ill, minority groups, children and youth, and the elderly. Although more restricted than in some proposals, these priority cohorts still exceed 50 percent of the U.S. population. Analyses of resource shortages that emphasize maldistribution as the principal problem generally lead to selective strategies rather than to the more traditional solution of increasing the overall pool of human resources. Since several administrations and Congresses have viewed maldistribution as a delimited problem, federal training funds have been steadily reduced for over a decade.

Kimmel (1978) identifies four types of resource maldistribution: structural, frictional, demographic, and dynamic. Structural maldistribution results from basic changes in the service delivery system, while frictional maldistribution results from imbalance in supply and demand for services in the normal labor market. Demographic maldistribution occurs as a consequence of shifts in the locus of care—shifts that result from changes in population patterns. Dynamic maldistribution, a normal condition, is the result of any combination of the other three forces.

Measuring maldistribution is beset with the same problems as other human resource analyses and projections. Kimmel (1978) states unequivocally that "measuring maldistribution *technically* in any precise manner is now impossible" (p. 83). He describes as analytic constraints the relative, variable, culturally defined, or professionally influenced data about the incidence and prevalence of health problems; the severe lack of knowledge about the comparative effectiveness of various treatment modalities and settings; the inherent limitations of problem or disease classification systems; the absence of reliable and tested case-finding methods; and the scarcity of hard data on utilization of services and outcomes of treatments.

Several factors influence attempts to solve the problem of

maldistribution (Kimmel, 1978). They include general population shifts, the state of the economy, the nature of specialized labor markets, social and cultural values, preferences as to home and work locations, personal decisions about life-styles, the principal goals of the profession, and cost and availability of services.

The maldistribution thesis assumes that if health professionals are available, they will automatically be more accessible. Although availability must precede accessibility, it certainly does not guarantee the latter. Thus, there is a high ratio of physicians to population in major American cities, but many urban poor still lack access to medical care. Numerous factors influence accessibility including cultural, social, and ethnic ones. The capacity of patients to pay for services, travel and waiting time, and loss of wages are equally important. The caregiver's productivity and efficiency also affect accessibility.

Two sets of influences affect professionals' choice of location and specialty. One set pertains to the individual's personal, social, and cultural characteristics, as well as to his family background, geographical origin, and educational experience prior to professional training. The second set of influences include the individual's experience at the site of professional training as well as real and perceived economic opportunities.

Supply and demand considerations are much more complex than maldistribution per se since adequacy issues can never be studied by reference to a single profession alone. For example, the roles that registered nurses can play is affected by the availability of physicians, licensed practical nurses, social workers, and a variety of health technicians. Similarly, many functions performed by physicians can be enhanced, complemented, or performed by nurse practitioners, generalist nurses, physicians' assistants, optometrists, dentists, pharmacists, podiatrists, social workers, and others. In the mental health field, the supply and demand of psychologists and social workers can be examined in a similarly complex manner (Mitnick and Kole, 1978).

A variety of factors will affect future resource patterns. Certainly the enactment of a national health insurance program, in either an incremental or comprehensive form, would significantly impact on the supply of health manpower. The growing enrollment of patients in Health Maintenance Organizations (HMOs) is another factor of note. Role restructuring among professionals and gender shifts are potent influences on resource patterns. New technologies can also have a substantial effect. Pharmacological developments in the late 1950s contributed to the emptying of many of our tuberculosis sanitariums and have significantly reduced the censuses of public mental hospitals. If a true shift of focus to primary and secondary prevention were to occur, it too could be extraordinarily important. Political factors must also be weighed. The hostility to big government and its expenditures evident in the 1980 national elections promises to profoundly alter our way of life and our use of human services. Alternatively, the increasing political strength of the elderly and minorities and their demands for more and better services for themselves may have some countervailing influence.

The strategies currently used to influence the distribution of professional resources are many and sometimes even contradictory. Funds can be given or withheld for any particular profession, training program, or residency position. For example, third-party reimbursement procedures can be manipulated to enhance or inhibit the financing of specific residencies, the support of various professions, and the legitimacy of particular diseases and emotional conditions.

The National Health Service Corps scholarships obligate recipients to undertake a period of service following completion of training as a condition for having their educational loans forgiven. Thus, low- and middle-income students are provided strong economic incentives to practice for designated time periods by specialty and geography according to federal priorities. Some states have similar incentives for professionals. Although the program's effectiveness remains uncertain, it clearly is inequitable. It creates angry recipients since professionals with personal resources can practice what and where they wish. Those lacking personal resources face the equivalent of indentured servitude.

Despite the social inequity, questionable constitutional-ity, and lack of data regarding the efficacy of payback programs, the defunct Mental Health Systems Act (1980) included similar provisions. The act obligated any individual receiving a federally funded clinical traineeship for psychology, psychiatry, nursing, or social work to provide mental health services at a site designated by the secretary of the Department of Health and Human Services. Failure to perform the required service would cause the individual to incur heavy financial penalties.

Another approach to resolving imbalances in the geographical and specialty distribution of professionals is to rely on the natural forces of supply and demand. Classical market theory suggests that if the supply of health resources exceeds demand, professionals will change clinical specialty or move to less well-served geographical areas. As is evident from policy directives in recent years, federal policy makers have rejected this economic principle. They may be correct in doing so, but they have acted without valid empirical data to go by. In fact, the theory has never been adequately tested since there are no major American examples of mental health professionals being in a significantly surplus position over a long period of time. Furthermore, there are contrary examples from the health field. Vermont has a fine medical school, is a rural state with high taxes, few natural resources, and a limited economic base, and is located at some distance from major cultural and economic centers. Nevertheless, in 1978 Vermont had 184 active nonfederal physicians engaged in patient care per 100,000 population, a ratio exceeded only by California, Connecticut, Maryland, Massachusetts, and New York.

Selected Human Resource Issues

Shortages of trained and qualified mental health professionals abound nationwide. In 1978, more than 1,500 budgeted but unfilled psychiatric positions existed in state-affiliated mental health facilities (Department of Health and Human Services, 1980). The President's Commission on Mental Health (1978) expressed alarm about this century-old problem. The reasons for it are many and well known. It is noteworthy that over the last two decades the policy debate has gradually shifted from asking how to make the public mental hospital a viable component of the service delivery system, to emphasizing the mental hospital's residual role, and finally to devising ways of systematically closing the mental hospital system and transferring its resources and assets to community-based programs. Although nationally the inpatient daily census has been reduced over 70 percent, "phasing down" still remains the policy in most states, and wishful thoughts continue to be expressed about using the nearly 300 existing institutions as "backup" facilities.

The National Association of State Mental Health Program Directors (1978) has criticized university training programs for not effectively preparing their graduates for work in public mental health hospitals. However, few educators believe in perpetuating the system, and they cannot easily be motivated to train future professionals to function in settings that they view as anachronistic. There is no reason to believe that the staffing patterns espoused for public mental hospitals will ever be met unless the supply of professionals substantially exceeds demand in all programs using such personnel. Only then is it likely that some professionals will accept positions in state hospitals pending other options.

The President's Commission on Mental Health (1978) explored several alternative means to meet the professional manpower shortage in state-supported programs and facilities. Among the potential options are to have payback provisions for medical students under P.L. 94-484, which would include service in state mental hospitals; higher salaries for physicians working in them; promotion of continuing education; postgraduate teaching fellowships designed to increase the number of educators with special skills and competence in the problems encountered in public facilities; career ladders in state hospitals; contract mechanisms with the private sector; and the employment of physician assistants, children's health associates, and nurse practitioners for medical services to patients.

It may well be that closure is the only satisfactory solution to the chronic shortage of competent public mental hospital personnel. Professionals will work in such hospitals but with what degree of competence and for how long? If quality patient care is the goal, the public mental hospital had no past, it certainly has no present, and its future is even more problematic. To give just one example, the deputy secretary for mental health in Pennsylvania, Dr. Scott H. Nelson, reported that two thirds of the full-time staff psychiatrists at one state mental hospital were "seriously mentally ill." In Pennsylvania's sixteen state mental hospitals he found that "many of [the doctors] could not get a job elsewhere because they have personality problems or serious documented, psychiatric disorders—manic depression and schizophrenia" (Sobel, 1981, p. C2).

Community Mental Health Centers (CMHCs). By 1980, 763 comprehensive community mental health centers had made services available to about one half of the nation's population. For adequate national coverage, NIMH estimated that 1,350 centers would be needed (Department of Health and Human Services, 1980). The clinical efficacy of CMHCs remains uncertain, however. Although there is no reason to believe that they are inherently dysfunctional, after two decades they are still seeking an appropriate role within the human services system. Resource issues for the CMHCs are several. A key one is their gradual loss of psychiatrists, which Bass and Cravens (1978) ascribe to: (1) competition from other mental health settings; (2) less challenging clinical roles; (3) greater financial rewards in alternative roles; and (4) cost considerations (psychiatrists are paid more than other mental health professionals). Other resource gaps in CMHCs include the problem of recruiting competent executives who combine administrative and clinical skills and of securing professionals who can effectively bridge the gap between the general human services industry and the CMHC.

If the centers assume leadership roles in the community-based management of the chronically mentally ill, a lower staff-patient ratio of psychiatrists and other professional personnel may not be a problem in and of itself. The personal, familial, social, housing, and vocational needs of this particular client group may appropriately be subsumed under case management and task-centered casework practices more common to social work. The extraclinical services nestled under the concept of community support systems and appropriately developed through community organization and community development methods are likewise the usual and customary responsibility of social workers. However, to the degree that CMHCs provide emergency and crisis care, medication, long-term psychotherapy, and so on, highly trained and skilled psychiatrists, psychologists, and psychiatric nurses must also be recruited to their staffs.

Credentialing. Accreditation, licensure, and certification are the three principal means by which professional competence is signified. But the accreditation process has come under fire. As our social and educational institutions have become more complex, their boundaries more permeable, and the environmental demands on them more intense and conflicting, it is not surprising that complaints are increasingly being made about the private accreditation process. In social work, for example, accreditation has become, in part, an interest group phenomenon, leading to significant displacement of vital professional goals. Another factor in this development is a small but growing and influential federal and state bureaucracy that prefers to see accreditation managed by the public sector.

Moreover, the *Adams* v. *Califano* case, which began as a rather standard civil rights case, has stimulated proposed remedies in the credentialing process that are relevant to mental health personnel as well. Crystal Lloyd-Campbell of the Harvard Law School concluded that "the implications . . . are vast. . . . The traditionally autonomous functions that characterize academia . . . such as admissions policies, faculty selection, curriculum, and academic standards . . . are at stake in the outcome of this situation" (quoted in Arnold, 1980, p. 18). To achieve equal opportunity for all applicants, the federal Office of Civil Rights and the court order require a statewide rather than a college-by-college solution. The net result would be a statewide plan approved at the gubernatorial level, more bureaucracy, increased hierarchy, and reduced collegial authority. The faculty in professional schools and programs could lose considerable control over admissions and curriculum. Although the current case is directed to a single state university in North Carolina, it is a part of a ten-state effort, and the plaintiffs have pressed to extend the remedies nationally into private as well as public institutions of higher education (Arnold, 1980).

Nevertheless, the certification of professionals by the associations to which they belong continues to survive and expand, mostly by specialty, despite legal attacks. The number of health certification programs probably approaches 100 (Health Resources Administration, 1979b). The Bureau of Health Manpower of the U.S. Department of Health and Human Services has, in fact, entered into several contracts with certifying bodies to develop national comprehensive qualifying examinations. By 1979, ten health professions with approximately 720,000 practitioners had been covered by this program. The department has "called for a national voluntary system for allied health certification, national standards for credentialing selected health occupations, criteria for future state licensure decisions, improved licensure procedures, competency measurement, and assurance of continued competence " (Health Resources Administration, 1979b, p. 32).

Additional problems exist with regard to state-operated licensure procedures for all the core mental health professions except medicine. To practice, psychiatrists must meet the same basic requirements as other physicians, but only about 50 percent of the practicing psychiatrists are board certified (Mitnick and Kole, 1978). Psychologists and social workers are relative newcomers to licensure, and state-by-state enactment of appropriate legislation for them has been a long and arduous task. Opposition in psychology has come principally from psychologists with only master's degrees and graduates from nonaccredited programs. Ironically, after psychologists finally achieved licensure or certification in all fifty states, sunset legislation began to diminish this total, and statutory credentialing procedures are now lacking in several states. In social work some opposition has come from black social workers who postulate that state licensure may discriminate against them. The major sources of difficulty, however, have come from inertia, from state civil service bureaucrats who resent this imposition on their "right" to determine competence, from politicians wanting to control expenditures, and from general public suspicion of psychologists and social workers.

Nurses are possessed of their own unique problems in demonstrating psychiatric competency. The same examination is used for all nursing applicants, regardless of their educational achievement. An effort to upgrade requirements and to identify two separate classes of nurses is creating a major turmoil in American nursing circles.

Credential renewal (relicensure and/or recertification) has also become a spritely topic in the 1980s. Updating of competence has become legitimated and required in many states. As the half-life of knowledge is reduced, renewal is increasingly necessary and required. Continuing education is often the prescribed means, and it has become a significant growth industry. But it is also marked by conflicts of interest because of perceived revenue potential.

Minorities. The current federal policy is to proclaim that there is an abundance of health professionals except in certain geographical areas but that there is a general undersupply of racial and ethnic minority professionals. Although efforts to resolve problems of maldistribution seem, in part, a rationalization after the fact to control or reduce expenditures, the shortage of minority health professionals is very real, and solutions are critical. In his 1978 review, Clark found a minority psychiatrist to minority population ratio of only 1 to 17,000, although about 13 percent of psychiatrists in training are from minority populations (Department of Health and Human Services, 1980).

Psychology is similarly disadvantaged with regard to minorities. The proportion of all doctorally trained human service psychologists in 1977 with ethnic or racial minority backgrounds was only 2 percent. In 1980, however, the student bodies of doctoral training programs supported by NIMH in clinical, school, and community psychology included 16 percent ethnic or racial minorities (Department of Health and Human Services, 1980).

In contrast, the proportion of ethnic and racial minority students currently enrolled in schools of social work generally resembles the minority proportion of the total U.S. population, although it slipped slightly in the 1975-1979 period (Council on Social Work Education, 1981). With regard to psychiatric nursing, the proportion of minorities is substantial, but still below the proportion of minorities in the general population (Department of Health and Human Services, 1980). In 1977, 7.5 percent of the total nursing work force were minority members. For those admitted to basic nursing education in 1978, 11.1 percent were minorities (Health Resources Administration, 1979b).

The picture of gender distribution is more complicated. Nursing has traditionally been a female profession, although the proportion of males entering it has slowly increased. Social work, nearly two-thirds female, is becoming even more female in composition. Psychiatry and clinical psychology, generally male fields in the past, have recruited more females in recent years and, like other caregiving professions, are becoming more balanced by gender.

Through the remainder of this century, the persisting issue will be how to recruit and train an adequate supply of racial and ethnic minorities for psychiatry and clinical psychology and of males for nursing and social work. It is likely that nursing and social work will easily meet responsible objectives for racial and ethnic minorities while clinical psychology and psychiatry will substantially increase the number of females entering into professional training programs.

In some respects, the Hispanic population has the most favorable demographic prospects. This population has a substantially lower median age than both the general and black populations; moreover, the cohort of white eighteen year olds is expected to steadily decline in the mid 1990s. These patterns should put both Chicanos and Puerto Ricans into a seller's market. A decade or so later, there should be a burgeoning pool of Hispanic mental health professionals.

This relatively optimistic prognosis depends on a number of factors. It assumes that urban public schools will halt their decline and demonstrate an improved capacity to provide an adequate education for people from diverse cultures who speak different languages. The prognosis also assumes that graduate business schools and law schools will lose some of their current popularity among minority college graduates. Another expectation is that even though Hispanic minorities will continue to experience difficulties during the next several years, because of linguistic and cultural differences, in the long run their path to professional training will be much more direct and successful than that for other minorities. The struggle for the latter group will be a much more lasting one. It also is expected that white American females can become fully competitive with males more quickly in mental health services than in other professions; discrimination directed toward women is the most solvable of the many invidious strains negatively impacting on American society. Last, but certainly not least, unencumbered financial assistance must be made available to enlarge the population entering and completing college. Similarly, the professional schools must be given the fiscal support necessary to keep them viable and competitive. Given a large student pool and adequate financial aid, all the professional schools will increase their ethnic and minority student bodies.

Trends in Private Practice. A development that has engendered considerable interprofessional conflict is the desire of psychologists, social workers, and nurses to practice independently and to receive third-party fees without medical supervision of their activities. Although this development is generating much friction, it must be placed in perspective. Even among psychiatrists, only a minority practice privately on a full-time basis. In recent studies, the number of psychiatrists exclusively in private practice was found to range from 10 to 23 percent (Department of Health and Human Services, 1980). It is likely that similar results would be found for the other mental health professions even if reimbursement opportunities were made more readily available to them. For example, among recent NIMH-supported graduates in clinical psychology, only 2.7 percent entered private practice (Department of Health and Human Services, 1980).

As eligibility for third-party coverage is spread among more potential clients, the upper socioeconomic bias usually evident in private practice will become less manifest. Cost-effectiveness studies are equivocal, but they generally show that private practice therapy has a lower per capita cost than agency-based interventions. Of course, private practitioners do not provide community education, training, consultation, research, client advocacy, and other nonrevenue-generating services.

In the marketplace of a pluralistic society, it should be possible to accommodate a variety of service delivery mechanisms as long as they meet prescribed standards. But there are important questions needing attention. Will the competition stimulated by freedom of choice laws drive rates down? What will be the effect of expanded private practice on organized nonprofit public and private settings? Will the private practitioners skim off the more interesting clients with better prognoses? If they do, what will be the implications for staffing and operating organized programs? The trend to private practice is inevitable. For nursing and social work, especially, it will be an important step toward improved professional status, assuming that in the competitive marketplace the services of nurses and social workers are sufficiently attractive to generate viable practices.

Third Party-Reimbursement. Directly affecting the trend toward private practice are such questions as whether all four core professions—psychiatry, psychology, social work, and nursing—should be covered. For what services should they be reimbursed? Under what organizational arrangement? Under whose supervision, if any? The ultimate answers to these questions will determine the viability of mental health professions, their status, the livelihood of many of their practitioners, and the therapeutic interventions that are utilized.

The decision in recent years by third-party payers to reimburse some outpatient services on a limited basis has facilitated the growth of these services. Conversely, the reluctance of third-party payers to reimburse providers of day hospital care has seriously limited this intervention's utilization. What are the likely results of including or not including personal services under the health rubric? Is it likely that primary prevention will succeed through the services of health practitioners? Other than during the acute withdrawal stage, is alcoholism a medical problem? Is there any evidence that mental health practitioners have been more effective in treating alcoholics than have other human service professionals or Alcoholics Anonymous? Identical questions, of course, can be posed for the field of drug dependence. As was noted earlier, effective habilitation of the chronically mentally ill indeed requires a variety of nonmedical interventions. Thus even successful integration of all four core mental health professions under the health umbrella may be a mixed blessing. The medical model is not without its complications.

Planning for Human Resources

The availability of adequate human resources for the 1980s depends upon proper planning, but this task is fraught with complex political and economic strains.

In addition to the factors discussed earlier, a number of additional concerns will affect this planning process. A key one is the misguided decision by NIMH to give responsibility for mental health manpower planning to state governments on the assumption that human resource development should relate to service needs. In theory, this would make for more effective preparation, distribution, utilization, and retention of personnel. Although this proposition seems reasonable on the surface, its dangers are many. First, specialists in professional education do not work for state mental health authorities and do not abide by similar priorities. Second, the principal human resource problem according to many state mental health directors is their inability to hire and retain professional personnel for state mental hospitals—a backward view at best and probably highly dysfunctional at worst. Third, state mental health authorities are concerned with maldistribution of personnel, and this leads them to focus on relatively small geographical units. This perspective is valid perhaps to some degree for community colleges that train generic human services workers, but it has limited validity for university-based graduate professional schools that must maintain a national perspective to be maximally effective.

Unionization, especially in American nursing, is another symptom of extraordinary change that must be incorporated into the planning process. Are the interests of the professions and organized labor really compatible? Will anomalies continue to occur because of contradictory goals? Again, as concern for public protection grows, increasingly stringent licensure laws are posited. Simultaneously, however, sunset legislation is becoming more popular, and state licensure programs are among the first to be critically examined and eliminated.

Early in the chapter, I reviewed various formulas used by the federal government (and increasingly by state governments) to establish quantitative parameters in policy making for human resources. They are useful devices but are still unvalidated. To maximize their potential, we must be sensitive to and understand their limitations. Experimentation needs to continue on their potential for planning, but these efforts should be recognized as research and development rather than as the basis for major public policy. Informed judgment remains essential in the planning process.

One of the major themes of the President's Commission on Mental Health (1978) was the integration of mental health services into the general health care system. The commission urged the training of primary care providers in mental health care, and, in turn, the placement of mental health professionals in primary care programs. For this to succeed, we need improved and equitable reimbursement systems, but these can be implemented only after the underlying and fundamental resistance of many providers to dealing with the mentally ill has been overcome. A step in this planning process would be more research into human resources. We need to better understand the nature of positive incentives (present policy focuses primarily on negative incentives), the benefits and costs of mental health care, ways to improve measures of quality, the implications of alternative reimbursement mechanisms, the effects of regulatory procedures, and methods of linking these findings to populations at risk. In effect, we need a systems view of human resource development that will bind its many-faceted components together and establish meaningful goals for each rather than for only one or two.

References

Alcohol, Drug Abuse, and Mental Health Administration. *Report of the ADAMHA Manpower Policy Analysis Task Force,* Vol. I. Rockville, Md.: Alcohol, Drug Abuse, and Mental Health Administration, 1978.

Arnold, C. R. "Federal Intrusion into the Academy: The Landmark UNC Case." *The Green Sheet,* 1980, *15,* 17-20.

Bass, R. D., and Cravens, R. B. "Manpower Issues in Community Mental Health Programs." In *Report of the ADAMHA Manpower Policy Analysis Task Force.* Vol. 2. Rockville, Md.: Alcohol, Drug Abuse, and Mental Health Administration, 1978.

"Careers: Beating Inflation." *New York Times,* Oct. 12, 1980, p. 15.

Clark, L. B. "Alcohol, Drug Abuse, and Mental Health Manpower Issues Involving Racial and Ethnic Minorities." In *Report of the ADAMHA Manpower Policy Analysis Task Force.* Vol. 2. Rockville, Md.: Alcohol, Drug Abuse, and Mental Health Administration, 1978.

Comings, L. "Alcohol, Drug Abuse, and Mental Health Manpower: Legislative Considerations." In *Report of the ADAMHA Manpower Policy Analysis Task Force.* Vol. 2. Rockville, Md.: Alcohol, Drug Abuse, and Mental Health Administration, 1978.

Council on Social Work Education. *Statistics on Social Work Education in the United States.* New York: Council on Social Work Education, 1981.

Department of Health and Human Services. *Personnel Needs for Mental Health Services: Report to the Senate.* Washington, D.C.: Department of Health and Human Services, 1980.

Hall, T. L. "Estimating Requirements and Supplies: Where Do We Stand?" In *Pan American Conference on Health Manpower Planning.* Scientific Publication No. 279. Washington, D.C.: Pan American Health Organization, 1974.

Health Resources Administration. *Health Professions Legislation—Areas Under Consideration.* Hyattsville, Md.: Health Resources Administration, 1979a.

Health Resources Administration. *Report on Health Personnel in the United States.* Health Resources Studies, Department of Health, Education, and Welfare Publication No. (HRA) 80-651. Washington, D.C.: U.S. Government Printing Office, 1979b.

Kimmel, W. A. "Maldistribution of Alcohol, Drug Abuse, and Mental Health Manpower: Executive Summary of a Concept Paper." In *Report of the ADAMHA Manpower Policy Analysis Task Force.* Vol. 2. Rockville, Md.: Alcohol, Drug Abuse, and Mental Health Administration, 1978.

Klerman, G. L. "Policy Analysis and Recommendations Concerning Clinical/Services Manpower and Training Activities of ADAMHA." Rockville, Md.: Alcohol, Drug Abuse, and Mental Health Administration, 1977.

Liptzin, B. "Supply, Demand, and Projected Need for Psychiatrists and Other Mental Health Manpower: An Analytic Paper." In *Report of the ADAMHA Manpower Policy Analysis Task Force.* Vol. 2. Rockville Md.: Alcohol, Drug Abuse, and Mental Health Administration, 1978.

Mental Health Systems Act, P.L. 96-398, 1980.

Mitnick, L., and Kole, D. M. "Discussion Paper on Credentials and Quality Assurance." In *Report of the ADAMHA Manpower Policy Analysis Task Force.* Vol. 2. Rockville, Md.: Alcohol, Drug Abuse, and Mental Health Administration, 1978.

National Association of State Mental Health Program Directors. "Manpower Issues in State and County Mental Hospitals." In *Report of the ADAMHA Manpower Policy Analysis Task Force.* Vol. 2. Rockville, Md.: Alcohol, Drug Abuse, and Mental Health Administration, 1978.

Orzack, L. H. "Educators, Practitioners, and Politicians in the European Common Market." *Higher Education,* 1980, 307-323.

President's Commission on Mental Health. *Report to the President.* Vol. I. Washington, D.C.: U.S. Government Printing Office, 1978.

Price, D. D. S. "R and D Productivity." *Science,* 1981, *211.*

Sobel, D. "State Psychiatric Hospitals Forced to Change or Close." *New York Times,* Feb. 10, 1981.

Stambler, H. V. "Health Manpower–the Right Number." In

Health Manpower Issues—A Presentation at the White House. Hyattsville, Md.: Health Resources Administration, 1976.

Summary Report of the Graduate Medical Education National Advisory Committee to the Secretary. Department of Health and Human Services Publication No. (HRA) 81-651. Vol. 1. Hyattsville, Md.: Health Resources Administration, 1980.

Zubkoff, M. (Ed.). *Health: A Victim or Cause of Inflation?* New York: Prodist, 1977.

Chapter 23

Social and Behavioral Sciences in Medical School Curriculum

James R. Allen

The functions of the physician are to relieve, to prevent, and to cure disease. During the past seventy years, however, we have become progressively more preoccupied with the biological mechanisms of disease—a preoccupation best understood as a consequence of a model of medicine that has contributed much to our therapeutic powers, and has therefore come to dominate our professional ideology (Engel, 1971, 1977).

In his influential study of medical education more than seventy years ago, Flexner (1910) advocated mastery of the scientific method and its application to all dimensions of medicine. However, his recommendations have been interpreted in a way that has emphasized unifactorial etiology, physiochemical explanations, and mind-body dualism. This particular version of the "medical model" seems to have evolved, at least in part, from a concession made to Christian orthodoxy. The Church's permission to study the intact human body included a tacit interdiction against the corresponding investigation of man's mind and behavior. It coincided with the development of the basic principles of post-Renaissance science. As advanced by Galileo, Descartes, and Newton, these principles were analytical, and they utilized a linear model of cause and effect. In medicine, this fostered a metaphor of the body as a machine and a conceptualization of disease as a consequence of breakdown in that machine. With the introduction of antibiotic and antipsychotic medications, the wisdom of this approach seemed confirmed.

In science, a model is revised or abandoned if it fails to account for all data. A dogma, in contrast, requires that discrepant data either be forced into the model or be excluded. Current biomedical dogma has assumed that disease is best understood in terms of deviation from measurable, biological variables, and the diagnosis of disease has preempted medical attention. When his work-up fails to uncover biological malfunctioning, however, the physician is often ill prepared to cope with symptoms that are no less "real" simply because they are psychosocial in origin. Grief, for example, has not usually been considered in the framework of disease. Yet many grieving people consult physicians because of somatic symptoms. When does grief become a disease?

It is ironic that those who dismiss many emotional problems as "mere problems in living," and therefore as ill suited for medical management, do so by attributing other medical disorders to "pure" biological causes. Surely, however, the physician who cares for the patient with hypertension must have the same sensitivity to psychosocial matters as the physician who cares for the schizophrenic patient. The hypertensive patient, no less than the schizophrenic one, has feelings and ideas about his illness and is responsive to familial and social pressures. The mere prescription of medication, exercise, and diet provides no assurance of improved outcome. In fact, the chances are great that the patient will not take his medication and follow his treatment regimen unless they make sense to him, unless he sees his aims and those of his physician as congruent, and unless the treatment's impact on his daily routines is compatible with his life-style. Furthermore, the course of his illness may be mitigated by his social support systems or it may be exacerbated by social stresses. His relationship with his physician may influence his medication requirements; it certainly will influence whether or not he takes the medication. Thus, the role of the family physician or internist is little different from that of the psychiatrist in that both need to be cognizant of psychosocial factors and interpersonal relationships and both must be sophisticated in the use of community resources. The physician's roles include, and always have included, those of educator and of psychotherapist.

The inclusion of psychodynamic, sociocultural, and behavioral approaches in the physician's thinking is not in opposition to standard and essential steps in biomedical diagnosis but rather is an extension of that practice. Rational treatment directed to biochemical indexes alone does not necessarily restore the patient to health, even in the face of documented correction of biochemical abnormality. Flexner himself nowhere implied that "scientific study" was to exclude the psychosocial. He noted: "The physician's function is fast becoming social and preventive rather than just individual and curative" (1910, p. 17). Flexner went on to stress that "the scientific character of the procedure depends not on where or by what means facts are procured. . . . The essence of science is method—the painstaking collection of all relevant data" (p. 17). It is difficult not to conclude that Flexner's report has yet to be fully implemented.

Two thousand years ago, Hippocrates of Cos, whose oath many physicians still take, taught that no physician, however skilled in detecting bodily dysfunction, could provide adequate treatment without an awareness of the patient's personality and interpersonal relationships, as well as of the environmental precipitants of illness. In the first chapter of his *Precepts,* he attributed illness not only to organic causes, as did the exclusively organic school of Knidos, but also to "excessive indulgences or repressions of appetites—disappointments in love and war—sustained tension in the race for fame and fortune—and fear and superstitions." The Hippocratic "medical model" was not biomedical.

A Practical Rationale

Quite apart from theoretical and historical justifications, there are today at least five major trends in medicine that necessitate the inclusion of behavioral and social sciences in the undergraduate curricula of our medical schools.

First, primary care providers have long been accorded priority in evolving national health policy. Of the 15 percent or so of the population who suffer from mental disorders each year in the United States, four times as many are treated by primary caregivers as by mental health specialists. In addition, primary care physicians play a major supportive role for patients coping with "problems in living."

Recent studies report that the prevalence of psychiatric disorder encountered in general medical practice is between 4 and 88 percent of all patients seen (Houpt and others, 1980). The vast majority of these studies report a rate between 4 and 20 percent, the variations reflecting differences in the criteria used to identify psychiatric morbidity and in the settings in which the studies were conducted. Despite this variability, the majority of recognized psychiatric disorders encountered in general medical practice are not "mere problems in living." Blumenthal and Dielman (1975), for example, found that the depressions treated by primary care providers profoundly affect the ability of patients to perform major role functions. In terms of medical resources, these patients make about twice as many visits to the physician as those without psychiatric disorders and require more general medical services, such as x rays and laboratory tests, than other patients. In addition, the treatment of these patients often places an emotional burden on nonpsychiatric physicians, who report that they feel inadequately trained to treat them.

At present, we lack good basic descriptive data on treatment—even a simple record of the number and kinds of treatments currently being provided by various practitioners. Unfortunately, the federal government has encouraged expansion of the primary care sector without an authoritative major study to guide its effects. Formal psychotherapy, however, is reported to be utilized in 2 percent of all visits to nonpsychiatric physicians. Because of the large number of patients seen by this group, these visits amount to 27 percent of all the time devoted to psychotherapy (Gori and Richter, 1978).

The importance of the primary care physician in the delivery of mental health services is likely to increase. Fewer medical school graduates are choosing psychiatry as a specialty, and newly enacted federal regulations have closed the doors to foreign medical graduates, who traditionally filled half the positions in the public mental hospitals. In addition, psychiatric manpower is poorly distributed, both in terms of geography and in terms of those who have social and economic access to it. Finally, the deinstitutionalization movement has spurred the return of state hospital patients to the community and, if they are lucky, into the care of primary physicians.

Second, there are clear relations between life-style and physical illness. Five of the six leading causes of death in the United States today (diseases of the heart and blood vessels, cancer, accidents, cirrhosis of the liver, and diabetes mellitus) are related to life-style, as are the major causes of disability (cardiovascular disease, chronic obstructive pulmonary diseases, and accidents). Over the last three decades, the United States invested an unprecedented portion of national resources in the study and care of diseases, but the health and longevity of Americans during that time did not show commensurate improvement. Indeed, a 1967 study suggested that neither an increase nor a decrease in disease care expenditures would likely have any impact on life expectancy (see Houpt and others, 1980).

The most important diseases today are caused by a variety of factors. Of these, the most significant seem to be personal and social habits, such as improper diet, drug abuse, lack of exercise, environmental pollution, and unsafe driving and working conditions. But the most effective preventive measures seem to be those that require the least personal effort, as in the case of public health management of water, sewage, food, and fluoridation. More difficult to institute are those in which the individual himself is responsible.

According to current estimates, fifty-five million Americans smoke cigarettes. Of the forty million who are overweight, fifteen million are 30 percent or more overweight. Nine to ten million Americans drink excessively. Half our diets are deficient in one or more of the basic nutrients. The serum cholesterol of 20 percent of American adults exceeds 260 mg/100 ml. Half the population makes appointments with physicians and does not keep them (Green, 1975).

Health education has been the chief tool of the general medical sector's response to these life-style hazards. Unfortunately, health care education seems more effective in raising awareness and motivation than in assisting people actually to make and sustain changes in living patterns. Commonly prescribed drug treatments and traditional psychiatric approaches have proved inadequate, a fact that has led many physicians to become reluctant even to encourage life-style modification. The techniques that seem to offer the greatest promise of effective meaningful change are behavioral techniques based on social learning theory (Pomerleau, Boss, and Crown, 1975). These approaches use three broad strategies: stimulus control, reinforcement control, and self-control. It would seem that these techniques should occupy a major place in today's medical curricula. They do not.

Third, there is growing awareness of patient nonadherence to medical regimens. About 50 percent of patients do not take their drug prescriptions as directed, and these errors and omissions create a serious health threat in an estimated 44 percent (Steward and Cluff, 1975). Hypertension, for example, is estimated to cause approximately sixty thousand deaths in the United States annually, in part through its role in a million and a half heart attacks and cerebrovascular accidents. Only about half of approximately eleven million people identified as having hypertension comply with hypertensive regimens, despite the fact that the disease can be controlled through drugs in 80 to 85 percent of cases (Kasl, 1975).

The primary determinates of nonadherence are situational, involving the characteristics of the regimen (the greater the complexity, the higher the rate of nonadherence), the characteristics of the disease (the nonadherence rate is higher for symptomatic and chronic illnesses), and the doctor-patient relationship (the adherence rate correlates with continuity of care and with physician empathy and warmth). In their review of 250 studies comparing educational, behavioral, and combined educational-behavioral approaches, Sackett and Haynes (1977) concluded that educational strategies alone are consistently less effective than combined strategies that incorporate stimulus control, the tailoring of a drug regimen to a patient's daily life, and the utilization of contingency contracting, social support, and encouragement. These topics have become a significant part of medical school curricula.

Fourth, during the past fifteen years, there has been a flood of studies describing the changing status of health services and medical education in this country—the Coggeshall report in 1965, the report on the Graduate Education of Physicians in 1966, the Health Manpower Report of 1967, the Carnegie Commission report of 1970, the Millis Report of 1971, and the Health Professions Assistance Act of 1976. All produced a substantial amount of evidence upon which to base recommendations for improving training as well as the delivery systems of the health sector.

While community psychiatry has had its slogans, it also has had its substance, and it has been a precursor of a number of the trends that are changing the delivery of both general health and mental health care. It has been a means for encouraging consumer participation, citizen involvement, community linkage, and multidisciplinary treatment teams. Not only has it improved the accessibility of services and broadened entitlement to care, but it has increased sensitivity to "nonmedical" influences on behavior and has served, for active involvement in the social arena, as a laboratory to study outreach, prevention, rehabilitation, and comprehensiveness of service delivery. These changes will have significant repercussions for medical education—repercussions that are just beginning to be felt and that are as likely to be felt in family practice, internal medicine, and pediatrics as in psychiatry.

Fifth, by its very success, contemporary biomedicine has been driven toward a confrontation with basic human values.

The physician must make decisions that are based on moral values as well as on clinical skills. Since the early 1970s, there has been a significant growth of interest in the teaching of human values and humanities to students in medicine. The first humanities department in a medical school was established at Pennsylvania State University at Hershey in 1967. Since 1972, the Institute on Human Values and Medicine has published three compilations of teaching programs in the humanities. The most recent, published in 1976, included twenty-nine medical schools (McElhinney, 1976).

Psychiatry has traditionally been the only clinical discipline in medicine concerned primarily with the study of man and the human condition. The current upsurge of interest in primary care and family medicine, however, clearly reflects a disenchantment with approaches to disease that neglect the individual character of the patient. While behavioral and social scientists, as well as a variety of humanists, have made some limited excursions into medical schools, it is mainly upon psychiatry that the responsibility to take the whole patient into account has fallen.

Undergraduate Medical School Curricula

What kinds of knowledge does a surgeon, a pediatrician, or a family practitioner need in order to be a good doctor? What skills, conceptual knowledge, and attitudes should medical students have acquired by the time they have finished their basic medical education? What is the core cluster of skills and knowledge that all physicians must have? When is the best time to teach these skills, and how are they best taught? These and related questions beset educators in every medical school.

In each school, the curriculum reflects the concepts, personalities, and territorial skirmishes of its faculty. Each school has a variety of students; some are interested in a trade-school approach to medicine, others in broader educational issues, but each has his own best way of learning. In addition, it would probably take fifteen years to teach medical students all that they need to know—and at least half that information would be obsolete by the time they were graduated.

In most medical schools, "internal medicine" is the standard against which other specialties are measured. Following the lead of pediatrics, the American Board of Internal Medicine (1979) recently developed and published criteria for clinical competence in internal medicine. Its task force defined the major variables involved in the clinical encounter as (1) attitudes and habits, (2) interpersonal skills, (3) motor and technical skills, and (4) intellectual abilities. It specifically requires that the physician provide comprehensive and continuing care, be sensitive to psychosocial factors, be alert to the patient's emotional needs, communicate effectively, and educate his patients in health maintenance.

Psychiatry, as a formal discipline, is a relative newcomer to medical education. The first chair of psychiatry, so designated, was that occupied by Johann Christian Heinroth in Leipzig in 1811, and American psychiatric teaching had its origin in the work of Benjamin Rush at about the same period. In the first half of this century, however, there were few academic departments of psychiatry, and those that did exist were usually divisions in departments of medicine. Psychiatric influence in the medical curriculum, if it existed at all, consisted of a few lectures or demonstrations of psychiatric syndromes. After World War II, however, departments of psychiatry began to assume a major role in preclinical medical education. This development was the result of several forces: the enactment of the National Mental Health Act; the Russell Sage Foundation residency programs, which provided opportunities for social and behavioral scientists to be brought into medical schools; the establishment of psychiatric services in general hospitals; the availability of federal matching funds for the building of psychiatric services in general hospitals; and the fact that, under the pressures of the war, anthropologists, psychologists, sociologists, and psychiatrists had learned to work together. In 1958, the National Institute of Mental Health began to offer support for the expansion of teaching programs that would lead to a broader understanding of human behavior as it relates to health and illness. In 1960, part two of the examination of the National Board of Medical Examiners included a section on clinical psychiatry. Finally, in the late 1960s, five schools followed Robert

Strauss' lead in experimenting with separate departments of human behavioral science at the University of Kentucky, but this movement has not grown. The recognition of the importance of the material, however, led to the establishment of a section on behavioral sciences in part one of the National Board examination in 1971.

Today, there are departments of psychiatry in all medical schools in the country. Psychiatrists usually teach in both the basic sciences and the clinical areas, a fact that differentiates them from other clinical instructors. Not infrequently, psychiatry is among the largest departments in the school. In most schools, it is responsible for teaching in the following areas: (1) the biological, psychological, and social forces that influence illness and the treatment of it; (2) normal development and behavior; (3) interviewing skills; (4) complexities of the doctor-patient relationship; (5) psychopathology and clinical psychiatric syndromes; (6) treatment and management of common behavioral problems, including marital problems, child abuse, sexual dysfunction, and death and dying; (7) psychiatric and mental health resources; and (8) referral practices.

Although some medical schools are better than others, all are carefully accredited and, therefore, are not likely to survive unless they demonstrate a respectable level of quality. This has led to a remarkable uniformity in curricula. The curriculum of the first year usually focuses on normal development during the life cycle and on general topics in the behavioral sciences. Psychiatrists often teach medical interviewing, perhaps as part of a course in physical diagnosis. In the second year, most departments of psychiatry cover psychopathology and the major psychiatric syndromes. The third or fourth year is likely to include a clinical clerkship in psychiatry, generally of six weeks duration, but ranging from four to eight weeks. Psychiatry has been a leader in moving toward the community, in utilizing multidisciplinary teams, and in reducing unnecessary hospitalizations.

The examinations of the National Board of Medical Examiners (1980) serve as a cognitive rite of passage in most medical schools. The areas of behavioral and social science presently examined in part one are behavioral biology, individual behavior, interpersonal and group behavior, and culture and society. The areas examined in the psychiatry section of part two are personality theory; social, community, and family relationships; assessment techniques; psychopathology; social and psychological aspects of nonpsychiatric illness; intervention techniques; and ethical and legal issues (National Board of Medical Examiners, 1980).

In one of the few published attempts to achieve a consensus about the composition of an ideal core curriculum, the American Psychiatric Association (1969) conducted a survey of forty-eight psychiatric department chairmen. The most frequently mentioned topics included community psychiatry, interviewing skills, the doctor-patient relationship, psychology, psychopharmacology, genetics, and drug abuse. Although many psychiatric educators have also made specific proposals, most of these have two serious deficiencies: They lack "in the field" appraisal of their clinical applicability and relevance, and they do not consider future needs and national priorities. Moreover, curricula designed by even the most experienced psychiatrists may not be attuned to the needs of the nonpsychiatric physician.

There is also considerable evidence that psychiatric educators have not yet succeeded in selecting curricula that seem relevant to their students. Studies of medical students show they have less interest in psychiatry at the end of the fourth year than at the beginning of medical school. Castelnuevo-Tedesco's survey (1967) of 110 recent graduates of American and Canadian medical schools, for example, revealed that almost half did not think that their courses prepared them adequately to deal with the psychological problems encountered in medical practice.

Several recent studies have been made to determine what aspects of psychiatry are relevant for nonpsychiatric physicians. The results are in close agreement and could provide the basis for a core curriculum in psychiatry appropriate to those medical students who enter nonpsychiatric areas. When the chairmen of 112 departments of psychiatry were questioned, however, a number of discrepancies were noted. The psychiatrists placed much emphasis on the diagnosis and treatment of schizophrenia.

Perhaps this is because most students traditionally have been taught psychiatry as an inpatient service. General physicians ranked understanding of psychosomatic disorders high, but psychiatrists did not. This may reflect frustration with teaching in an area where basic principles are not clear. Few psychiatrists rated an understanding of alcoholism as highly important, but the nonpsychiatric physicians did. Knowledge of mental health resources and how to refer a patient are of great concern to primary care physicians, but not to psychiatrists, who spend all their time working in the mental health system. Psychiatrists ranked geriatric psychiatry very low, although general physicians see an ever-increasing percentage of people over sixty-five years of age (Fine and Therrien, 1977).

Interpersonal Skills. In response to increasing recognition of the role of interpersonal and interviewing skills in patient satisfaction, cooperation, and adherence to therapeutic regimens, as well as in therapeutic outcomes, there has been a rapid growth in the number and variety of teaching programs in these areas. Indeed, almost all medical schools now have specific courses in interviewing skills, although eighty percent of them are less than five years old. This rapid implementation of programs seems to reflect an attitudinal change toward the place of social and behavioral sciences in medical education (Fine and Therrien, 1977). Most programs teach techniques of listening, responding, and data gathering, along with psychological interventions such as demonstrating empathy. Less than one third teach any specific type of counseling or how to give information to patients. Ninety percent use videotape technology for teaching or for assessing, but only about one third use an outcome index for evaluation.

While existing research indicates short-term benefit, there are few data to suggest how long these newly learned skills are retained. Less than 1 percent of the programs provide follow-up during the clinical years (Pacoe and others, 1976). There have been few attempts to teach and to evaluate interpersonal skills at the postgraduate level, except in departments of psychiatry and, more recently, in family practice. It has been shown that internal medicine residents could be trained to devote more time to psychosocial issues, to respond more effectively to emotionally charged material, and to show an increased level of empathy, even though the interviews remain primarily medical; the board now requires satisfactory performance as a qualification for admission to its certifying examination (Futcher, Sanderson, and Tusler, 1977).

Consultation and Liaison. The past ten years have brought an explosion of interest in consultation-liaison psychiatry. Caplan's (1970) development of consultation theory and technique during the early 1960s, along with later applications of general systems theory, enabled liaison consultants to develop intervention techniques and educational strategies that could be directed toward a wide variety of health care providers. The major impact of these programs is at the level of the residents and ward staff, although Reifler and Eaton (1978) in their NIMH report noted that highly rated programs actively involved medical students. To the degree that such programs are successful in increasing sensitivity to the psychosocial aspects of patient care, in helping patient care that is comprehensive both longitudinally and in cross section to become the norm, and in approaching Caplan's definition of community mental health, to that degree these programs will encourage holistic medical care.

Since medical students learn much from the residents with whom they work, it is entirely possible that they may learn the most practical applications of the behavioral sciences in departments other than psychiatry. This seems especially likely if the discipline of psychiatry, in its attempt to "return to (bio)medicine," limits itself to a very narrow spectrum of "biological markers" and neo-Kraepelinian interests, and if the new standards of the Joint Commission on Accreditation of Hospitals transform community mental health centers into social service agencies.

Areas of Neglect. Medical schools traditionally have emphasized the mechanisms of disease and curing, along with the preeminent role of the physician. Rehabilitation medicine, in contrast, emphasizes the fact that comprehensive care requires sustained team emphasis. There is considerable overlap between the two approaches, and both are essential for good health care, with the appropriate balance depending on the setting. But despite increased interest in family medicine, which proclaims interest in treating the whole family as an interrelated system and in delivering primary care by dealing with the needs of the whole person, medical students receive little training specifically devoted to care of the chronically ill, and physicians, therefore, have little knowledge of or interest in long-term approaches. Certainly, the physician whose training has emphasized single diagnosis will have neither the inclination nor the training to become actively involved in a team-oriented treatment program for the patient with many problems.

An even more basic problem is the ambivalent, if not blatantly negative, attitude of physicians toward the chronically ill and the elderly. While this attitude seems to be intensified during the socialization process of medical school, it also reflects the attitudes of our society. Perhaps, it is rooted in our own fears of death and our attempts to deny the fact of our own aging. It is important that students perceive rewards in the treatment of the patient who requires long-term care. If students are able to play a role in the return of the patient to his own home and to plan for and evaluate his maintenance at home, such an experience will make the concept of comprehensive care more understandable. At present, however, only 32 out of 114 medical schools offer geriatrics as an elective course, and none make it a requirement. Yet, an intensive study of twenty-seven senior medical students at Case Western Reserve University indicated that they would find personal satisfaction in treating such patients (Halstead and Halstead, 1978).

As of 1975, some 119 medical schools in the United States had eschewed the establishment of geriatrics as a medical specialty. None of them had a chair of geriatrics, and none required its students to visit a nursing home, although two thirds of every dollar spent on health care is spent on the population over sixty-five. There are more patients in nursing homes than in hospitals. The University of Michigan Medical Center, in contrast, does have a geriatric program that provides training for medical students. Its goals are to create an awareness of the special characteristics and needs of the ill elderly, to change the attitudes of students toward aging and to interest them in comprehensive medical and psychiatric care of the elderly, to develop their awareness of gerontology as a legitimate and important field of knowledge, and to introduce the gerontologist as a clinical provider rather than as a lecturer.

Another area currently overlooked in medical education is that of alcoholism. The problem of excessive use of alcohol exemplifies the overlap of medical illness, influence of life-style, and mental disorder. Overall, alcoholics have a mortality rate that is two to three and one-half times the expected rate. Alcohol abuse also has adverse effects on people other than the alcoholic himself. For example, the fetal alcohol syndrome (mental retardation, as well as cardiovascular and cranial-facial defects) may result from alcohol consumption by pregnant women. Roughly 50 percent of fatal traffic accidents are alcohol related, and alcohol was implicated in over one third of all crimes in the United States in 1975. It is therefore hardly surprising that an estimated nine million American alcohol abusers incur direct medical costs of approximately $12 billion annually and account for 19.9 percent of annual hospital care expenses. The total economic cost of alcoholism, including health care, lost production, fire losses, accident losses, and crime and social responses, as well as of alcohol-related medical illnesses, has been estimated at over $44 billion (Houpt and others, 1980).

Because of the many interdependent causes of alcoholism, the alcoholic patient and his family may need a complex form of treatment. Multidisciplinary, comprehensive treatment programs have generally produced more favorable results than programs that use only one modality (Houpt and others, 1980). These facts have important implications for medical education—implications that have not yet been integrated into curricula. The concept of integrated health and mental health care, along with the fact that nonpsychiatric physicians require greater competence in the psychological management of their patients and in working cooperatively with mental health professionals, has been neglected. Similarly, mental health professionals traditionally lack skill in the treatment of patients with somatic symptoms and physical illness, in behavioral approaches to life-style modification, and in working collaboratively with the general physician. Unfortunately, national endorsement of single, integrated health care settings is unlikely in view of the current emphasis on private practice. We also need to alter our present reimbursement mechanisms: Consultation and collaboration with health and social service professionals need to be reimbursed, even though a patient is not seen. As long as these practices continue unchanged, it is unlikely that medical school curricula will ever be satisfactory.

Because medical education in drug abuse and alcoholism has been scanty, and because medical students tend to acquire negative attitudes toward patients with these problems, the National Institute on Drug Abuse and the National Institute on Alcohol Abuse and Alcoholism established the Career Teacher Training Program in Addictions. A 1976 survey of drug abuse and alcoholism teaching in 105 schools revealed that few schools teach much about these problems. The average school spent .6 percent of curriculum time for instruction in both alcoholism and drug abuse (Pokorny, Putnam, and Fryer, 1978). In view of the fact that alcoholism alone is regarded as one of the nation's major health problems, this is inadequate.

Educational Evaluation

Although behavioral scientists are known for their sophisticated methodologies, they have not yet developed good means for evaluating the effectiveness of their own teaching. Most evaluation techniques measure how well students like courses rather than how well courses fulfill their objectives. There are three stages to the education experience: input, the process of learning, and output. Each of these can and should be the focus of systematic evaluation. Without consideration of the other two, information gathered from any one may lead to erroneous conclusions. There is, however, a long and unquestioned tradition in most educational institutions of attributing student achievement to the effectiveness of instructors and student failure to the inadequacy of the student.

The output of instruction has typically been the primary

if not the exclusive focus of attention, to the exclusion of evaluation of incoming students, selection processes, teaching methods, the student learning environment, student learning styles, and psychosocial factors that support or distress the student. Most medical instruction has been focused on teaching knowledge and skills, although students are asked in their medical practice to break many previously maintained behavioral taboos and face a series of potentially traumatic situations. Too frequently, their instructors and role models act as if personal experiences are not important or should not be discussed, lest they distract from learning to care for patients. But the way in which the student resolves these issues may determine, at least in part, his or her later effectiveness and happiness as a physician.

Even the focus on outcome evaluations has been restricted. Usually, it has been limited to cognitive material, which is the most easily evaluated. We have not invested the effort to devise methods that can adequately assess effective and systematic data-gathering and problem-solving skills, the capacity to establish basic trust and sharing relationships, effectiveness in initiating one's own learning, or the effects of student learning on later clinical practice. Many techniques of evaluation are not really methods of evaluation at all, but methods of scoring. The only objective aspect of so-called objective tests is the process of scoring, because determination is made in advance as to which responses will be treated as correct. The selection of questions, the response options, and even the options that will be regarded as correct involve highly subjective decisions. For many educators, ambiguity and uncertainty are unwelcome, but it is this very avoidance of ambiguity and uncertainty that often detracts from quality.

Formal evaluation of medical student competence today draws heavily on the results of National Board Examinations, but these examinations probably are not an adequate criterion for measuring qualifications for the practice of medicine. For example, these examinations contain detailed questions about psychiatric theory; what a student should learn in medical school is not just psychiatric theory, however, but how to work with patients who are troubled. Perhaps even more disconcerting is the fact that the multiple-choice approach presumes an immutable base of common, factual knowledge that does not exist even in the basic sciences.

The most valid measures of skill, on a short-term basis, are based on the observation of actual behavior, such as live or videotaped interviews and chart audits. Unfortunately, the most frequently reported skill measures are based on global, subjective impressions. However, scales have been developed for reliably rating skills in interviewing and for systematically scoring chart notes in order to evaluate skills in recognizing and managing psychosocial problems. Where actual behavior is difficult to measure directly, patient management problems, tests of empathic interviewing, and the students' written responses to filmed patient interviews have been used. Meyer Morrison, for example, has developed a videotape-based test at the Mt. Sinai School of Medicine, involving four major taped interviews and four one-minute sections. The test is able to differentiate third-year students who are finishing different programs and to distinguish second-year students from third-year students who have taken the basic psychiatry clerkships.

We expect medical students to develop certain desirable and "professional" attitudes. This hope is sometimes quite unrealistic. Indeed, the existing literature suggests that physicians have a rather negative attitude toward psychiatric patients. General practitioners, for example, are reported to view neurotics as "weak, foolish, twisted, complicated, and ineffectual," and senior medical students have described the typical emotionally ill patient as "someone whose ambiguous complaints are apt to make diagnosis uncertain and whose resistance to getting well is apt to nullify treatment." Indeed, some studies have suggested that after a basic course in the behavioral sciences, students may see both psychiatric patients and psychiatrists as less than desirable and as generally unlike themselves—but very much like each other. Training in certain limited areas, such as taking a sexual history, has rather frequently been observed to produce self-reported attitudinal changes and demonstrable behavioral changes when a student performs that specific task. Unfortunately, these courses are usually not closely related to the rest of the curriculum.

Major problems in the routine assessment of attitude change are the difficulty in translating common attitude change goals into specific, measurable objectives and the paucity of validated measures. A useful and appealing strategy for measuring attitude change involves recasting these goals into behavior change goals and then measuring the attainment of these changes. For example, if a goal is to increase the student's receptivity to concepts of holistic health care, the evaluator can identify such behavioral indicators as adequate use of consultation services, appropriate referral, psychosocial management, and adequate charting of the psychosocial history, and then determine whether these have been carried out. Ultimately, however, the most valid methods of assessing an educational program have to do with the impact it has on the quality of care that its graduates deliver.

A Shortage of Dinosaurs?

Fox (1978) stated recently that behavioral science is, in most medical schools, no more an accepted or integrated part of the curriculum than it was twenty-five years ago. Yet, many of the trends currently changing the face of medicine and medical education in the United States—the primary care emphasis on longitudinal responsibility, the integration of the physical, social, and psychological aspects of health, and the attempt to coordinate medical services and make them more accessible, as well as increased emphasis on consumer involvement and participation and the right to care—evolved in the area of community psychiatry. Topics such as crisis stabilization, the role of coping mechanisms and support groups, care of the dying and the grieving, and the importance of prenatal nutrition and early mother-child bonding are now part of general medical knowledge and, as such, are rapidly becoming part of the undergraduate curriculum. The real success, however, is that these topics are no longer necessarily taught by psychiatrists or mental health workers. Like good consultants or good parents, they have been most successful when they are no longer needed.

It is ironic that at a period when mental health concepts are infiltrating the general field of health care, the specialty of psychiatry is rejoicing in its "return to (bio)medicine" and is rejecting a biopsychosocial approach. Exciting indeed are recent breakthroughs in psychophysiology and neuropharmacology. Historically, however, whenever the biological bases of a disease have been elucidated, that disease (for example, pellagra or general paresis of the insane) has become the province of internal medicine.

Student interest in psychiatry has plummeted (Nielsen, 1979). Indeed, it is predicted that by 1990, psychiatry and child psychiatry will be the only shortage specialities in the United States. This shortage has been hailed with cries of alarm by psychiatric officials. Yet, if psychiatry concentrates on a narrow range of biological and traditional activity, the shortage may well be comparable to our shortage of dinosaurs.

References

American Board of Internal Medicine. "Clinical Competence in Internal Medicine." *Annals of Internal Medicine,* 1979, *90,* 402-411.

American Psychiatric Association. *A Report of a Conference on Psychiatry and Medical Education.* Washington, D.C.: American Psychiatric Association, 1969.

Blumenthal, M. D., and Dielman, T. E. "Depressive Symptomatology and Role Function in a General Population." *Archives of General Psychiatry,* 1975, *32,* 985-991.

Brown, B. S., and Regier, D. A. "How NIMH Now Views the Primary Care Practitioner." *Practical Psychology for Physicians,* 1977, *32,* 12-14.

Caplan, G. *The Theory and Practice of Mental Health Consultation.* New York: Basic Books, 1970.

Castelnuevo-Tedesco, P. "How Much Psychiatry Are Medical Students Really Learning?" *Archives of General Psychiatry,* 1967, *21,* 668-675.

Engel, G. L. "The Need for a New Medical Model: A Challenge for Biomedicine." *Science,* 1971, *196,* 129-136.

Engel, G. L. "The Care of the Patient: Art or Science?" *Johns Hopkins Medical Journal,* 1977, *141,* 222-232.

Fine, V. K., and Therrien, M. E. "Empathy in the Doctor-Patient Relationship: Skill Training for Medical Students." *Journal of Medical Education,* 1977, *52,* 752-757.

Flexner, A. *Medical Education in the United States and Canada. A Report to the Carnegie Foundation for the Advancement of Teaching.* Bulletin No. 4. Boston: Updyke, 1910.

Fox, R. "Is There a New Medical Student?" *Transactions of the College of Physicians of Philadelphia,* 1978, *45,* 206-211.

Futcher, P. H., Sanderson, E. V., and Tusler, P. A. "Evaluation of Clinical Skills for a Specialty Board During Residency Training." *Journal of Medical Education,* 1977, *52,* 567-577.

Gori, G., and Richter, B. J. "Macroeconomics of Disease Prevention in the United States." *Science,* 1978, *200,* 1124-1130.

Green, L. W. "Diffusion and Adoption of Innovations Related to Cardiovascular Risk Behavior in the Public." In A. J. Enelow and J. B. Henderson (Eds.), *Applying Behavioral Science to Cardiovascular Risk.* New York: American Cancer Association, 1975.

Halstead, L. S., and Halstead, M. S. "Chronic Illness and Humanism: Rehabilitation as a Model for Teaching Humanistic and Scientific Health Care." *Archives Physical Medicine and Rehabilitation,* 1978, *59,* 53-58.

Houpt, J. L., and others. "The Role of Psychiatric and Behavioral Factors in the Practice of Medicine." *American Journal of Psychiatry,* 1980, *137,* 37-48.

Kasl, S. V. "Social-Psychological Characteristics Associated with Behaviors Which Reduce Cardiovascular Risk." In A. J. Enelow and J. B. Henderson (Eds.), *Applying Behavioral Science to Cardiovascular Risk.* New York: American Cancer Association, 1975.

McElhinney, R. (Ed.). *Human Values Teaching Programs for Health Professionals.* Philadelphia: Society for Health and Human Values, 1976.

National Board of Medical Examiners. *Bulletin of Information and Description of National Board Examinations.* Philadelphia: National Board of Medical Examiners, 1980.

Nielsen, A. "The Magnitude of Declining Psychiatric Career Choice." *Journal of Medical Education,* 1979, *54,* 313-317.

Pacoe, L., and others. "Training Medical Students in Interpersonal Relationships." *Journal of Medical Education,* 1976, *51,* 743-750.

Pokorny, A., Putnam, N., and Fryer, J. "Drug Abuse and Alcoholism Teaching in U.S. Medical and Osteopathic Schools." *Journal of Medical Education,* 1978, *53,* 816-824.

Pomerleau, O., Boss, F., and Crown, V. "Role of Behavior Modification in Preventive Medicine." *New England Journal of Medicine,* 1975, *292,* 1277-1288.

Reifler, B., and Eaton, J. S. "The Evaluation of Teaching and Learning by Psychiatric Consultation and Liaison Programs." *Psychosomatic Medicine,* 1978, *40,* 99-107.

Sackett, D. L., and Haynes, R. B. *Compliance with Therapeutic Regimens.* Baltimore, Md.: Johns Hopkins University Press, 1977.

Steward, R. B., and Cluff, L. E. "A Review of Medication Errors and Compliance in Ambulant Patients." *Clinical Pharmacologic Therapy,* 1975, *13,* 463-468.

Vida, F., Korsch, B., and Marris, M. "Gaps in Doctor-Patient Communication—Patients' Response to Medical Advice." *New England Journal of Medicine,* 1969, *280,* 535-540.

Chapter 24

Primary Care and Mental Health Training in Community Settings

George L. Adams

In the three decades that followed the end of World War II, the history of medicine in the United States was characterized by impressive gains in scientific knowledge, by the proliferation of medical specialities, and by the clustering of physicians in urban medical centers upon which they depended in order to practice a technologically sophisticated and increasingly expensive type of medicine (Coggershall, 1965; Willard, 1966; Millis, 1971). Concurrently, there was an alarming decline in the ratio of general and family practitioners to the overall population, especially in the inner cities and in small rural communities—

Note: Work on this chapter was supported by National Institute of Mental Health Grant No. 1T21 MH 14863 and by the Hogg Foundation for Mental Health Grant No. 33-06533. The author hereby acknowledges the many significant contributions made to this endeavor by all the members of the Houston Primary Care Community Mental Health Training Consortium, and especially by Charles C. Cheney, who coordinated the development of the final report to the granting institutions.

which in many instances had no resident physician at all (Stone, 1976). These factors created a maldistribution and fragmentation of medical resources that restricted the availability and accessibility of health care services throughout the nation (National Health Council, 1975; Gray, 1976).

Inaccessibility, lack of availability, uneven quality, and the high cost of health care characterized a mounting national health care crisis. As a result, consumer advocates, legislators, and medical leaders called for a serious reappraisal of health care priorities and a refocusing of medical training to redress this situation (National Institute of Medicine, 1978). One approach utilized in the attempt to resolve the inadequacies of the medical system was to increase the manpower pool of primary care physicians. Examples of steps taken in this direction included the establishment of the Board of Family Practice in 1969 and the initial passage in 1971 of federal legislation to finance family practice training. Moreover, the Health Professions Educational Assistance Act (1976) set the goal of having 50 percent of all residency training positions in the primary care professions by 1980.

Despite a general acknowledgment of the prevailing shortage of primary care physicians, however, clarification was required as to what constitutes primary care medicine and how its practitioners should be trained. Perhaps the most generally accepted description of primary care was that offered by Alpert and Charney (1974), who distinguished three basic characteristics of primary care medicine: (1) It is "first contact" medicine; (2) it assumes "longitudinal responsibility" for the patient, regardless of the presence or absence of disease; and (3) it serves as the "integrationist" for the patient. In other words, the primary care physician represents the patient's initial link with the health care system, maintains long-term responsibility for the patient's health rather than for the short-term duration of the patient's illness, and coordinates all aspects of patient care—physiological, psychological, and sociological—when other health resources are involved. The primary care physician may perform these functions either as an individual practitioner or as a member of a primary care team. Petersdorf's (1975) delineation of the primary care physician's role touched upon the points noted by Alpert and Charney, but stressed the personalized, supportive relationship of the primary care physician in providing comprehensive care for the patient and in helping the patient to gain access to other specialists in the health delivery system. General practice, family practice, general pediatrics, and internal medicine were considered primary care fields. In addition, Pearson (1975) viewed obstetrics/gynecology as a primary care discipline.

Considerable controversy, however, surrounded the question as to whether psychiatry represented a primary care discipline. Whereas some (Fink and Oken, 1976; Oken and Fink, 1976) argued that *general* psychiatry is a primary care field as defined by Alpert and Charney, others (Council of Medical Specialty Societies, 1975; Fink and Strosnider, 1976; Hudson and Giacalone, 1975) contended that all psychiatric practice is highly specialized—that is, it is not characterized by comprehensive (psychological *and* physiological) care or by integration of patient care. Regardless of the differing stances that medical authorities took on this question, they nonetheless all pointed out that mental health and psychosocial aspects of patient care are integral to the practice of primary care medicine.

Antedating and parallel to the development of the primary care field was the rise of the community mental health movement. In order to rectify the inadequacies and inequalities of a national mental health care system whose services to the economically disadvantaged were essentially limited to prolonged institutionalization in state facilities, the Community Mental Health Centers Act was passed by Congress in 1963. The purpose of this act was to establish programs to provide community-oriented prevention, early detection and treatment of illness, and rehabilitation and supportive care for the chronically ill (Musto, 1977). Mental health providers who became involved in the delivery of community mental health services included not only the four basic disciplines of psychiatry, psychiatric nursing, psychology, and social work but also such other diverse fields as occupational therapy and expressive arts therapy (Moffic and others, 1979). Moreover, by 1975, paraprofessionals (for example, caseworkers, alcoholism and drug counselors, sociotherapists) had come to comprise as much as 50 percent of the staffs of community mental health centers (Wolford, 1975).

Despite the optimism that attended the births of the primary care and community mental health movements, progress in these fields had by 1975 only partially met initial commitments. Moreover, although some tangible gains were being achieved in terms of primary care manpower development and the implementation of certain modes of community mental health care, the continuing proliferation of separate health and mental health service delivery systems and educational institutions had led to fruitless competition for scarce resources, as well as to the duplication and further specialization of services and training (National Institute of Medicine, 1978; Dener, 1974; Borus, 1978). It had become broadly recognized that primary care providers were usually the first point of contact for those with either physical or mental disorders and that recipients of care often simultaneously utilized both health and mental health resources. Nevertheless, the primary care and mental health movements generally remained isolated from one another while developing along parallel tracks (Borus, 1976; Coleman and Patrick, 1976).

One study estimated that primary care providers devoted as much as 70 percent of their time to their patients' emotional difficulties and treated a spectrum of psychological problems that ranged from the stresses of modern life to the emotional concomitants of physical illness and severe psychotic disorders (Borus, 1976). Yet the available mental health expertise required to effectively deal with these problems was often limited. Seldom were mental health professionals incorporated into primary care settings; interagency referral mechanisms between primary care and mental health care systems were usually intricate and obstacle ridden, if they existed at all; and physicians and other primary caregivers generally did not possess the skills necessary to handle the psychosocial aspects of patient care (Borus, Janowitch, and Kieffer, 1975; Borus, 1971).

The delivery of community mental health services was characterized by difficulties ranging from the complexity of establishing and maintaining effective preventive care to issues of interagency coordination in the hospitalization and aftercare of the mentally ill, including the reintegration of patients returning from state hospitals into their families and communities (Scherl and English, 1969; Holland, 1977). Moreover, the failure of mental health centers to offer services appropriate to the specific sociocultural characteristics of consumer populations sometimes seriously impeded the provision of care to minority groups (Kline, 1969; Phillipus, 1971).

It was noted that the capacity of primary care settings and community mental health care centers to provide optimal mental health services was often constrained by limitations in the training experiences of their staff members (Borus, 1976). In the course of their biologically oriented training, physicians and other primary care providers generally received little psychological education, and that which they gained was seldom relevant and applicable to primary care delivery (Lipsett, 1975; Lazerson, 1976; Drossman, 1977-1978). Further, health and mental health professionals usually had not acquired prior first-hand knowledge of primary care and community mental health services or flexibility in interpreting the roles and functions of their various disciplines in the provision of comprehensive care (Drossman, 1977-1978; Banta and Fox, 1972; Brenneis and Laub, 1973; Morrison, Shore, and Grobman, 1973). Indeed, in spite of the attention given to fostering interdisciplinary approaches to care delivery, the more salient developments in this area were, for the most part, centered on questions of which discipline should assume leadership and on methods of mediating status and role conflicts rather than on the development of anticipatory guidance and preparatory practicum education in teamwork (Borus, 1978; Tichy, 1974, 1975-1977; Wise and others, 1974; Zusman and Lamb, 1977; Lammert, 1978; Rae-Grant and Marcuse, 1968; Cummins, Smith, and Inui, 1980).

Moreover, the standard training of both primary care providers and mental health professionals was seldom focused on meeting community-oriented needs. That is, their education usually did not equip them with the psychosocial and cross-cultural perspectives required to readily comprehend and appropriately address the problems encountered when providing neighborhood-based primary care and mental health care services to historically underserved segments of the population, including the poor, children, the elderly, and minority groups (Zwerling, 1975). In recognition of this fact, psychosocial and cross-cultural considerations began to receive attention in training and practice: The National Council on Social Work Education determined in 1971 that ethnic and cultural content would henceforth be mandatory for social work training institutions to receive accreditation; about twenty schools of nursing added transcultural components to their curricula; and a number of community psychology and community psychiatry programs introduced psychosocial and cross-cultural material into their educational endeavors (Moffic and others, 1979). Yet, in the main, health and mental health training programs failed to integrate sociocultural content thoroughly into core curricula while simultaneously providing trainees with complementary, in-depth, clinical instruction in community-based centers serving predominantly low-income, minority populations (Bradshaw, 1978; Garcia, 1971; Leininger, 1978; Martinez, 1977).

Thus on the national level, the prevalent use in 1975 of such descriptors as "continuous," "coordinated," and "holistic" were less representative of achieved realities than of future goals in primary care and community mental health service delivery and training (Holtzman, 1980; Beigel, 1980).

Metropolitan Houston

During the period from 1965 to 1975, Houston mushroomed from a city of 750,000 to a metropolis of over two million persons, its economy fueled by the petrochemical and construction industries and its Sunbelt prosperity attracting immigration from northern cities as well as from the rural South and the Mexican borderlands. By 1975, metropolitan Houston had become virtually coterminous with Harris County. While affluent suburban communities proliferated in adjacent counties, densely populated black ghettos and Mexican-American barrios deteriorated within the inner city—cut off by the geographical barriers of canals, freeways, and railroad yards, as well as by ethnic minority status and poverty, from the benefits of Houston's burgeoning economic growth. Reflecting, indeed exemplifying, national trends in health-related service, research, and education, Houston could boast of being home to one of the largest and most scientifically sophisticated medical complexes in the United States, encompassing a broad variety of specialized institutions geared to special research and training pursuits and private patient care rather than to coordinated services for underserved segments of the surrounding urban society.

A high degree of duplication, competition, and fragmentation also characterized local public sector health care delivery. Publicly funded health delivery systems included both county and city public health departments, in addition to the Harris County Hospital District (HCHD). Established in 1965, HCHD administered two hospitals (one of which contained limited psychiatric facilities) and seven primary care clinics in low-income neighborhoods of the Greater Houston area and represented the major source of health care services for the "medically indigent." The HCHD primary care clinics had the responsibility of delivering the widest possible range of medical services to the communities in which they operated. In an effort to provide effective care for their patients, the clinics also served a number of mental health functions, which included addressing the emotional problems that accompany physical illness, providing somatic therapies (for example, psychopharmacological agents) to moderately disturbed patients, and screening and referring complex psychiatric problems to secondary and tertiary mental health facilities. However, due to the high proportion of mental health problems coming to the primary care settings, the lack of personnel trained to deal with these mental health factors, and the complexity of the interagency referral process, the primary care clinics were hampered in their ability to provide comprehensive physical and emotional care to their patients.

Community mental health care was provided in the main by the Mental Health and Mental Retardation Authority of Harris County (MHMRA), established in 1967, which operated a network of mental health services—including ten ambulatory mental health units—throughout the city and surrounding county. The MHMRA community mental health units had the principal mission of reducing the necessity of admitting patients to state mental hospitals and of maintaining aftercare for patients returning from such hospitals, all of which were located in distant Texas cities. Because of the great demands that this task imposed on the personnel and fiscal resources of the community mental health units, they were restricted in their capacity to deliver a broad spectrum of preventive services, provide a variety of psychotherapeutic and counseling services to less seriously disturbed individuals, develop community-oriented consultation and education programs, and establish effective in-service training and continuing education for their staff members. The community mental health units also found it difficult to integrate their services with those of HCHD clinics, even when community mental health and primary care components were housed in the same physical structures.

Thus, although HCHD and MHMRA were mandated to provide services for the public sector of Houston's greater metropolitan area, these separately administered agencies were hard pressed to accomplish their respective medical and mental health service functions and to coordinate their efforts in the provision of comprehensive care in neighborhood settings, due to rapidly increasing service needs, fiscal constraints, and rigid bureaucratic infrastructures.

Formed in 1969 (concurrently with the HCHD Community Medicine Service), the Department of Community Medicine of Baylor College of Medicine (BCM) set out to provide the medical staff for the HCHD Neighborhood Health Program, which included all the HCHD community-based primary care clinics. Also, the BCM Department of Community Medicine assumed a major role in primary care training when it undertook to coordinate the rotations of internal medicine residents, pediatric residents, and medical students in the HCHD neighborhood clinics, established a generic prototype primary care residency program, and created a Division of Family Practice. However, by 1975, the Department of Community Medicine had still not achieved one of its long-standing objectives: in-depth instruction of the trainees under its egis in the assessment and management of the emotional problems commonly encountered in primary care practice, as well as education in the psychosocial and cross-cultural parameters of primary care.

The BCM Department of Psychiatry, including its Division of Psychology, undertook to give its trainees an understanding of mental health and mental illness within an overall social framework. However, prior to 1975, the department had not established an ongoing community mental health training thrust that combined complementary didactic and practicum education.

The University of Houston Graduate School of Social Work was established in 1967 and was fully accredited by the Council on Social Work Education in 1970. By 1975, it had formed close working relationships with a variety of professional organizations, community groups, and almost fifty social service agencies, both public and private, that provided field settings for practicum training. But even though students in the graduate school who participated in the social treatment track were provided with a wide range of field training experiences, they had limited opportunity for didactic and practicum education in medical social work, much less in primary care/mental health settings. Moreover, although the students received classroom instruction in ethnic and cultural issues and had field experiences in working with minority populations, these dual aspects of sociocultural training were in the main separate and disjointed rather than complementary and integrated.

The University of Texas School of Nursing at Houston began the clinical teaching of baccalaureate nursing students in 1972, and in 1975 the school was in the process of developing a graduate program, one component of which would be psychiatric nursing. Issues that had not been resolved in curriculum planning, however, included the possible utilization of ambulatory health care clinics as field training sites and the implementation of a core concentration in the theoretical and applied principles of community mental health nursing.

Thus, Baylor College of Medicine, the University of Houston Graduate School of Social Work, and the University of

Texas School of Nursing at Houston all shared the goal of providing the highest quality professional education to their trainees, who, it was anticipated, would to varying degrees apply their acquired knowledge and skills to meeting community service needs. Yet, as of 1975, the various training programs of these institutions did not give trainees the opportunity to gain in-depth preparatory experience in learning to work together in neighborhood primary care/community mental health settings and to utilize interdisciplinary approaches in rendering culturally congruent care to economically disadvantaged minority populations.

Houston Consortium

In recognition of these national generic issues and in response to local circumstances, an interinstitutional, interagency, and interdisciplinary consortium was formed in Houston in January 1976 to create an experimental mental health training and service delivery program geared to primary care community settings serving underprivileged populations. The Houston Primary Care Mental Health Training Consortium was composed of three educational institutions and two service agencies: Baylor College of Medicine (the Department of Psychiatry—including its Community and Social Psychiatry programs and Psychology Division—and the departments of Community Medicine, Internal Medicine, and Pediatrics); the University of Houston Graduate School of Social Work; the University of Texas School of Nursing at Houston; the Mental Health and Mental Retardation Authority (MHMRA) of Harris County; and the Harris County Hospital District (HCHD).

The Houston Consortium set forth the following training goals:

1. To develop, implement, and evaluate an interdisciplinary educational model and generic mental health curriculum geared to comprehensive primary care delivery.
2. To allow mental health trainees to develop skills in delivering mental health services both as fully integrated members

of a primary care team and as members of a secondary mental health team in primary care settings.

3. To enable primary health caregivers and trainees to acquire mental health skills that would help them to better serve their patients.
4. To allow health caregivers (including mental health caregivers) and trainees to develop psychosocial and cross-cultural perspectives in the delivery of comprehensive primary health care and secondary mental health care in primary care neighborhood clinic settings.
5. To develop interdisciplinary working skills in primary care settings.

During the consortium's planning year (1975-1976), cooperative relationships were formed, and a prospectus outlining the consortium's training goals and objectives was compiled and submitted to the National Institute of Mental Health (NIMH). In recognition that–should NIMH respond positively to the prospectus–considerable work would be required to implement a primary care mental health program by July 1977, the consortium sought and was awarded a one-year grant by the Hogg Foundation for Mental Health in order to facilitate the coordination of preparatory activities. NIMH did in fact react favorably to the consortium's prospectus, and in June 1976 two of its representatives visited Houston and made constructive recommendations regarding submission of a formal grant proposal to NIMH.

The Houston Consortium's developmental year (1976-1977) was devoted to writing a formal grant proposal to NIMH, to developing an interdisciplinary training model and generic curriculum, and to recruiting prospective faculty members to provide instruction to primary care/mental health trainees in the program. The promulgation and securing of local approval for the proposal entailed complicated, time-consuming negotiations at both the executive and operational levels of all the independent organizations involved. Representatives of NIMH again visited the consortium in the fall of 1976 and made cogent recommendations to which the consortium responded with a detailed proposal addendum regarding programmatic clarifications and budgetary modifications. Program syllabus design was the subject of ongoing, intensive efforts on the part of the Consortium Curriculum Committee during the spring of 1977. The consortium received official notification of a three-year (1977-1980) grant award from NIMH in April 1977. Completion of the 1977-78 academic year consortium program syllabus and recruitment of a full complement of prospective faculty members were achieved by June 1977.

The program was initiated in July 1977 at Casa de Amigos Neighborhood Health Center. This field training site was selected for several reasons. First, its mission was to provide comprehensive services appropriate to the needs of the low-income, predominantly Mexican-American population of the surrounding community. Second, it housed both primary care (HCHD) and mental health service (MHMRA) components within one structure. Third, plans were underway for primary care to be delivered through dyadic teams (one for pediatric and the other for adult care) composed of physicians, physician extenders, nurses, and nutritionists. Finally, trainees from two of the consortium's participating educational institutions were already rotating through this facility. Consortium Training Program didactic activities were scheduled for Wednesday mornings at Baylor College of Medicine.

The program's trainees included residents in psychiatry, pediatrics, and internal medicine; medical students; and graduate students in psychology, social work, and psychiatric nursing. The primary care residents and medical students were to serve as members of the primary care teams. Also, graduate psychiatric social work and nursing trainees were to be integrated into the primary care pediatric and adult teams to provide mental health assessment and most of the mental health services for patients, as well as to link the two teams in addressing family mental health problems. Psychiatric residents and clinical psychology interns were to be grouped into a secondary mental health care team within the framework of the neighborhood center's mental health unit and serve (1) to provide liaison, consultation, and backup services on complex psychiatric problems for the primary care teams, (2) to deliver preventive and aftercare services to the mental health unit's psychiatric patients, and (3) to render consultation and educational services to community helping organizations.

Instruction was provided by an interdisciplinary (psychiatry, primary care, psychology, social work, nursing, anthropology, sociology), bilingual (English-Spanish), and bicultural core faculty representing the consortium's participating educational institutions. Faculty members supervised, taught, and served as role models for all trainees. Further, the faculty provided in-service training and continuing education to the neighborhood center's primary care and mental health personnel and served as a resource for community organizations. Arrangements were also made for supplemental teaching contributions by members of the consortium's educational institutions and service agencies.

The fact that the dyadic pediatric and adult medicine primary care teams were not fully implemented, along with the reluctance of some clinical personnel to let others share in the decision-making process, initially impeded the integration of consortium social work and nursing faculty members and trainees into the primary care service delivery process. Yet the social work and nursing students came to play increasingly viable, if essentially referral-oriented, roles, especially during the program's third year. Also, due to a variety of organizational, interdisciplinary, and interpersonal difficulties, the secondary mental health team composed of psychiatry and psychology trainees did not become fully operational until the program's third year. However, despite an initial division of labor in which the psychiatric residents concentrated on rendering aftercare services to the mental health unit's patients while the psychology interns focused on providing backup and consultation to the primary care clinic, the secondary mental health team eventually assumed the form originally intended. Its members demonstrated their ability to interchange roles in the delivery of a broad range of direct and indirect services to the mental health and primary care components of the field training site. Moreover, the availability of the on-site core faculty and the long-term trainee placements in the field training site gave the mental health trainees of all disciplines in-depth experience in the provision of mental health services in a primary care/community mental health setting. In contrast, the pediatric residents, medical residents, and medical students who participated in the Consortium Training Program did so for limited periods of time. Yet during their rotations in the field training site they—like the Casa de Amigos primary care clinic staff members—had the opportunity to work closely with the program's interdisciplinary core faculty and mental health trainees and to take part in on-site, clinically oriented didactic activities.

The development, implementation, and yearly assessment and realignment of the training program syllabus formed a painstaking and difficult process but one necessitated by the goal of creating a generic mental health curriculum design for a *pot pourri* of trainees at different levels of education in separate disciplines. The final product fell short of being truly generic, since it entailed separate didactic instruction efforts for primary care and mental health trainees. And the dual-track format finally arrived at for the mental health trainees represented a compromise that was considered acceptable to most, but ideal for none, of the disciplines concerned. For example, trainees in some mental health disciplines, such as social work, tended to find merit in interdisciplinary education, whereas others, such as psychiatric residents, preferred selective instruction tailored to their perceived specific needs. Moreover, the establishment of seminars and case conferences at Baylor College of Medicine instead of at the consortium field training site—as well as the maintenance of a conjoint didactic program for mental health trainees with experiential placements in differently oriented clinical settings—worked against the achievement of complementarity in practicum and didactic instruction. Nonetheless, the consortium training program was successful in developing curriculum components that proved useful to this educational endeavor and that were utilized to enhance the separate training efforts of the respective participating institutions, programs, and disciplines. Examples in point would be the interdisciplinary primary care mental health case conferences held in the field training site; seminars focusing on sociocultural, programmatic, and political and legal aspects of service delivery; and site visits to community-based, municipal, and state-level organized care settings.

The consortium, in light of lower than anticipated support for evaluation endeavors, concentrated its efforts at assessment on the following: (1) consortium and program functions and processes, (2) mental health trainee cognitive gains, (3) mental health trainee attitudinal changes, and (4) the operational process of service delivery provided in the field training site. The documentation of consortium and program activities provided a major source for the consortium's final report and might serve as a partial basis for future analysis of the project's impact. The measurement of trainees' cognitive gains proved to be problematic and yielded mediocre results, suggesting that significant cognitive gains are less readily attainable—and measureable—in a practicum-oriented training endeavor than in a more academically based program. The assessment of trainees' attitudinal changes—which were difficult to evaluate—revealed virtually no pre- and postexperience test shifts, thus indicating that the trainees' basically multidisciplinary rather than interdisciplinary orientations stayed constant throughout their consortium training program experiences. The efforts to evaluate the nature and quantity of primary care/mental health services rendered through the Consortium Training Program at Casa de Amigos were hindered by lack of resources, but they did obtain data that demonstrated that a considerable degree of service was provided to the patient population through an essentially training-oriented endeavor.

A particularly noteworthy outcome of the Houston Consortium Program was that a significant proportion of trainees indicated that they had decided to select careers in areas of national need: primary care and public sector mental health. Moreover, a number of former consortium trainees have found professional placements wherein they are already contributing to primary care/community mental health efforts in Houston and other communities.

Conclusion

The Consortium Training Program had significant ramifications for health and mental health education and service delivery in Harris County. Indeed, the formation of the Houston Consortium in itself had important implications as an effort to coordinate various systems—including diverse public and private educational institutions, public service agencies, and professional disciplines—in order to better address local health and mental health needs through a comprehensive community service-oriented training project.

The establishment of the Consortium Training Program at Casa de Amigos Neighborhood Health Center augmented the mental health capability of its primary care and community health components, enhanced the scope of services provided in the community setting, and bridged institutional barriers that separated the primary care and mental health units. The efforts contributed by the core faculty members and mental health trainees were a major source of mental health service delivery in the provision of comprehensive primary care, and they enabled the community mental health unit not only to increase its capacity to prevent hospitalization and improve aftercare but also to provide preventive and consultative services within the neighborhood health center. The participation of the faculty members and mental health trainees lent cross-cultural and psychosocial dimensions to the treatment of all patients. In addition, the faculty implemented a program of mental health in-service training and continuing education for staff personnel of the service components of the neighborhood health center. Thus, implementation of the Consortium Training Program at Casa de Amigos made truly coordinated, comprehensive, and culturally congruent services available to persons in their own community: All mental health services except hospitalization became readily accessible in the neighborhood setting, and local resources became part of an extensive community mental health network. And, based upon their experiences with the consortium, the staffs of the Casa de Amigos primary care and mental health units and two of the educational institutions (Baylor College of Medicine and the University of Houston) made arrangements to continue interagency cooperation in patient care and in-service training after the official termination of the consortium project.

Furthermore, as of June 1980, separate contractual arrangements were formed between Baylor College of Medicine and MHMRA on the one hand and between the University of Houston Graduate School of Social Work and MHMRA on the other. These contracts provided for the active participation of psychiatric and social work full-time clinical faculty and trainees, as well as medical students, at five (and of psychology faculty and trainees, at two) out of ten adult community mental health units—three of which are housed in the same facilities as HCHD neighborhood clinics. Advances made in comprehensive primary care mental health training and care delivery at Casa de Amigos —inluding in-service training, interagency case conferences, and mental health liaison and consultation—have been extended to other sites and will serve to further integrate and coordinate the delivery of health and mental health services in Harris County.

The planning, development, and establishment of this primary care/mental health training project entailed complicated, time-consuming negotiations and renegotiations at both the executive and operational levels of all the independent organizations involved. Further, the absence of a common degree of commitment, inconsistent representation and participation by member organizations, and the inability of some constituent institutions to meet extramural obligations led to the overallocation of responsibility to—and overassumption of authority by—the most administratively accountable component of the Houston Consortium in terms of project development, implementation, evaluation, and day-to-day procedures. For more efficient management, a primary care/mental health project should encompass a limited number of constituent elements, all contained within the organizational framework of one educational institution with preexisting service agency linkages. Project directorship should reside within one administrative entity that (1) is accountable to an executive officer committed to the success of the project and (2) holds a supraordinate and neutral position relative to the project's departmental, programmatic, and disciplinary components. If no local established organizational structure is in place to form the framework for a primary care/mental health educational effort, a consortial endeavor should be undertaken by independent institutions (and different disciplines), provided they share the following: common educational *and* community concerns, commensurate initial risks *and* potential benefits, balanced degrees of authority *and* responsibility, and complementary explicit *and* implicit understandings of project goals and objectives. Moreover, careful attention should be given to assessing the internal organizational viability of prospective consortial partners to ensure that they are capable of meeting external obligations vis-a-vis effective representation and participation in the project.

Despite constant efforts to establish a generic mental health curriculum, the Houston project was not able to achieve a didactic format that equally met the expressed needs of each of the disciplines represented by the heterogeneous mix of consortium trainees. Yet a certain degree of consensus was reached by trainees in regard to the relative usefulness of some educational material. For example, the didactic presentations and discussions on interdisciplinary teamwork proved almost universally to be more frustrating than informative, whereas examinations of clinical issues and the sociocultural dimensions of normal and abnormal behavior were generally perceived as relevant. Therefore, the attempt to create a generic curriculum that would be *equally* useful for trainees in a broad range of primary care and mental health fields is a frustrating pursuit not suggested for other projects. The devotion of time and effort to teaching about—as against role modeling—interdisciplinary teamwork would seem to be especially fruitless. Nevertheless, despite initial resistance on the part of the Casa de Amigos service agency personnel and the fact that true primary care teams were not fully developed in the field site, the practicum training model was established in close approximation of its intended form, was judged by most trainees to provide a valuable educational experience, and eventually won the approval and support of agency staffs.

Therefore, based on the Consortium Training Program experience, it is recommended that primary care/mental health educational efforts focus on patient care issues and be concentrated in the field training sites, with instruction provided, in order of importance, through (1) faculty role modeling and supervision, (2) interdisciplinary case conferences, and (3) specific didactic sessions that deal with a mixture of pragmatic clinical and sociocultural considerations in patient care. These activities could also serve as an in-service training vehicle for agency staff and foster interagency dialogue and cooperation. Additional didactic efforts would be best pursued under the separate purviews of the participating disciplines and conducted in their respective academic departments and programs.

The consortium's evaluation efforts were hindered by inadequate financial support for research staff and activities. This lack of funds partially accounted for the imprecision in design and procedural difficulties, the severe time constraints, the turnover in personnel, and the lack of continuity in thrust and follow-through that plagued many of the project's evaluation activities. If a project is to achieve effective program evaluation, sufficient financial support should be provided, and early consensual commitment to the focuses and methods of evaluation is necessary. The development and implementation of evaluation techniques, and the analyses of findings, should be the principal—if not the sole—responsibility of qualified personnel who can without interference devote their full efforts to the kinds of painstaking and time-consuming pursuits required for meaningful objective research.

The Houston project showed that mental health services can be integrated into a primary care setting to render comprehensive patient care and that effective training can be provided within a comprehensive care setting. It is recommended that, insofar as possible, mental health services and primary care delivery be integrated and that primary care and mental health trainees receive at least a portion of their professional education in such a comprehensive care context.

The project demonstrated to field training site service agency personnel that training and care delivery can be complementary, and it provided a mechanism for bridging cross-agency administrative barriers in the delivery of comprehensive care. Moreover, this project served to enhance Harris County's coordination of primary care and mental health service delivery systems. To the degree that such interinstitutional, interagency projects promise to be cooperative and integrative in function, they should be pursued in other communities in the interest of promoting local efforts to pool resources and to better coordinate training and service delivery in the fields of primary care and mental health. The experiences of the Houston Primary Care Mental Health Training Consortium can profitably be drawn upon by other locales in which a need is recognized for a cooperative effort to enhance primary care/mental health training and service delivery.

References

Alpert, J. J., and Charney, E. *The Education of Physicians for Primary Care.* Department of Health, Education, and Welfare Publication No. 74-3113. Washington, D.C.: U.S. Government Printing Office, 1974.

Banta, D. A., and Fox, R. C. "Role Strains of a Health Care Team in a Poverty Community." *Social Science and Medicine,* 1972, *6,* 697-722.

Beigel, A. "A New Continuity of Care Perspective: The Relationship of Community Mental Health and Primary Care." In G. L. Adams and C. C. Cheney (Eds.), *Proceedings of the Houston Consortium Community Mental Health/Primary Care Regional Workshop.* Houston, Tex.: Baylor College of Medicine, 1980.

Borus, J. F. "The Community Mental Health Center and the Private Medical Practitioner: A First Step." *Psychiatry,* 1971, *34,* 274-288.

Borus, J. F. "Neighborhood Health Centers as Providers of Primary Mental Health Care." *New England Journal of Medicine,* 1976, *295,* 140-145.

Borus, J. F. "Issues Critical to the Survival of Community Mental Health." *American Journal of Psychiatry,* 1978, *135,* 1029-1035.

Borus, J. F., Janowitch, L. A., and Kieffer, F. "The Coordination of Mental Health Services at the Community Level." *American Journal of Psychiatry,* 1975, *132,* 1177-1181.

Bradshaw, W. H. "Training Psychiatrists for Working with Blacks in Basic Residency Programs." *American Journal of Psychiatry,* 1978, *135,* 1520-1524.

Brenneis, C. B., and Laub, D. "Current Strains for Mental Health Trainees." *American Journal of Psychiatry,* 1973, *130,* 41-43.

Coggershall, L. T. *Planning for Medical Progress Through Education.* Evanston, Ill.: Association of American Medical Colleges, 1965.

Coleman, J. V., and Patrick, D. L. "Integrating Mental Health Services into Primary Medical Care." *Medical Care,* 1976, *14,* 654-661.

Council of Medical Specialty Societies. *Report of the Ad Hoc Committee to Draft a Statement on Primary Care.* Chicago: Council of Medical Specialty Societies, 1975.

Cummins, R. O., Smith, R. W., and Inui, T. S. "Communication Failure in Primary Care: Failure of Consultants to Provide Follow-Up Information." *Journal of the American Medical Association,* 1980, *243,* 1650-1652.

Dener, B. "The Insanity of Community Mental Health: The Myth of the Machine." *International Journal of Mental Health,* 1974, *3,* 104-126.

Drossman, D. A. "Can the Primary Care Physician Be Better Trained in the Psychosocial Dimensions of Patient Care?" *International Journal of Psychiatry in Medicine,* 1977-1978, *8,* 169-184.

Fink, P. J., and Oken, D. "The Role of Psychiatry as a Primary Care Specialty." *Archives of General Psychiatry,* 1976, *33,* 998-1003.

Fink, F. J., and Strosnider, J. S. "The Place of Psychiatry and Behavioral Science in the Education of Primary Care Physicians." *Psychiatric Opinion,* 1976, *13,* 21-26.

Garcia, A. "The Chicano and Social Work." *Social Casework,* 1971, *52,* 174-178.

Gray, P. D. Personal communication, Oct. 20, 1976.

Health Professions Educational Assistance Act, (S. 3239, H.R. 5546), 1976.

Holland, B. C. "An Evaluation of the Criticisms of the Community Mental Health Movement." In W. E. Barton and C. J. Sanborn (Eds.), *An Assessment of the Community Mental Health Movement.* Lexington, Mass.: Lexington Books, 1977.

Holtzman, W. H. "Community Mental Health and Primary Care: Texas Perspectives." In G. L. Adams and C. C. Cheney (Eds.), *Proceedings of the Houston Consortium Community Mental Health/Primary Care Regional Workshop.* Houston, Tex.: Baylor College of Medicine, 1980.

Hudson, J. I., and Giacalone, J. J. "Current Issues in Primary Care Education: Review and Commentary." *Journal of Medical Education,* 1975, *50* (supplement), 211-233.

Kline, L. Y. "Some Factors in the Psychiatric Treatment of Spanish Americans." *American Journal of Psychiatry,* 1969, *125,* 1674-1681.

Lammert, M. H. "Power, Authority, and Status in Health Systems: A Marxian-Based Conflict Analysis." *Journal of Applied Behavioral Science,* 1978, *18,* 321-323.

Lazerson, A. M. "The Psychiatrist in Primary Medical Care Training: A Solution to the Mind-Body Dichotomy?" *American Journal of Psychiatry,* 1976, *133,* 964-966.

Leininger, M. (Ed.). *Transcultural Nursing: Concepts, Theories, Practices.* New York: Wiley, 1978.

Lipsett, D. R. "Some Problems in the Teaching of Psychosomatic Medicine." *International Journal of Psychiatry in Medicine,* 1975, *6,* 317-329.

Martinez, J. (Ed.). *Chicano Psychology.* New York: Academic Press, 1977.

Millis, J. *A Rational Public Policy for Medical Education and Its Financing.* New York: National Fund for Medical Education, 1971.

Moffic, H. S., and others. "Training in Community Mental Health." *Community Mental Health Review,* 1979, *4,* 1-11.

Morrison, A. P., Shore, M. F., and Grobman, J. "On the Stresses of Community Psychiatry and Helping Residents to Survive Them." *American Journal of Psychiatry,* 1973, *130,* 1237-1241.

Musto, D. F. "The Community Mental Health Movement in Historical Perspective." In E. W. Barton and C. J. Sanborn (Eds.), *An Assessment of the Community Mental Health Movement.* Lexington, Mass.: Lexington Books, 1977.

National Health Council. *Report on National Health 1974-1975 Regional Workshops on Health Manpower Distribution.* New York: National Health Council, 1975.

National Institute of Medicine. *Manpower Policy for Primary Health Care.* National Academy of Sciences Publication No. 2764. Washington, D.C., 1978.

Oken, D., and Fink, P. J. "General Psychiatry: A Primary Care Specialty." *Journal of the American Medical Association,* 1976, *235,* 1973-1974.

Pearson, J. W. "The Obstetrician and Gynecologist: Primary Physician for Women." *Journal of the American Medical Association,* 1975, *231,* 815-816.

Petersdorf, R. G. "Issues in Primary Care: The Academic Perspective." *Journal of Medical Education,* 1975, *50* (supplement), 5-13.

Phillipus, M. "Successful and Unsuccessful Approaches to Mental Health Services for an Urban Hispanic Population." *American Journal of Public Health,* 1971, *61,* 820-830.

Rae-Grant, A. F., and Marcuse, D. J. "The Hazards of Teamwork." *American Journal of Orthopsychiatry,* 1968, *38,* 408-416.

Scherl, D. J., and English, J. T. "Community Mental Health and Comprehensive Health Service Programs for the Poor." *American Journal of Psychiatry,* 1969, *125,* 1666-1674.

Stone, B. "Country Doctors." *Houston Post,* Apr. 4-6, 1976.

Tichy, M. K. *Health Care Teams: An Annotated Bibliography.* New York: Praeger, 1974.

Tichy, M. K. (Ed.). *Health Team News, I-II.* Bronx, N.Y.: Institute for Health Team Development, Montefiore Hospital and Medical Center, 1975-1977.

Willard, W. *Meeting the Challenge of Family Practice.* Chicago: American Medical Association, 1966.

Wise, H., and others. *Making Health Teams Work.* Cambridge, Mass.: Ballinger, 1974.

Wolford, J. L. "Paraprofessional Training and Role." In A.

Freedman, H. Kaplan, and B. Sadock (Eds.), *Comprehensive Textbook of Psychiatry.* Vol. 2. Baltimore, Md.: Williams and Wilkins, 1975.

Zusman, J., and Lamb, R. "In Defense of Community Mental Health." *American Journal of Psychiatry,* 1977, *134,* 887-892.

Zwerling, I. *Racism, Elitism, Professionalism.* New York: Jason Aronson, 1975.

Chapter 25

People Helping People: Beyond the Professional Model

Phyllis Rolfe Silverman

Over the past century we have been witness to the growth of secular institutions with the mandate to ameliorate and, if possible, to cure the emotional dilemmas people face. Until this century these issues were in the domain of theologians and philosophers. Today they are the responsibility of mental health professionals and the agencies and institutions in which they work. These professionals do not represent a single theoretical frame of reference but instead advocate various helping modalities.

Almost every decade of the century has seen the rise to eminence of a different modality. Each has its own ideology, a point of view about what it can accomplish and how (Davis, 1938; Strauss and others, 1964). Some modalities have been attempts to implement new knowledge about human behavior, others to organize new patterns of delivery of service. We have seen, for example, the ascendancy of psychoanalysis, behavior modification, gestalt therapies, psychopharmacology, the community mental health movement, preventive psychiatry, and the paraprofessional movement. With each new modality yet another population of troubled people has been included in those who might benefit from treatment by the mental health system. Each new modality has been accompanied by new excitement and by the hope that it can make up for the deficiencies of other methods and service delivery systems. At the same time, each innovation has been criticized by those dubious about its actual benefits. Today there is similar excitement, as well as similar arguments, about the mutual help movement in which people help people and the sufferer turns to himself and similar others to find a solution to their common problems.

This chapter will examine the reasons for this growing interest in mutual help and its implications for mental health practice. The first part of the chapter will define mutual help and contrast it with the kinds of help offered by professional helping systems. The subsequent sections will point to times when mutual help may indeed be the help of choice. Finally, the chapter will close with a discussion of the implications of these findings for professional practice. It is the premise of this paper that no one modality can provide all the answers. It is necessary to understand each modality for what it can do and cannot do to help people and to determine under what circumstances each modality may interface with the others for the benefit of its consumers.

What Is Mutual Help?

The terms *support, self-care, self-help,* and *mutual help* are often used interchangeably. These terms are applied haphazardly to professionally led groups, to educational programs that teach people self-care, and to member-run organizations. In fact, each of these offers a different experience with different consequences for the participants. But to the extent that each provides participants with an opportunity to share their common concerns and solutions, it approximates a mutual help exchange.

A *support group* such as one offered to hospital patients with handicapping illnesses or to families of ill children is typically led by a professional and therefore is not a mutual help group. The professional is responsible for the group's continuity and development and does not rely on the experiential knowledge of the members; moreover, the participants are generally not offered the opportunity to become helpers in turn or to control resources. *Self-care* programs, which are found in nursing homes, rehabilitation units, and so on, are also led by professionals and have the goal of teaching people new skills in caring for themselves. People come as consumers, and while a certain degree of mutuality and sharing may develop among participants, there is no expectation that the consumers will become helpers or take charge of the program, nor will the helping program rely primarily on knowledge developed from the participants' personal experiences. These self-care programs may become occasions to translate technical information into lay terms to facilitate its application. The term *self help* can best be reserved for self-directed study with the end of improving one's own situation. Finally, a *mutual help* exchange is characterized by a helping interaction that takes place between people because they share a common problem.

Characteristics of Mutual Help Groups. When people come together in some formal way to find or exchange solutions to common problems, they form mutual help groups. Such groups are highly specialized "agencies" that generally focus on a single issue that their constituents have in common. They become organizations when the groups regularize their practices and formalize membership. In these organizations, members control the resources of the group as well as plan and carry out programs (Killilea, 1976; Gartner and Riessman, 1977; Silverman, 1978).

Each organization develops its own techniques for helping members. There are a wide range of services offered by mutual help groups: outreach programs, informational and educational meetings, social activities, small-group and one-on-one discussions in person and on the telephone, newsletters, advocacy, and public education. Helpers are chosen because they are willing to use their own experience as the basis for helping someone else. Indeed, knowledge gained from one's own experience is highly valued (Borkman, 1976). In a society where professional knowledge is given precedence, knowledge gained from experience is often not appreciated. Helpers are themselves members of the groups and are involved in reciprocal and mutual relationships with those they help; hence it is a question of *mutual help* rather than of *self-help* (Lenneberg and Rowbatham, 1970). People who are recipients of service can become helpers in turn. The focus of help is on promoting well-being or adapting to change.

Since participants frequently change their relationship to the organization, either by becoming helpers to new members, by assuming administrative or other leadership positions in the group, or simply by leaving, most groups experience a high turnover of membership and leadership. In contrast to most human service agencies they are often unstable. They can go through periods when no new leadership emerges. And, with their shoestring budgets, these groups remain active only as long as there are members to do the work. The most successful and long-lived groups are part of a national organization, which provides program information and organizational guidance for local affiliates. The number of groups with a national constituency is growing. The best known of these groups with strong central organizations are Alcoholics Anonymous, La Lêche League (Silverman and Murrow, 1976), and Recovery, Inc. (Raiff, 1979). Among the newer national groups are Concerned United Birthparents (for men and women who have surrendered a child for adoption) and the National Coalition for Battered Women.

Members' prior experiences dictate the types of organizational models that the groups develop. Most people have belonged to "clubs" at various stages in their lives. They are familiar with Robert's *Rules of Order.* They elect officers and generally follow a traditional, hierarchical organizational model. In some instances, however, group members have had bad experiences with bureaucratic agencies and institutions and consequently have chosen a quite different structure. The Mental Patients Liberation Movement and the Gray Panthers, for example, are run by consensus, each member having equal authority and the chair being rotated among members at each meeting. These groups have sacrificed a certain amount of efficiency in order to ensure that each member has an opportunity to participate fully in every decision. Their national organizations are loose federations of local groups (Silverman, 1980). Whether they have formal or informal structures, however, most meetings of mutual help groups are small, and organizational rules are, for the most part, disregarded to the end that the mutual help group may achieve a less restrictive bureaucratic structure compatible with its goals, values, and striving for autonomy.

Mutual Help Groups and Mental Health Services Systems. The factors that most clearly distinguish mental health service systems from mutual help groups are reflected in the way services are organized, in the relationships of the consumer as client or patient to the systems or groups, and in the criteria for choosing helpers. Formal mental health service systems have a mandate from the community to treat particular problems. Professionals are society's licensed caregivers, with their own special areas of expertise. Society needs experts, people who concern themselves full time with solving problems, whether they are politicians, physicians, social workers, scientists, or funeral directors. This division of labor is the only way to maintain a viable society. However, once there is a need to standardize service, certain problems inevitably occur. A bureaucracy is set up with procedures that tend to depersonalize the participants. Professionals come to have a vested interest in maintaining their positions as experts and in maintaining a population of people who continue to need their services. Staff typically relate to one another in hierarchical order, with each position regulated by specific rights and duties.

The allocation of resources within the agency and the decisions about the work of the agency are the concern of the staff or the governing board. Generally, new services are planned by board members, professional planners, and clinicians whose decisions are based on their professional expertise, gained from training and work experience. The patients' perceptions of their needs or priorities may be considered, but patients are not in charge (Freidson, 1970). Although the Community Mental Health Center Act of 1976 mandated consumer representation on the boards of directors of these centers, it is the mental health professionals working in the centers who make the clinical decisions, based on their professional training (Borkman, 1976). But in mutual help groups, consumers, as members of the organization, control the resources, making all decisions about what is appropriate help. These groups are fluid organizations, with structures that allow for a good deal of mobility in the system to accommodate a transient membership and with flexible boundaries for changing activities and programs.

In formal human service systems, including mental health service agencies, an individual defines himself as having a problem and seeks out an expert to help him with it. The decision about the help he should receive is not up to the troubled individual. The professional makes the rules about what is appropriate help. Formal agencies set up institutional barriers to screen out people they feel they cannot help. These barriers often take the form of elaborate diagnostic processes that precede the decision to accept a given individual for treatment. The focus is on looking for dysfunction and repairing or curing it (Silverman, 1969). In service systems in which professionals work, the relationship between the expert and the patient is always unequal. One person is always the helper, and the other is always being helped. The expert knowledge that forms the basis for helping remains, to a large extent, remote and mysterious to the patient. In fact, the concept *patient* implies that the individual is defective and therefore in many ways dependent on the expert to whom he has applied for assistance. The relationship is circumscribed by the time and place in which interactions can occur. These are usually in office settings and during standard office hours. As Hurvitz (1974) points out, the psychotherapist is not a role model, does not set personal examples, and is presumed normal; he does not identify with his patient. When the patient is cured, he must leave the system.

In contrast, in mutual help groups the "expert" is simply a fellow sufferer; he is a role model who identifies with the person he is helping, and the helping relationship is reciprocal rather than one sided. As a result of being helped in mutual help groups, the individual can stay on to help others. Unlike the professional service systems that focus on people's deficiencies, in mutual help groups the focus is not on members' deficits but on how they are like others in this particular situation or typical for people with this condition.

It is obvious that mutual help groups and professional service systems are not competing modalities. Each may be appropriate for different situations or different aspects of a situation, and they are not necessarily mutually exclusive helping modalities. A mutual help experience may be essential when the troubled person needs to be one among peers and needs to learn about how other people cope with a similar problem. In practice, most people who form mutual help groups, or who are attracted to them, are facing major changes in their life situations for which their typical adaptive strategies are inadequate. They report a need to learn to deal with the world in new ways (Silverman, 1980, forthcoming). They are not necessarily ill or emotionally disturbed but are in a time of transition or change for which they are ill prepared.

Mutual Help and Transition States

What is there about being in transition that makes mutual help groups attractive? A critical transition generally seems to unfold in three stages (Silverman, 1966): First, there is an event, or series of events, that has a disequilibrating effect on an individual and taxes his ability to cope. This event or series of events may be part of the normal life cycle and associated with developmental processes, or the events may be unanticipated—for example, natural disasters or accidents. Second, adaption to the event takes place over time (White, 1974). There is a process that has a beginning and an end, between which the individual does the "work of transition." This work can itself be divided into phases, each of which has its own tasks. Third, the transition involves status changes for the affected individuals, necessitating a redefinition of the roles they perform in their social networks (Rappaport, 1963). Tyhurst (1957) notes that the key issue for people in transition is how to negotiate the social and psychological circumstances of being in the state of moving from one status to another.

Tyhurst (1957) and Bowlby (1961) describe transitions

as involving three stages: impact, recoil, and accommodation. Others have extended these to four or five stages (Kubler-Ross, 1969; Weiss, 1976). During *impact* the individual is numb or dazed. There is a sense of disbelief that a change has really occurred. Marris (1974) attributes this to what he calls a conservative impulse; the individual does not want to believe that a change has occurred or that further change will be required, and so he works at keeping things as they were. The second stage, *recoil,* is characterized by a growing recognition of the reality of the change, as well as by a growing frustration and tension that results from the inability to continue to live as if no change had taken place (Silverman and Silverman, 1979). Parkes (1971) talks of a crisis in meaning, when it is no longer possible to live by the old rules. In every change there has to be some grieving for what is lost (Marris, 1974). During *accommodation* the individual will find a new direction and, in part, a new identity into which some of the past can be assimilated (Pincus, 1975; Silverman and Silverman, 1979; Anderson, 1974; Marris, 1974; Levinsohn and others, 1978). Incorporating elements of the past into new roles helps people bridge the gap between past and future.

The work of transition is to move from one stage to the next. In order to understand how individuals cope with a critical transition, it is as necessary to know the stage of transition they are at as it is to have their past history. To effectively aid a person in transition, the help offered must be synchronous with the phase of transition the individual is in (Silverman, 1966, 1971). As a result of observations of the widow-to-widow program from 1966 onward, I documented how a mutual help experience enhanced the ability to cope with a transition (Silverman, 1974). I noted that the help offered to the new widows differed at each phase of the transition. Initially, the contact with another widow helped the new widow to see herself in that role. She was then able to grieve and, finally, as a result of the network of new friends she made, she was able to learn how to shift her identity from wife to widow (Silverman, 1970, 1972, 1974). Movement in critical transition periods seems to be facilitated by a mutual help experience because people are provided with learning opportunities that offer pertinent information, they learn from peers, and there is an opportunity for role mobility, that is, to move from the role of recipient to that of helper.

Learning Opportunities. White (1974) suggests that adaptation involves learning and that the adaptive strategies people develop are affected by the learning opportunities available to them. When an individual faces a critical change, there is no reason to believe that he will know what to do without a prior orientation or a current educational opportunity. Hamburg and Adams (1967) reported that effective coping with transitions that involved major illness or life cycle role change was related to the availability of pertinent information. The Community Support Systems Task Force of the President's Commission on Mental Health (1978) found that access to guidance and information is an essential aspect of an individual's helping network, whether it is a matter of coping effectively with problems of daily living or with major transitions. There are very few educational opportunities available in our society that help people learn how to deal with critical transitions. One of the few places where such expertise is concentrated is in a mutual help organization. For example, it was only in the widow-to-widow program that a woman was able to obtain the information that she needed to make the psychological transition from wife to widow (Silverman, 1972).

Pertinent Information. Hamburg and Adams (1967) list the various types of information people seek in new situations, namely, information about diagnosis, treatment, ways of dealing with loss, and how to learn new roles. For this broad range of information to be of value, however, it has to be relevant to the specific needs of people. Most people in transition feel isolated by their situation. They often report that professional knowledge is based on an incomplete view of their situation. In part, this is due to the fact that professionals are outsiders, not living with the situation on a daily basis. They do not always understand. In addition, professional knowledge is often based on limited samples and extreme cases. For example, when I first began my work with the widowed, bereavement was seen as a crisis that could be resolved in six weeks. The widows I worked with reported it often took two years before they saw a future for themselves. More recent work with battered women calls attention to the problem of attributing the battering to a woman's masochism instead of the reality of her situation (Davidson, 1978). The most pertinent information battered women needed was from others who knew the reality of their situation, and from whom they could learn how to manage their predicament and change their lives.

Learning from Peers. New information becomes easier to digest and assimilate as a result of the special relationship that develops between people who share a common experience. In a small sample of members of three mutual help groups—the Kidney Transplant and Dialysis Association, the Cured Cancer Club, and the Spina Bifida Association of Massachusetts—I found that people who joined these groups did so out of a pressing need to find someone else who had had a similar experience (Silverman and Smith, forthcoming). They reported a need to talk with someone who could understand and share their feelings and who could show them that there were other ways of coping with their new situation.

From a follow-up study of the original widow-to-widow program, data were available on every new widow under the age of sixty-five in the Boston community in which the program operated over a two-and-one-half year period, and in particular from those women who refused the offer of help (Silverman, 1971). I found that most of those who had refused help had friends or relatives who were widows. Their existing social and helping networks were able to meet their needs. These findings raise the question of whether people who do not affiliate have different needs or whether they do not affiliate because they already have others in their network who have experienced a similar illness or condition and with whom they can share their concerns. The help offered by a mutual help group would then be redundant.

Bandura (1977) noted that learning in crises or emotionally laden situations can be enhanced if it takes place in a peer context. Reporting on a study of affiliative tendencies in college students during periods of anxiety, Schacter (1959) observed that subjects chose to be alone when under stress rather than with people who did not share their experience. He concluded that whatever the needs aroused by a particular anxiety, the allaying of it demanded the presence of others in a similar situation. Is this process a continuation of what takes place during adolescence? It is accepted (Kagan and Coles, 1973) that peers play an important role in the manner in which adolescents cope with developmental issues. I would suggest that, faced with a new situation, a person must obtain relevant new information in order to cope. Moreover, the ability to use this information is affected by the availability of someone who has gone through the experience—someone with whom the individual can identify. This may be a continuation of an adaptive strategy established in adolescence, if not even earlier in the life cycle (Kagan and Coles, 1973).

Role Mobility. Not only is the need to find "someone like me" central to making a critical transition, but the opportunity to change roles and become a helper seems important as well. Lieberman, Borman, and others (1979) surveyed both members of Mended Hearts and heart surgery patients not affiliated with the organization to determine how participation in it had affected adjustment to their illness. They found that significant differences appeared between the two groups only in the case of retired men who were very active in the organization. Those who became helpers made the best adjustment to the aftermath of open heart surgery. The role of the helper tends to foster competency in the helper, even more than the fact that being helped by someone with whom they can identify tends to minimize a sense of weakness or incompetence in the persons needing help.

The factors that facilitate coping with a transition seem to be reflected in a three-part progression identified by Lifton (1973) in a study of mutual help experiences of returning Vietnam veterans: "The first [factor] is that of *affinity*, the coming together of people who share a particular (and in this case overwhelming) historical personal experience, along with a basic perspective on that experience, in order to make some sense of it. The second principle was that of *presence*, a kind of being there or full engagement and openness to mutual impact—no one ever being simply a therapist against whom things are rebounding. The third was that of *self-generation,* the need on the part of those seeking help, change, or insight of any kind to initiate their own process and conduct it largely on their own terms so that, even when calling in others with expert knowledge, they retain major responsibility for the shape and direction of the enterprise. Affinity, presence, and self-generation seem to be necessary ingredients for making a transition between old and new images and values, particularly when these relate to ultimate concerns, to shifting modes of symbolic immortality" (pp. 77-78).

Similar elements can be found in the way Alcoholics Anonymous divides its helping process into Recovery, Unity, and Service. To achieve *recovery* the individual must identify himself as an alcoholic. He becomes involved because he finds at least one person to whom he can relate. This person makes him feel less alone, and he therefore becomes more willing to see himself as one of the group. The second step, *unity,* occurs when he expands his identification with the group to accept the program and its fellowship and mutuality. *Service* involves becoming a helper or, for some, a leader in the organization. By being able to help others, AA sees the recovered alcoholic as being able to sustain his sobriety over time. This is consistent with findings that the people in mutual help organizations who are helped the most are the ones who stay to become helpers.

A parallel can be drawn between the way a mutual help exchange unfolds and the stages of transition described earlier. The drawing of this parallel seems a good way of summarizing the unique aspects of mutual help in aiding people through transitions.

Impact/Affinity/Recovery. In the first stage of a transition, people typically refuse to accept their new situation. Their ability to make an accommodation depends on their allowing the numbness to dissipate and on recognizing at some level that a new reality exists. This becomes easier to do when someone is available who has been in the same situation, is now living a "normal" life, and is even able to help others. An affinity develops that makes its possible for a bond to grow between them within the mutual help organization. New members are then less fearful about their new situation.

The willingness of new members to talk with such a helper is an indication of their readiness to consider making a transition, that is, to learn now to accept their new status and role designation. For example, a woman agreeing to talk about her widowhood with another widow is now beginning to let the numbness lift and to see that this designation may apply to her. She still may not be ready to call herself a "widow" and accept the full meaning of her husband's death for her current life. But in the new exchange she will find guidelines. The first questions she will ask are, "What happened to you? How did you get here?" The helper must be prepared to retell her story.

Recoil/Presence/Unity. In the recoil phase of transition, help consists of the provision of specific information about the condition and/or new role and about how to deal with it effectively. The person in transition is able to accept this information because of the sense of unity that has developed. Either in one-to-one contact or at group meetings, advice is offered about how to deal with a problem or what to expect from the situation that the sufferer is experiencing. A framework is provided for the problem. Not only does the individual come to understand what she is experiencing currently, but she may get anticipatory guidance about other problems that will arise. For example, a newly bereaved woman does not know that she will ever be able to stop crying or ever feel joy again. She learns how others have dealt with the problem, and they share with her their "tricks of the trade" (Goffman, 1963). Such interactions serve to expand her coping repertoire and options.

The content of the help will inevitably differ with the problem. The information offered has to relate to the specific transition; nevertheless, "once people have found a way of talking to each other, what is it that is talked about? Much of what mutual aid is about is the small things. It's not the big deal, the surgery (that is, the important life-saving experience or whatever else it might be), it's the small survival kind of things . . . it is the small things that make up the essence of daily life" (Lenneberg, 1971).

Accommodation/Self-Generation/Service. Accommodation is a period when individuals' feelings have "quieted down," and they are beginning to integrate all the knowledge they have obtained into new identities. They use this time to practice new behavior patterns, new ways of dealing with themselves and the world. Accommodation can be likened to an active apprenticeship period. During this time, the moral support of the group may be essential for success as individuals attempt to integrate the past with the present.

In this period, the individual moves out of "new-member" status and becomes aware of and responsive to other people's needs. The option of becoming a helper is now available to him. Not only is the need to find "someone like me" central to making a critical transition, but the opportunity to change roles and become a helper seems essential as well. In order to be helpful in turn, either in an informal exchange or as part of an organized effort, the helper has to control resources and be able to integrate the knowledge gained from his experience into the helping activity. The context in which the help is offered becomes critical. It is not only the type of help that distinguishes mutual help from professional help; it is the setting in which the work is carried out and the helper's relationship to that system. I hypothesize that at times of critical transitions in an individual's life where no opportunity for a mutual help experience exists, the individual will create one to fill the gap.

Implications for Professional Practice

I began this chapter by pointing out the way that professional practice has changed over the years. A helping modality may be discovered or developed and quickly adopted. Often it is integrated into current practice before it is tested and just as often it is co-opted into and changed by the system, which then goes on as before. For example, when it was first proposed that psychiatric clinics become community mental health centers, the proposed change was designed to bring help to people in their own communities. The Joint Commission on Mental Illness hoped to make help more relevant. Beyond agencies changing their names, however, little was done to change agency practice or professional education to implement the recommendations. In part, the direction of the recommended change was to eliminate the medical model for delivering services (Schwartz and Schwartz, 1964). This has not happened.

A decade later the paraprofessional movement (Pearl and Riessman, 1965) represented yet another effort to make mental health and human services more relevant and accessible to potential consumers. The paraprofessionals were indigenous to the communities they served, and it was anticipated they would be able to use their experiential knowledge on behalf of their fellow residents and provide new modalities of help. Instead they were absorbed by the agencies, and the people they helped became their clients or patients. The workers were agency staff and became concerned with formalizing their education to facilitate their mobility in the system. They are now simply another level of professional worker in the agency—distinguished from others by their lack of advanced education.

Many people are now looking to mutual help groups to provide models for humanizing the mental health system and to expand the range of services offered (Gartner and Riessman, 1977; Levy, 1976; President's Commission on Mental Health, 1978). Hence, we are seeing a repetition of the phenomena noted in the preceding paragraphs. However, unlike the paraprofessional or the community mental health movements, the mutual help movement includes many different organizations that have already developed the structures and skills needed to be autonomous. These serve as models for the new groups that develop. As a consequence, it may be more difficult to simply coopt or incorporate mutual help organizations into professional service systems.

Most of the interaction between formal human service agencies and mutual help groups has been characterized by tension and even competition. Members of mutual help organizations have often had poor experiences with formal helping systems and at times have denigrated the services that these systems offer, encouraging members to rely on each other for any and all assistance they may require. This is in part because, historically, professionals have often attempted to co-opt mutual help organizations or to impose the authority of professional knowledge alone so that now many mutual help organizations consider them to be intruders (Katz, 1961; Collins and Pancoast, 1976). For example, some mutual help groups have turned to professional agencies to provide them with additional resources and organizational stability. But instead of cooperation, there was often a struggle for control (Kleiman and others, 1976), and some of the mutual help groups lost their identity. This in some ways is inevitable since few professional agencies can justify sponsoring organizations with officers and rules for services not subject to review by the agencies (Silverman, 1980). It was no accident that the original widow-to-widow program sponsored by the Laboratory of Community Psychiatry (LOCP) was successful. The LOCP was a freestanding research institution with no clinical responsibilities. The widow-aides did not have to account to clinicians for the services they chose to offer. Clinicians were not in positions that were competitive with those of the aides, nor were clinicians role models for the aides. At the same time, however, most mutual help groups do not dissipate their energy in being antiprofessional. In fact many mutual help groups—for example, La Lêche League, the Ostomy societies, and Recovery, Inc.—are actively involved with professional helping systems as well. Their concern is with effective collaboration and with helping their members become competent consumers of needed services.

Baker (1977) noted that the two systems, professional help and mutual help, compete for clients, political sanctions, financing, volunteers, and information. Huey (1977) identified a source of tension resulting from the professional's need to maintain a superordinate position as "expert." Differences in perspective about the value of the help offered is another cause of tension. Professionals sometimes judge mutual help to be superficial because it does not involve restructuring or rebuilding the participant's personality. In addition, professionals often see continuous participation in the mutual help group as an indication of dependency rather than as a demonstration of newfound strength to help others (Silverman, 1978). Further, professionals traditionally value objectivity and detachment and are uncomfortable with the level of personal involvement exhibited by members of mutual help groups. Finally, professionals feel that credentials are required to work with people who are experiencing serious personal difficulties.

There are many incentives for professionals, in spite of these reservations, to become involved with mutual help groups. To be eligible for federal funding, community mental health agencies have been mandated, in the past, to develop widow-to-widow programs as part of their consultation and education programs. The President's Commission on Mental Health (1978) recommended that agencies reach out to mutual help groups to provide them with technical assistance, to develop directories of groups in their communities, and to set up clearinghouses where potential consumers can learn about groups and groups can learn about each other. Books are being written to teach professionals how to organize groups (Silverman, 1980). But further research is needed to determine how this activity impacts on mutual help organizations.

Professionals have to be cautioned to consider their interventions very carefully, and the kind of technical assistance offered requires particular scrutiny. These efforts could become vehicles for absorbing groups into formal mental health service systems. I would suggest that before professionals begin to work with mutual help organizations, they need to examine their own attitudes. They need to be sure that they are respectful and appreciative of the values of these other systems of care and what they can accomplish (Silverman, 1978, 1980). Once professionals are clear in their own minds that they come to consult and facilitate rather than to bring "enlightenment," they need to develop a model for collaborating that meshes with this goal. I have proposed a model (Silverman, forthcoming) in which the professional's role is that of a linking agent. The linkages are made between mutual help groups in need and resources (people, ideas, and materials) that could help to solve their problems. A linking agent is a consultant who has the task of building awareness and understanding of a body of information in the consultee, in this case a mutual help organization. As it turns out, however, the most relevant information that groups need is available from other mutual help groups. Therefore the linking agent's primary task is to link groups directly with each other or to provide them with relevant information gathered from other groups when members of different groups cannot meet directly with each other. There are three stages in this process:

1. Organizations discover that their problems are not unique and that there are commonalities across divergent organizations.
2. Sharing their experiences of successful and unsuccessful solutions, organizational representatives engage in a mutual learning exchange, identify with each other, and provide models for each other on how to implement new knowledge.
3. Together organizational representatives search for additional answers, solutions, and techniques: mutual helpers helping each other in the task of organizational development.

The reader will recognize that this is a replica of the mutual help experience of individual members within their respective organizations. The role of the professional as a linking agent is (1) to make it easier for members of different groups to meet with each other; (2) to help them to mobilize appropriate resources; (3) to legitimate group-to-group learning, using experiential rather than professional knowledge; and (4) to catalyze the sharing of members' skills in group process and organizational development. Above all, professionals have to know when to step back and let groups take over this process for themselves. The role of the linking agent is one of several roles that professionals can play if they wish to work with mutual help organizations as collaborators to enhance the growth of this informal system of help and at the same time maintain its integrity (Silverman, 1980).

The mutual help movement is in its ascendancy at a time when people find themselves facing critical transitions with no precedents on which to base their coping strategies. This is not an antiprofessional movement. It is a movement that sees professionals as having their place among many other sources of help. It takes helping *beyond professionalism.*

References

Anderson, R. "Notes of a Survivor." In S. B. Troup and W. A. Greene (Eds.), *The Patient, Death, and the Family.* New York: Scribner's, 1974.

Baker, F. "The Interface Between Professional and Natural Support Systems." *Clinical Social Work Journal,* 1977, *5,* 139-148.

Bandura, A. *Social Learning Theory.* Englewood Cliffs, N.J.: Prentice-Hall, 1977.

Borkman, T. "Experiential Knowledge: A New Concept for the Analysis of Self-Help Groups." *Social Service Review,* 1976, *50,* 445-456.

Bowlby, J. "Processes of Mourning." *International Journal of Psychoanalysis,* 1961, *42,* 317-340.

Collins, A., and Pancoast, D. L. *Natural Helping Networks.* Washington, D.C.: National Association of Social Workers, 1976.

Davidson, T. *Conjugal Crime.* New York: Hawthorn Books, 1978.

Davis, K. "Mental Hygiene and the Class Structure." *Psychiatry,* 1938, *1,* 55-56.

Freidson, E. "Dominant Professions, Bureaucracy, and Client Service." In W. Rosengren and M. Lefton (Eds.), *Organizations and Clients.* Columbus, Ohio: Merrill, 1970.

Gartner, A., and Riessman, F. *Self-Help in the Human Services.* San Francisco: Jossey-Bass, 1977.

Goffman, E. *Stigma: Notes on the Management of Spoiled Identities.* Englewood Cliffs, N.J.: Prentice Hall, 1963.

Hamburg, D. A., and Adams, J. E. "A Perspective on Coping: Seeking and Utilizing Information in Major Transitions." *Archives of General Psychiatry,* 1967, *17,* 277-284.

Huey, K. "Developing Effective Links Between Human Service Providers and the Self-Help System." *Hospital and Community Psychiatry,* 1977, *28,* 767-770.

Hurvitz, N. "Peer Self-Help Psychotherapy Groups: Psychotherapy Without Therapists." In P. Roman and H. Trice (Eds.), *The Sociology of Psychotherapy.* New York: Jacob Aronson, 1974.

Kagan, J., and Coles, R. (Eds.). *12 to 14: Early Adolescence.* New York: Norton, 1973.

Katz, A. H. *Parents of the Handicapped.* Springfield, Ill.: Thomas, 1961.

Killilea, M. "Mutual Help Organizations: Interpretations in the Literature." In G. Caplan and M. Killilea (Eds.), *Support Systems and Mutual Help: Multidisciplinary Explorations.* New York: Grune & Stratton, 1976.

Kleiman, M. A., and others. "Collaboration and Its Discontents: The Perils of Partnership." *Journal of Applied Behavioral Sciences,* 1976, *12,* 403-409.

Kubler-Ross, E. *On Death and Dying.* New York: Macmillan, 1969.

Lenneberg, E. Personal communication, 1971.

Lenneberg, E., and Rowbatham, J. L. *The Ileostomy Patient.* Springfield, Ill.: Thomas, 1970.

Levinsohn, D., and others. *The Seasons of a Man's Life.* New York: Knopf, 1978.

Levy, L. H. "Self-Help Groups: Types and Psychological Processes." *Journal of Applied Behavioral Science,* 1976, *12,* 310-313.

Lieberman, M. A., Borman, L. D., and others. *Self-Help Groups for Coping with Crisis: Origins, Members, Processes, and Impact.* San Francisco: Jossey-Bass, 1979.

Lifton, R. J. *Home from the War.* New York: Simon & Schuster, 1973.

Marris, P. *Loss and Change.* New York: Random House, 1974.

Parkes, C. M. "Psycho-Social Transitions: A Field of Study." *Social Science and Medicine,* 1971, *5,* 101-115.

Pearl, A., and Riessman, F. *New Careers for the Poor.* New York: Free Press, 1965.

Pincus, L. *Death and the Family.* New York: Random House, 1975.

President's Commission on Mental Health. *Report to the President.* Vol. 2. Washington, D.C.: U.S. Government Printing Office, 1978.

Raiff, N. "Recovery, Inc.: A Study of a Self-Help Organization in Mental Health." Unpublished doctoral dissertation, University of Pittsburgh, 1979.

Rappaport, R. "Normal Crises, Family Structure, and Mental Health." *Family Process,* 1963, *11,* 68-80.

Schacter, S. *The Psychology of Affiliation.* Stanford, Calif.: Stanford University Press, 1959.

Schwartz, M., and Schwartz, C. *Social Approaches to Mental Patient Care.* New York: Columbia University Press, 1964.

Silverman, P. R. "Services for the Widowed During the Period of Bereavement." In *Social Work Practice.* New York: Columbia University Press, 1966.

Silverman, P. R. "Service to the Widowed: First Steps in a Program of Preventive Intervention." *Community Mental Health Journal,* 1967, *1,* 37-44.

Silverman, P. R. "The Client Who Drops Out: A Study of Spoiled Helping." Unpublished doctoral dissertation, Florence Heller Graduate School, Brandeis University, 1969.

Silverman, P. R. "The Widow as Caregiver in a Program of Preventive Intervention." *Mental Hygiene,* 1970, *54,* 540-545.

Silverman, P. R. "Factors Involved in Accepting an Offer of Help." *Journal of Thanatology,* 1971, *1,* 161-171.

Silverman, P. R. "Widowhood and Preventive Interaction." *The Family Coordinator: Journal of Education, Counseling and Services,* 1972, *21,* 95-102.

Silverman, P. R. "Helping Each Other." In P. R. Silverman and others (Eds.), *Widowhood.* New York: Health Sciences, 1974.

Silverman, P. R. *Mutual Help Groups: A Guide for Mental Health Workers.* Publication No. (ADM) 78-646. Rockville, Md.: National Institute of Mental Health, 1978.

Silverman, P. R. *Mutual Help Groups: Organization and Development.* Beverly Hills, Calif.: Sage, 1980.

Silverman, P. R. "The Mental Health Consultant as Linking Agent." In D. Beigel and A. H. Naparstek (Eds.), *Community Support Systems and Mutual Help: Building Linkages.* New York: Springer, forthcoming.

Silverman, P. R., and Murrow, H. G. "Mutual Help During Critical Role Transitions." *Journal of Applied Behavioral Science,* 1976, *12,* 410-418.

Silverman, P. R., and Smith, D. "Helping Mutual Help Groups for the Physically Disabled." In A. Gartner and F. Reissman (Eds.), *Mental Health and the Self-Help Revolution.* New York: Human Sciences, forthcoming.

Silverman, S. M., and Silverman, P. R. "Parent-Child Communication in Widowed Families." *American Journal of Psychotherapy,* 1979, *33,* 428-441.

Strauss, A., and others. *Psychiatric Ideologies and Institutions.* New York: Free Press, 1964.

Tyhurst, J. S. "The Role of Transition States—Including Disasters—in Mental Illness." In Walter Reed Army Institute of Research (Eds.), *Symposium on Preventive and Social Psychiatry.* Washington, D.C.: U.S. Government Printing Office, 1957.

Weiss, R. S. "Transition States and Other Stressful Situations." In G. Caplan and M. Killilea (Eds.), *Support Systems and Mutual Help.* New York: Grune & Stratton, 1976.

White, R. W. "Strategies of Adaptation: An Attempt at Systematic Description." In G. V. Coelho, D. A. Hamburg, and J. E. Adams (Eds.), *Coping and Adaptation.* New York: Basic Books, 1974.

Chapter 26

Audiovisuals in Mental Health Education: A Quantum Leap

Edward A. Mason

Although the term *audiovisuals* has become synonymous with the modern classroom, it only minimally conveys the transformation in teaching that access to the visual image has generated. Recognition of the value of film and video in professional education has been growing rapidly. Audiovisuals are available for illustrating diagnostic categories, therapeutic techniques, family dynamics, crisis behavior, developmental stages, ethical issues and, it seems, almost any aspect of psychological assessment or mental disorder. Recent developments in electronic equipment have made it increasingly possible for every professional to be a filmmaker, every institution a television producer. Video, in particular, is being used in a growing variety of ways for localized, intrainstitutional applications, with users more and more taking advantage of its capacity for instant replay. As a psychiatrist and film and video producer, as well as an educator of professional, paraprofessional and preprofessional mental health workers, I would like to offer a few comments about some of the current and future key issues in this field. These comments are directed primarily to users of audiovisuals but also to the mental health professional who is or may become a producer.

Audiovisuals have become an accustomed aspect of teaching at all levels, and they are especially effective when integrated into traditional instruction (Romano, 1955). Current entry-level students have found from personal experience what research findings demonstrated some time ago: Information is retained longer when it is reinforced by audiovisuals (Nelson, 1952), and learning can often be accomplished in significantly less time by using instructional technology (Wendt and Butts, 1960). Most studies have measured media effectiveness in terms of increases in skills or information. Since the acquisition of sensitivity to human behavioral cues is more difficult to measure objectively, it has not received the attention of researchers. However, from the point of view of convinced users, the value of audiovisuals is undisputed.

Another important contribution of film or video is its special helpfulness at an early stage of learning a new skill or technique. For any level of training, a role model demonstrating actual use of the technique can crystalize the gestalt of that skill in action. For example, in teaching professionals his technique of consultee-centered case discussion, Caplan found that the film *An Example of Mental Health Consultation* (Mason, 1966) prepared his students to move on more securely from seminar to actual consultation. Still another way in which audiovisuals can support the education of mental health workers is in providing a broader context for their work. As an illustration, childcare workers shown *Boys in Conflict* (Mason, 1969) found validation for their own work because they saw their counterparts in the film facing the same difficulties as they did in managing emotionally disturbed children. More than the spoken or written word, successful audiovisuals transmit complex interactions that permit the student to engage in an active learning process.

The proliferation of professionally produced, prepackaged programming and the increased availability of filming and taping equipment for use by mental health workers and organizations have both posed new problems for the mental health professions. With regard to programming, the central issue is how to obtain information about access to, and evaluation of the growing flood of available material. With regard to program production, the issues have to do, first, with the selection and maintenance of hardware, and, second, with decisions about what kinds of material to record and how to record it for maximum effectiveness. An overriding issue affecting both prepackaged material and local production efforts is the question of how to properly protect the privacy and confidentiality of people who are filmed or videotaped.

Film Versus Video

In the 1960s, technical developments in the 16mm movie industry opened the way for a new style of filming (sometimes called *cinema verité*) that used synchronous sound and hand-held, very mobile cameras that supposedly minimized the subjectivity of the filmmaker and represented actuality. This made it possible to film in any location and to portray ordinary people engaged in their day-to-day activities. Many important mental health documentaries would have been impossible without the access and mobility that this equipment made possible. But it was not until video equipment became available at moderate costs that institutions began to purchase portable television units. In fact, as with many other desirable technical developments, soon every department wanted its own unit (individual departments now often have multiple units). With such proliferation comes the incentive for more ways to use video and for more persons to try their hand at making tapes.

The rapid advances in video have created the impression for some people that film is already out of date. This is far from true, particularly since 16mm facilities are the only ones available worldwide. Film has a certain polish and technical quality that continues to make it the production medium of choice for many entertainment as well as educational filmmakers. Film is sharper and offers a wider exposure range than the video camera, and it provides a more satisfactory image on a large screen, a feature that, in combination with a darkened room, induces an intensified involvement with what transpires on the screen.

In contrast, video has problems of incompatibility in respect to sizes of tape and differences between European and American technical standards. However, video has a tremendous advantage over film in that whatever is recorded can be instantly played back. This makes it an ideal medium for assisting in the supervision of therapists, as well as for teaching special therapeutic techniques. Alger has demonstrated how he uses the video camera in *Family Circle* (Diedrich, 1978) to capture family interaction for immediate playback. The feedback of verbal exchanges or behavioral cues can be a potent stimulus for family understanding. With video one can play and replay a segment at varying speeds immediately after recording it to take advantage of the therapeutic moment. With special equipment it is also possible to slow the playback for microanalysis of the material.

Another area for video use is in community health efforts. The availability of mass-produced home entertainment equipment, bringing costs within reach of many agencies, has made possible videotapes about concerns particular to a single community. When completed, these tapes naturally appeal to the residents of that community, but it is as much in the production as in the screenings that communication between agencies opens up and community action is mobilized. The lack of technical skill in making tapes seems not to detract from the benefits of this process. In Ypsilanti, Michigan, three agencies collaborated to form "Viewpoint," a community video educational project whose director believes there may even be advantages in having "homespun quality" (Weal, 1979).

Utilization of Existing Software. Since both video equipment and programming are becoming more available and more widely used, there is more need for information about "software" (films, tapes, and cassettes). Most mental health educators start with catalogues from local public film and tape libraries, including institutional, governmental, and commercial sources. In addition, they might request catalogues from distributors or libraries specializing in mental health materials (such as the Pennsylvania Cinema Register at Pennsylvania State University; the Extension Media Center at the University of California, Berkeley; the American Psychiatric Association in Washington; the Concord Films Council in Ipswich, Great Britain; or the National Centrim Voor Geestelijke Volksgezondheid in Utrecht, Holland). However, none of these has a complete listing of everything that has been produced. The National Information Center for Educational Media at the University of Southern California issues a listing every three years that has more entries but unfortunately less information about each than other more helpful services. The Mental Health Materials Center issues *The Selective Guide to Audiovisuals for Mental Health and Family Life Education* (Neher, 1979), which truly is a beacon shining through the fog. Without it, many good materials would remain in obscurity. Evaluative comments and creative suggestions for use are an integral part of each listing. Furthermore, to fill the gap between editions, Neher writes a quarterly supplement called *Sneak Previews.*

Through the use of AVLINE, an on-line data bank at the National Library of Medicine, information is available at many computer terminals throughout the United States on audiovisuals in the medical and mental disorder fields. With the cooperation of the American Association of Medical Colleges, about 150 new programs are evaluated monthly by qualified specialists. The completeness of the descriptions and evaluations makes the information a valuable resource. To illustrate, I recently requested information about audiovisuals on the topic of "Interview, psychological" and received eighty-nine entries, all appropriate—a comprehensive if not definitive list. Perhaps no data bank can keep up with every production, but at least techniques of information retrieval have advanced. No longer is one forced to order a film or tape with only the producer's publicity as a guide.

There are various sources of independent reviews besides those already mentioned. The *Community Mental Health Journal* and *Hospital and Community Psychiatry* regularly publish reviews of recent films and tapes, as do such other periodicals as *Film News.* The Education Film Library Association evaluates films in the health field and sponsors the noted American Film Festival for nontheatrical films and tapes.

Creating New Programming. Just as two decades ago, the need for materials to train professionals fostered the expansion of my role as teacher to that of producer, so too will many users of mental health audiovisuals now become producers. Often beginning with recordings for clinical supervisory conferences, educators are extending their efforts to make more permanent audiovisuals for use by others. In this movement my experience recommends two cautions: Attention must be paid to the maintenance of quality and to the protection of the human rights of participants.

There is danger in any mass swing of popularity that expectations will outreach performance, and certainly that is a possibility with video. Many professionals report that institutions buy new equipment that soon gathers dust, unused after the first glow because it demanded too many technical skills. Quality videotapes are not as simply obtained as is sometimes thought. Advertisers would have us believe that all we have to do is "push a button." Even if we are skeptical enough to plan on hiring assistants with technical skills, there are hurdles in collaboration. For example, mental health specialists must learn that simply delivering a lecture to the camera will make for a dull tape, and production experts must learn that subtle content may be more important than perfect lighting.

The fact that it is so easy to record on videotape tends to encourage letting the tape run on. The producer is always initially fascinated with the raw material, every flaw and pearl of it, but the viewer needs to see an edited version to appreciate the points being made and not to become lost in material that is redundant, confusing, or excessive. In order to be effective, a film or tape must hold the audience's attention. That demands quality of content as well as style of presentation and skill in editing.

Whether mental health audiovisuals should show fictional or actual patients has been a matter of concern for several decades. At first the question was focused on which method most effectively conveyed the desired information. Professional trainees were disdainful of acted films, which were considered primarily for "entertainment," and they reacted negatively to them in training settings. Therefore, the trend was toward documentary filming. Now, two developments are of concern to every professional educator. One is the explosion of electronic equipment that makes it possible for every professional to be a television producer and every patient or client a film subject. The other is the growing awareness of patients' rights, along with considerations of confidentiality. Contemporary concerns about informed consent have made many audiovisual producers turn to acted tapes and films to avoid the dangers of exposure and embarrassment that may accompany the distribution of live action materials. But learning and research are more effectively built on a foundation of accurate, documented material. Often, as with infants and young children, there can be no substitute for the real thing.

A Classic Among Audiovisuals. One of the world's outstanding series of documentaries is *Young Children in Brief Separation* (Robertson, 1967-1976). I would like to comment in some detail on the content of these films because they have made remarkable research data on child behavior available and they have been universally successful as training materials. They have contributed significantly at all levels of professional experience, and many are available in several different languages.

Climaxing a lifetime of study and teaching about the impact of separation on young children and the factors that can aggravate or mitigate such an experience, Robertson with his wife, Joyce, observed five children between one and one-half and two and one-half years of age who, because their mothers had been hospitalized, were temporarily deprived of their usual source of love and care. Four of the children were taken into the Robertsons' own home under what can only be described as ideal conditions of foster care. Kate, at twenty-nine months, responded at first in a reserved but cheerful way, and her anxiety only began to appear after a week with the Robertsons. After Kate returned from a visit to her mother, more feeling broke through as she said, "I *found* my Mummy," and she had her first tantrum. When finally reunited with her mother, she was able to resume a warm relationship, although she showed some anger and irritability. At a six-month follow-up visit she readily recalled her experience, and this might lead one to believe that it had had no serious impact. Yet Kate's visit to a daycare center two weeks after reunion with her mother had precipitated an extended attack of breathlessness that probably arose from fear of another separation. Only with such detailed studies can one appreciate the possible consequences of separation for a young child even when the outcome is considered good.

More troubling is evidence of the failure of foster care in a residential nursery for the fifth child, John. In contrast to Jane, who was also seventeen months old but was cared for by the Robertsons, he was dramatically affected by the strange environment, multiple caretakers, unsupportive peers, and the separation from his mother. There are no actors who could convey the distress and the anger that caused John to turn away from his mother on reunion, though perhaps a good actress could recreate the misery his mother shows when he rejects her. This powerful film should always be used in conjunction with at least one—but preferably three or four—of the others in order to illustrate the effect of variables such as age of the children and their experience of care after separation, and to broaden the viewer's perception to include issues of personality development, parenting, institutional procedures, and separation. Not only is this easiest in a group that has established a climate that encourages discussion, but far more can be derived from the rich material in these films by having the opportunity over time to explore their various dimensions.

The issue of confidentiality in this series is not crucial for the most part, since four of the children were seen under ideal circumstances and reacted with what can only be described as normal behavior. In the case of John, however, viewers have been critical of the childcare residence, of the parents for leaving him there, and even of the Robertsons for not intervening in the child's behalf. It is unlikely that the child will be harmed by this exposure since he is no longer readily recognizable. He has changed as he has grown, and he was not identified by last name or residence. Yet the question must always be raised: Do the benefits outweigh the risks in showing a particular family's problems to the public?

Sensitive Issues

The human rights issue is especially critical when it comes to filming those identified as having a mental illness. To demonstrate basic psychopathology to medical students, nurses, and psychologists, there is a series of videocassettes called *The Electronic Textbook of Psychiatry and Neurology* (Ryan, 1974-1975). Four of the twenty-three so far available deal with schizophrenia and show excerpts of actual patient interviews, with commentary by experts pointing up characteristic features of schizophrenia and therapeutic techniques. The producers sell these tapes only to accredited medical institutions able to assure the producers that they will restrict the audiences to "professionals in training in the mental health sciences." Even though these tapes are black and white and technically not very polished, they provide readily accessible and valuable teaching material. The opposite approach has been taken by other producers. The University of Southern California has produced the *Simulated Psychiatric Patient Interviews* (Snibbe, Johnson, and Evans, 1980) in which actors do a credible job of conveying the impression of psychiatric disorders. Produced in color, these films have a contemporary appeal and flair.

For demonstrating a special program or technique, I believe it is usually most convincing if the actual subjects are filmed. One of my own films, *We Won't Leave You* (Mason, 1975), shows a six-year-old during her experience with one-day surgery in a program at Massachusetts General Hospital that tries to reduce psychological trauma by minimizing parent-child separation. The film has been used by health professionals to encourage interest in duplicating this service elsewhere and by parent groups to show how a hospital staff can foster the welfare of the family. It would be difficult, although not impossible, to find a director and actors who could give an acted version the same impact. And, in this case, although the family exposes itself to the public, the fact that there is no stigma attached to a hernia operation means that there is limited possibility of embarrassment.

In cases of child abuse, however, the delicacy of the subject matter calls for caution. *The Sexually Abused Child: Identification/Interview* (Cavalcade Productions, 1978) was produced to show how a teacher might interview a young girl whom she suspected of being a victim of abuse. Intended to develop the skill and sensitivity of the interviewer, it serves as a focus for discussions about such questions as whether or not to interview the child, in what setting an interview should take place, how to reassure the child, and what to do with the information gained. In this film the characters are actors, and the audience accepts the minor loss of realism in deference to protection of the privacy of the child and her family. It is my belief here that even if the audience were strictly limited to professionals, concern for the discomfort of the subject might constitute a heavy barrier to viewing. Paradoxically, the very protection of privacy can build anxiety in the viewer. Conveying the suggestion that such interviews are highly delicate and difficult to carry out may undermine the goal of the film: to help teachers master a natural hesitancy to undertake this kind of interview.

Live or Acted. Another purpose of audiovisuals is the presentation of more complex material than could be presented "live"—consideration of a clinical syndrome, for example, that involved many individuals in multiple locations or of a psychological issue extending over time and into sociological, legal, or ethical territory. For example, *Tourette Syndrome: The Sudden Intruder* (Addis, 1978) demonstrates not only the strange and troublesome aspects of this condition and its impact on family and others but also the course of the therapy. It would be difficult to communicate on the same level if actors were used. Here the subtle, sometimes quite peripheral, data in the film give it authenticity. At the same time, however, authenticity was maintained in *The Eye of the Storm* (Peters, 1970) in which an Iowa teacher reenacted an experiment about prejudice in her third-grade class. The teacher divided the students according to eye color and assigned "superiority" on the first day to the "blue eyes" and on the following day to the "brown eyes." The visible evidence of the effect on these children of this artificially created method of discrimination is convincing proof of the significance of prejudice for self-image and personality development. Even though not new to the experiment, the pupils respond convincingly in the film.

In another example, the classic *Hillcrest Family* (Van Vlack, 1968), four well-known family therapists were recorded in separate interviews with a family. Each also was filmed discussing his assessment with a therapist who had been working with the family. As difficult as multiple interviews must have been for the family, the result was invaluable for training during a decade when family therapy was first beginning to flourish. Finally, in a film made for television, the documentation of problems in the deinstitutionalization of mental patients becomes much more vivid because the viewer knows that what he is seeing really happened. *Anyplace But Here* (Spain, 1979) follows several discharged Creedmoor Hospital patients into the community; Bill Moyers as commentator and Dr. Bill Werner, the hospital director, sensitively discuss the problems of budget and community resistance, as well as the possibility of helping patients return to useful lives.

Generally, I believe that a film or tape is not an end in itself. I see the purpose of audiovisuals as not only to engage the audience during viewing but to lead to some active process that will have a significant impact on the viewers' attitudes, behavior, or knowledge. I am referring to a discussion among the viewers and/or with a subject expert that explores and emphasizes the content most pertinent to that audience. It may bring about new understanding as various ideas are expressed, or it may consolidate group feeling as viewers find they share goals. Professionals in training, as well as the lay public, may find themselves intrigued by the account of the psychotherapy of a young woman with a multiple personality in *Sybil* (Petrie, 1976), a film made for television, or by the motion picture about the psychotherapy of a suicidal adolescent in *Ordinary People* (Redford, 1980). Each film uses the advantages of fiction to get the audience emotionally involved. Many medical settings have used "entertainment" films such as these to explore professional issues and to capitalize on these learning opportunities.

Informed Consent. If films and tapes involving real patients are to be made, means must be found to protect patient rights as much as possible. Consent must be obtained from every person filmed; to be fully informed, the subjects should be told (1) what will be expected of them, (2) the aim of the film, (3) the intended audience, (4) that refusal to participate will not deny them treatment, and (5) that participation can be discontinued at any time. A desirable safeguard is the omission of last names or geographical identification even when the audience is restricted. Further safeguards could include the presence of an impartial observer when consent is being obtained and the availability of a professional advisory panel to view the completed film or tape and raise questions about the propriety of any sequence that might bring harm to the participants. All these precautions should be taken even when the completed audiovisual is intended to be restricted to professional audiences.

Material to be shown to the general public imposes even more critical demands for informing the participants fully. They should be told whether the material will appear on television (commercial, educational, cable, or closed circuit) and in what types of educational settings it will be shown, as well as in which parts of the world. The risks taken by participants include the possibility of embarrassment, economic loss, prejudice, shame, teasing, rejection, or even attack, yet few are able to be fully aware of all such dangers before filming. Although many producers refuse to give up authority over content, the best protection would be achieved by requiring a second consent from every participant after he or she had viewed the finished product. Even if it is only for their information rather than approval, a showing of the completed work prepares the participants for the reactions of others who may see it. Such an act is also an expression of the producer's appreciation of and respect for the participants. I would note in passing that many of the subjects of my films have found the experience a gratifying one, sometimes of major personal significance.

There are special problems when a production involves children or adults who are not competent to sign consent agreements. It is my practice to ask each person to sign even if a parent or guardian must legally also give permission. For an institutionalized patient, the approval of both a therapist and a representative of the administration should also be obtained. These measures are advisable to conform to the spirit of contemporary concerns about human rights. So far, few of these issues have reached the courts. In probably the most publicized case, the film *Titicut Follies* (Wiseman, 1967) was found to be appropriate only for professional audiences in Massachusetts, where it was filmed (*Commonwealth of Massachusetts* v. *Wiseman,* 1969). The court also found that Wiseman did not comply with agreed-upon conditions in obtaining consent and did not exclude those incompetent to understand and give such consent. Also "there is collective, indecent intrusion into the most private aspects of the lives of these unfortunate persons." However, showings to "specialized audiences may be of benefit to the public interest, to the inmates themselves, and to the conduct of an important state institution." In other states the film can be shown publicly, and its widespread fame has drawn attention to the plight of institutionalized, criminally insane.

For every film or video production, someone must assess the risk-benefit ratio. Even though a producer believes that individual or social benefits justify the risks, it must be realized that such a person is only human and that personal interests may obscure judgment. Therefore, an advisory committee should be given the responsibility of overseeing the aims, methods, and results of audiovisuals involving actual patients. Many documentaries that deal with individual and family psychopathology are being made and shown publicly. Perhaps these will not only inform the public about therapeutic progress but will also remove some of the stigma still associated with mental illness.

A Look Toward the Future

The ascendance of the television medium certainly seems likely to continue. In spite of some incompatibility, equipment will keep on improving and becoming more attractive and accessible. As the market expands, prices will tend to decline, and video receivers will be found in every classroom, seminar, and conference center. But I believe that the software will change more dramatically than the hardware. The prerecorded videocassettes now available are largely feature-length entertainment, but I foresee expanded marketing of specialized educational materials as more and more homes and organizations purchase equipment.

The appearance of the videodisc has been heralded as another contribution to video potential; perhaps it will offer improvements over the present system of distributing and playing back prerecorded programs. At present, however, many potential purchasers are waiting to see which of the competing playback systems will succeed in the marketplace. The features of videodiscs and videocassettes are comparable; if they can be made cheaply enough, in quantity, they may sell for less than it now costs to *rent* programs. This will allow more professionals to establish their own libraries and avoid the delays of rentals and in shipping that currently handicap distribution. Both formats offer the possibility of two sound tracks and rapid access to any segment of them. These are especially useful features for training purposes; a program can have two language sound tracks, stereo sound or instructional material at different levels. Electronic attachments also allow slow and fast motion, the use of stop frames and automatic repeat, and selected review or location of a specific part of a disc; soon attachments will convert players into self-paced, interactive, tutorial-remedial, and teaching-learning machines.

Although not as many of these features apply to film projection, it is unlikely this format will become obsolete, even if some persons have been predicting the demise of the optical reproduction of picture and sound for a decade. The number of projectors in existence still is greater than the number of video playback decks. Perhaps in several decades all classic and archival films will be available in electronic form, but for the near future films will continue to hold a place of importance.

The greatest opportunity for the future, I believe, lies in the dissemination of the materials produced. Videodiscs and videocassettes will be cheaper and more accessible, but cable and microwave transmission of live programs will also multiply. Broadcasts via satellite will aim material to specific target audiences and will make conferences, lectures, and professional instruction available in even the most remote locations.

Another exciting development will be linked to progress in the use of teletext. This is a technology that transmits data via normal broadcasting signals; at present it is used mostly in business and industry. There also are two-way systems being developed in Great Britain, France, and Canada, as well as in the United States, that allow a viewer to request information from a computer databank. Perhaps future developments will also make possible the viewing of motion pictures from audiovisuals stored in a central library. This would allow the ultimate in assistance to an instructor to efficiently preview, use, or review material.

But just as people have had to learn to use and not to be controlled by the telephone, future advances in technology will have to be integrated with sound educational techniques and skills. Teaching still represents the combination of an art and a skill. Technical revolutions only point up the need for careful assessment of teaching requirements, goals, and results in order that nonprint materials, like printed materials, will be a creative addition to learning.

References

Addis, B. *Tourette Syndrome: The Sudden Intruder.* 16mm film. Los Angeles: Behavioral Sciences Media Lab, University of California, 1978.

Cavalcade Productions. *The Sexually Abused Child: Identification/Interview.* 16mm film. Schiller Park, Ill.: MTI Teleprograms, 1978.

Commonwealth of Massachusetts v. *Wiseman,* 356 Mass. 251 (1969).

Diedrich, B. *Family Circle.* Videocassette. New York: I.E.A. Productions, 1978.

Mason, E. A. *An Example of Mental Health Consultation.* 16mm film. Boston: Harvard Medical School, 1966.

Mason, E. A. *Boys In Conflict.* 16mm film. Boston: Harvard Medical School, 1969.

Mason, E. A. *We Won't Leave You.* 16mm film or videocassette. Boston: Harvard Medical School, 1975.

Neher, J. (Ed.). *The Selective Guide to Audiovisuals for Mental Health and Family Life Education.* (4th ed.) Chicago: Marquis Academic Media, 1979.

Nelson, C. M. "Effectiveness of Sound Motion Pictures in Teaching a Unit on Sulfur in High School Chemistry." *School Science and Mathematics,* 1952, *52,* 8-10.

Peters, W. *The Eye of the Storm.* 16mm film. Middletown, Conn.: Zerox Films, 1970.

Petrie, D. *Sybil.* Los Angeles: Lorimar Productions and NBC Television, 1976.

Redford, R. (Producer). *Ordinary People.* 35mm film. New York: Paramount Pictures, 1980.

Robertson, J. *Young Children in Brief Separation.* Five 16mm films. Suffolk, England: Concord Films Council, 1967-1976.

Romano, L. *The Role of Sixteen-Millimeter Motion Pictures and Projected Still Pictures in Science Unit Vocabulary Learnings at Grades Five, Six, and Seven.* Unpublished doctoral dissertation, University of Wisconsin, 1955.

Ryan, J. H. *The Electronic Textbook of Psychiatry.* Videocassette. New York: New York State Psychiatric Institute, 1974-1975.

Snibbe, J., Johnson, C. W., and Evans, L. *Simulated Psychiatric Patient Interviews.* Videocassette. Los Angeles: School of Medicine, University of Southern California, 1980.

Spain, T. *Anyplace But Here.* 16mm film. New York: Carousel Films, 1979.

Van Vlack, J. D. *The Hillcrest Family: Studies in Human Com-*

munication. 16mm film. Philadelphia: Eastern Pennsylvania Psychiatric Institute, 1968.

Weal, E. " 'Home-Made' Videotapes Spur M. H. Awareness." *Innovations,* Summer 1979.

Wendt, P. R., and Butts, G. K. *A Report of an Experiment in the Acceleration of Teaching Tenth-Grade World History with the Help of an Integrated Series of Films.* Carbondale, Ill.: General Publications, 1960.

Wiseman, F. *Titicut Follies.* 16mm film. Boston: Zipporah Films, 1967.

Epilogue: Personal Reflections by Gerald Caplan

It is natural for a teacher to be proud of the achievements of his former students, even though it is clear that their success must be ascribed to their own merits and not to his. My pride in this book derives, however, from my belief that I originally played a part in helping its writers draw the cognitive maps that have guided their later explorations. I rejoice that my students and colleagues feel that I was a catalyst in promoting their endeavors and that they have therefore seen fit to honor me in this volume. I accept with gratitude the honor they do me.

I last wrote a personal epilogue in 1968. It was the final chapter in my daughter Ruth's book, *Psychiatry and the Community in Nineteenth-Century America* (Caplan, 1969). On that occasion I used the opportunity to make predictions about likely developments in community mental health, based on analyzing the implications for our times of factors that Ruth demonstrated to have been operating over the previous century. I will use the present opportunity for the same kind of reflections.

In 1969 many readers felt that my predictions were overly gloomy and pessimistic: At the height of the popularity and active expansion of the community mental health center movement, I prophesied an impending decline. In 1981 some readers may feel that I am being overly optimistic, because at a time when the popularity of community-based services is rapidly deteriorating, I once again invoke the metaphor of the pendulum, or of the ocean tide, and confidently predict that within a few years our community philosophy will return to favor among the general public and among those leaders who disburse public funds.

In 1968 I did not base my predictions only on the analogy of the pendulum or the tide but also on identifying and evaluating specific features in the implementation of community programs similar to those that my daughter had shown to have been recurrently significant in the nineteenth century. I have set myself the same tasks in this chapter.

Creative Developments in Theory and Practice

I believe that the community mental health movement, despite its current unpopularity among decision makers in Washington and in several state capitals, is basically in good condition because its concepts and techniques are continuing to be developed actively and creatively and have not crystalized into a static dogma and canon of orthodox practices. This activity is abundantly demonstrated in the various chapters of this book. In my own areas of special interest it is shown by my recent move beyond the crisis model to support systems theory, and beyond the consultation method to methods of collaboration and mediation. Moreover, these developments in theory and practice are not products of armchair speculation; rather, they are solidly based on well-designed research projects or on explorations and evaluations of innovative operations by myself and others in the many localities where our services continue to be supported at a time when community funds are in short supply.

I have documented this thesis in a number of recent papers. For instance, in a recent issue of the *American Journal of Psychiatry* (Caplan, 1981) I published a review of current scientific thinking about the mastery of stress and the implications of this for the prevention of bodily and mental illness. In that paper I summarized a number of well-controlled empirical studies, including some with an experimental design that repeatedly validated the finding that a high level of social support prevents increased vulnerability to disease consequent on the experience of high stress. I also proposed a detailed explanation for this finding by focusing on the cognitive and problem-solving deterioration that is usual in individuals exposed to high stress, as a result of the deleterious effect of emotional arousal and its biochemical correlates. I ascribed the benefits of social support to the lowering of emotional tension and the supplementation of the stressed individual's eroded cognitive and problem-solving capacities.

My paper documents a major advance in our understanding of the pathogenic effects of stress and provides research-based directives for preventing certain types of disease by promoting support systems that provide essential guidance for the individual, as well as assistance with emotional mastery. These directives contrast with our former community mental health prescriptions. Although now seen to have been sound in principle, they were mostly based on clinical experience and intuition, and were not sufficiently precise, especially in failing to emphasize the crucial importance of cognitive elements in overcoming stress. Moreover, although my article on mastery of stress certainly does not negate the importance of crisis intervention, it widens the preventive field significantly by extending our focus to include situations of long-term stress, which may be no less pathogenic than short-term ones.

A similar development from vague global concepts to more specific ideas that provide precise prescriptions for action is demonstrated in another paper that I published last year (Caplan, 1980a). This paper proposes a revision of the model of primary prevention that guided our previous practice in community mental health. It focuses on two main sets of variables: (1) a list of biopsychosocial risk factors that have been shown by empirical research to be regularly associated with an increased incidence of psychopathology in index groups as opposed to control groups not exposed to these risks and (2) a set of intervening variables that determine whether exposed individuals will indeed become sick. These variables include a personality factor (often called "competence") that is a complex of constitutional and experiential traits manifested by "self-efficacy"—the individual's expectation that he can master his life problems by his own efforts and with the help of others—and a repertoire of learned skills for solving social and physical problems. The other major intervening variable, which represents, as it were, competence in action, is expressed by the behavior of the individual under stress, as he is influenced by his social supports. This model provides us with additional concrete guidance for understanding and organizing intervention points. These efforts include reducing biopsychosocial risks, improving self-efficacy and problem-solving skills, improving methods of intervention in crises, and promoting support systems, particularly in populations at special risk.

Once again, we see how advances are taking place in theory that will enable us to refine and extend our practice methodology and to replace attempts at global amelioration of the social and material environment with interventions focused on specific factors. This precision should in the future enable us to evaluate the results of our interventions by an experimental design, as is already being done in testing the effect of social support in certain stress situations (Caplan, 1981).

Another promising feature in current developments is the rapidly growing number of serious researchers in many different fields who are devoting themselves to studies that have relevance to the control of mental disorders. Mona Kornberg and I have reviewed the recent professional literature with a bearing on our preventive model in childhood. The publication that emerged took up almost an entire issue of the new *Journal of Prevention* and included a review of 659 articles (Kornberg and Caplan, 1980). The support systems literature is also vast and rapidly growing. Marie Killilea (1976), in her article on supportive aspects of mutual help organizations, reviewed 220 publications. Since then there has been an accelerating interest in that field, and a comprehensive review of support systems today would have to take into account a huge number of studies.

The literature on practice methodology has not grown as rapidly. Unfortunately, many creative practitioners do not publish. But I am at present embarked on some very interesting developments that are taking me and my colleagues far beyond the techniques that have been current in community mental health centers over the past fifteen years. In crisis intervention, our main advance has been linked with the recognition of the importance of supporting strategic withdrawal in individuals in the early stages of crisis, and sometimes for weeks or months afterwards, rather than urging them actively to confront their life problems and to proceed apace with their "worry work" or their "grief work." This recognition is in part the result of our clinical experience, which has increased our respect for the capacity of stressed individuals to assess intuitively the amount of psychological burdens they can bear and to defend themselves by denial, evasion, and isolation until they feel they can begin to deal effectively with the psychological impact of their environmental problems. It is also based on such research findings as those of our Harvard studies on conjugal bereavement, which show that mourning and "grief work" take much longer to accomplish than we used to think (Glick, Weiss, and Parker, 1974). And in part it is based on an important paper by Wallerstein and Kelly (1974), which showed that adolescents who reacted by strategic withdrawal during the period when their parents were in the throes of divorce often adapted better in the long run to this problem without damage to their mental health than those who faced the traumatic situation at the time with open eyes and became personally involved and upset.

The second advance in methodology is the development within the last few years of support systems practice. A short time ago, I prepared two lectures describing a whole range of support system techniques for use in adult psychiatry and in child psychiatry; when I delivered these lectures in different centers in the United States and Canada, I found that many other practitioners were actively pioneering and experimenting along similar lines.

The third area of methodological innovation is the attempt to modify the method of mental health consultation for use outside the boundaries of institutions in mediating between feuding factions in a community, whether to prevent violence or to overcome blockages in communication that interfere with the utilization of community services. I discussed my early explorations of this issue in 1970 in one of the final chapters of my book on mental health consultation (Caplan, 1970), and my book *Arab and Jew in Jerusalem* (Caplan, 1980b) describes a seven-year project in which I acted as a mediator in conflicts between Jewish providers of human services and Arabs who were potential service recipients.

The fourth, and possibly the most important, area of methodological exploration lies in the extension of consultation by mental health specialists to areas outside institutions. Instead of restricting ourselves to improving the functioning of other professionals in dealing with the psychosocial aspects of their cases, we can seek to build partnerships that provide opportunities for us to intervene directly with clients in nonmental health settings by sharing professional responsibility for patient care with our hosts. In a forthcoming article in the *Journal of Prevention* (Caplan and others, in press), I make a preliminary analysis of some basic issues in the development of such collaboration as a defined set of techniques. I believe that the next few years will see many practitioners focusing their efforts on accomplishing for mental health collaboration the same task of definition, explication, and evaluation that we have carried out over the past twenty years with the method of mental health consultation.

Population Orientation

As far back as the 1960s, Baker and Schulberg (1967) isolated five categories that their analysis of the professional literature led them to believe were central to the ideology of the community mental health movement. These were population focus, primary prevention, social treatment goals, comprehensive continuity of care, and total community involvement. This list has stood the test of time. We might now add a few refinements, such as emphasizing that the population for whose members the service program accepts responsibility should be circumscribed, either by living in a bounded geographical area or by membership in a defined collectivity—for instance, all the workers in an organization, all the patients in a hospital, or all the students in a school. We might add secondary and tertiary prevention to primary prevention. We might specify the need for penetration by mental health specialists into human services systems outside the boundaries of mental health institutions and agencies, along with the need for such techniques as consultation and collaboration to achieve this. We might also add the need to recognize and accept the realities of life in our society, and in particular the need to pay attention to legal, economic, social, cultural, and political systems. And most important, we might add the need to understand that human well-being —and services to improve it—depend on multifactorial open systems of biopsychosocial forces in a continual interplay between individuals and their social and material environments.

But the significant point is that neither the original list of categories nor those refinements that might be added on the basis of the past fourteen years of experience in community mental health specify elements that are restricted to the community mental health center as a service modality or even, except as an illustration, to mental health as such. The ideology is generic in nature and could be applied just as easily to almost any other aspect of the human services field of health, education, and welfare. In fact, I see no reason to attach to this ideology the name *community mental health*; perhaps a more appropriate label would be the *population orientation.* This name would emphasize the widespread significance of the ideology and would highlight the degree to which it differs from the individual-patient orientation that has been characteristic, for example, of psychiatry during those recurring periods of history when that profession has restricted its responsibility to patients who seek and are accepted by it for treatment of illness.

It may also be emphasized that apart from the use of the phrase *community agents* in the fifth category of the Baker and Schulberg (1967) list to designate caregiving professionals with whom mental health specialists should work, the notion that the community is the framework within which community mental health must operate is not mentioned. The term *community* implies the existence of a circumscribed system, consisting of people with a shared history and culture, usually living within geographic boundaries, that is organized to identify and solve the problems of its members by means of a planned network of interacting institutions. This definition was probably in the minds of those who drafted the community mental health center legislation, with its focus on bounded catchment areas and a central service center. But the ubiquity of such communities was rapidly shown by experience to be a myth, except in small-town settings or in relatively small neighborhoods in large cities. The consequences of the artificial attempt to carve up the maps of big cities into catchment area "communities" of 75,000 to 200,000 inhabitants have been among the reasons for the widespread disenchantment with community mental health programs. And yet it can be seen that the community mental health center as a service delivery modality was not an inevitable outcome of the core ideology. Nor were various other counterproductive elements of the community mental health movement, such as grandiose promises of a mental health utopia and the staffing of centers with clinical workers who lacked political sophistication and skills and were also untrained in population theory and practice.

Indeed, very little of the present unpopularity of community mental health can be ascribed to its ideology, and this ideology will probably continue in the future, as in the past, to be attractive to the man in the street, to political leaders, and especially to planners in the human services delivery field. Incidentally, I believe that the development of our ideology and certainly the impetus for President Kennedy's "Message Relative to Mental Illness and Mental Retardation" (1963) and P.L. 88-164 were influenced not only by psychiatrists who were imbued with the population orientation but also by certain human services planners—for example, the program analysts of the Bureau of the Budget, whose attitudes to the development of federal services for the mentally ill were very much in line with their ideas about the planning of other services in the health and welfare field. And although the popularity of community mental health centers has decreased, I see no indication of this happening in those other health and welfare services that are based to an equal degree on the population ideology. Rather, I believe that our own present fall from favor is a segmental issue, related to undue speed in the development of the community mental health center program and to such operational shortcomings as I have previously mentioned. The population orientation itself continues to influence developments in the rest of the human services field, and it seems to me inevitable that the community mental health movement will eventually be brought back into line with these developments.

Spread of Population-Oriented Educational Programs. Even though a major shortcoming of the federal and state legislation that established community mental health centers was a lack of provision for training line workers in the new concepts and skills essential for effective community work, the past twenty years has seen the widespread development by local initiative of programs of community mental health education. The first of these were the Harvard Visiting Faculty Seminar and the Inter-University Forum for Educators in Community Psychiatry, which provided an opportunity for educating teachers in psychiatric residency programs. Training in population-oriented concepts and skills was subsequently introduced in most programs for psychiatric residents, and this was soon followed by the introduction of similar programs in departments of psychology and schools of social work and nursing. At the present time there is also a move in many medical schools to develop similar courses for medical students. Such courses have been available for many years in schools of public health.

The multiplication of these programs in the relevant professional schools has greatly contributed to molding the concepts and values of the new generation of psychiatrists, psychologists, social workers, physicians, and nurses and has introduced into each of these professions an explicit awareness of their common commitment to the control of illness, including mental illness, in populations. It is ironic that the increased flow of population-oriented professionals into our field is occurring at a time when the community mental health center movement is itself in decline. Ten years earlier this flow might well have enabled these centers to become effective. Nevertheless, I believe that although many young professionals will give up their population orientation when they fail to find jobs in community mental health centers, some will almost certainly succeed in finding jobs in other service facilities that will allow them to utilize their particular concepts and skills, and they will therefore maintain their ideological commitment.

Diversification of Service Delivery Patterns. It must be said to the credit of those who framed community mental health center legislation and the governmental regulations for implementing the legislation that they provided sufficient flexibility for many alternative patterns of service delivery, in addition to the standardized community mental health center. In particular, they permitted the obligatory functions of centers to be spread over a number of community agencies bound together by formal agreements; and, at the same time, the outreach services of the centers made it possible to promote patterns of decentralized mental health service delivery within the framework of other human services institutions. Federal and state community mental health center funds have therefore been used to pay for the employment of mental health specialists in a variety of health, education, and welfare institutions such as general hospitals, health maintenance organizations, and neighborhood health centers, as well as for the staffing of community hot lines, emergency medical services, rehabilitation programs, crime prevention programs, and programs to combat addiction. In many of these settings, the mental health workers have proved their value, and the institutions have transferred them to their own payrolls.

Many community mental health specialists, in fact, have never worked in formally designated community mental health centers but only in alternative population-oriented service systems, and the funding for their operations has always come from other sources than community mental health center legislation. I myself have been working for the past four years inside a general hospital, where I established with hospital funds a department of child psychiatry that is committed to serving the mental health needs of a community catchment area, as well as the mental health needs of all children being investigated or treated for physical illnesses in the hospital's wards. My population-oriented ideology and skills have been equally utilized in both settings. There is nothing new in this. Erich Lindemann, when he moved from the Harvard School of Public Health to the Harvard Medical School in 1954, promoted a population orientation in the Department of Psychiatry at Massachusetts General Hospital. There he pioneered the modification of the concepts and skills that he had developed in his community program at the Wellesley Human Relations Service for use inside the hospital. He tried to deal not only with the community of patients but with the community of the hospital staff and the intrahospital social system, as he had become accustomed to do in dealing with the social systems of community agencies and with the field of social forces in the town of Wellesley.

Inertia of Numbers. One practical result of P.L. 88-164 and related legislation, along with various actions of the federal government, has been a vast outpouring of funds for the erection and staffing of community mental health centers. Between 1965 and 1977 this amounted to $1.85 billion. Although I do not presently have access to data later than those contained in the President's Commission on Mental Health (1978), my educated guess is that about 600 federally financed community mental health centers are currently in operation. To this number must be added the more than 500 centers that have been erected and staffed by means of state and local funds. In 1963 federal planners estimated that 2,000 community mental health centers would be required to satisfy the catchment area needs of the entire country. So we see that more than half this target has been achieved.

In addition, there has been a large expenditure of funds by other branches of federal and state government for population-oriented local mental health services in programs of primary medical care, welfare programs, school services, rehabilitation efforts, and programs for reduction of alcoholism and drug abuse and for crime prevention. The result has been a phenomenal growth in population-oriented mental health programs, many of which are housed in newly constructed buildings in large centers of population.

In the past, when the pendulum of popularity swung away from population-oriented programs, a quick change occurred in local services because the number of community facilities was small and it took little effort to close or modify a few programs and so alter the entire picture. But the present establishment of a great number of mental health centers, distributed in relation to population concentrations, has produced an unprecedented situation. Once established, each center develops its vested interest groups of staff, clients, and local political supporters, including community professionals and agencies that derive benefits from it. Such a center can be closed only with great difficulty. The loss or reduction of federal support may stop the building of new centers and may slow down the population-oriented development of others, but the nationwide network of community mental health centers is by now too large to be drastically affected within the next few years. Before that happens, I believe that the pendulum of political popularity will begin to swing back toward a population orientation.

Urban and Rural Contrasts

Disenchantment with community mental health centers is concentrated in large cities, where the catchment areas are often no more than artificial copies of communities. Moreover, there are often protagonists in these areas who are sophisticated in grantsmanship and influential in Washington, so that their lobbying leads to quick and massive flows of federal funds. This results in the building and staffing of centers more rapidly than the population can make full use of them and before staff with the necessary skills can be recruited. The result has usually been lack of satisfaction of population needs, a situation often aggravated by the inflated promises of lobbyists, eager to achieve quickly their goals in Washington without regard to the need to develop the active collaboration of the local population, to investigate its felt needs, and to articulate adequately with local caregivers, all of which take a long time.

The situation has often been quite different in regions

where people live mostly in small towns. Especially in the central and southern states, a spirit of local conservatism has reduced the drive to solicit funds from Washington and even from the state governments. Although the people in these areas are usually not unsophisticated or deficient in political power and influence, they often choose not to ask the central government to intervene in a problem and thus to give it control over their local services. They suspect that their own wishes about types of programs and speed of development will be sacrificed, or at any rate not given due weight, in centralized decisions molded by the political forces in Washington or the state capital. In such regions, the geographically bounded community is a valid concept, and the community mental health center is sensitive to the needs of the population. Linked with a relatively small number of other caregiving agencies in an intercommunicating network, the rural or small town mental health center has over the past ten to fifteen years proved in practice to be a valuable model of service delivery.

The centers in such regions have been largely financed by local taxes and voluntary funds. This means that the centers have been developed only after the community has organized itself to tailor services designed specifically to satisfy its needs. It also means that the centers have been built slowly and that the programs have often been started in makeshift premises that could be molded to the demands of local reality before being replaced by new buildings. It means that staff have been recruited slowly, so that even if they initially did not have the required skills, they could be given the time to learn on the job. On the whole, new staff in such programs have been younger and more idealistic than those working in metropolitan centers. I have traveled widely in such small-town regions and have given seminars for center staffs. I have found that although they often have less impressive paper credentials than their big-city counterparts, they have usually acquired greater population-oriented skills and sophistication because they have been molded by the local community forces, particularly by the constant surveillance of community leaders who keep them in line with the felt needs of the population in order to ensure that scarce local funds are being profitably expended.

Not only has the community mental health center proved a successful service pattern in such small towns, as shown by the continuing willingness of local authorities and some state governments to continue to finance them from public funds, but this situation is not much affected by changes in Washington political fashions. In fact, I have the impression that the community mental health movement in rural states got off to a slow start because of reluctance to go along with ideas coming out of Washington. If anything, it has probably picked up speed, now that it is seen to be moving in the opposite direction from that of federal and state authorities.

Professional Opposition

Opposition to the population ideology has long characterized the politically dominant groups in the psychiatric professions. These elites have been committed to an individual-patient ideology, whether their professional philosophy has been dominated by psychoanalytic and psychodynamic ideas, by a focus on individual, group, or family treatment, or by a primary interest in biological processes. Their attitudes and influence were expressed in the report of the Joint Commission on Mental Illness and Mental Health in 1961 that recommended increasing governmental support for existing psychiatric institutions and programs without significant changes in patterns of service delivery. These recommendations were set aside by President Kennedy in his 1963 message to Congress and in the community mental health center legislative acts. However, the flow of federal funds to new community service programs did not change the attitudes of the psychiatric elites. On the contrary, it probably added bitterness and disappointment to their traditional hostility, and they have continued in their opposition to a population approach. Their political influence was evident in the rapid neutralization of the recommendations for federal support of programs of primary prevention that emerged from the President's Commission on Mental Health (1978). And I believe that they have also exerted influence on Washington decision makers to reduce support for community mental health centers.

On the one hand, it is unlikely that the opposition of this group will lessen significantly in the near future, since it is firmly rooted in professional vested interests and in an ideology. On the other hand, it seems that this front is not as solid as it used to be. The junior and middle-level ranks of academic psychiatry, which is one of the strongholds of the psychiatric elites, have been influenced by the Peace Corps program and by the training programs in community mental health that have been organized in most medical schools. The Inter-University Forum for Educators in Community Psychiatry and the Harvard Visiting Faculty Seminar influenced a number of key academic psychiatrists. A number of senior psychiatrists in medical schools have also changed to a population orientation after studying in schools of public health or after being personally involved in organizing local community mental health programs. And I have been impressed during visits to a number of medical schools that serve rural hinterlands where community mental health centers have proved their value by the increased openness nowadays to population-oriented concepts, even in departments with a reputation for excellence in individual-patient approaches.

And so, I believe that as the present psychiatric leadership retires, it may in many places be succeeded by people who will be less staunchly opposed to a population ideology. And there are several university departments of psychiatry, even in such metropolitan areas as Boston, New York, Chicago, San Francisco, and Los Angeles, in which senior faculty are already committed to a population orientation.

Taking the broadest view possible, what conclusions can be drawn about the future of community mental health? There are at least eight:

1. Despite the current reduction in the political popularity of community mental health and in central government funding of community mental health centers, many of these centers continue to operate successfully, particularly in small towns and rural areas. Many are supported from local and state funds, and many will probably continue to be financed by state governments when federal funding is cut off or rechanneled.

2. The basic ideology of the community mental health movement emerges from its population orientation and is not

necessarily linked with the community mental health center pattern of service delivery.

3. Researchers and practitioners committed to a population orientation have developed concepts and skills that are being successfully utilized in a variety of human services settings outside community mental health centers. There is every indication that they will continue to be so used in the future and to be financially supported by public funds, despite the recent fall from popularity of community mental health centers.

4. Community mental health centers often proved unsuccessful in metropolitan areas. Such centers will probably eventually be replaced by services that focus on neighborhoods or that are integrated within primary medical care facilities, such as neighborhood health centers and health maintenance organizations, as well as general hospitals.

5. Planners in health, education, and welfare are increasingly committed to a generic population orientation, and this will eventually result in steps to integrate mental health specialists within many service delivery systems or to revive sponsorship of autonomous population-oriented psychiatric facilities that will satisfy felt local needs and be articulated with other community services.

6. The pendulum swing away from population approaches on this occasion has not had such a deleterious effect on community mental health programs as on previous occasions over the past 150 years.

7. I believe that population-oriented mental health services will recover their nationwide popularity and financial support by central government agencies within a relatively short period, possibly within about ten years.

8. I predict that the population ideology will continue to increase in popularity in medical schools, in schools of social work and nursing, and in departments of psychology and that this will lead to the stimulation of relevant research and to the training of the many community practitioners who will be needed when the community mental health movement regains its appeal to federal and state funding agencies. Meanwhile, it would be valuable for population-oriented academic departments to organize outreach continuation education for the

staffs of those community programs that continue to operate successfully in small-town and rural areas, as well as neighborhood mental health centers in big cities.

References

Baker, F., and Schulberg, H. C. "The Development of a Community Mental Health Ideology Scale." *Community Mental Health Journal*, 1967, *3*, 216-225.

Caplan, G. *The Theory and Practice of Mental Health Consultation.* New York: Basic Books, 1970.

Caplan, G. "An Approach to Preventive Intervention in Child Psychiatry." *Canadian Journal of Psychiatry*, 1980a, *25*, 671-682.

Caplan, G. *Arab and Jew in Jerusalem: Explorations in Community Mental Health.* Cambridge, Mass.: Harvard University Press, 1980b.

Caplan, G. "Mastery of Stress: Psychosocial Aspects." *American Journal of Psychiatry*, 1981, *138*, 413-420.

Caplan, G., and others. "Patterns of Cooperation of Child Psychiatry with Other Departments in Hospitals." *Journal of Prevention*, in press.

Caplan, R. B., in collaboration with Caplan, G. *Psychiatry and the Community in Nineteenth-Century America.* New York: Basic Books, 1969.

Glick, I. O., Weiss, R. S., and Parker, M. C. *The First Year of Bereavement.* New York: Wiley, 1974.

Killilea, M. "Mutual Help Organizations: Interpretations in the Literature." In G. Caplan and M. Killilea (Eds.), *Support Systems and Mutual Help.* New York: Grune & Stratton, 1976.

Kornberg, M. S., and Caplan, G. "Risk Factors and Preventive Intervention in Child Psychopathology: A Review." *Journal of Prevention*, 1980, *1*, 71-133.

President's Commission on Mental Health. *Report of the Task Panel on the Nature and Scope of the Problems.* Appendix, Vol. 2. Washington, D.C.: U.S. Government Printing Office, 1978.

Wallerstein, J. S., and Kelly, J. B. "The Effects of Parental Divorce: The Adolescent Experience." In E. J. Anthony and C. Koupernick (Eds.), *The Child in His Family: Children at Psychiatric Risk.* New York: Wiley, 1974.

Chronological Bibliography of Gerald Caplan

1937

Caplan, G. "Investigation of the Nerve Endings in the Pericardium of the Dog." Manchester University Library, 1937.

Caplan, G. "Investigation on Muscle Pain in Man." Manchester University Library, 1937.

1941

Caplan, G. "Nonconvulsive Faradic Shock Therapy." *British Medical Journal,* 1941, *1,* 479.

1945

Caplan, G. "Experience with a Simplified Apparatus for the Electrical Induction of Convulsions." *Journal of Mental Science,* 1945, *91,* 200.

Caplan, G. "Studies on Electric Shock Therapy in Neuropsychiatry." Unpublished Master's thesis, Manchester University Library, 1945.

Caplan, G. "Treatment of Epilepsy by Electrically Induced Convulsions." *British Medical Journal,* 1945, *1,* 511.

1946

Caplan, G. "Electrical Convulsion Therapy in the Treatment of Epilepsy." *Journal of Mental Science,* 1946, *91,* 784.

Caplan, G. "Fractures of Dorsal Vertebrae in Epilepsy and Convulsion Therapy." *Journal of Mental Science,* 1946, *92,* 766.

1947

Caplan, G. "Electronarcosis." *Lancet,* Sept. 6, 1947, 368-369.

1948

Caplan, G., and Bowlby, J. "Aims and Methods of Child Guidance." *Health Education Journal,* 1948, *6.*

Caplan, G. "Electronarcosis–An Improvement in Technique by the Use of Pentothal and Curare." *Proceedings of the Royal Society of Medicine,* 1948, *41,* 584-585.

1950

Caplan, G. "Electronarcosis" (in Hebrew). *Harefua,* Oct. 1950, *39,* 69.

Caplan, G. "The Treatment of Emotionally Disturbed Children and Child Guidance Services." *Child Care in Israel* (Jerusalem), 1950, p. 183.

1951

Caplan, G. "A Public Health Approach to Child Psychiatry." *Mental Hygiene,* 1951, *35,* 235.

Caplan, G. "Education of Teachers in Mental Health Principles" (in Hebrew). *Megamot,* Apr. 1951, p. 227.

Caplan, G. "Mental Hygiene Problems of Immigrants and Transplanted Persons." *Proceedings of the 4th International Congress of Mental Health,* 1951.

Caplan, G. "Mental Hygiene Work with Expectant Mothers—A Group Psychotherapeutic Approach." *Mental Hygiene,* 1951, *35,* 41.

Caplan, G. "Prophylactic Child Guidance" (in Hebrew). *Megamot,* July 1951, p. 314.

1952

Caplan, G. "Mental Hygiene Contributions to the Resettlement of Immigrants in Israel." *Mental Hygiene,* 1952, *36,* 607-617.

Caplan, G. "The Disturbance of the Mother-Child Relationship by Unsuccessful Attempts at Abortion." *Courier of the International Children's Center,* 1952, *11,* 193-201.

1954

Caplan, G. "A Public Health Approach to Child Psychiatry." *Nordisk Medicin* (Oslo), 1954, pp. 51-78.

Caplan, G. "Clinical Observations on the Emotional Life of Children in the Communal Settlements in Israel: Problems of Infancy and Childhood." *Transactions of the 7th Conference of the Josiah Macy, Jr., Foundation,* 1954, pp. 91-120.

Caplan, G. "Preparation for Healthy Parenthood." *Children,* Sept. 1954, pp. 171-175.

Caplan, G. "The Disturbance of the Mother-Child Relationship by Unsuccessful Attempts at Abortion." *Mental Hygiene,* 1954, *36,* 67-80.

Caplan, G. "The Mental Hygiene Role of the Nurse" (in Hebrew). *Megamot,* Sept. 1954.

Caplan, G. "The Mental Hygiene Role of the Nurse in Maternal and Child Care." *Nursing Outlook,* 1954, *2,* 14-19.

Rosenfeld, J. M., and Caplan, G. "Techniques of Staff Consultation in an Immigrant Children's Organization in Israel." *American Journal of Orthopsychiatry,* 1954, *24,* 45-62.

1955

Caplan, G. (Ed.). *Emotional Problems of Early Childhood.* New York: Basic Books, 1955.

Caplan, G. "Recent Trends in Preventive Psychiatry." In G. Caplan (Ed.), *Emotional Problems of Early Childhood.* New York: Basic Books, 1955.

Caplan, G. "The Role of the Social Worker in Preventive Psychiatry." *Medical Social Work,* 1955, *4,* 144-160.

1956

Caplan, G. "An Approach to the Study of Family Mental Health." *Public Health Reports,* 1956, *71,* 1027-1030.

Caplan, G. "Book review: *Mental Health and Mental Disorder* by A. M. Rose and others." *Psychosomatic Medicine,* 1956, *18,* 102.

Caplan, G. Book review: *Social Science in Medicine* by L. W. Simmons and H. G. Wolff. *Psychiatry,* 1956, *19,* 105-107.

Caplan, G. *Mental Health Aspects of Social Work in Public Health.* Berkeley: University of California Press, 1956.

Caplan, G. "Mental Health Consultation in Schools." In *The Elements of a Community Mental Health Program.* New York: Milbank Memorial Fund, 1956.

1957

Caplan, G. "Detection in Pregnancy of Future Disturbed Mother-Child Relationships: Ways to Forestall Future Emotional Disturbances." Lecture reported by the *Hawaii Health Messenger,* 1957, *18* (6).

Caplan, G. "Psychological Aspects of Maternity Care." *American Journal of Public Health,* 1957, *47,* 25-31.

Caplan, G. "Psychological Aspects of Maternity Care." *Bulletin of Maternal Welfare,* Nov.-Dec. 1957, pp. 18-22, 29.

Caplan, G. "Psychological Aspects of Maternity Care." In *Some New Approaches to Maternity Care.* Department of Health, Education, and Welfare Publication, 1957.

1958

Caplan, G. "Book review: *Four Basic Aspects of Preventive Psychiatry–Report of 1st Institute of Preventive Psychiatry at the State University of Iowa.*" *American Journal of Public Health,* 1958, *48,* 684.

Caplan, G. "Clinical Observations on the Emotional Life of Children in the Communal Settlements in Israel." In C. F. Reed, I. E. Alexander, and S. S. Tompkins (Eds.), *Psychopathology: A Source Book.* Cambridge, Mass.: Harvard University Press, 1958.

Caplan, G. "Mental Health Consultation in Preventive Psychiatry." *A Crianca Portuguesa,* 1958, *42,* 479-489.

1959

Caplan, G. "An Approach to the Education of Community Mental Health Specialists." *Mental Hygiene,* 1959, *43,* 268-281.

Caplan, G. "Book review: *The Psychodynamics of Family Life* by N. Ackerman." *International Journal of Group Psychotherapy,* 1959, *9,* 376-377.

Caplan, G. "Concepts of Mental Health and Consultation." Children's Bureau Publication No. 373, Department of Health, Education, and Welfare, 1959.

Caplan, G. "Practical Steps for the Family Physician in the Prevention of Emotional Disorder." *Journal of the American Medical Association,* 1959, *170,* 1497-1506.

Hamovitch, M. D., Caplan, G., Hare, P., and Owens, C. "Establishment and Maintenance of a Mental Health Unit." *Mental Hygiene,* 1959, *43,* 412-421.

1960

Caplan, G. "Emotional Implications of Pregnancy and Influences on Family Relationships." In H. C. Stuart and D. G. Prugh (Eds.), *The Healthy Child.* Cambridge, Mass.: Harvard University Press, 1960.

Caplan, G. "Patterns of Parental Response to the Crisis of Premature Birth." *Psychiatry,* 1960, *23,* 365-374.

Caplan, G. "The Roots of Human Relationships: Mother and Infant." In H. C. Stuart and D. G. Prugh (Eds.), *The Healthy Child.* Cambridge, Mass.: Harvard University Press, 1960.

Parad, H. J., and Caplan, G. "A Framework for Studying Families in Crisis." *Journal of Social Work,* 1960, *5,* 3-15.

1961

Caplan, G. *An Approach to Community Mental Health.* New York: Grune & Stratton, 1961.

Caplan, G. "An Approach to the Study of Family Mental Health." In I. Galdston (Ed.), *The Family: A Focal Point in Health Education.* Montpelier, Vt.: Capital City Press, 1961.

Caplan, G. "Book review: *Symposium on Preventive and Social Psychiatry,* Walter Reed Army Institute of Research." *Mental Hygiene,* 1961, *45,* 290-291.

Caplan, G. *Common Problems of Early Childhood.* Atlanta: Maternal and Child Health Service, Public Health Nursing Service, Georgia Department of Public Health, 1961.

Caplan, G. "Concluding Discussion." In G. Caplan (Ed.), *Prevention of Mental Disorders in Children: Initial Explorations.* New York: Basic Books, 1961.

Caplan, G. "Curriculum Content." In *Mental Health Teaching in Schools of Public Health.* New York: Columbia University Press, 1961.

Caplan, G. "General Introduction and Overview." In G. Caplan (Ed.), *Prevention of Mental Disorders in Children: Initial Explorations.* New York: Basic Books, 1961.

Caplan, G. (Ed.). *Prevention of Mental Disorders in Children: Initial Explorations.* New York: Basic Books, 1961.

1962

Caplan, G. *Manual for Psychiatrists Participating in the Peace Corps Program.* Washington, D.C.: Medical Program Division, Peace Corps, 1962.

Caplan, G., and Cadden, V. *Adjusting Overseas—A Message to Each Peace Corps Trainee.* Washington, D.C.: Peace Corps, 1962.

1963

Caplan, G. "Book review: Recent Research Looking Toward Preventive Intervention, Proceedings of the Third Institute on Preventive Psychiatry." *Social Casework,* 1963, *44,* 94.
Caplan, G. "Conception, Pregnancy, and Childbirth." In A. Deutsch and H. Fishman (Eds.), *Encyclopedia of Mental Health.* Vol. 1. New York: Franklin Watts, 1963.
Caplan, G. "Opportunities for School Psychologists in the Primary Prevention of Mental Disorders in Children." *Mental Hygiene,* 1963, *47,* 525-539.
Caplan, G. *Principles of Preventive Psychiatry.* New York: Basic Books, 1963.
Caplan, G. "Psychological Aspects of Pregnancy." In H. Lief and others (Eds.), *The Psychological Basis of Medicine Practice.* New York: Harper & Row, 1963.
Caplan, G. "Types of Mental Health Consultation." *American Journal of Orthopsychiatry,* 1963, *33,* 470-481.

1964

Caplan, G. "A Conceptual Model for Primary Prevention." In D. A. van Krevelen (Ed.), *Child Psychiatry and Prevention.* Bern, Switzerland: Verlag Hans Huber, 1964.
Caplan, G. "Book review: *Psychological Development in Health and Disease* by G. L. Engel." *Mental Hygiene,* 1964, *48,* 672.
Caplan, G. "Current Issues Relating to the Education of Psychiatric Residents in Community Psychiatry." *Proceedings of 3rd Annual Conference, Mental Health Career Development Program.* Public Health Service Publication No. 1245. Bethesda, Md.: National Institutes of Health, 1964.
Caplan, G. "The Role of Pediatricians in Community Mental

Health (with Particular Reference to the Primary Prevention of Mental Disorders in Children)." In L. Bellak (Ed.), *Handbook of Community Psychiatry and Community Mental Health.* New York: Grune & Stratton, 1964.

Mason, E. A., and Caplan, G. "Working with the Peace Corps—A Training Opportunity in Social Psychiatry." *Mental Hygiene,* 1964, *48,* 172-176.

1965

Caplan, G. "Book review: *The Growth and Development of the Prematurely Born Infant* by C. P. Drillien." *American Journal of Mental Deficiency,* 1965, *69,* 593-594.

Caplan, G. "Community Psychiatry—Introduction and Overview." In S. E. Goldston (Ed.), *Concepts of Community Psychiatry: A Framework for Training.* Public Health Service Publication No. 1319, Department of Health, Education, and Welfare, 1965.

Caplan, G. "Current Issues Relating to the Training of Psychiatric Residents in Community Psychiatry." In S. E. Goldston (Ed.), *Concepts of Community Psychiatry: A Framework for Training.* Public Health Service Publication No. 1319, Department of Health, Education, and Welfare, 1965.

Caplan, G. "Opportunities for School Psychologists in the Primary Prevention of Mental Disorders in Children." In N. M. Lambert (Ed.), *The Protection and Promotion of Mental Health in Schools.* Public Health Service Publication No. 1226. Department of Health, Education, and Welfare, 1965.

Caplan, G. "Problems of Training in Mental Health Consultation." In S. E. Goldston (Ed.), *Concepts of Community Psychiatry: A Framework for Training.* Public Health Service Publication No. 1319, Department of Health, Education, and Welfare, 1965.

Caplan, G., Mason, E. A., and Kaplan, D. M. "Four Studies of Crisis in Parents of Prematures." *Community Mental Health Journal,* 1965, *1,* 149-162.

1966

Caplan, G. "Crisis in the Family." *Medical Opinion and Review,* 1966, *1,* 21-23.

Caplan, G. "Elements of a Comprehensive Community Mental Health Program for Adolescents." In *Psychiatric Approaches to Adolescence.* International Congress Series No. 108. The Netherlands: Excerpts Medica Foundation, 1966.

Caplan, G. "Foreword." In H. R. Huessy (Ed.), *Mental Health with Limited Resources.* New York: Grune & Stratton, 1966.

Caplan, G. "Some Comments on 'Community Psychiatry and Social Power.' " *Social Problems,* 1966, *14,* 23-25.

Caplan, G., and Cadden, V. "The Turning Points of Life." *McCall's,* Oct. 1966, pp. 114-115, 185-186.

Caplan, G., and Lebovici, S. "Introduction." In *Psychiatric Approaches to Adolescence.* International Congress Series No. 108. The Netherlands: Excerpts Medica Foundation, 1966.

Caplan, G., and Lebovici, S. (Eds.). *Psychiatric Approaches to Adolescence.* International Congress Series No. 108. The Netherlands: Excerpts Medica Foundation, 1966.

1967

Caplan, G. "Growing Up and Society." In *Proceedings of the White House Conference on Health.* Washington, D.C.: Department of Health, Education, and Welfare, 1967.

Caplan, G., and Cadden, V. "How to Deal with a Crisis." *Reader's Digest,* Jan. 1967, pp. 80-83.

Caplan, G. "Preface." In N. Paul, *A Chance to Grow.* Boston: WGHB Radio, 1967.

Caplan, G., and Caplan, R. B. "Development of Community Psychiatry Concepts." In A. M. Freedman and H. I. Kaplan (Eds.), *Comprehensive Textbook of Psychiatry.* Baltimore, Md.: Williams and Wilkins, 1967.

Caplan, G., and Gruenbaum, H. "Perspectives on Primary Prevention." *Archives of General Psychiatry,* 1967, *17,* 331-346.

1968

Caplan, G. "Opportunities for School Psychologists in the Primary Prevention of Mental Disorders in Children." In E. Miller (Ed.), *The Foundation of Child Psychiatry.* Oxford, England: Pergamon Press, 1968.

Caplan, G. *Principios de Psiquiatria Preventiva.* Buenos Aires: Paidos, 1968.

Caplan, G. "The Nature and Problems of Evaluation in Community Mental Health." In L. Roberts (Ed.), *Comprehensive Mental Health: The Challenge of Evaluation.* Madison: University of Wisconsin Press, 1968.

Caplan, G., and Cadden, V. "Lessons in Bravery." *McCall's,* Sept. 1968, pp. 85, 151-153, 158.

Schulberg, H. C., Caplan, G., and Greenblatt, M. "Evaluating the Changing Mental Hospital: A Suggested Research Strategy." *Mental Hygiene,* 1968, *52,* 218-225.

1969

Caplan, G. "Foreword." In S. E. Golann, *Coordinate Index Reference Guide to Community Mental Health.* New York: Behavioral Publications, 1969.

Caplan, G., and Lebovici, S. (Eds.). *Adolescence: Psychosocial Perspectives.* New York: Basic Books, 1969.

Caplan, G., Macht, L., and Wolf, A. *Manual for Mental Health Professionals Participating in the Job Corps Program.* Document No. JCH 330-A. Washington, D.C.: Office of Economic Opportunity, 1969.

Caplan, R. B., in collaboration with Caplan, G. *Psychiatry and the Community in Nineteenth-Century America.* New York: Basic Books, 1969.

1970

Caplan, G. "Community Psychiatry and Illegitimacy." In P. M. Steinmetz and J. E. Teele (Eds.), *The Unwed Mother.* Boston: United Community Services of Metropolitan Boston, 1970.

Caplan, G. "Schools and the Challenge of Change." In S. Alexander and D. Lancaster (Eds.), *Schools and the Challenge of Change.* Pittsburgh: United Mental Health Services of Allegheny County, 1970.

Caplan, G. "Summation." In S. Alexander and D. Lancaster (Eds.), *Schools and the Challenge of Change.* Pittsburgh: United Mental Health Services of Allegheny County, 1970.

Caplan, G. *Theory and Practice of Mental Health Consultation.* New York: Basic Books, 1970.

Spivack, M., Weiss, R. S., Caplan, G., Sheldon, A. P., and Schulberg, H. C. *Mental Health Implications of the Organization of the Large-Scale Physical Environment.* Hearings Before the Select Committee on Nutrition and Human Needs of the U.S. Senate (91st Congress, 2nd session on Nutrition and Human Needs). Washington, D.C., 1970.

1972

Caplan, G. "Sex Problems in Happy Marriages." *Redbook,* July 1972, pp. 120-123.

Caplan, R. B., Caplan, G., Richards, D., and Stokes, A. P. *Helping the Helpers to Help.* New York: Seabury Press, 1972.

1973

Caplan, G. "An Outpouring of Love for Shirley Temple Black." *McCall's,* Mar. 1973, pp. 48, 50, 52, 54.

1974

Caplan, G. *Support Systems and Community Mental Health: Lectures in Concept Development.* New York: Behavioral Publications, 1974.

Caplan, G. (Ed.). *The American Handbook of Psychiatry.* Vol. 2. New York: Basic Books, 1974.

Caplan, G. "When Stress Becomes Too Much." In *Coping with Stress.* Chicago: Blue Cross Association, 1974.

1975

Caplan, G. "A Multimodal Approach to Primary Prevention of Mental Disorders in Children." In L. Levi (Ed.), *Society, Stress, and Disease.* Vol. 2: *Childhood and Adolescence.* Oxford, England: Oxford University Press, 1975.

Caplan, G. "Beyond Consultation: A Support Systems Approach." In *Proceedings of a Conference on Innovations in Mental Health Consultation to Clergy.* Ann Arbor, Mich.: Washtenaw County Community Mental Health Center, 1975.

Caplan, G. "In Memorium–Erich Lindemann, 1900-1974." *American Journal of Psychiatry,* 1975, *132,* 3.

Caplan, G. "Support Systems in Times of War" (in Hebrew). In *The Individual and the Community in Times of Emergency.* Jerusalem: Ministry of Interior, 1975.

1976

Caplan, G. "Foreword." In H. Parad, H. L. P. Resnick, and L. Parad (Eds.), *Emergency and Disaster Management.* Bowie, Md.: Charles Press, 1976.

Caplan, G. "Introduction and Overview." In G. Caplan and M. Killilea (Eds.), *Support Systems and Mutual Help: Multidisciplinary Explorations.* New York: Grune & Stratton, 1976.

Caplan, G. "Organization of Support Systems for Civilian Populations." In G. Caplan and M. Killilea (Eds.), *Support Systems and Mutual Help: Multidisciplinary Explorations.* New York: Grune & Stratton, 1976.

Caplan, G. "Spontaneous or Natural Support Systems." In A. H. Katz and E. I. Bender (Eds.), *The Strength in Us: Self-Help Groups in the Modern World.* New York: Franklin Watts, 1976.

Caplan, G. "The Family as Support System." In G. Caplan and M. Killilea (Eds.), *Support Systems and Mutual Help: Multidisciplinary Explorations.* New York: Grune & Stratton, 1976.

Caplan, G., and Killilea, M. (Eds.). *Support Systems and Mutual Help: Multidisciplinary Explorations.* New York: Grune & Stratton, 1976.

1980

Caplan, G. "An Approach to Preventive Intervention in Child Psychiatry." *Canadian Journal of Psychiatry,* 1980, *25,* 671-682.

Caplan, G. "Individual and Group Reactions to Stress" (in Hebrew). *Ha-Oref* (Tel-Aviv), Apr.-May 1980, pp. 41-43.

Caplan, G., and Caplan, R. B. *Arab and Jew in Jerusalem: Explorations in Community Mental Health.* Cambridge, Mass.: Harvard University Press, 1980.

Kornberg, M. S., and Caplan, G. "Risk Factors and Preventive Intervention in Child Psychopathology: A Review." *Journal of Prevention,* 1980, *1,* 71-133.

1981

Caplan, G. "Mastery of Stress: Psychosocial Aspects." *American Journal of Psychiatry,* 1981, *138,* 4.

Caplan, G. "Partnerships for Prevention in the Human Services." *Journal of Primary Prevention,* 1981, *2,* 3-5.

Caplan, G., and others. "Patterns of Cooperation of Child Psychiatry with Other Departments in Hospital." *Journal of Primary Prevention,* 1981, *2,* 40-49.

Menahem, S., Lipton, G. L., and Caplan, G. "The Psychologically Orientated Pediatrician and the Provision of Psychoanalytic Psychotherapy." *Child Psychiatry and Human Development,* 1981, *12,* 67-81.

1982

Caplan, G. "Epilogue: Personal Reflections." In H. C. Schulberg and M. Killilea (Eds.), *The Modern Practice of Community Mental Health: A Volume in Honor of Gerald Caplan.* San Francisco: Jossey-Bass, 1982.

Name Index

Abrahams, R. B., 72-73, 334-357
Acock, A., 257-258, 261
Adams, G. L., 82, 491, 508, 587-610
Adams, J. E., 174, 204, 619, 629
Addis, B., 642, 647
Adler, D., 44, 84
Adler, N. E., 490, 512-513
Ahearn, F. L., 399, 416, 417
Albee, G. W., 127, 140, 143-144
Aldrete, J., 491, 510-511
Alexander, F., 12
Alexander, J. F., 441, 443
Allard, M. A., 475, 482
Allen, J. R., 81, 565-586
Allinsmith, W., 457, 461
Alpert, J. J., 588-589, 606
Ames, A., 167, 196
Anderson, J. L., 195, 199
Anderson, R., 618, 629
Anderson, S., 96, 119
Andrews, G., 181, 196
Anthony, W., 526, 535
Antze, P., 259-260, 261
Applebaum, P., 60, 84
Archer, J., 183, 204
Arieti, S., 77, 84
Armor, D., 250, 261
Armstrong, L., 475, 483
Arnold, C. R., 554-555, 562
Arthur, R. J., 222-223, 229
Ashbaugh, J., 61, 84
Attkisson, C. C., 266, 272, 286, 501, 507, 509, 524, 536
Attneave, C. L., 183, 212, 420, 444
Austin, M. J., 255, 256, 261
Authier, J., 508, 509
Averill, J. R., 173, 207
Avery, B. J., 280, 286

Bachrach, L., 59-60, 67, 69, 70, 84-85
Backer, T., 524, 535
Bahn, A. K., 107, 119
Baker, A. P., 252, 256, 261

Baker, F., 56-57, 92, 246-264, 489, 509, 530, 538, 626, 629, 655, 656, 666
Baldwin, J. A., 107, 119
Balint, M., 6, 7
Bandura, A., 620, 629
Banta, D. A., 591, 606
Barker, R. G., 181, 196, 456, 462
Barnes, J. A., 178, 196
Bass, R. D., 80, 85, 553, 562
Bassuk, E. L., 236, 244, 248, 262
Baumheir, E. C., 469, 482
Beck, D. F., 422, 441
Becker, E., 349, 354
Becker, H. A., 166, 196
Beery, W. L., 182, 190, 211
Beigel, A., 592, 606
Belle, D., 179, 196
Bender, E. I., 52, 89, 187, 206
Bennett, C. L., 115, 121
Berg, R. L., 337, 354
Bergner, L., 78, 85
Berkman, L. F., 139, 144, 179, 182, 196
Berkman, P. L., 337, 356
Berlin, I., 63, 85
Berlin, R., 80-81, 85
Berlin, T. N., 455, 462
Bernard, H., 55, 89
Bertelsen, A., 108, 122
Bessell, H., 449, 462
Bhrolchain, M. A., 180, 197
Bibring, G., 13-14, 15
Bindman, A. J., 71, 372-396
Bion, W., 6, 7
Birren, J. E., 336, 354
Blenker, M., 341, 354
Bloch, S., 102, 119
Block, W. E., 251, 262
Bloom, B. L., 42, 50-51, 85, 126-147, 193, 421, 441, 446, 448, 462
Bloom, J., 81, 86
Bloom, M., 354, 448, 457, 462
Blumenthal, M. D., 568, 584
Boggs, E., 72, 85
Boggs, E. M., 379, 396
Bond, G., 187, 208, 523, 537
Bond, L., 140, 144
Bonney, M. E., 448, 463-464
Bordow, S., 183, 196
Borkman, T., 186, 197, 613, 616, 629
Borman, L. D., 52, 90, 621, 630
Borus, J. F., 42-43, 66, 85, 491, 493, 494-495, 509, 590, 591, 606-607
Boss, F., 570, 586
Bott, E., 178, 197
Boulding, K., 238, 244
Bowen, M., 430, 432, 433, 442
Bower, E. M., 446, 447, 462
Bowlby, J., 6, 7, 37, 165, 177, 178, 197, 617-618, 629, 668
Bradburn, N., 150, 161
Braddock, D., 72, 85
Bradshaw, W. H., 458, 462, 592, 607
Brassard, J. A., 179, 199
Braun, P., 70, 85
Braverman, J., 459, 462
Breeskin, J., 251, 262
Brenneis, C. B., 591, 607
Brenner, M. H., 96, 119
Brinton, J., 29
Brodie, H., 77, 84
Brodie, H. K. H., 174, 204
Brody, E. B., 96, 122
Brody, E. M., 339, 354
Bromet, E., 521, 522, 538
Bronfenbrenner, U., 181, 197, 446, 447, 455, 457, 462
Broskowski, A., 61-62, 66-67, 86, 265-288, 479, 482, 486-513
Brown, B. S., 584
Brown, G. W., 108, 109, 115, 119, 125, 180, 181, 197, 217, 227
Brown, V., 419, 442
Bruhn, J. G., 182, 197
Budman, S. D., 66-67, 77, 86, 423, 442, 495-496, 497, 509-510
Budson, R. D., 183, 197
Burke, J. D., 486*n*, 488, 491, 510
Burnand, G., 150, 161
Burns, B. J., 488, 491, 496, 504, 510
Burns, J. M., 269, 287
Buros, O., 524, 535
Bursten, B., 44, 86
Busk, P., 449, 465
Butcher, J. N., 422, 442
Butler, R. N., 344, 348, 355, 356
Butts, G. K., 634, 649
Byrne, D. G., 181-182, 205

Cabot, R., 186
Cadden, V., 24, 38, 173, 198, 673, 675, 676
Callahan, J., 354, 355
Campbell, A., 149-150, 161
Campbell, D., 528, 535
Cancro, R., 101-102, 119
Cannon, W. B., 165, 176, 197
Cantril, H., 167, 198, 205
Capildeo, R., 183, 198
Caplan, A. S., 4
Caplan, D., 1-2
Caplan, G., x-xi, xii-xiii, 2, 11, 15, 17, 19, 20, 24, 26, 30-31, 32, 34, 35, 36, 37-38, 39, 46, 50, 51, 52, 54, 63, 64, 65, 73, 74, 75, 77, 83, 86, 89, 127, 131, 137, 138, 144, 146, 149, 161, 164-165, 170, 171, 173, 175, 177, 181, 186, 188, 193, 198-199, 207, 209, 211, 219, 227, 252, 262, 289, 291-293, 298, 305-306, 311, 340, 342, 355, 360, 366, 371, 373, 396, 399, 400, 416, 419, 426, 440, 443, 445, 446, 447, 448, 450, 452, 462-463, 477, 482-483, 577, 584, 650-679. *See also* Subject Index entry
Caplan, R. B., 33, 34, 35, 38, 39, 184, 188, 199, 252, 349, 355, 650-651, 666, 675, 676, 677, 679
Caplan, S. Z., 1
Caplan-Moskovich, R. B., 1-39
Caplovitz, D., 150, 161
Carmines, E. G., 100, 125
Carter, B. D., 452, 463
Carter, D., 524, 535
Carter, J. E., 44
Cartwright, A., 195, 199
Cassel, J. C., 137, 138-139, 144, 176, 181, 182, 183, 199, 206, 209, 339, 355
Castellon, R. S., 399, 416
Castelnuevo-Tedesco, P., 575, 584
Catalano, R., 96, 107, 120
Cazares, P. R., 452, 463
Cedar, T. B., 474, 483
Celentano, D., 179, 208
Charney, E., 588-589, 606
Cheney, C. C., 587*n*
Chu, F. D., 256, 262
Chun, K., 524, 535
Cibulka, J., 57, 93
Clark, L. B., 556, 562
Clarkin, J., 65, 87
Cleary, P., 524, 535
Cluff, L. E., 570, 586
Cobb, S., 149, 161, 176, 177, 181, 199, 202, 524, 535
Cochran, M. M., 179, 199
Coggershall, L. T., 571, 587, 607
Cohen, D., 337, 345, 355
Cohen, F., 490, 512-513
Cohen, M., 526, 535
Cohen, R. E., 75, 397-418
Coleman, J. V., 171, 199, 495, 510, 590, 607
Coleman, R. F., 452, 463
Coles, R., 621, 630
Colletta, N. C., 179, 199
Collins, A. H., 182, 186, 188, 200, 626, 629
Colmen, J. G., 169, 201
Comings, L., 542, 562
Comrey, A., 524, 535
Conley, R. W., 373, 396
Connolly, T., 517, 535
Converse, P., 149-150, 161
Cook, T., 528, 530, 535, 537
Cooley, C. H., 148-149, 151, 161
Cooper, J. E., 102, 107, 110, 119, 125
Cooper, S., 449, 463
Costa, P. T., 349, 356
Court, C., 183, 198
Cowen, E. L., 446, 448, 456, 463
Cox, G., 272, 273, 287
Cravens, R. B., 553, 562
Crocetti, G. M., 109, 122
Crogg, S. H., 183, 200
Cronbach, L. J., 256, 262
Crown, V., 570, 586
Cumming, E., 341, 355
Cummings, N., 491, 510
Cummins, R. O., 591, 607
Curle, A., 169, 200
Curtis, W., 46, 47, 61, 86
Curtis, W. R., 186, 200
Cutter, D., 81, 86
Cypress, B. K., 140, 144-145

Datel, W., 525, 535
Davenport, J., 469, 472, 483
Davenport, J., III, 469, 472, 483
Davidson, T., 620, 629
Davis, K., 611, 629
Dean, A., 53, 86, 176, 181, 200, 208
de Araujo, G., 183, 200
DeFleur, M., 257-258, 261
deGoza, S., 173, 205
Delgaudio, A. C., 258-259, 262
Demone, H. W., Jr., 56, 79, 230-245, 540-564
Dener, B., 590, 607
Derogatis, L., 524, 535
DeRosis, H. A., 454, 463
Derr, J. M., 482
Descartes, R., 566
Deutsch, J., 517, 535
Dewey, J., 149, 162
DeWild, D. W., 127, 145
Diedrich, B., 636, 648
Dielman, T. E., 568, 584
DiMatteo, M. R., 194, 200
Dinitz, S., 113, 115, 123
Dinkel, N., 531, 535
Dinkmeyer, D., 455, 463
Dixon, W. J., 112, 119
Dohrenwend, B. P., 97, 100, 108, 110, 111, 112, 119-120, 136, 145, 181, 191-193, 200, 238, 244, 400, 417
Dohrenwend, B. S., 97, 108, 110, 111, 119-120, 136, 145, 181, 191-193, 200, 203, 238, 244, 400, 417
Dooley, D., 96, 107, 120
Douvan, E., 187, 213
Drossman, D. A., 591, 607
Drucker, P. F., 275, 287
Dubos, R., 142, 145
Duhl, L., 23
Dunbar, E., 475, 483
Duncan-Jones, P., 157, 181-182, 205
Dunham, H. W., 105, 120
Dydhalo, N., 457, 465

Earls, F., 503-504, 510
Eaton, J. S., 577, 586
Eaton, J. W., 255, 262
Eaton, W. W., 48, 87, 110, 120, 181, 200
Eckenrode, J., 181, 200-201
Edwards, D., 529, 535
Egbert, L. D., 173, 201, 218, 227
Ehrlich, R., 491, 508, 511
Eisdorfer, C., 337, 345, 355
Eisenberg, L., 129, 132, 137, 140, 145
Eliot, T. D., 166, 201
Ellsworth, R., 525, 528-529, 535-536
Emerson, W. R. P., 186, 201
Endicott, J., 48, 87, 98, 107, 124, 518, 524, 536
Engel, G. L., 176, 201, 565, 584
English, J. T., 23, 169, 201, 208, 591, 609
Ennis, B., 58, 87
Ensel, W., 53, 86, 181, 208
Erickson, G. D., 183, 201
Erikson, E. H., 165, 201
Erikson, K. T., 399, 402, 417
Evans, L., 641, 648
Ewalt, J. R., 27-28, 29, 32

Fair, E., 481*n*, 483
Fairweather, G. W., 183, 186, 201
Feifel, H., 349, 355
Feigner, J. P., 98, 120
Feld, S., 187, 204
Feldman, S., 62-63, 87, 268, 287
Felix, R. H., 24, 26
Fenton, F. R., 116, 120
Fields, S., 344, 355
Filstead, W., 529-530, 536
Fine, P., 183, 201
Fine, V. K., 576, 585
Fink, F. J., 589, 607
Fink, P. J., 80-81, 87, 589, 607, 609
Finlayson, A., 183, 201
Fischer, A., 49, 92
Fischer, C. S., 182, 202
Fischer, M., 108, 122
Fisher, C., 351, 355
Fishman, H. C., 430, 443
Fitzgerald, R., 218, 227
Flaherty, E., 531, 535
Flax, J. W., 467, 469, 473, 474, 477, 483
Fleiss, J. L., 97, 120, 124
Flexner, A., 565, 567, 585
Flomenhaft, K., 424, 442

Folkman, S., 175, 202
Follette, W., 491, 510
Ford, M., 60, 87
Ford, R. C., 449, 465
Forgays, D., 140, 145
Fox, R., 583, 585
Fox, R. C., 591, 606
Framo, J., 430, 439, 442
Frances, A., 65, 87
Frank, J. D., 113, 120
Frank, R., 61, 80, 87, 516, 536
Frederick, C. J., 400, 417
Freidson, E., 182, 202, 258, 262, 615, 629
French, J., 12, 524, 535
French, J. R. P., Jr., 181, 202, 207
Freud, A., 6, 7
Freud, S., 149, 162, 172, 202, 247
Friedlander, K., 6, 7
Fritz, C. E., 399, 417
Froland, C., 182, 187, 202
Frydman, M. I., 181, 202
Fryer, J., 580, 586
Fryers, T., 109, 125
Futcher, P. H., 577, 585

Gage, R. W., 482
Galileo, G., 566
Gans, S., 492, 493, 510
Garcia, A., 592, 607
Gardner, E. A., 107, 120
Gardner, G., 14
Garrison, J., 183, 202
Garrison, V., 183, 202
Gartner, A., 52, 74, 87, 187, 202, 613, 625, 629
Gennep, A. van, 169, 202, 224, 228
Gerson, S., 236, 244, 248, 262
Gerstel, N., 179, 202-203
Gettings, R. M., 381, 396
Giacalone, J. J., 589, 608
Gibson, M., 78, 88
Gilbert, D., 249, 262
Gilbert, J. P., 96, 120-121
Gilchrist, L., 504, 510
Gildea, M. C. L., 454, 463
Glaser, E., 524, 535
Glass, A. J., 167, 203
Glass, G., 490, 491, 505, 512
Glasscote, R. M., 50, 88, 346, 355-356
Glick, I. O., 654, 666
Glidewell, J. E., 454, 463
Goetzel, V., 236, 245
Goffman, E., 623, 629
Goldberg, D., 96, 121
Goldberg, E., 179, 203
Goldberg, I. D., 48, 92, 126, 146, 488, 506, 510, 512
Goldberger, J., 95, 121
Golden, R. R., 193, 203
Goldman, F., 14-15, 27
Goldman, H., 68, 88
Goldman, W., 45-46, 88
Goldstein, C., 268, 287
Goldston, S. E., 50, 89, 129, 145, 445, 463
Goodhart, D., 522, 539
Goodstein, L., 63, 88
Goplerud, E., 490, 510
Gordon, J. E., 15, 108, 123
Gordon, J. S., 344, 356
Gore, S., 176, 181, 191, 200-201, 203, 206
Gorham, D., 524, 537
Gori, G., 569, 585
Gottlieb, B. H., 52, 88, 139, 145, 179, 182, 203
Gove, W. R., 98, 121
Gracey, C., 445*n*
Grad, J., 188, 195, 211
Grady, M., 78, 88
Granovetter, M. S., 180, 203
Gray, P. D., 588, 607
Green, L. W., 570, 585
Greenblatt, M., 676
Gregg, C. H., 179, 199
Griffin, C. L., 447, 458-459, 463, 465
Griggs, J. W., 448, 463-464
Grimes, J. W., 457, 461
Grobman, J., 591, 608
Gross, H. W., 251, 262-263
Gruenbaum, H., 675
Gruenberg, E. M., 52, 68, 72, 88, 115, 121, 128, 131, 139, 141, 145, 182, 183, 189, 190, 193, 195, 203-204
Grunberg, E., 114, 122
Gudeman, J. E., 355-356
Guerra, F., 491, 510-511
Gump, P., 456, 462

Gurin, G., 187, 204
Gussow, Z., 184, 204
Gutheil, T., 60, 84
Gutwirth, L., 53, 88, 179, 205

Hagedorn, H., 491, 511, 524, 536
Hagens, J. H., 218, 228
Hall, T. L., 545, 562
Halstead, L. S., 578, 585
Halstead, M. S., 578, 585
Hamburg, B. A., 74, 88, 172, 173, 174, 176, 181, 204, 205
Hamburg, D. A., 172, 173, 174, 204-205, 619, 629
Hammer, M., 53, 88, 179, 205
Hamovitch, M. D., 671
Hankin, J., 489-490, 505, 511
Hansell, N., 68, 114, 115-116, 121, 177, 183, 186-187, 189, 205, 358-371, 415, 417
Hanushek, E. A., 106, 121
Hare, P., 671
Hargreaves, W., 524, 536
Harrington, M., 467, 483
Harris, L., 336, 356
Harris, T. O., 108, 109, 119, 180, 181, 197, 217, 227
Harshbarger, D., 56, 79, 230-245
Harty, M., 530, 536
Hassinger, E. W., 468, 471, 483
Hatfield, A. B., 183, 205
Hausman, C. P., 345, 356
Hausman, W., 63, 88
Haynes, R. B., 571, 586
Hays, R., 194, 200
Heinroth, J. C., 573
Heller, K., 52, 88-89
Helming, M., 96, 124
Henderson, A. S., 152, 153, 157, 162, 178, 180, 181-182, 205
Henderson, S., 53, 89
Henry VIII, 2
Henry, W. E., 341, 355
Hersch, C., 251, 263
Herz, M. I., 116, 121
Herzog, A. N., 95*n*, 107, 110, 122
Hill, R., 170, 205
Hinton, J., 221, 228
Hippocrates of Cos, 567
Hirsch, B., 55, 89
Hirschowitz, R. G., 63, 312-333
Hobbs, N., 247, 263
Hockey, L., 195, 199
Hoffer, W., 6
Hogarty, G., 525, 536
Holahan, C. J., 51, 89, 338, 356
Holland, B. C., 591, 608
Hollander, R., 57, 82, 89, 247, 263
Hollen, L., 491, 508, 511
Hollingshead, A. B., 97-98, 121, 249-250, 263
Hollister, W. G., 449, 464
Holmes, T., 181, 205
Holst, E., 182, 207
Holtzman, W. H., 592, 608
Homans, G., 149, 162
Hopkins, B. R., 282, 287
Horton, C., 492, 493, 510
Horwitz, L., 530, 536
Houge, D., 268, 287
Houpt, J. L., 490, 511, 568, 569, 579, 585
House, J. S., 149, 150, 162, 181, 207
Howard, G., 529, 536
Howard, L. A., 251, 263
Howell, J., 268, 287
Hudson, J. I., 589, 608
Huey, K., 626, 629
Hurvitz, N., 616, 629-630

Inui, T. S., 591, 607
Iscoe, I., 139, 145, 458, 464
Ittleson, W. H., 167, 205

Jackson, D. A., 224, 229
Jackson, E. J. R., 182, 190, 211
Jackson, J. E., 106, 121
Jacobson, G. F., 171, 205
James, D., 173, 205
James, S., 182, 206
Janis, I. L., 172-173, 206, 322, 333
Janowitch, L. A., 590, 607
Janowitz, M., 149, 162
Jaques, E., 324, 333
Jayaratne, S., 428, 442
Joffe, J. M., 140, 144
John, D., 493, 511
Johnson, C., 445*n*
Johnson, C. W., 641, 648
Johnson, L. B., 379
Jones, J. D., 476, 483

Jones, K., 490, 491, 505, 511
Jones, M. A., 182, 206, 422, 439, 441, 442, 443
Jones, R., 96, 121
Joslin, E., 186
Juel-Nielsen, N., 109, 121, 337, 356

Kadushin, A., 452, 464
Kagan, J., 621, 630
Kagey, J. R., 139, 145
Kahn, R. L., 179-180, 181, 202, 206
Kain, J. F., 106, 121
Kamerman, S. B., 350, 356
Kamis-Gould, E., 49, 91
Kaplan, B. H., 176, 181, 183, 206, 209
Kaplan, D. M., 170-171, 198, 206, 207, 424, 441, 442, 674
Kapp, F. T., 399, 417-418
Kasl, S. V., 570, 585
Kastenbaum, R., 349, 356
Katz, A. H., 52, 89, 182, 187, 206, 207, 626, 630
Katz, M., 525, 536
Kaufman, M. K., 454, 463
Keill, S., 67, 89
Kellam, S. G., 74, 89, 454-455, 457-458, 464
Kelly, J. B., 654, 666
Kelly, J. G., 456, 464
Kennedy, D. A., 451, 464
Kennedy, J. F., 25, 40, 378, 379, 396, 657, 663
Kenny, D. A., 104, 121
Kent, M. W., 140, 145
Keppler-Seid, H., 517, 520, 536-537
Kesselman, M., 101-102, 119
Kessler, L., 488, 510
Ketterer, R., 78, 89
Kieffer, F., 590, 607
Killilea, M., ix-xiii, 29, 31, 36, 38, 40-94, 163-214, 477, 482-483, 613, 630, 653, 666, 678
Killworth, P., 55, 89
Kimmel, W. A., 548-549, 563
Kiresuk, T. J., 96, 121
Kissinger, H., 272, 273-274, 287
Kitching, E. H., 3, 4, 5, 6
Klebanoff, L. B., 71, 372-396
Klee, G. D., 96, 122
Kleiman, M. A., 626, 630
Klein, D. C., 50, 89, 171, 206
Kleinbaum, D. G., 182, 206
Klerman, G. L., 141, 147, 250, 261, 543, 563
Kliman, A. S., 403, 417
Kline, L. Y., 591, 608
Kohler, M., 74, 87
Kole, D. M., 549, 555, 563
Konan, M., 475, 483
Koos, E. L., 170, 206
Kornberg, M. S., 89, 131, 146, 193, 207, 653, 666, 679
Korsch, B., 586
Koss, M. P., 422, 442
Kouzes, J. M., 274-275, 287
Kramer, M., 64, 72, 89-90, 190, 207
Krupinski, J., 107-108, 121-122
Kubler-Ross, E., 349, 356, 618, 630
Kuhn, T., 246-247, 263
Kulka, R. A., 187, 213
Kulp, C., 183, 202
Kuriloff, P., 449, 464

Lalonde, M., 130, 146
Lamb, H. R., 43, 51, 90, 94, 140, 146, 236, 245, 591, 610
Lammert, M. H., 591, 608
Langbein, L. I., 106, 122
Langsley, D. G., 43, 90, 171, 207, 424, 425, 441, 442
Langston, J., 487, 511
Langston, R. D., 251, 263
LaRocco, J. M., 181, 207
Larsen, D., 525, 537
Laub, D., 591, 607
Lavrakas, F., 445*n*
Lawton, M. P., 339, 356
Lazarus, A. A., 428, 442
Lazarus, H. R., 218, 228
Lazarus, R. S., 173, 175, 202, 207
Lazerson, A. M., 591, 608
Leavell, H. R., 14, 27
LeBon, G., 149, 162
Lebovici, S., 675, 676
Lee, R. H., 450, 466
LeFave, H. G., 114, 122
Leff, J. P., 108, 122
Leighton, A. H., 46, 47
Leighton, B., 182, 213
Leighton, D. C., 101, 103, 107, 111, 122

Leininger, M., 592, 608
Lemkau, P. V., 109, 122
Lemle, R., 448, 449, 464
Lenneberg, E., 614, 623-624, 630
Leopold, R., 23
Leutz, W. N., 182, 207
Levin, L. S., 182, 207
Levine, C. H., 276, 277, 278, 287
Levine, D. S., 338, 356
Levine, S., 183, 200
Levinsohn, D., 618, 630
Levinson, D., 249-250, 260, 262, 263, 264
Levinson, H., 63, 289-311, 313, 319, 322, 326, 333
Lévi-Strauss, C., 181, 207
Levy, L. H., 47, 48, 95-125, 184, 207, 625, 630
Lewin, K., 181, 207
Lewis, M. I., 348, 356
Liberman, R., 182, 208
Lichtman, A. J., 106, 122
Lieberman, M. A., 52, 90, 187, 208, 339, 356, 523, 537, 621, 630
Lifton, R. J., 399, 417, 621-622, 630
Light, R. J., 96, 120-121
Lin, N., 53, 86, 176, 179, 181, 200, 208
Lin, T., 108, 122
Lindemann, E., 12-13, 14, 15, 18, 26, 32, 39, 166-167, 171, 183, 206, 208, 223, 228, 399, 400, 417, 660
Lindenthal, J. J., 181, 209
Lippitt, G. L., 296, 311
Lipsett, D. R., 591, 608
Lipson, A., 183, 200
Lipton, G. L., 679
Liptzin, B., 79, 90, 546, 563
Litwak, E., 183, 208
Lloyd-Campbell, C., 554
Long, N., 493, 511
Longest, J., 475, 483
Lord, G., 532, 538
Lorr, M., 524, 537
Lounsbury, J., 46, 90
Lowenkopf, E., 504, 511
Lowenthal, M. F., 337, 356
Lund, S. H., 96, 121
Lutz, W., 139, 145
Lyerly, S., 525, 536

Mabe, P., 533, 538
McAuliffe, W., 520, 537
MacBride, A., 180-181, 213
McElhinney, R., 572, 585
McGuire, T., 61, 80, 90
Machotka, P., 424, 442
Macht, L., 493, 512, 676
Macindoe, I., 268, 287
McKelvey, J., 475, 483
McKinlay, J. B., 182, 208
MacMillan, D., 183, 208
McPheeters, H. L., 129, 146
McQueen, D. V., 179, 208
McTighe, J., 277-278, 287
Maddison, D. C., 181, 208
Majchrzak, A., 514, 537
Makiesky-Barrow, S., 53, 88, 179, 205
Mann, P. A., 137, 146
Mannhein, K., 167, 208
Marcuse, D. J., 591, 609
Marks, E., 66-67, 86, 491, 497, 512
Marmor, J., 422, 442
Marris, M., 586
Marris, P., 216, 228, 322, 333, 618, 630
Martinez, J., 592, 608
Masnick, R., 517, 537
Mason, E. A., 82, 170-171, 198, 206, 633-649, 674
Massey, F. J., Jr., 112, 119
Masters, R. J., 346, 357
Matus, R., 50, 90
Mawson, D., 225, 228
Maynard, H., 183, 186, 201
Mazer, M., 472, 473, 483
Mead, G. H., 149, 162
Mechanic, D., 439, 442
Mednick, S., 50, 90
Menahem, S., 679
Mendoza, L., 182, 187, 213
Menninger, W. W., 169, 208
Menzies, I. E. P., 324, 333
Mersh, S., 381, 396
Merton, R., 181, 208
Meyer, A., 181, 208-209
Meyers, J. K., 181, 209, 450, 464
Michaels, J. J., 15
Mico, P. R., 274-275, 287

Mikawa, J. K., 96, 122
Miles, D. G., 355-356
Miller, M., 337, 357
Miller, S., 518, 537
Millis, J., 571, 587, 608
Mills, G. W., 142, 146
Mintzberg, H., 271, 272, 275, 276, 287-288
Minuchin, S., 430, 432, 443
Mischler, E. G., 109, 122
Mitchell, J. C., 178, 209
Mitnick, L., 549, 555, 563
Moffic, H. S., 589, 592, 608
Monroe, R. R., 96, 122
Moos, R. H., 182, 209, 457, 466, 526, 537
Moreno, J. L., 181, 209
Morical, L., 477-478, 484
Morrill, R., 495, 512
Morrill, W. A., 479, 484
Morris, J. N., 99, 122
Morrison, A. P., 591, 608
Morrison, J. K., 57, 91, 253-254, 263
Morrison, M., 582
Mosteller, F., 96, 120-121
Moyers, B., 643
Mueller, D. P., 53, 90, 179, 209
Muller, A., 134, 146
Multari, G., 452, 464
Mumford, E., 490, 491, 505, 512
Murphy, J., 525, 535
Murphy, J. M., 102, 123
Murray, H. A., 181, 209
Murrow, H. G., 614, 631
Musto, D. F., 589, 609
Myers, J. K., 48, 90, 98, 99, 108-109, 123, 124-125, 518-519, 539

Nagi, S., 336, 357
Neher, J., 637, 648
Neigher, W., 532, 539
Nelson, C. M., 634, 648
Nelson, R. C., 450, 464
Nelson, S. H., 553
Nesser, W., 182, 209
Neugarten, B. L., 343, 357
Neuhring, E., 50, 90
Nevid, J. S., 57, 91, 253-254, 263
Newman, F., 524, 535
Newton, I., 566
Neilsen, A., 81, 91, 584, 585
Nielsen, M., 354
Nixon, R. M., 42, 233
Noren, J., 270, 288
Northman, J. E., 252, 261
Nuckolls, K. B., 181, 183, 209

O'Brien, G., 66, 91, 267, 286
Offutt, J., 268, 287
O'Flaherty, H., 491, 510
Ogburn, K. D., 455, 463
Ojemann, R. H., 73, 91, 448, 464-465
Oken, D., 589, 607, 609
Oktay, J., 489-490, 505, 511
Olarte, S., 517, 537
O'Neil, T., 222-223, 229
Opton, E. M., 173, 207
O'Reilly, J. J., 4, 6
Orzack, L. H., 541, 563
Osborne, P., 272, 273, 287
Otto, J., 526, 537
Overall, J., 524, 537
Owens, C., 671
Ozarin, L. D., 75-76, 467-485

Packard, R., 280, 286
Pacoe, L., 576, 586
Pancoast, D. L., 182, 186, 200, 626, 629
Papp, P., 434, 443
Parad, H. J., 77, 137, 146, 170, 209, 419-444, 672
Parad, L. G., 137, 146, 419, 421, 422, 443
Pardes, H., 65, 67, 79, 91, 420, 443
Park, R. E., 167, 209
Parker, M. C., 654, 666
Parkes, C. M., 54, 169-170, 210, 215-229, 618, 630
Parloff, M., 524, 539
Parsons, B. V., 441, 443
Pasamanick, B., 113, 115, 123
Paschall, N., 525, 539
Patrick, D. L., 495, 510, 590, 607
Patterson, R. D., 72-73, 334-357
Pattison, E. M., 179, 183, 210
Paul, B., 15, 27
Paul, N., 430, 443
Paykel, E. S., 109, 123, 181, 210, 217, 229

Pearl, A., 625, 630
Pearlin, L. I., 175, 210
Pearse, I. H., 142, 147
Pearson, J. W., 589, 609
Penk, W., 529, 537
Pepper, M. P., 181, 209
Perlmutter, F. D., 50, 93, 128, 146
Perrow, C., 269, 288
Peters, W., 642, 648
Petersdorf, R. G., 588-589, 609
Peterson, R., 270, 288
Peterson, W. D., 450, 464
Petrie, D., 643, 648
Phillipus, M., 591, 609
Piasecki, J., 49, 91
Pincus, A., 67, 91, 497, 498, 499, 512
Pincus, H. A., 65, 91, 420, 443
Pincus, L., 618, 630
Pinel, P., 247
Pitt, N. W., 450, 464
Platt, S., 182, 210
Plunkett, R. J., 108, 123
Pokorny, A., 580, 586
Polak, P., 439, 442, 443
Pollack, P., 525, 535
Pomerleau, O., 570, 586
Porritt, D., 180, 183, 196, 210
Pratt, J. H., 185-186, 210
Prevost, J., 267, 286
Price, D. D. S., 547, 563
Price, R. H., 52, 88-89, 140, 146
Pricener, P., xiii
Proger, S. H., 186, 210
Prosen, H., 63, 88
Prugh, D., 14
Prunty, H. E., 453, 458, 465
Putnam, N., 580, 586

Quinn, R. P., 181, 206

Rabkin, J. G., 110, 123, 181, 211
Rae-Grant, A. F., 591, 609
Rahe, R. H., 181, 205, 217, 222-223, 229
Raiff, N., 614, 631
Ramsay, R. W., 225, 229
Rapoport, L., 171, 211
Rapoport, R. V., 169, 171, 211
Rappaport, R., 617, 631
Reagan, R., 45, 267, 541, 542
Reddaway, P., 102, 119
Redford, R., 643, 648
Redl, F., 419, 444
Redlich, F. C., 97-98, 121, 249-250, 263
Rees, J. R., 6, 7
Regan, J., 445*n*
Regier, D. A., 48, 64, 92, 93, 98, 99, 123, 126, 146, 488, 505, 512, 584
Reich, T., 96, 123
Reichardt, C., 530, 537
Reiff, R., 142, 146
Reifler, B., 577, 586
Reinherz, H. Z., 50, 73, 74, 445-466
Reiss, S., 457, 465
Resnick, H. L. P., 137, 146, 419, 443
Reul, M. R., 469, 484
Richards, D. E., 199, 677
Richardson, M., 71, 93
Richter, B. J., 569, 585
Rickman, J., 6, 7
Reissman, C. K., 179, 202-203
Riessman, F., 52, 74, 87, 182, 187, 202, 211, 613, 625, 629, 630
Rinder, M., 449, 464
Robertson, J., 639-640, 648
Robertson, J., 639-640
Robins, E., 98, 124
Robins, L., 48, 92, 519, 537
Robins, S. S., 483
Robinson, W. S., 105-106, 123
Rodgers, W., 181, 202
Rogawski, A. S., 78, 92
Rogers, C., 449-450, 465
Rogers, W., 149-150, 161
Rolf, J. E., 140, 145
Romano, L., 634, 648
Rose, F. C., 183, 198
Rose, S. M., 247-248, 263
Rosen, A., 517, 537
Rosen, B. M., 117, 123
Rosen, J., 140, 144
Rosen, S., 183, 202
Rosenblatt, P. C., 224, 229
Rosenfeld, A., 64, 93
Rosenfeld, J. M., 11, 39, 171, 211, 669
Rosenthal, A., 26
Roth, L., 59, 92

Roth, M., 337, 357
Rowbatham, J. L., 614, 630
Rowitz, L., 102, 105, 122
Rubin, J., 70, 92
Rubinstein, D., 424-425, 444
Rueveni, U., 420, 444
Rush, B., 573
Rustad, K., 449-450, 465
Ryan, J. H., 641, 648
Ryan, W., 138, 146

Sackett, D. L., 571, 586
Sainsbury, P., 188, 195, 211
Salasin, J., 474, 483
Salber, E. J., 182, 190, 211
Salmon, T., 167, 211
Sanders, D. H., 183, 186, 201, 211
Sanderson, E. V., 577, 585
Sartorius, N., 107, 125
Satore, R. L., 450, 464
Saunders, C. M., 221, 229
Scarpitti, F. P., 113, 115, 123
Schacter, S., 620-621, 631
Schainblatt, A., 532, 537
Scheff, T. J., 98, 123
Scherl, D. J., 591, 609
Schlesinger, H., 490, 491, 505, 512
Schlosberg, A., 254-255, 264
Schniewind, H., 503-504, 512
Schooler, C., 175, 210
Schuckit, M. A., 337, 357
Schulberg, H. C., ix-xiii, 40-94, 246, 250, 251, 252, 256, 258, 261-262, 264, 514-539, 655, 656, 666, 676, 677
Schulman, J. L., 449, 453, 465
Schulsinger, F., 50, 90
Schur, E. M., 98, 100, 123
Schutz, A., 196, 211
Schwab, J. J., 96, 103, 123
Schwartz, C., 625, 631
Schwartz, M., 625, 631
Scotch, N. A., 109, 122
Sechrest, L., 533, 538
Sehnert, K. W., 344, 357
Seidman, S. B., 451, 464
Selye, H., 176, 211
Shanas, E., 334, 357
Shapiro, J. H., 182, 186, 211
Shapiro, L. E., 101-102, 119
Sharaf, M., 249-250, 264
Sharfstein, S., 42, 92
Shaw, M. S., 218, 229
Sheinfeld, S., 532, 538
Sheldon, A. P., 677
Shepherd, M., 108, 124
Sher, K., 52, 88-89
Sherman, S., 420, 428, 444
Shields, P., 284, 288
Shils, E. A., 149, 162
Shneidman, E. S., 221, 229
Shore, J., 81, 86
Shore, M. F., 591, 608
Showstack, J., 531, 538
Shriver, S., 24
Shure, M. B., 138, 147, 448, 449, 454, 466
Signell, K. A., 450, 455, 466
Silverman, P. R., 82-83, 182, 183, 184, 187, 188, 211-212, 611-632
Silverman, S. M., 618, 632
Silverman, W. H., 453, 466
Simmel, G., 149, 162
Simon, B. B., 339, 356
Simon, H. A., 272, 288
Sinclair, I. A. C., 218, 229
Singer, T. L., 453, 458, 465
Skodol, A., 48, 92
Sluss, T. K., 182, 195, 204
Smith, D., 620, 632
Smith, R. W., 591, 607
Snibbe, J., 641, 648
Snow, H. B., 115, 121
Snow, J., 95, 124
Snyder, S. H., 362, 371
Sobel, D., 553, 563
Sorensen, A., 124
Sorensen, J., 524, 536
Spain, T., 643, 648
Speck, R. V., 183, 212, 420, 444
Spencer, L., 493, 512
Spitzer, R. L., 48, 87, 92, 97, 98, 100, 107, 124, 518, 536
Spivack, G., 448, 454, 466
Spivack, M., 677
Srole, L., 49, 92, 101, 103, 107, 111, 124, 467, 484
Stambler, H. V., 546-547, 563-564
Standley, C. C., 108, 122
Steidl, J. H., 428, 430, 444
Stein, L., 69, 70, 92, 93, 183, 212, 525, 527, 538, 539

Steward, R. B., 570, 586
Stewart, A., 114, 122
Stoddard, S., 350, 357
Stokes, A. P., Jr., 199, 677
Stone, A., 58, 92
Stone, B., 588, 609
Stone, G. C., 490, 512-513
Stout, C., 182, 212
Strauss, A. L., 194, 212, 249-250, 258, 264, 611, 632
Strauss, R., 574
Streuning, E. L., 116, 120, 181, 211
Stringer, L. A., 454, 466
Stroller, A., 107-108, 121-122
Stromgren, E., 124
Strosnider, J. S., 589, 607
Sturt, E., 107, 125
Sugarman, N. A., 282, 288
Sullivan, M., 445*n*
Syme, S. L., 139, 144, 179, 182, 196
Szasz, T. S., 100, 101, 124, 253, 264
Szelenyi, I., 183, 208

Talbott, J., 69, 92-93
Talbott, J. A., 167, 212
Tartakoff, H., 15
Taube, C. A., 48, 64, 92, 93, 126, 146, 488, 512
Ten Hoor, W., 70, 93, 183, 187, 212, 520-521, 538
Tessier, L., 116, 120
Test, M. A., 69, 70, 92, 93, 183, 212, 525, 527, 538, 539
Therrien, M. E., 576, 585
Thomas, L. A., 453, 458, 465
Thomas, W. I., 165-166, 167, 212
Tichy, M. K., 591, 609
Tichy, N. M., 332, 333
Tischler, G., 517, 538
Titchener, J. L., 399, 417-418
Todd, D. M., 139, 145
Tolsdorf, C. C., 179, 180, 183, 212
Toynbee, A., 349, 357
Tracy, G. S., 184, 204
Treusch, P. E., 282, 288
Trickett, E., 78, 88
Trickett, E. J., 457, 466
Trist, E. L., 6, 169, 200
Troop, J., 218, 229
Trotter, S., 256, 262
Tuke, S., 247
Turner, J., 70, 93, 183, 187, 212, 520-521, 538
Tusler, P. A., 577, 585
Tweed, D., 475, 483
Tweeten, L., 469, 484
Tyhurst, J. S., 167, 169, 212-213, 399, 400, 418, 617-618, 632
Tyroler, H., 182, 209

Uhlmann, J., 469, 484
Umana, R. F., 441, 444

Vachon, M. L. S., 180-181, 213
Vaillant, G. E., 324, 325, 333
Vallance, T., 477, 484
Vallé, R., 182, 187, 213
van Gennep, A., 169, 202, 224, 228
Van Vlack, J. D., 643, 648-649
Varenhorst, B., 74, 88
Vayda, A. M., 50, 93, 128, 146
Vega, W., 182, 187, 213
Venables, P., 50, 90
Veroff, J., 187, 204, 213
Vickers, G., 328, 333
Vida, F., 586
Vischi, T., 490, 491, 505, 511
Visotsky, H. M., 173, 213
Vitalo, R., 526, 535
Vivace, J., 139, 145
Volkan, V., 225, 229
Vorwaller, C. J., 280, 286

Wagenfeld, J., 469-470, 485
Wagenfeld, M. O., 75-76, 93, 467-485
Walker, E., 506, 513
Walker, K. N., 180-181, 213
Walker, W. L., 181, 208
Wallace, A. F. C., 167, 213
Wallack, S., 354, 355
Wallerstein, J. S., 654, 666
Walsh, R. P., 224, 229
Warren, D. I., 182, 213
Waskow, I., 524, 539
Watson, G. S., 134, 147
Watzlawick, P., 430, 444
Weal, E., 636, 649
Weinberg, J., 346, 357
Weiner, R., 42, 93
Weinstein, S., 80-81, 87

Weisbrod, B. A., 61, 70, 93, 96, 124, 527, 539
Weisman, A. D., 349, 357
Weiss, R. S., 53-54, 148-162, 170, 178, 180, 186, 213, 618, 632, 654, 666, 677
Weissman, M. M., 48, 90, 98, 99, 108-109, 123, 124-125, 141, 147, 518-519, 525, 539
Wellman, B., 182, 213
Wendt, P. R., 634, 649
Werner, B., 643
Wershow, H. J., 350, 357
West, M., 71, 93
Wexler, J. P., 428, 430, 444
White, R. W., 172, 214, 324, 333, 617, 619, 632
White, S., 62, 93, 284, 288, 491, 508, 511
Wilks, A., 134, 147
Willard, W., 587, 609
Williams, H. B., 399, 417
Williams, J., 48, 92
Williamson, G. S., 142, 147
Willis, G. L., 186-187, 205
Willner, S. G., 338, 356
Wilson, N., 518, 537
Windle, C., 57, 93, 514, 517, 520, 525, 532, 536-537, 539
Winer, L. G., 445*n*
Wing, J. K., 107, 109, 115, 125
Wing, L., 108, 125
Winslow, W., 80-81, 94
Wise, H., 591, 609
Wiseman, F., 645, 649
Witzke, D., 251, 262
Wolf, A., 676
Wolff, H. G., 176, 214
Wolff, S., 251, 262
Wolford, J. L., 590, 609-610
Woodburn, P. K., 128, 146
Woy, J., 517, 520, 536-537

Yarvis, R., 425, 444
Yeaton, W., 533, 538
Yee, T. T., 450, 466
Yessian, M., 46, 47, 86

Zador, P. L., 134, 147
Zautra, A., 522, 539
Zeller, R. A., 100, 125
Zilboorg, G. A., 247, 264
Zinober, J., 531, 535
Zubkoff, M., 542, 564
Zusman, J., 43, 51, 90, 94, 140, 146, 591, 610
Zwerling, I., 504, 511, 592, 610

Subject Index

Aarhus, Denmark, epidemiology in, 108
Accountability. *See* Evaluation
Accreditation: issue of, 554; of services for mentally retarded, 386-389
Accreditation Council for Mental Retardation and Developmental Disabilities (AC MRDD), 387-389, 395
Accreditation Council for the Mentally Retarded, 386
ACTION, programs for elderly by, 343
Action for Independent Retirement (AIR), 343
Adams v. *Califano*, and credentialing, 554
Adaptation: of chronically mentally ill, 360-365; and disaster victims, 400
Administration on Aging, 345
Administrators: decision processes by, 273-274; as integrators, 283-286; knowledge, attitudes, and skills needed by, 270-271; leadership and management by, 265-288; limited control by, 274-280; principles for, 285-286; school, and primary prevention, 453; training of, 62
Advocacy: for mentally retarded, 383-384; in rural areas, 480-482
Affective disorders, chronic: background of services for, 359; and medication to assist adaptation, 363-365; rates of, 108-109
Affective education, for children, 449
Affiliation, relationships of, 157-158
Affirmative action, for community mental health centers, 232, 240
Aggregation bias, in epidemiology, 105-107

Alabama: mentally retarded in, 392; rural areas in, 476
Alaska, Native Health Service of, 22
Alcohol, Drug Abuse, and Mental Health Administration (ADAMHA), 497, 534, 543, 544-545, 562
Alcoholics Anonymous, 184, 259, 260, 560; as mutual help group, 614, 622
Alcoholism, neglect of, in medical education, 579-580
Alzheimer's Senile Dementia Family Groups, 184
American Academy of Pediatrics, 387
American Association of Medical Colleges, 637
American Association of Medical Social Workers, 19
American Association of Retired Persons (AARP), 343
American Association on Mental Deficiency (AAMD), 374, 386, 387
American Automobile Association, 493
American Board of Internal Medicine, 573, 584
American Motorcyclist Association, 134
American Nurses Association, 387
American Occupational Therapy Association, 388
American Psychiatric Association, 48, 65, 69, 84, 98-99, 359, 371, 387, 575, 584, 637
American Psychological Association, 388
American Public Health Association, 131, 139, 144
Amniocentesis, issues of, 391
Anticipatory guidance: and Caplan, 17, 19, 23, 173, 219; and transitions, 218-222
Area Agency on Aging, 476
Arizona, Indian Health Service in, 22
Aroostook CMHC, interagency collaboration by, 478
Assessment. *See* Evaluation
Attachment, relationships of, 157
Attachment theory, and social support, 177-178
Audiovisuals: analysis of, 633-649; background of, 633-635; classic example of, 639-641; effectiveness of, 634; film versus video for, 635-641; future of, 646-647; human rights issues and, 638-639, 641-642; informed consent for, 639, 644-645; issues in, 641-645; and live or acted issue, 642-644; new programming in, 638-639; periodicals for, 637; software utilization in, 636-638
Australia, social support research in, 178

Bangor, Maine, and rural services, 476
Basic Books, 26
Baylor College of Medicine (BCM), 595-596, 598, 600, 602-603; Department of Community Medicine of, 594-595; Department of Psychiatry of, 595
Behavior, value system effects on, 257-259
Behavioral Repertoire, 525
Belief system. *See* Value system
Bennington County (Vermont), rural services in, 476
Beth Israel Hospital, 13-14
Biology, in prevention, 130, 132
Bishop-to-Bishop program, 183-184
Bi-State Mental Health Foundation, and community advocacy, 481-482
Block grants, potential benefits of, 266
Board of Family Practice, 588
Bonding: for chronically mentally ill, 365-367; professional role in, 368
Bonds: characteristics of, 155; in friendship; 154; in marriage, 154-155; relationships and, 154-159; in work relationship, 154
Boston: crisis research in, 166, 399; disaster intervention near, 407-

416; program for elderly in, 346, 347-348; self-help groups in, 183, 185-186; service linkage in, 494-495; widow-to-widow program in, 183, 620
Boston Health Department, 17
Boston Lying-in Hospital, 14
Boston State Hospital, ideology in, 258
Boston Visiting Nurse Association, 17-18
Bowman et al. v. *Commonwealth of Pennsylvania*, 392
Brevard, North Carolina, and rural services, 475
Brief family crisis therapy: analysis of, 419-444; background for, 419-420; case examples of, 433-438; characteristics of, 430; and community care, 438-441; in community mental health, 77; conceptual framework for, 425-430; crisis intervention distinct from, 421; development of, 420; eclecticism in, 428-430; research on, 424-425, 441; steps in, 432; therapeutic principles for, 430-432; time limits for, 421-424
Brief Psychiatric Rating Scale, 524
British Psychoanalysic Society, 15
Budget Reconciliation Act, 488
Buffalo Creek, and disaster victims, 399, 402
Bureau of Community Health Services (BCHS), 498

California: elderly in, 344; human resources in, 551; newism in, 255; research in, 430
California at Berkeley, University of: Extension Media Center at, 637; School of Social Welfare at, 19-20
California State Health Department, 20
Canada: planning in, 114; prevention in, 130; teletext in, 647
Caplan, G.: and anticipatory guidance, 17, 19, 23, 173, 219; bibliography of, 667-679; biography of, 1-39; childhood of, 2; and clinics, 4-5, 14; and community mental health centers, 25-26, 64, 83; and consultation, 11-12, 17-18, 22, 32-33, 63, 74, 171, 183-184, 289, 291-293, 298, 452, 577, 634, 654-655; and convulsion therapy, 4, 5; and crisis research, 16-17, 32, 75, 77, 164-165, 419, 422, 654; education of, 2-3; and grantsmanship, 28; in Israel, 8-13, 28, 35, 37, 171; lecture series by, 19-21; and multidisciplinary teams, 18-19; personal reflections by, 650-666; and population orientation, 10-11, 22-24, 65, 655-661; and primary prevention, 6, 9-10, 15, 46, 50, 73, 445, 450, 652-653; and stress mastery, 54, 171, 651-652; and support systems theory, 35-37, 52, 138, 177, 340, 652, 653, 654; and training institutes, 25-26, 31-32; training of, 4, 6-7, 14-15; in United Kingdom, 8, 21-22; in United States, 13-37. *See also* Name Index entry
Caplan Electroconvulsive Apparatus, 5
Career Teacher Training Program in Addictions, 580
Carnegie Commission report, 571
Carter administration, 45, 547
Casa de Amigos Neighborhood Health Center, 598, 600, 601, 602-603, 604
Case definition, issues in, 97-102
Case-study consultation: benefits of, 297-298; consultant role in, 295-296; formal report in, 296-297; outline for, 293-299
Case Western Reserve University, and geriatrics, 578
Causal attribution, threats to, 528-530
Causation, correlation and, 104-107
Cavalcade Productions, 642, 647
Cefn Coed Mental Hospital (United Kingdom), 5
Certification, issues in, 555

Change: anticipation of, consultation in, 318-321; background of, 312-313; consultant's role in, 330-332; consultation for, 63; defense, resistance, and mastery related to, 323-326; and grief, 322; leadership processes for, 327-330; loss in, and tasks of, 322-323; modulation of, 327-330; organizational, consultation for, 312-333; principles of consultation for, 321-330; requisite supplies for, 326-327; in school environment, 457-459; sequential, 319, 328-329; and strategic retreats, 330-331. *See also* Transitions
Charrette, concept of, 458
Chicago: primary prevention in school in, 454-455, 457-458; schizophrenia in, 110
Chicago, University of, crisis research at, 166
Chicago Council for the Jewish Elderly, 346-347
Child Psychiatry Congress, 7
Children, as primary prevention targets, 448-450
Children's Medical Center (Boston), 14
Chronically mentally ill: adaptation of, medications to assist, 360-365; analysis of services for, 358-371; background of services for, 358-360; bonding for, counseling with, 365-367; community mental health services for, 43, 67-71, 81; services needed by, 359-360; spin-off groups for, 367; stretched format of services for, 370-371; support systems for, 367-370
Citizens Committee for New York City, 345, 355
Class, social, and epidemiology, 98, 105, 110
Client Satisfaction Questionnaire, 525
Clientele, evaluation of appropriateness of, 518-519. *See also* Patients
Clinical consultation, focus of, 291
Collaboration, relationships of, 157-158
Colorado: assessment of effort in, 518; brief family crisis therapy in, 439
Colorado, University of, crisis intervention research at, 137
Committee on Preventive Psychiatry, 26, 39
Commonwealth Fund, 28
Commonwealth of Massachusetts v. *Wiseman,* 645, 648
Communication: in family, 426, 434, 437; principles of, 319-320
Community, concept of, 657
Community Adjustment Form, 525
Community mental health: analysis of transitions in, 40-94; background of, 1-94; boundary problem of, 42-43; brief family crisis therapy in, 77; for chronically mentally ill, 43, 67-71, 81; conceptual changes in, 46-55; consultation in, 77-78, 289-311; creative developments in, 651-655; for disaster intervention, 74-75, 397-418; for elderly, 72-73, 334-357; and environment, 55-63; epidemiological strategies in, 47-49, 95-125; future of, 664-666; judicial decisions on, 58-60, 72, 391-395, 554, 645; legislation on, 41-46; and the mentally retarded, 71-72, 372-396; population orientation in, 655-661; primary care related to, 589-591; and primary prevention, 49-52, 445-466; principles of, 95-229; professional opposition in, 663-664; and program evaluation, 78-79, 514-539; program models for, 64-79; resource development for, 79-84, 540-649; resources diminishing for, 60-63; in rural areas, 75-76, 467-485; and social support systems, 52-55, 148-162, 186-187; technologies in, 76-78; urban and rural contrasts in, 661-663
Community mental health centers

(CMHCs): affirmative action for, 232, 240; and block grants, 241; consultation for, 63, 299-304; and environment, 55, 61-62; evaluation of, 514-539; extent of, 660-661; federal funding for, 42; and human resources, 553-554; ideology and social values of, 56-58; leadership and management for, 265-288; linkages of, 494-495, 496, 497, 498, 506; mission changes for, 238; and mutual help groups, 83; options of, for future, 267-268; program models in, 64, 66, 71, 72-73, 76, 78; staffing patterns in, 80-81; and third-party payment, 236

Community Mental Health Centers Act of 1963 (P.L. 88-164): Amendments to, 514, 531, 615; and Caplan, 25, 27; and development of centers, 41-42, 45, 67, 77; and evaluation, 514, 519; and mentally retarded, 378-379; and population orientation, 657, 660; and primary care training, 589; and rural services, 479

Community Mental Health Ideology (CMHI) Scale, 250-251, 252, 259

Community Neighborhood Health Center, and disaster relief, 408

Community-Oriented-Programs-Environment Scale, 526

Community stability, and social support, 182

Community Support Programs, and evaluation, 520-521, 522

Community Support System Core Service, and interagency cooperation, 478

Competence: social, and prevention, 138, 139; training in, for children, 448-449

Comptroller General of the United States, 256, 262

Concerned United Birthparents, 614

Concord Films Council, 637

Connecticut: disaster victims in, 402; epidemiological study in, 48, 98, 249, 518-519; human resources in, 551; mentally retarded in, 376

Consultant: knowledge needed by, 298-299; pressures on, 331-332; role of, 291-293, 295-296, 330-332; and role strain, 305-311

Consultation: application of, 299-304; background of, 289-293; and Caplan, 11-12, 17-18, 22, 32-33, 63, 74, 171, 183-184, 289, 291-293, 298, 452, 577, 634, 654-655; case discussion of, 321-330; case-study outline for, 293-299; clinical orientation to, 290-293; in community mental health, 77-78; and crisis theory, 171; for defense, resistance, and mastery, 323-326; and diminishing resources, 63; for disaster relief workers, 405-406, 414-415; earlier intervention case of, 316-317; early intervention case of, 318-321; ethics in, 299; late intervention case of, 313-315; and leadership, 304-305; for leadership processes, 327-330; on loss and tasks of transition, 322-323; and medical education, 577; organizational, 289-311; for organizational change, 312-333; problem-solving approach to, 453; for programs for elderly, 342-343; for requisite supplies, 326-327; role strain in, 305-311; for teachers, 452-453; types of, 289-291

Consumer participation, trends toward, 57-58

Convening activities, for bonding assistance, 368

Coordination: background of, 486-513; developing and maintaining, 499-504; efforts toward, 488-491, 492; epidemiology and treatment research for, 505-506; future needs in, 504-509; generic models of, 492-494; models for, 491-498; organizational and financial research for, 506-507; professional training and devel-

opment for, 507-509; setting-specific models of, 494-498; variables in, 499-504. *See also* Linkages
Coping: analysis of, 172-175; cognitive processes and, 174-175; crisis theory and social support related to, 163-214; defined, 172; development of theory and practice of, 172-175; emotion-focused and problem-focused, 175; with everyday stress, 175; inventories of, 172; with severe illness, 173-174
Coping with the Overall Pregnancy Experience (C.O.P.E.), 184
Corning, New York, disaster victims in, 403
Corning Glass Works, 403
Corporate configuring: advantages of, 282-283; concept of, 280-281; and diminishing resources, 62; legal aspects of, 282; for mental health services, 280-283
Correlation, causation and, 104-107
Cost-benefit analysis, and diminishing resources, 61
Cost containment, and staffing patterns, 80
Cost offset, effect of, 490-491, 505, 507
Costs of health care, and elderly, 351-354
Council for Exceptional Children, 388
Council of Medical Specialty Societies, 589, 607
Council on Social Work Education, 557, 562, 592, 595
Counseling, for chronically mentally ill, 365-367
Counseling Center, multifocal services of, 476
Counselors, and social support, 150, 158-159
Courts. *See* Judicial decisions
Credentialing, and human resources, 554-556
Creedmoor Hospital, 643
Crisis: defined, 164-165, 450; strategic withdrawal from, 654. *See also* Brief family crisis therapy
Crisis intervention, brief therapy distinct from, 421
Crisis theory: analysis of, 164-170; and Caplan, 16-17, 32, 75, 77, 164-165, 419, 422, 654; coping and social support related to, 163-214; development and practice of, 165-170; and disaster victims, 75, 399, 400; distinctions in, 170; and intervention programs, 170-171; and prevention, 137; primary prevention linked to, 450; and social support system, 53, 187-190; and time use, 422-424; and transition states, 167-170
Cured Cancer Club, 620
Custodial Mental Illness (CMI) Scale, 249

Dangerousness, and judicial trends, 58
Death: fear of, 220-221; as part of life, 349-350
Decision processes, of administrators, 273-274
Defense, concept of, 324
Deinstitutionalization: assumptions in, 69-71; and community mental health environment, 59-60, 68-71; of mentally retarded, 72; trends in, 236-237
Demopolis, Alabama, and rural services, 476
Denmark: epidemiology in, 108; institutes in, 21
Denver, brief family crisis therapy in, 439
Department of Health and Social Security (United Kingdom), 114-115, 119
Department of Mental Health (Israel), 8
Depression, in elderly, 337
Depressive disorders, rates of, 108-109
Developmental disabilities: background of, 379-380; services for, 372-396
Developmentally Disabled Assistance and Bill of Rights Act, 393

Diagnosis, and intervention, in organizations, 289-311
Diagnostic and Statistical Manual of Mental Disorders (DSM-III), 48, 65, 75, 99, 102, 111, 119
Diagnostic Interview Schedule (DIS), 48, 49, 99, 519
Director. *See* Administrators
Disaster Relief Act of 1974 (P.L. 93-288), 74-75, 397, 417
Disaster victims: adaptation and, 400; analysis of services for, 74-75, 397-418; background of, 397-400; case example of services for, 407-416; conceptual framework regarding, 400-401; and crisis caretakers, 404-405, 414-415; and crisis theory, 75, 399, 400; emotional reactions by, 411-412; in follow-up period, 412-415; guidelines for interventions with, 404-406; information gathering on, 401-403, 407; initial action plan for, 403-404, 407-408; intervention activities for, 409-410; intervention model for, 401-407; and linking activities, 407-408; loss and bereavement related to, 399, 400; and medication needs, 410-411; phase-appropriate help for, 406; reaction phases of, 399, 410-415; and social support, 400; and stress, 75; triage for, 404, 409-410

East Boston/Dorchester program for elderly, 346, 347-348
Eastern Montana Community Mental Health Center, and transportation problems, 474-475
Eastern Washington University, rural practitioner training at, 477
Eclecticism, in brief family crisis therapy, 428-430
Ecological fallacy, in epidemiology, 105-106
Ecological model: application of, 342-351; and elderly, 338-342
Economic Development Division Staff, 469
Education Film Library Association, 637-638
Education for All Handicapped Act (P.L. 94-142), 73, 381-382, 383, 447
Education of the Handicapped Act (P.L. 91-239), 378, 381-382, 383
Effectiveness, evaluation of, 519-523
Effort, evaluation of, 516-519
Elderly: active, 343; analysis of services for, 72-73, 334-357; application of ecological model for, 342-351; background of services for, 334-336; coordinated, comprehensive programs for, 346-349; defined, 334; demography of, 335-336; depression in, 337; dying as part of life for, 349-350; ecological perspective on, 338-342; and environmental changes, 339; in Europe, 350-351; formal and informal helpers for, 345-346; and health care costs, 351-354; health status of, 336-338; organic brain syndrome in, 337-338; physical support systems for, 341-342; self-care and self-help for, 344-345; social disengagement by, 341; social support needs of, 73, 340-341
Elementary and Secondary Education Act, amendments to, 377, 381-382
Emmanuel Church, 186
Emotional support: concept of, 150-151; conclusions about, 160-161
English Zionist Federation, 8
Environment: and community mental health, 55-63; concept of, 176; in prevention, 130, 131; school, and primary prevention, 455-459; school, change of, 457-459; variables in, 456-457
Epidemiologic Catchment Area (ECA) Program, 48, 99-100, 103, 117, 519
Epidemiology: of affective disorders, 108-109; analysis of, 47-49, 95-125; background of, 95-97; and case definition, 97-102;

changing strategies in, 47-49; concept of, 95; correlation and causation in, 104-107; methods of, 95-96; of nonpsychotic disorders, 111-113; planning and evaluation related to, 113-118; and point of onset definition, 102-103; and population at risk, 104; and rates of mental disorder, 107-113; reliability and validity in, 100; of schizophrenia, 109-111; and social class, 98, 105, 110; and social support, 182; and stress, 101, 109, 110-111; usefulness of, 96-97; and value judgments, 102
Epilepsy Foundation of America, 388
Episcopal church, consultation with, 33, 36, 183-184
Ethics: in audiovisuals, 638-639, 641-642; in consultation, 299; of evaluation, 531-532
Europe: elderly in, 350-351; social support studies in, 149, 178
European Economic Community, and human resources, 541
Evaluation: analysis of, 78-79, 514-539; background of, 514-516; conducting, 527-532; data collection instruments for, 524-527; of effectiveness, 519-523; of effort, 516-519; of environmental conditions, 526-527; ethics of, 531-532; fiscal issues in, 532; of impact, 520-521; and informed consent, 531-532; levels of, 515-516; of medical education, 580-583; of mental health services, 115-118; need for, 514-515; outcome, 519-520; outcome indexes in, 522-523; perspective of, 530-531; and policy implications, 532-534; of psychiatric status, 524; research designs for, 527-530; of satisfaction with treatment, 525; of social adaptation, 524-525; of target populations, 521-522; of vocational performance, 525-526
Evaluation Research Society, 532
Expectancies, and mental retardation, 376
Expert, concept of, 191

Falk Fund, 28
Family: as client, 431, 440. *See also* Brief family crisis therapy
Family Service Agency, 403
Federal Assistance to State-Operated and Supported Schools for Handicapped (P.L. 89-313), 377
Federal government: and human resources policy, 540-545; role of, related to mental retardation, 377-380, 388; and rural areas, 479-480
Field theory, and social support, 181
First Friends, 366
Florida, leadership in, 279-280, 283-284
Florida Health Study, 103
France, teletext in, 647
Freedom, principle of, 58-59
Friend, concept of, 154
Friendly visitor, and mutual help groups, 185-186
Friendship, bonds of, 154
Functional support, concept of, 150
Funding: constraints on, consequences of, 233-234; management of cutbacks of, 276-278; paradoxes in cutbacks of, 277; policies of, and mental health services, 232-233, 235, 237-238

General Accounting Office, 69, 87
General hospital, and mental health linkage, 67
Genetic disorders, prevention of, 132
Geriatrics, training in, neglect of, 578-579
Gheel, bonding in, 366
Global Assessment Scale, 524
Graduate Education of Physicians report, 571
Graduate Medical Education National Advisory Committee (GMENAC), 547, 564

Grant Foundation, 28
Gray Panthers, 343, 614
Grief: and change, 322; loss related to, 218; posttransition guidance for, 223-227; and social support, 166-167, 183
Group for the Advancement of Psychiatry, 26, 39, 69, 88
Guggenheim Memorial Foundation, John Simon, 148*n*

Hadassah Hebrew University Medical School, 8-9, 13; Department of Child Psychiatry at, x, 37
Harris County Hospital District (HCHD): Community Medicine Service of, 594; Neighborhood Health Program of, 594; and primary care training, 593, 594, 596, 598, 603
Harris County, Texas, primary care training in, 592-606
Harvard University: bereavement studies at, 183; Department of Public Health Practice of, 14; Department of Social Relations of, 13; Family Guidance Center of, 419, 425; Family Health Clinic of, 14, 18; Law School of, 35; Medical School of, x, xi, 13, 26-27, 28; School of Public Health of, xi, 12-13, 14, 15, 16, 18, 21, 26-27, 28, 29, 30, 34, 419, 425; Visiting Faculty Seminar at, 29-31, 658, 664
Hawaii, Health Department of, 22
Hays, Kansas, and rural services, 476
Head Start, 378, 449
Health: as process, 142; status of, for elderly, 336-338
Health Activation Course, 344
Health care organization, in prevention, 130, 131, 143
Health care services, linked with mental health services, 486-513
Health disorders, mental health disorders related to, 488-490
Health field, concept of, 130
Health Maintenance Organizations (HMOs): and elderly, 353; and human resources, 550; linkages with, 490, 494-496, 497, 507
Health Manpower Report, 571
Health Opinion Survey (HOS), 103
Health Professions Educational Assistance Act of 1976, 571, 588, 608
Health promotion: prevention distinct from, 129-130; and social support, 190-191
Health Resources Administration, 543, 544, 555, 557, 562-563
Health Services Administration, 497
Help receiving, relationships of, 157-159
Helper therapy, and social support, 182
Helpers: formal and informal, for elderly, 345-346; informal, and social support, 182
High Plains Comprehensive CMHC, multifocal services of, 476
Hiroshima, disaster victims at, 399
Hogg Foundation for Mental Health, 587*n*, 597
Homeostasis, and crisis theory, 165
Hospice: and anticipatory guidance, 220-221; and elderly, 349-350
Houston, primary care training in, 592-606
Houston, University of, Graduate School of Social Work of, 595-596, 603
Houston Primary Care Mental Health Training Consortium, 82, 587*n*, 596-606
Human Development Program, 449
Human resources: analysis of, 540-564; bureaucratic stances on, 542-543; and community mental health centers, 553-554; and credentialing, 554-556; factors in patterns for, 549-550; federal policy objectives for, 540-545; federal reports on, 543-545; issues of, 551-560; maldistribution of, 547-549; and medical education, 565-586; and minorities, 556-558; planning for, 560-561; in private practice, 558-559;

projection models for, 545-547; supply and production trends in, 547-551; and third-party payment, 558, 559-560; training of, in community settings, 587-610
Human service ideology, 57
Human Service Ideology (HSI) Scale, 252-253, 256

Ideology, conceptual changes in, 56-58. *See also* Value systems
Illinois: planning in, 114; social support survey in, 150. *See also* Chicago
Illness, severe: coping with, 173-174; and social support, 194-195
Incidence, concept of, 128
Infection, prevention of, 132
Information helpers: for elderly, 345-346; and social support, 182
Information: on disaster victims, gathering, 401-403, 407; leadership, and processing of, 271-274; sources of, 272-273
Informational support, concept of, 150
Informed consent: for audiovisuals, 639, 644-645; and evaluation, 531-532
Injuries, prevention of, 133-134
Inpatient Multidmensional Psychiatric Scale, 524
Institute for Creative Aging, 344
Institute on Human Values and Medicine, 572
Internal Revenue Service (IRS), 281, 282
International Association for Child Psychiatry and Allied Professions, 7, 26
Inter-University Forum for Educators in Community Psychiatry, 31, 658, 664
Intervention: diagnosis and, in organizations, 289-311; levels of, 142
Involutional melancholia, population at risk for, 104
Ireland, Republic of, mental health services in, 22
Israel: Caplan in, 8-13, 28, 35, 37, 171; immigration stress in, 171

Johnson administration, 240, 547
Joint Commission on Accreditation of Hospitals (JCAH), 284, 386, 388, 389, 577
Joint Commission on Mental Illness and Health, 24, 44, 243, 245, 378, 625, 663
Judge Baker Clinic, 14
Judicial decisions: on community mental health, 58-60, 72; on credentialing, 554; on informed consent, 645; on mentally retarded, 391-395

Kansas, rural services in, 476
Kappa coefficients, 97
Katz Adjustment Scale, 525
Kentucky, University of, medical education at, 574
Kidney Transplant and Dialysis Association, 620
Kin-type alliances, relationships of, 157-158

Labeling, and case definition, 98
Laboratory of Community Psychiatry (LOCP), xi, 27-29, 32, 34, 186, 218, 219, 626
La Lêche League, 184, 614, 626
Lasker Mental Hygiene and Child Guidance Center (Israel), 9, 10
Leadership: background of, 265-267; for change, 327-330; for corporate configuring, 280-283; information processing for, 271-274; long-range perspective on, 267-274; management compared with, 268-271; for mental health centers, 265-288; in organizations, 304-305; in planning, 271; principles of, 285-286; for process integration, 283-286
Least restrictive environment, concept of, 59
Legislation, on community mental health, 41-46
Levels of Functioning Scale, 524
Libertarian Mental Health Ideology (LMHI) Scale, 253-254
Libertarian values, in community mental health, 57, 58-59
Licensure, issues of, 555-556

Life-style: of family, 426; issues of, and medical education, 569-570; in prevention, 130-131, 133-134
Linkages: of health services and mental health services, 486-513; and mutual help groups, 627-628; in rural areas, 479; triage, 497. *See also* Coordination
Lithium, adaptation assisted by, 360, 364-365
London: elderly in, 350; epidemiology study in, 108, 109
Los Angeles, elderly in, 344
Loss: background of, 215-217; and crisis theory, 166-167; and disaster victims, 399, 400; grief related to, 218; and social support, 215-229

Maine: interagency collaboration in, 478; rural services in, 476
Make Today Count, 184
Management: of cutbacks, 276-278; of expansion and diversification, 278-280; issues in, 239-244; leadership compared with, 268-271
Management information systems, 271-272
Managers, issues for, 62-63
Managua, Nicaragua, disaster victims in, 399-400, 403
Manchester, University of, social support research at, 178
Manchester Grammar School, 2
Manchester Royal Infirmary, 3
Manchester University, Caplan at, 3, 5
Mania, rates of, 108
Manpower. *See* Human resources
Marriage: bonds in, 154-155; and stress, 153, 161; as transition, 169
Maryland, human resources in, 551
Massachusetts: Episcopal church in, 33; human resources in, 551; informed consent case in, 645; mental health policy in, 23; mentally retarded in, 374, 375, 381, 382-383, 384, 392-393; rural areas in, 472. *See also* Boston
Massachusetts General Hospital, 13, 18, 185, 186, 641, 660
Mastery, requisite supplies for, 326
Maternal and Child Health and Mental Retardation Planning Amendments of 1963 (P.L. 88-156), 378
Matrix design, and diminishing resources, 62
Mature Temps, 343
Medicaid: and chronically mentally ill, 70-71; and client choice, 234; and elderly, 348, 349, 351-352, 353, 354; and locus of care, 64-65
Medical education: analysis of, 565-586; audiovisuals in, 633-649; background of, 565-567; and consultation and liaison, 577; current relevance of, 583-584; currriculums in, 574-576; evaluation of, 580-583; in interpersonal skills, 576-577; and life-style issues, 569-570; neglected areas in, 577-580; and patient nonadherence, 570-571; population orientation in, 658-659; and primary care providers, 568-569; psychiatry in, 573-574; and status of health services, 571; trends in, 568-572; undergraduate curriculum in, 572-580; and values, 571-572
Medical sector, and professional staff, 81-82
Medicare: and elderly, 344, 351-352, 353, 354; and locus of care, 64-65
Medications: for chronically mentally ill, 360-365; for disaster victims, 410-411; patient responsibility for, 361-362
Mended Hearts, 184, 621
Mental disorders: epidemiology of, 95-125; preventable, 131-134; prevention of, 126-147; rates of, 97, 107-113
Mental health, social support related to, 148-162
Mental Health and Mental Retardation Authority of Harris County

(MHMRA), and primary care training, 593-594, 596, 598, 603
Mental Health Materials Center, 637
Mental health services: assumptions about, in 1970s, 230-232; and block grants, 241; for chronic patients, 358-371; and client choice, 234-235; context changes for, 230-333; corporate configuring for, 280-283; for disaster victims, 397-418; and discrimination against elderly, 348; domains of, 274-275; for elderly, 334-357; evaluation of, 514-539; expansion and diversification of, 278-280; extent of need for, 47; for families in crisis, 419-444; and funding policies, 232-233, 235, 237-238; general health linkage with, 66-67; health care services linked with, 486-513; human resources for, 540-564; ideological changes in, 248-256; issues for, 238-244; leadership for, 265-288; for mentally retarded and developmentally disabled, 372-396; mutual help groups compared with, 615-617; and planning, 113-115, 237; and professional problems, 242; public policy impact on, 230-245; quality of, 386-389; remedicalization of, 43-44, 57, 81; in rural areas, 467-485; in schools, 445-466; for specific populations, 334-539; and strain toward revision, 56; stretched format of, 370-371; and third-party payers, 235-236; training for, in community settings, 587-610; utilization of, and social support, 182; and value systems, 246-264
Mental Health Study Act of 1955, 24
Mental Health Systems Act of 1980 (P.L. 96-398): and development of community mental health, 45, 50, 78; and evaluation, 514, 517, 520; and health care system linkages, 487-488; and human resources, 543, 544, 548, 551, 563; and leadership, 265; and rural areas, 467, 479, 482
Mental Patients Liberation Front, 83, 614
Mental Research Institute, 430
Mental Retardation Amendments of 1967, 379
Mental Retardation Facilities and Community Mental Health Centers Construction Act of 1963 (P.L. 88-164). *See* Community Mental Health Centers Act
Mentally ill. *See* Patients
Mentally retarded: accreditation of services for, 386-389; advocacy for, 383-384; analysis of services for, 71-72, 372-396; background of, 372-374; community clinical nursery schools (CCNS) for, 374-377; courts and, 391-395; defined, 374; federal government role and, 377-380, 388; individualized educational plan for, 383; legal rights of, 381-383; medical and developmental models of, 389-391; and parent power, rights, and advocacy, 380-384; parents of, at risk, 375; prevalence of, 373-374; program audits for, 388-389; in public institutions, 390; service delivery for, 384-386; service quality for, 386-389; university-affiliated facilities for, 379
Merthyr Tydfil General Hospital (United Kingdom), 5
Michigan: evaluation costs in, 532; video education project in, 636
Michigan, University of, Medical Center of, 578-579
Midtown Manhattan study, 101, 103, 107, 111, 112, 518
Midtransition guidance, for psychosocial transitions, 222-223
Milbank Memorial Fund, 183, 209
Military psychiatry, and social support theory, 167-168
Ministration, requisite supplies for, 326
Minorities, and human resources, 556-558

Mitre Corporation, 474
Modeling, requisite supplies for, 326-327
Monoamine oxidase inhibitors, adaptation assisted by, 364
Montana, rural services in, 474-475
Morgantown, West Virginia, interagency collaboration in, 479
Most therapeutic environment, concept of, 60
Mt. Sinai School of Medicine, videotaped test at, 582
Multitone Company, 5
Mutual help groups: accommodation/self-generation/service in, 624; analysis of, 611-632; background of, 611-612; characteristics of, 259-260, 613-615; for chronically mentally ill, 369-370; concept of, 612-617; as coping resources, 184-185; history of, 185-186; impact/affinity/recovery in, 622-623; information pertinent to, 619-620; and learning opportunities, 619; and linkages, 627-628; mental health services compared with, 615-617; and peer learning, 620-621; and professionals, 624-629; recoil/presence/unity in, 623-624; recommendations on, 627-628; as resources, 82-83, 611-632; and role mobility, 621-622; and transitions, 617-624

National Alliance of Families of the Mentally Ill, 83, 184
National Ambulatory Medical Care Survey, 490
National Association for Retarded Citizens (NARC), 378, 381, 385-386, 388
National Association of Prevention Professionals, 49-50
National Association of Private Residential Facilities for the Mentally Retarded, 388
National Association of Social Workers, 388
National Association of State Mental Health Program Directors, 552, 563
National Board of Medical Examiners, 573, 574-575, 581, 585
National Centrim Voor Geestelijke Volksgezondheid, 637
National Clearing House on Aging, 336, 357
National Coalition for Battered Women, 614
National Council of Senior Citizens, 343
National Health and Welfare (Canada), 130
National Health Council, 588, 609
National Health Service Corps, 550
National Health Survey, 336
National Institute of Medicine, 588, 590, 609
National Institute of Mental Health (NIMH), 445*n*, 486*n*; and Caplan, 24, 25, 28; Center for Prevention recommended for, 50; Community Support Program (CSP) of, 70, 187, 248; and development of community mental health, 45, 48, 61, 66, 80, 90-91; and disaster victims, 397; Division of Biometry and Epidemiology of, 98, 486*n*, 517, 527; and Epidemiologic Catchment Area Program, 48, 99-100, 103, 117, 519; and epidemiology, 117; Human Aging Study of, 336; and human resources, 545, 547, 553, 556, 558, 560; and leadership, 266; and medical education, 573, 577; and rural areas, 474; and training in community setting, 587*n*, 597-598; and value systems, 241
National Institute on Alcohol Abuse and Alcoholism, 580
National Institute on Drug Abuse, 580
National League of Nurses, 19
National Library of Medicine, AVLINE of, 637
National Mental Health Act, 573
National Planning Committee on

Accreditation of Residential Centers for the Retarded, 386
National Society for Autistic Children, 388
National Task Force on Mental Health/Mental Retardation Administration, 62, 92
Need-response pattern, in family, 427-428
Neighborhood health centers (NHCs), linkages with, 487, 506
Netherlands: audiovisuals in, 637; institutes in, 21; mental health services in, 22
Neuroleptics, adaptation assisted by, 360-361
Neurosis, treatment of, and planning, 113-114
New Hampshire, mentally retarded in, 392
New Haven, epidemiological study in, 48, 98, 249, 518-519
New Jersey, mentally retarded in, 376
New York (city): epidemiology study in, 101, 103, 107, 110, 111, 112, 518; parents' group in, 454
New York (state): disaster victims in, 403; human resources in, 551; interagency collaboration in, 478; mentally retarded in, 392
Nicaragua, disaster victims in, 399-400, 403
Nixon administration, 241, 541, 542
Nonadherence, and medical education, 570-571
Nonpsychotic disorders, rates of, 111-113
North Carolina: credentialing case in, 554; rural areas in, 475
Northside CMHC (Tampa), 279-280, 283-284
Norway: institutes in, 21; mental health services in, 22; social support research in, 178
Nova Scotia study, 101, 107, 111
Nurturance, relationships of, 157-158
Nutritional deficiencies, prevention of, 132-133

O'Connor v. *Donaldson,* and right to treatment, 60
Oklahoma, community advocacy in, 481-482
Onset, defining point of, 102-103
Organic brain syndrome, in elderly, 337-338
Organization: consultation for change in, 312-333; diagnosis and intervention in, 289-311; diagnostic role in, 310-311; leadership in, 304-305
Organization development, as consultation method, 290
Organizational diagnosis, and diminishing resources, 63
Ostomy groups, 184, 626
Outward Bound, 173
Oxford English Dictionary, 164, 209

Palo Alto, California, research in, 430
Panel on Mental Retardation, 378
Paradigm, concept of, 246-247
Paraprofessional movement, 625
Parents: of mentally retarded, 380-384; primary prevention role of, 453-455; and service delivery, 384-386
Patients: benefits of linkages to, 491-492; locus of care for, 48, 64; nonadherence of, and medical education, 570-571; psychosocial aspects of, 566-567; responsibility of, for medication, 361-362; rights of, 232. *See also* Chronically mentally ill
Peace Corps: and anticipatory guidance, 173; and crisis theory, 168-169; influence of, 664; and psychiatric consultation, 23-24, 26, 27
Pennhurst State School suit, 72, 392, 393-394
Pennsylvania: human resources in, 553; mentally retarded in, 72, 384, 392, 393-394

Pennsylvania State University: medical education at, 572; Pennsylvania Cinema Register at, 637
Personal Adjustment and Role Skills Scale, 525
Phenylketonuria, 391
Planned short-term treatment (PSTT), described, 421-423
Planning: leadership in, 271; of mental health services, 113-115, 237
Poisoning, prevention of, 131
Ponca City, Oklahoma, community advocacy in, 481-482
Population at risk, defining, 104
Population orientation: and Caplan, 10-11, 22-24, 65, 655-661; in community mental health, 655-661; educational programs in, 658-659; of program models, 65-66
Postdisaster crisis counseling, defined, 397-398
Posttransition guidance, for psychosocial transitions, 223-227
President's Commission on Mental Health: and brief family crisis therapy, 430, 443; and chronically mentally ill, 359, 371; Community Support Systems Task Force of, 619; and development of community mental health, 44-45, 47, 50, 52, 59, 66, 83, 91; and epidemiology, 112; and health care linkage, 487, 512; and human resources, 543, 547, 551, 552, 561, 563; and mutual help, 625, 627, 630; and prevention, 140, 146; and public policy impact, 242-243, 245; reflections on, 660, 663, 666; and rural areas, 467, 469, 477, 482, 484; and school settings, 446, 465; and social support, 176, 181, 187, 188, 210
President's Committee on Mental Retardation, 379
Presque Isle, Maine, interagency collaboration in, 478
Prevalence, concept of, 127
Prevention: advances and obstacles in, 126-147; background of, 126-127; concepts in, 127-131; and crisis theory, 137; disorders susceptible to, 131-134; general disease paradigm of, 136-137; health promotion distinct from, 129-130; research on, 140-141; and social competence, 138, 139; and social systems support, 138-139. *See also* Primary prevention
Primary care: community mental health related to, 589-591; defined, 588-589
Primary care health programs (PCHPs): and interagency collaboration, 479; linkages with, 498
Primary care training: background of, 587-592; in community settings, 587-610; conclusions on, 602-606; consortium for, 596-601; goals in, 596-597; recommendations on, 605
Primary prevention: advantages of schools as settings for, 446-448; amount of, 50; background of, in schools, 445-446; barriers to, 140-143; and Caplan, 6, 9-10, 15, 46, 50, 73, 445, 450, 652-653; and childhood psychopathology model, 50; children as targets of, 448-450; and community mental health, 49-52; concept of, 128, 446; and conceptual changes, 49-52; crisis theory linked to, 450; and environment of school, 455-459; future objectives of, 461; future of, 139-143; future programs for, 460-461; general disease paradigm of, 51; in organizational change, 312-333; paradigm shift in, 134-139; parental role in, 453-455; research needed for, 52; and school administrators, 453; in schools, 73-74, 445-466; and social support, 193; status and future of, 459-461; and stress, 51, 136-138; and teachers, 451-453. *See also* Prevention
Problem-solving mechanisms, in family, 426-427

Professional and Technical Workers for Alyah (PATWA), 8
Professional staff: bonding role of, 368; boundary-spanning, 503; in community mental health centers, patterns of, 80-81; and community mental health ideology, 251; continuing education for, in rural areas, 477; coordination training for, 507-509; development of, 79-84; and funding cutbacks, 276-277; and medical sector, 81-82; and mutual help groups, 624-629; opposition of, 663-664; recruitment and retention of, in rural areas, 475-478; socialization of, 238; training of, for brief family crisis therapy, 439-440. *See also* Human resources; Medical education; Primary care training
Program models: for community mental health, 64-79; population focus of, 65-66
Programs, evaluation of, 517-518
Project Head Start, 378, 449
Psychiatric networks, and social support, 183
Psychiatric Status Schedule (PSS), 100
Psychiatry: in medical education, 573-574; as primary care, 589
Psychoanalytic Institute: Boston, 15; Chicago, 12; London, 6, 15
Psychosocial transition, defined, 217. *See also* Transitions
Public Health Service Act, 50
Public Law 88-156, 378
Public Law 88-164. *See* Community Mental Health Centers Act
Public Law 89-313, 377
Public Law 91-239, 378
Public Law 93-288, 74-75, 397, 417
Public Law 93-380, 383
Public Law 94-63, 42, 479, 480
Public Law 94-142, 73, 381-382, 383, 447
Public Law 94-484, 552
Public Law 95-49, 378
Public Law 96-398. *See* Mental Health Systems Act
Puerto Rico, mental health services in, 22

Reagan administration, 45, 51, 70-71, 233, 237, 241, 266, 488, 514
Recovery, Inc., 184, 259, 260, 366; as mutual help group, 614, 626
Red Cross, and disaster victims, 404-405, 408, 409
Rehabilitation: concept of, 127; rituals of, 225
Rehabilitation medicine, neglect of, 577-578
Relationships: bonds and, 154-159; primary and secondary, 151; provisions of, to social support, 151-154; types of, 156-157, 159-160
Remedicalization: implications of, 44; of mental health services, 43-44, 57, 81
Rennie v. *Klein*, and right to refuse treatment, 60
Research Diagnostic Criteria (RDC), 98-99
Resistance, concept of, 325
Resources: for community mental health, 79-84, 540-649; diminishing, and administrative solutions, 60-63; human, 540-564; mutual help groups as, 82-83, 611-632; training of, 565-610
Retarded. *See* Mentally retarded
Ritual: and crisis theory, 169; for psychosocial transitions, 224-225
Rogers v. *Okin*, and right to refuse treatment, 60
Role network, in family, 426, 434-435
Rouse v. *Cameron*, and right to treatment, 60
Rural areas: analysis of, 75-76, 467-485; barriers to service in, 473; community advocacy in, 480-482; demography of, 468-469; interagency collaboration in, 478-479; personnel recruitment and retention for, 475-478; satellites in, 474; services in, 473-482; social organization

in, 471; social support in, 477; sociology of, 468-473; transportation in, 474-475; values as source of stress in, 472; values in, 469-471
Russell Sage Foundation, 573

St. Christopher's Hospice, 350
St. Louis County, parents' groups in, 454
Saskatchewan, planning in, 114
Satisfaction, life, and social support, 149-150
Scandinavia: depression in, 109; mentally retarded in, 376
Schedule for Affective Disorders and Schizophrenia (SADS), 48, 98-99, 518
Schizophrenia: background of services for, 358-359; and bonding, 366; brief family crisis therapy for, 435-438; and community care, 68; and floating affects, 362; and instruction, 362-363; management of, and social support, 183; and medication to assist adaptation, 360-363; mislabeling of, 102, 110; population at risk for, 104; rates of, 109-111; treatment for, 113, 115-116
School: environment of, and primary prevention, 455-459; as gatekeeper, 447; mental health services in, 445-466
SCL-90, 524, 529
Secondary prevention, concept of, 128
Self-care programs: concept of, 613; for elderly, 344-345
Self-concept, for children, 449-450
Self-help: concept of, 613; for elderly, 344-345
Seminars for the Separated, 186
Senior Actualization and Growth Exploration (SAGE), 344
Service delivery: as culturally syntonic, 473; diversification of, 659-660; for mentally retarded, 384-386; value systems and, 246-264
Social breakdown syndrome: and evaluation, 115-116; and social support, 182-183
Social engineering, norm of, 57
Social impact statements, proposed, 241
Social networks: as coping resources, 183; defined, 179-180; functions of, 180; social support distinct from, 179; types of, 179
Social organization, and crisis theory, 165-166
Social space, and social support, 182
Social support: analysis of, 52-55, 148-162, 176-187; background on, 148-151; benefits of, 148-149; and bonding for chronically mentally ill, 366-367; and Caplan, 35-37, 52, 138, 177, 340, 652, 653, 654; and chronic illness, 194-195; conceptual changes in, 52-55; conclusions about, 159-161; coping and crisis theory related to, 163-214; crisis theory convergent with, 53, 187-190; defined, 177; and disaster victims, 400; and elderly, 73, 340-341; evaluative intervention model of, 194-195; functional, informational, and emotional, 150-151; future research on, 190-196; ideology role in, 259-261; in loss and transitions, 215-229; negative aspects of, 149-150; and primary prevention, 193; processes of, 53-54; program strategies for, 188-190; programming for, 183-187; provisions of relationships to, 151-154; relationships and bonds in, 154-159; in rural areas, 477; social network distinct from, 179; stimuli to theory of, 181-183; and stress, 153, 160-161, 181; and stress mastery, 54; structural characteristics of, 178-179; theory and practice of, 177-183
Sociometry, and social support, 181
Southern California, University of, audiovisuals at, 637, 641

Southwest Denver Mental Health Service, 439
Spina Bifida Association of Massachusetts, 620
Staff. *See* Professional staff
Sterling County, epidemiology studies in, 103, 518
Stone Foundation, 28
Strens, concept of, 449
Stress: and disaster victims, 75; and epidemiology, 101, 109, 110-111; everyday, coping with, 175; illness related to, 191-193; impact variables of, 176; and primary prevention, 51, 136-138; in rural areas, values as source of, 472; and social support, 153, 160-161, 181
Stress mastery: and Caplan, 54, 171, 651-652; and social support, 54
Stroke Clubs, 184
Suicide, brief family crisis therapy for, 433-435
Supplemental Security Income (SSI), 235
Support group, concept of, 612-613
Survey feedback, as consultation technique, 290
Swansea General Hospital (United Kingdom), 5
Synanon, 259, 260
Systemic disorders, prevention of, 133

Take Off Pounds Sensibly (TOPS), 184
Tampa, leadership in, 279-280, 283-284
Task Panel on the Nature and Scope of the Problems, 47, 93
Tavistock Clinic (United Kingdom), 6-7, 21-22
Teachers, as primary prevention targets and agents, 451-453
Technologies, in community mental health, 76-78. *See also* Audiovisuals
Tertiary prevention, concept of, 127
Texas, primary care training in, 592-606
Texas, University of, School of Nursing of, 595-596
Third-party payment: and human resources, 558, 559-560; and locus of care, 64; and mental health services, 235-236; and prevention, 143; in rural areas, 480; and services for elderly, 352-353
Time limits, for brief family crisis therapy, 421-424
Transitions: anticipatory guidance in, 218-222; communities for, 169; factors in coping with, 621-622; marriage as, 169; and mid-transition guidance, 222-223; and mutual help groups, 617-624; phases in, 167; and post-transition guidance, 223-227; psychosocial, 169-170, 217-218; rituals for, 224-225; and social support, 215-229; stages in, 617-618; work of, 618-619; and world model, 216-217. *See also* Change
Transportation, in rural areas, 474-475
Treatment, right to and right to refuse, 60
Trend Community Mental Health Center, and transportation, 475
Triage: for disaster victims, 404, 409-410; linkage, 497
Tricyclics, adaptation assisted by, 360, 364-365

Union of Soviet Socialist Republics, political dissidents as schizophrenic in, 102, 110
Unionization, and human resource planning, 560-561
United Cerebral Palsy Associations, 388
United Counseling Service, multifocal services of, 476
United Kingdom: audiovisuals in, 637, 647; and Caplan, 8, 21-22; diagnosis in, 107; elderly in, 349, 350, 351; epidemiology study in, 108, 109; evaluation in, 115; planning in, 114-115
U.S. Bureau of the Budget, 24, 657-658
U.S. Bureau of the Census, 335, 336, 484

U.S. Bureau of Developmental Disabilities, 380
U.S. Bureau of Labor Statistics, 544
U.S. Children's Bureau, 20
U.S. Court of Appeals, 393
U.S. Department of Agriculture, 475, 484; Cooperative Extension Service of, 478
U.S. Department of Commerce, 469
U.S. Department of Health and Human Services (DHHS), 69, 136, 147, 234-235, 543, 544, 551, 553, 556, 557, 558, 562; Bureau of Health Manpower of, 555; Steering Committee on the Chronically Mentally Ill of, 86
U.S. Department of Health, Education, and Welfare, 239-240, 542; Services Integration Projects of, 486-487, 492
U.S. Department of Labor, 469, 484, 543
U.S. District Court, 392, 393-394
U.S. Office of Civil Rights, 554
U.S. Office of Education, 377
U.S. Senate Special Committee on Aging, 351, 357
U.S. Supreme Court, 60, 72, 393-394
U.S. Surgeon General's Office, 69, 70
University Jewish Society (United Kingdom), 3
University Zionist Society (United Kingdom), 3
Utica, New York, interagency collaboration in, 478

Valley CMHC, interagency collaboration by, 479
Value systems: background of, 246-248; changes in, 248-256; of community mental health, 250-252; defined, 249, 470; effects of, on behavior, 257-259; and epidemiology, 102; of family, 426, 434; of human service, 252-253; humanistic, 249-250; libertarian, 253-254; and medical education, 571-572; and newism strained toward, 254-256; in rural areas, 469-472; and service delivery, 246-264; and social support, 259-261. *See also* Ideology
Vermont: human resources in, 551; rural areas in, 476
Vermont Conference on the Primary Prevention of Psychopathology, 49
Veterans Administration, 80
Victims. *See* Disaster victims
Virgin Islands, mental health services in, 22
Virginia, evaluation costs in, 532

Wabash Mental Health Center, consultation with, 300-304
Walter E. Fernald State School, 374
Washington, retarded persons in, 71
Washington University, rural practitioner training at, 477
Wellesley Human Relations Service, 12, 14, 18, 21, 171, 660
West Alabama Mental Health Center, personnel for, 476
West Virginia, interagency collaboration in, 479
West Virginia University, rural practitioner training at, 477
Western Michigan University, rural practitioner training at, 477
Whittier Street Field Training Program, 16, 18, 21
Widow-to-Widow, 183, 184, 193; as mutual help group, 618, 620, 626, 627
Willowbrook, suit concerning, 392
Windsor Locks, Connecticut, disaster victims in, 402
Winson Green Mental Hospital (United Kingdom), 4-5
Wisconsin at Menominee, University of, and rural peer counselor training, 477-478
Woodlawn Project, 74
Work relationship: bonds in, 154; and social support, 181
World Federation of Mental Health, 12
World model, and transitions, 216-217

Worry, work of, and coping, 172-173
Wyatt v. *Stickney:* and least restrictive environment, 59; and retarded persons, 72; and right to treatment, 60
Youngberg v. *Romeo,* 394*n*
Youth Aliya (Israel), 10-11
Ypsilanti, Michigan, video education project in, 636

Many community mental health practices developed within the past two decades are no longer suited to today's needs. The *modern* practice of community mental health must adapt to new exigencies—shrinking budgets, new legal requirements, shifting patterns of resource allocation, changing population needs, and rapid innovations in treatment methods, to name but a few. This book—written in honor of Gerald Caplan and his pioneering efforts in community mental health—describes the management, leadership, programs, delivery methods, and professional competencies essential to effective community mental health today. Twenty-six chapters prepared expressly for this volume incorporate the wide-ranging knowledge and recommendations of practitioners and scholars at the forefront of community mental health—including psychiatrists, psychologists, social workers, physicians, sociologists, specialists in public and allied health, and other human services professionals.

The volume provides a comprehensive assessment of changing trends, the latest techniques, and the most urgent needs in mental health treatment—whether extended through public or private centers, general health care organizations, or community